LIFE U[ ] ⟨⟩ W9-AIK-331

100 Questions & Answers About Fibromyalgia

Sharon Ostalecki, PhD

Helping Our Pain & Exhaustion, Inc. (HOPE), Novi, MI
Executive Director
American Pain Foundation
Michigan State Leader
Fibromyalgia: Fitting the Pieces Together
Executive Producer

Martin S. Tamler, MD, FAAPMR

William Beaumont Hospital, Royal Oak, MI
Physical Medicine & Rehabilitation Residency Program Director
Director of Subacute Rehabilitation
Director of Prosthetics and Orthotics
Director of the Electrodiagnostics Lab

JONES AND BARTLETT PUBLISHERS
Sudbury, Massachusetts
BOSTON   TORONTO   LONDON   SINGAPORE

LIFE UNIVERSITY LIBRARY
1269 BARCLAY CIRCLE
MARIETTA, GA 30060
770-426-2688

World Headquarters

Jones and Bartlett Publishers	Jones and Bartlett Publishers	Jones and Bartlett Publishers
40 Tall Pine Drive	Canada	International
Sudbury, MA 01776	6339 Ormindale Way	Barb House, Barb Mews
978-443-5000	Mississauga, Ontario L5V 1J2	London W6 7PA
info@jbpub.com	Canada	United Kingdom
www.jbpub.com		

Jones and Bartlett's books and products are available through most bookstores and online booksellers. To contact Jones and Bartlett Publishers directly, call 800-832-0034, fax 978-443-8000, or visit our website, www.jbpub.com.

Substantial discounts on bulk quantities of Jones and Bartlett's publications are available to corporations, professional associations, and other qualified organizations. For details and specific discount information, contact the special sales department at Jones and Bartlett via the above contact information or send an email to specialsales@jbpub.com.

Copyright © 2010 by Jones and Bartlett Publishers, LLC

All rights reserved. No part of the material protected by this copyright may be reproduced or utilized in any form, electronic or mechanical, including photocopying, recording, or by any information storage and retrieval system, without written permission from the copyright owner.

The authors, editor, and publisher have made every effort to provide accurate information. However, they are not responsible for errors, omissions, or for any outcomes related to the use of the contents of this book and take no responsibility for the use of the products and procedures described. Treatments and side effects described in this book may not be applicable to all people; likewise, some people may require a dose or experience a side effect that is not described herein. Drugs and medical devices are discussed that may have limited availability controlled by the Food and Drug Administration (FDA) for use only in a research study or clinical trial. Research, clinical practice, and government regulations often change the accepted standard in this field. When consideration is being given to use of any drug in the clinical setting, the healthcare provider or reader is responsible for determining FDA status of the drug, reading the package insert, and reviewing prescribing information for the most up-to-date recommendations on dose, precautions, and contraindications, and determining the appropriate usage for the product. This is especially important in the case of drugs that are new or seldom used.

Production Credits

Senior Acquisitions Editor: Nancy Anastasi Duffy
Editorial Assistant: Sara Cameron
Production Director: Amy Rose
Production Assistant: Tina Chen
Marketing Manager: Ilana Goddess

Manufacturing and Inventory Supervisor: Amy Bacus
Composition: Appingo Publishing Services
Printing and Binding: Malloy, Inc.
Cover Printing: Malloy, Inc.

All artwork courtesy of Sharon Ostalecki. Figure 3 courtesy of John Romans.

Cover Credits
Cover Design: Carolyn Downer, John Romans
Cover Images: © Stockbyte/Alamy Images; © Photos.com; © Stockbyte/age fotostock; © Victoria Alexandrova/Shutterstock, Inc.

Library of Congress Cataloging-in-Publication Data
Ostalecki, Sharon.
   100 questions and answers about fibromyalgia / Sharon Ostalecki, Martin S. Tamler.
     p. cm.
   Includes index.
   ISBN-13: 978-0-7637-6656-6
   ISBN-10: 0-7637-6656-9
   1. Fibromyalgia—Popular works. 2. Fibromyalgia—Miscellanea. I. Tamler, Martin S. II. Title. III. Title: One hundred questions and answers about fibromyalgia.
   RC927.3.O883 2009
   616.7'42—dc22

                           2008052306
6048

Printed in the United States of America
13 12 11 10 09 10 9 8 7 6 5 4 3 2 1

CONTENTS

Fibromyalgia is not technically a disease; a disease has known causes and the symptom process is understood. Fibromyalgia is a syndrome—a group of signs and symptoms that characterize a disorder. Fibromyalgia has been nicknamed "The Invisible Disease" because it is not perceptible to others. The face of fibromyalgia is every face, and unless you know what symptoms to look for, you cannot tell who has it and who does not.

Twenty years ago I spent my days searching for a reason for the pain that was taking over my life. Today I am a tenacious patient advocate working to bring awareness and education about a disorder that, although gaining recognition as a valid medical condition, is still a condition that causes physicians to close their practice to treating us because we present with a constellation of symptoms besides muscle and joint aching and pain.

Living with fibromyalgia can be difficult for not only do we live with pain, but many of us are handed a cocktail of condescension and doubts about our limitations. The crisis of confidence that follows can be contagious and soon affects every part of our being.

When I was diagnosed 20 years ago, the challenge was just that—getting a diagnosis. Today most patients see between 5 and 7 physicians to reach a diagnosis and, on average, it takes 1.9 to 2.7 years to reach a diagnosis. I was not that lucky. Before I was diagnosed I had the pleasure of meeting 37 medical practitioners and spent 12 years searching for a label to the pain that was my constant companion. At that time there was virtually no useful information that helped patients learn and understand the many faces of fibromyalgia. So, I learned by trial and error, and sadly, for the most part, our physicians had little information about a disorder they too could not understand. Chronic pain is not just about the patient but about the pain, isolation, and depression he or she suffers.

Professor Harald Breivik, President of the EFIC (European Federation of International Association for the Study of Pain Chapters) states, "Chronic pain is one of the most underestimated healthcare problems in the world today, causing major consequences for the quality of life of the sufferer and a major burden on the healthcare system in the Western world. The consequences of unrelieved pain are great." What has to happen around the world to improve the treatment of those suffering with chronic pain? I believe it starts with an understanding and awareness of the condition of disorders and diseases causing chronic pain. Chronic conditions do not resolve themselves and are little noticed or understood by an unknowing public that would prefer not to think about them. With chronic illness, every facet of a once-robust life is overtaken and redefined. From the ability to find and hold jobs to the capacity to build and sustain personal relationships, the facts of a sick person's world change dramatically. Still, we go on. We double the effort and we search for answers to our questions.

For the past 10 years Dr. Tamler and I have been involved in answering these questions through a lecture series focusing on the many facets of fibromyalgia. We have lectured internationally yet the questions asked always have a familiar sound to them, for they are the same no matter what the location: "What causes fibromyalgia?" "Is there a cure?" "How do I stop the pain?" "My doctor does not understand; what should I do?" "Why does it hurt so much?"

So, when your journey with fibromyalgia starts, it is essential that you have the knowledge to navigate through the maze of medical tests and terms, the familiarity with the newest medications, and the skills to communicate with your physician. The questions presented in this book are the questions that were the chorus at our lectures and in conversation with patients, or the questions I presented to the many physicians I encountered in my quest for a diagnosis. This book also includes comments from patients living with fibromyalgia. All were ready to share. Sometimes it was difficult for them, but they are extraordinary for their courage to help others with their thoughts.

Living with fibromyalgia in the early to mid 1990s was challenging just as it is today. But today there are thousands of physicians, scientists, universities, medical institutions, corporations, professional organizations, and government agencies that are working hard to ensure a better future for us. The FDA has recently approved Lyrica and Cymbalta for the treatment of fibromyalgia, and more drugs are soon to come. We salute the pharmaceutical companies for their persistence in developing drugs that target pain, memory loss, and sleepless nights—all the companions of fibromyalgia.

The prognosis of fibromyalgia is better than ever. The efforts of individuals, support groups, organizations, and medical professionals have improved the quality of life for people with fibromyalgia. Better ways to diagnose and treat fibromyalgia are on the horizon. The symptoms of fibromyalgia can vary in severity, and they often wax and wane, but most patients do tend to improve over time. By seeking new information, talking to others who have fibromyalgia, reevaluating daily priorities, making lifestyle changes, and working hard to keep a hopeful attitude, patients can continue to live life to the fullest. And for the newly diagnosed patient, we hope this book will ease your journey and answer many of the questions most of us once asked to achieve a better quality of life despite fibromyalgia.

Sharon Ostalecki, PhD

Preface

Forty million people in the world live with fibromyalgia. Why is this number so high?

When discussing the most important aspects of treatment for fibromyalgia, four basic components are always included: the need for enhanced sleep, stress reduction, exercise, and a well balanced diet incorporating protein, which is the building block for muscle repair. These common sense requisites should be perfected by every individual in the general population. But over time, as society has become hurried, as the world becomes more rushed and industrious, as individuals try to complete more activities in a shorter period of time, the basic principles of good health get neglected. Therefore, as people continue to remain stressed and neglect the necessities of sleep, exercise, and diet, the incidence of fibromyalgia will continue to grow.

Martin S. Tamler, MD, FAAPMR

FOREWORD

Although the world is full of suffering, it is also full of the overcoming of it.
—Helen Keller

I remember seeing the pleading look in her eyes. *Doctor, please help me make sense of everything that I am feeling.* How many times had I heard those words in my 8 years of private practice? Physicians referred me patients who had widespread pain, fatigue, and sleep problems. I remembered learning about fibromyalgia during my training in Physical Medicine and Rehabilitation. I struggled to provide my patients with information about this disorder—I wish I'd had this book!

Dr. Tamler and Dr. Ostalecki have created an easy-to-read, comprehensive text, organized in a question-and-answer format. They summarized recent drug trials and shared the thoughts of many fibromyalgia patients. This book contains a wealth of practical information such as: How can I avoid a flare? What should I expect at my first physical therapy visit? This manual will be a valuable resource for residents in training, medical practitioners, and patients.

Healing takes courage, and we all have courage, even if we have to dig a little to find it.
—Tori Amos

May this book give you courage to heal.

Tracy R. Johnson, MD
University of Texas Health Science Center San Antonio, TX
Assistant Professor
Physical Medicine and Rehabilitation Residency Program Director

ACKNOWLEDGMENTS

To write any book involves the generosity of many people: our friends who make helpful comments, our heroes and mentors who inspire us, and those who support us in many ways.

A special thanks to my friend and mentor, Dr. Martin Tamler. You embraced my vision for this book from the beginning and your support never wavered. Thank you for joining me in writing this book to help all the patients who share my journey of living with fibromyalgia.

The following physicians and healthcare providers have contributed information, and I am extremely grateful:

Dr. Kenneth Peters, MD, Chairman of Urology,
William Beaumont Hospital

Peter Ianni, PhD, Behavior Pain Psychologist

Loren DeVinney, PT, OMPT, Physical Therapist

Virginia Drouin-Berry, Certified Massage Therapist

Deborah A. Barrett, PhD

These acknowledgments would not be complete without recognizing the giving and caring physicians and medical professionals who guided me in my search for answers to understand fibromyalgia: Dr. Martin Tamler, Peter Ianni, and Loren DeVinney, my physical therapist and friend.

I am grateful to Jones and Bartlett Publishers for recognizing the importance of fibromyalgia education. The staff at Jones and Bartlett is a remarkable group of people to work with, open to ideas and suggestions.

A special thanks to my dear friend, Ginger, who always listens to my complaints of living with pain and guided me on the path to wellness. She is a blessing to those who are fortunate enough to be part of her practice.

Most important, all the patients I have come in contact with—you are the reason this book was written.

Sharon Ostalecki, PhD

No book is ever the product of one person's efforts and this collaboration was certainly no different. The information in this book is the result of many hours of labor by so many people dedicated to benefiting those individuals plagued with fibromyalgia. However, this project would never have become a reality without the help and suggestions of many supportive friends and colleagues.

My biggest thanks go to Dr. Sharon Ostalecki, whose vision of this book and its benefit to the fibromyalgia community is the sole reason for its existence. Thank you for your heartfelt and tireless dedication to the fibromyalgia community. Because of your commitment, thousands will forever benefit from your advocacy.

I would also like to acknowledge the debt I owe to my first mentors and colleagues: Robert K. Silbert, MD; Myron M. LaBan, MD; Joseph R. Meerschaert, MD; and Ronald S. Taylor, MD, who shaped my career and from whom my interest in fibromyalgia grew.

And to the readers for whom the work is intended—those with fibromyalgia, their family and friends, and all the clinicians that find a curiosity as to the contents of this book—it is with great hope and anticipation that this book will prove to be useful, beneficial, enlightening, interesting, and enjoyable for all.

Martin S. Tamler, MD

With a great deal of love, I dedicate this book to Matthew, Abigail, Isabella, Jacob, and "Papa," who are always there to help me in my journey with fibromyalgia. Also, to Renae, Philip, and Nick, who have learned to understand and accept that some days are not always the best when one lives with chronic pain.

Sharon Ostalecki, PhD

I dedicate this book to Trish, Ilyssa, Spencer, and Kendall, who unselfishly share me with the medical community and whose love, patience, and understanding have enabled me to better serve those who are truly in need. To you, those with fibromyalgia and those associated with its pain and suffering will be forever indebted.

Martin S. Tamler, MD

PART ONE

The Basics

What is fibromyalgia?

What are the symptoms of fibromyalgia?

How is fibromyalgia treated?

More . . .

Fibromyalgia

A chronic disorder characterized by widespread musculoskeletal pain, fatigue, and multiple tender points that occur in precise, localized areas, particularly in the neck, spine, shoulders, and hips.

Fibromyalgia has dramatic effects on the body and the mind of the patient. For decades, many patients have not been able to persuade their physicians to believe in the reality of their symptoms. The term fibromyalgia has been used in a disparaging way, and many healthcare professionals generally believe that the majority of symptoms experienced by fibromyalgia patients are either imaginary or a byproduct of depression. These same physicians believe, wholeheartedly, that this group of patients is "crazy, hypochondriacs and/or drug seeking." Additionally, most healthcare professionals, including physicians, find this patient population to be one of the most time-consuming and frustrating populations that they will see in their practice.

AN INTRODUCTION TO FIBROMYALGIA

1. What is fibromyalgia?

Syndrome

A group of symptoms as reported by the patient and signs as detected in an examination that together are characteristic of a specific condition

Soft tissue

The ligaments, tendons, and muscles in the musculoskeletal system.

Wax and wane

Refers to symptoms that come and go without definitive cause.

Fibromyalgia is a **syndrome**, or group of symptoms that occur together, rather than a disease. Fibromyalgia is characterized by chronic, widespread, musculoskeletal pain of at least 3 months' duration in all four quadrants of the body; stiffness; **soft tissue** tenderness; general fatigue; and sleep disturbances. The most common sites of pain include the neck, back, shoulders, pelvic girdle, and hands, but any body part can be affected. Fibromyalgia patients experience a range of symptoms that **wax and wane** over time. This condition falls into the category of muscular endurance disorders that result from exceeding the endurance capabilities of the **muscle**. Once this occurs, the interdigitating fibers of the muscle become mechanically locked into a position that produces pain. These pain-producing sites are known as **tender points**, and they can be found in virtually every muscle of the body. Any condition (i.e., infections, connective tissue disorders, trauma) that diminishes the endurance of the muscles can put an individual at increased risk of developing fibromyalgia. The use of the term fibromyalgia, however, is probably no more descriptive than using the term rash. When one thinks of the term rash, it immediately evokes the thought of a skin disorder. However, this term alone is inadequate to reveal the etiology of that skin disorder. Similarly, fibromyalgia refers to some muscle endurance disorder but fails to disclose the underlying cause of the syndrome. When a single muscle is overused, the muscle becomes locked down or stuck in a noncontracting state and is often referred to as a "charley horse." When a group or region of muscles experiences this phenomenon, it is designated as **myofascial pain** syndrome or regional fibromyalgia. When the problem becomes widespread, involving all four quadrants of the body (i.e., the right and left sides, both above and below the waist), then it is referred to as fibromyalgia.

2. List the underlying conditions that cause or perpetuate the low-endurance state of the muscle in fibromyalgia.

- Sleep disorders
- Stress and tension
- Endocrine problems (i.e., **thyroid** and parathyroid disorders)
- Neurologic disorders (i.e., radiculopathy, peripheral nerve entrapment, multiple sclerosis, myasthenia gravis)
- Myopathies and muscle deficiencies
- Infectious diseases
- Connective tissue diseases (i.e., lupus, **rheumatoid arthritis [RA]**)
- Nutritional deficiencies
- Chronic microtrauma (i.e., poor posture, repetitive motion)
- Macrotrauma (i.e., motor vehicle accidents, sudden impact injuries)
- Postoperative influences (i.e., immobility, spasm, muscle injury)
- Other conditions that lead to a deconditioned or debilitated state

The Basics

Muscle

A body tissue consisting of long cells that contract when stimulated and produce motion.

Tender points

Sites where the interdigitating fibers of the muscle become mechanically locked into a position that produces pain.

Myofascial pain

Pain and tenderness in the muscles and adjacent fibrous tissues (fascia).

Thyroid

A gland located beneath the voice box (larynx) that produces thyroid hormone. The thyroid helps regulate growth and metabolism.

Rheumatoid arthritis (RA)

A chronic disease characterized by stiffness and inflammation of the joints, loss of mobility, weakness, and deformity.

3. Can you list some of the muscle dysfunctions associated with fibromyalgia?

Individuals with fibromyalgia show a number of abnormal patterns in muscle physiology, such as the following:

- High basal levels of muscle tension even at rest
- Asymmetries: higher levels of muscle tension in the same muscle on one side of the body than on the other
- Coactivations: muscles that are not designed to function during a movement are found to tense during the activity
- Failure to recover after exertion: muscles do not return to relaxation following use
- Long-term atrophy of muscle tissue with shortening of muscle fibers and increased sensitivity

Many of these abnormalities make sense in terms of the patient's body reaction to the presence of pain. When human beings experience pain, they tense. A common example of this finding is the twisting of body posture defensively around a painful site in order to splint or brace the painful region. This causes the tensed torso and musculature to lose **flexibility**. Additionally, those in severe pain tend to avoid activity in an attempt to minimize pain. This results in a muscle disuse syndrome consisting of atrophy of muscle tissue, muscle deconditioning, and loss of flexibility and strength.

Flexibility

The ability of muscle to relax and yield to stretch forces.

4. Why did fibromyalgia remain invisible for so long?

One contributing factor is the fact that 80% to 95% of fibromyalgia sufferers are women. In fact, fibromyalgia is believed to be the most common cause of chronic musculoskeletal pain in women aged 20 to 50. Like other conditions predominantly acquired by women, its symptoms have often been attributed to hypochondria. In the 1950s and 1960s in the United States, fibromyalgia was often considered a "manifestation of psychogenic rheumatism," (Barrett, 2000) and patients were considered hysterical. Until recently, many physicians classified people who complained of the pain and fatigue as malingerers. Even with growing evidence of the physical reality of fibromyalgia, the gendered nature and virtual invisibility of this condition can result in insensitive and (at worst) nontherapeutic doctor–patient relations.

The gendered nature of fibromyalgia can also negatively impact men with the disorder. Because fibromyalgia is defined as a "women's condition," men with symptoms confront separate issues of credibility. Not only can the physical diagnosis be overlooked in men, as with breast cancer or eating disorders, but there is the added psychological impact as males face the additional burden of contending with weak, painful muscles in light of societal ideals of masculine strength and independence.

Jerry's comment:

I would like to bring up a common grievance among fibromyalgia sufferers: We are not always taken seriously because we don't look as sick as we feel—if we look sick at all. Because of that, some people don't believe that we are suffering. I know now that not looking as sick as you feel, and having some people not believe you, is not the hardest part of fibromyalgia. You must know and understand that some people either don't want to or can't understand what you're going through.

Like any difficult situation, your attitude is the key. In this case, the glass can either be half empty or half full. Although some days I felt miserable and no one could tell, on a good day I felt like a million bucks. And it was in this latter situation that not looking like the scourge of the Earth wasn't so bad.

5. Is awareness of fibromyalgia increasing?

Awareness of fibromyalgia is definitely growing and will continue to do so. One of the most important recent contributions to this increased awareness has been the U.S. Food and Drug Administration's (FDA) approval of Lyrica® (pregabalin) in

Even with growing evidence of the physical reality of fibromyalgia, the gendered nature and virtual invisibility of this condition can result in insensitive and (at worst) nontherapeutic doctor–patient relations.

The Basics

2007 and Cymbalta® (duloxetine) in 2008. History reveals that a similar phenomenon occurred with the management and treatment of depression during the 1980s. Before the release of Prozac, depression was a disorder rarely discussed or treated by most physicians. After the release of Prozac and subsequent similar medications (**select serotonin reuptake inhibitors [SSRIs]**), a greater understanding of depression developed, and the treatment of depression became commonplace for all physicians.

Prior to the pharmaceutical companies' involvement, one of the most significant contributions to the visibility of fibromyalgia was the creation of diagnostic criteria by the American College of Rheumatology (ACR) in 1990. In 1992, a second significant contribution came when medical experts from around the globe signed an international declaration that was endorsed by the **World Health Organization** which stated that fibromyalgia was "indeed a true medical problem." Although the clinical diagnosis of fibromyalgia is currently based on detecting 11 of 18 tender points (regions that are painful when manually **palpated** with 4 kg of pressure), increased sensitivity to pressure in this condition extends beyond tender points and involves the entire body. While the official diagnostic criteria rest on an examination by a physician with knowledge of "tender" points throughout the body, this "classification" system is probably best reserved for sorting patients in clinical research studies. This is because the disorder is dynamic, constantly changing; in some instances a patient having a good day may only have 8 tender point locations and on a bad day 15. Does that mean the disorder was coming and going? Of course not. As a result, the diagnosis should not rest solely on the ACR criteria. Although some physicians still refuse to accept that the bundle of symptoms commonly associated with fibromyalgia actually constitutes a real disease entity, a growing number of physicians now recognize and treat fibromyalgia. With further research and education this number will continue to grow.

Select serotonin reuptake inhibitor (SSRI)
A type of drug that is used to treat depression.

World Health Organization
The directing and coordinating authority for health within the United Nations' system.

Palpate
To touch or feel.

6. *How common is fibromyalgia?*

Fibromyalgia is the second most common rheumatologic disorder following osteoarthritis. It is the number one cause of severe, generalized musculoskeletal pain even when back pain is included on the list. Population-based studies have demonstrated that fibromyalgia affects approximately 2% to 7% of the population, with a very similar prevalence in at least five industrialized countries. This translates into approximately 6 to 21 million Americans who suffer from fibromyalgia. However, at any one time, 10% to 12% of the general population report chronic generalized musculoskeletal pain that cannot be traced to a specific structural or inflammatory cause. Such idiopathic widespread pain most often fits the classification criteria for fibromyalgia. Women are generally affected by fibromyalgia disorder eight to ten times more than men, and the syndrome most often develops during the reproductive years. Children can also suffer from fibromyalgia; however, in this age group, boys and girls are equally affected.

Jenny's comment:

We think of fibromyalgia as something that happens to other people, people we don't even know. How different it seems when it happens to you. Indeed, every case of fibromyalgia is unique. The onset of this disease is unique in each patient. Nonetheless, in the stories of individual patients certain patterns emerge or at least suggest themselves. For example, the onset of fibromyalgia often follows some serious injury or illness. Some people are genetically **predisposed** *to fibromyalgia so that they fall prey to it after an injury or illness. Another common theme is that, because there are so many mysterious symptoms and because the pain occurs in so many places, fibromyalgia is often misdiagnosed or regarded as "all in the patient's head." One thing is for sure: fibromyalgia always has a tremendous impact on the patient's life.*

Women are generally affected by fibromyalgia disorder eight to ten times more than men, and the syndrome most often develops during the reproductive years.

Predispose
Having factors that increase the risk of myofascial pain.

7. *What are the symptoms of fibromyalgia?*

Fibromyalgia literally means "condition of pain in the muscle fibers." The most prominent symptom of fibromyalgia is the presence of widespread muscle pain, often achy, gnawing or burning, either constant or recurrent, and varying in severity. Pain may wax and wane but is usually present all day and is made worse with increased activity, stress, and/or poor sleep. The muscle pain is often confusing to the patient and the health practitioner because the pain can fade and intensify, or even change location within the body, but this usually corresponds to the muscles that have been fatigued beyond their endurance capabilities. Muscles become tightened down into taunt fibrous bands. The stretch placed on **fascia** and musculotendinous fibers, as they draw inward toward the center and away from the origin and insertion of the muscle, produces the pain. The pain can begin at the site of an injury and then become systemic, spreading to all muscles of the body as accessory muscles become overused trying to compensate for other overexhausted muscles. The pain of fibromyalgia has been described as having "charley horses" scattered all over the body. As the pain worsens it can result in various combinations of numbness, tingling, and radiating pain. Over time the sensory system can develop **allodynia**, a painful response to a usually nonpainful stimulus. Allodynia differs from **hyperalgesia**, an extreme reaction to a stimulus that is normally painful. Both of these clinical features are usually present in fibromyalgia. In essence, all sensory stimuli reaching the brain's sensory processing centers is amplified or augmented to much greater levels than is normal or expected, resulting in extreme sensitivity to exertion, strain, or trauma, with many routine activities triggering intense and severe pain. Additionally, patients complain of heightened sensitivity to sounds, smells, and bright light.

The second most prominent symptom of fibromyalgia is moderate to severe fatigue. Because fibromyalgia is a muscle endurance disorder, exceeding one's endurance capability results in having no remaining energy to carry out routine functional activities.

Fascia

A fibrous membrane covering, supporting, and separating muscle and some organs of the body. Also known as soft tissue.

Allodynia

An altered sensation in which normally nonpainful events are felt as pain.

Hyperalgesia

An extreme reaction to a stimulus that is normally painful.

Furthermore, the pain and fatigue is accompanied by a confusing variety of seemingly unrelated complaints. Some of the other associated symptoms commonly observed in fibromyalgia include stiffness and arthralgias, imitating many arthritic processes; soft tissue swelling; muscle spasms; fatigue; sleep disturbances; anxiety; depression; irritable bowel syndrome; interstitial cystitis; headaches; temporomandibular **joint** dysfunction; chest pain, abdominal pain, and perineal pain depending on the location of the tender points that develop; restless legs syndrome; impaired memory and concentration; skin sensitivities; rashes; dry eyes and mouth; ringing in the ears; dizziness; visual difficulties (i.e., eye pain, sensitivity to light, blurred vision, and fluctuating visual clarity); **Raynaud's phenomenon**; neurological symptoms; impaired coordination; and, at times, sensitivity to medications.

8. What causes fibromyalgia?

The cause of fibromyalgia is not known but it's likely that a number of factors contribute to its development. Researchers have a number of theories about the causes or triggers of the syndrome. Some of the theories include:

- **Peripheral Sensitization (injury or trauma to either the musculoskeletal or nervous system)**
  This can lead to a phenomenon of peripheral sensitization of the sensory nervous system through nociceptive activation. This can be seen in such conditions as arthritic disorders; peripheral nerve damage, as in diabetic neuropathy or postherpetic neuralgia; and in sympathetic modulation as in reflex sympathetic dystrophy (complex regional pain syndrome).

- **Central Sensitization (neurological alterations)**
  Many researchers agree that fibromyalgia is a disorder of central processing with neuroendocrine/**neurotransmitter** dysregulation. In other words, fibromyalgia is a pain amplification syndrome. This central sensitization theory states that people with fibromyalgia have a lower threshold for pain due to increased brain sensitivity

The Basics

Joint
The point of connection between two bones or elements of a skeleton (especially if the articulation allows motion).

Raynaud's phenomenon
Discoloration of the fingers or toes due to emotion or cold in a characteristic pattern over time: white, blue, and red.

Central sensitization
A malfunction in the brain's pain recognition centers that causes people with fibromyalgia to experience pain instead of normal sensations.

Neurotransmitters
Chemicals in the brain, such as acetylcholine, serotonin, and norepinephrine, that facilitate communication between nerve cells (neurons).

Chronic fatigue syndrome

A condition of excessive fatigue, cognitive impairment, and other varied symptoms.

Temporomandibular joint (TMJ)

The connecting hinge mechanism between the base of the skull (temporal bone) and the lower jaw (mandible).

Some researchers theorize that disturbed sleep patterns may be a cause rather than just a symptom of fibromyalgia.

to pain signals. Researchers believe repeated nerve stimulation causes the brains of fibromyalgia patients to change. This change involves an abnormal increase in levels of certain neurotransmitters, which are chemicals in the brain that cause nerves to communicate, and is believed to result from overwhelming the "gated" protective mechanism of afferent sensory inputs into the dorsal root ganglion of the spinal column. Unfortunately, it is not known what initiates the process of central sensitization, but it is interesting to note that central sensitization is seen in other syndromes including irritable bowel syndrome (IBS), irritable bladder syndrome, chronic pelvic pain, **chronic fatigue syndrome**, tension headache, and **temporomandibular joint (TMJ)** dysfunction syndrome.

- **Sleep Disturbances**
  Some researchers theorize that disturbed sleep patterns may be a cause rather than just a symptom of fibromyalgia.

- **Changes in Muscle Metabolism**
  It has been suggested that deconditioned muscles and decreased blood flow to muscles may contribute to fatigue and decreased endurance. Endurance is a function of how efficient the body is at getting oxygen and nutrients to the muscle and then carting away the waste products. Therefore, anything that affects one of these variables can play a role in endurance. Metabolic alterations and abnormalities in the hormonal substance that influence nerve activity may also play a role.

- **Infectious Agents**
  Some researchers theorize that a viral or bacterial infection may trigger fibromyalgia. While it is not an exhaustive list, some of the agents implicated have included hepatitis C, Epstein-Barr virus, and Lyme disease.

- **Endocrine Disturbances**
  Thyroid disease is commonly associated with fibromyalgia and may play a contributing role in its cause.

- **Posttraumatic Stress**

  A smoothly functioning hormonal stress response system controlled by the hypothalamus-pituitary-adrenal (HPA) axis helps the body remain stable under physiological and psychological stress through the actions of three hormones. Fibromyalgia patients often show reduced function of the HPA hormone system. Some researchers also believe that in individuals with posttraumatic stress disorder (PTSD), the HPA axis response is dysregulated. Individuals with PTSD have low circulating levels of cortisol. In one study of motor vehicle accident victims, low cortisol levels immediately after the accident were associated with the development of PTSD and high cortisol levels were associated with the development of depression. Additionally, psychological trauma, resulting from childhood physical abuse or maltreatment, exerts enduring negative effects on the developing brain and induces a cascade of physiological effects, including changes in hormones and neurotransmitters in vulnerable brain regions.

- **Abnormalities of the Autonomic (Sympathetic) Nervous System**

  People with fibromyalgia appear to have a problem with a vast network of nerve pathways throughout the brain, spinal cord, and body known as the **autonomic nervous system**. The autonomic nervous system may be thought of as the "automatic" nervous system that runs the life support functions typically not under conscious control. These functions include heart rate, blood vessel contraction, sweating, salivary flow, and intestinal movements.

Autonomic nervous system

System of the brain that controls key bodily functions not under conscious control, such as heartbeat, breathing, and sweating.

- **Hormonal Influence**

  Researchers have found little correlation with the sex hormone estrogen despite the fact that fibromyalgia is more common in women than men. Many women find that their symptoms greatly improve during pregnancy. Additionally, fibromyalgia patients produce less cortisol in response to stress than do healthy people, possibly having to do with a defect in the HPA axis. When the body is deficient in cortisol, the symptoms of fibromyalgia are mirrored. However, it is not clear how important cortisol deficiency is in the onset or course of fibromyalgia, but it is known that giving patients corticosteroid medications does not improve the condition.

- **Genetic Influence**
  One theory suggests a genetic predisposition to developing an autonomic or central nervous system disorder (i.e., a disorder of the brain and spinal cord) that affects the response to severe pain.

One study reports a 5% to 10% incidence of hereditary transmission and suggests that the possible gene for fibromyalgia is linked with the human leukocyte antigen system (HLA). HLA is the name of the major histocompatibility complex in humans. This group of genes, related to immune system function in humans, resides on chromosome 6, and encodes cell-surface antigen-presenting proteins and many other genes. The proteins encoded by HLAs are the proteins on the outer part of body cells that are unique to that individual. The immune system uses the HLAs to differentiate self cells and non-self cells. Any cell displaying that person's HLA type belongs to that person and will not be destroyed by the body. Another study proposed that fibromyalgia is more common in people who have a family history of alcoholism and depression. Fibromyalgia and reduced pressure pain thresholds have been shown to aggregate strongly within families. An individual is 8.5 times more likely to develop fibromyalgia if they have a family member with fibromyalgia versus a family member with rheumatoid arthritis.

An individual is 8.5 times more likely to develop fibromyalgia if they have a family member with fibromyalgia versus a family member with rheumatoid arthritis.

9. Explain the autonomic nervous system and the sympathetic nervous system and its relationship to fibromyalgia pain.

Central nervous system

The brain and spinal cord.

The **central nervous system** is made up of the brain and spinal cord. The autonomic nervous system is a system of nerve fibers in the brain, spinal cord, and throughout the body that automatically controls regulatory processes such as heart rate, blood pressure, sweating, salivary flow, intestinal movements, body temperature, and various reflexes. The autonomic nervous system has two divisions—one that works like an accelerator and one that works like a brake. These divisions, or subsystems, are called the **sympathetic nervous system** and the parasympathetic nervous system. Generally, the sympathetic nervous system serves as the accelerator, stimulating activity, and the parasympathetic nervous system serves as the brake, inhibiting or slowing activity.

When a hyperresponsive prolonged general firing of the sympathetic nervous system occurs, it is known as the "fight-or-flight" response. It is the body's natural response system for dealing with dangerous situations. The response prepares humans for vigorous muscular activity to counter a perceived threat. It is usually triggered by trauma, fear, anger, or cold and prepares us to react physically and emotionally to a threatening situation. This activation is associated with specific physiological actions, both directly and indirectly, through the release of epinephrine (adrenalin) and, to a lesser extent, **norepinephrine** from the adrenal glands. These reactions include:

- Acceleration of heart and lung action
- Inhibition of stomach and intestinal action
- General effect on the sphincters of the body
- Constriction of blood vessels in many parts of the body
- Liberation of nutrients for muscular action
- Dilation of blood vessels for muscles
- Inhibition of lacrimal gland (responsible for tear production) and salivation
- Dilation of pupil
- Relaxation of bladder
- Inhibition of erection
- Auditory exclusion (loss of hearing)
- Tunnel vision (loss of peripheral vision)

Sympathetic nervous system

The part of the autonomic nervous system that raises blood pressure and heart rate in response to stress.

Norepinephrine

A neurotransmitter found mainly in areas of the brain that are involved in governing autonomic nervous system activity, especially blood pressure and heart rate.

In fibromyalgia, nerve fibers become hypersensitive and more active than normal, resulting in activation of the "fight-or-flight" response.

In fibromyalgia, nerve fibers found in both the central nervous system and the sympathetic division of the autonomic nervous system become hypersensitive and more active than normal, resulting in activation of the "fight-or-flight" response. As a result, any or all of the listed responses can occur. In fact, evidence suggests that the higher incidence of fibromyalgia in females is due to sex-linked differences in the responsiveness of the autonomic and central nervous system. The other major system activated in the **acute** stress response is the HPA axis.

10. What is the role of serotonin?

Serotonin is an inhibitory neurotransmitter that, along with GABA, norepinephrine, and insulin-like growth factor-1 (ILGF-1), modulates or dampens pain responses. Without adequate quantities of these substances in the central nervous system, perceived pain intensifies and the level of pain tolerance diminishes. Additionally, a deficiency of serotonin induces several biochemical abnormalities that best explain many of the signs and symptom of fibromyalgia. This was best demonstrated by administering parachlorophenylalanine, a selective enzyme inhibitor of serotonin synthesis, which produced symptoms of hyperalgesia and myalgia similar to those seen in fibromyalgia.

Serotonin not only dampens pain responses but is also believed to trigger stage 4 sleep, induce smooth muscle contraction (i.e., bowel peristalsis), and preserve the general well-being of the brain by preventing anxiety and depression. Medications that elevate serotonin, such as the SSRIs and **tricyclic antidepressants**, are commonly suggested for the treatment of fibromyalgia. Data does exist that reveals the relative power of each of the antidepressants to elevate serotonin levels. Unfortunately, these medications only allow circulating molecules of serotonin to exist in the body for longer periods of time but do not increase serotonin production. The only method known to increase the manufacturing of serotonin is exercise.

Acute

Condition of short duration that starts quickly and has severe symptoms.

Serotonin

A neurotransmitter within the central nervous system.

Tricyclic antidepressants

A group of drugs used to relieve symptoms of depression. These drugs may also help relieve pain.

11. What is the role of DHEA?

When levels of serotonin are inadequate to trigger stage 4 sleep, this stage of sleep is bypassed. Consequently, dehydro-epiandrosterone (**DHEA**), a vital chemical responsible for initiating the cascade of events that result in muscle tissue repair, falls to low levels in the body. It is believed that DHEA is only produced during stage 4 of sleep. When this chemical is not made, essential **protein** repair processes fail to take place. This results in gradual deterioration of basic proteins that make up the **immune system**, muscle, and enzymes necessary for digestion and cellular function. Laboratory levels of DHEA sulfate can be measured to determine whether DHEA needs to be supplemented. The normal reference range for a 25- to 50-year-old female would be 150 to 250 mcg/100ml. It has been shown that 74% of fibromyalgia patients will respond to micronized DHEA when levels are normalized.

12. What causes the pain in fibromyalgia?

There are mechanical reasons and chemical reasons for the pain. First, if you stretch or pull a soft tissue structure such as a tendon, **ligament**, or muscle, it will hurt proportional to the force of pull applied. For example, bend your thumb backward, and it will be painful. In fibromyalgia, the interdigitating fibers in muscle draw into center and get locked or stuck, forming the tender point. The attachment sites of the muscle found at the ends of muscle are, therefore, placed into a rigid "tug of war" stretch producing the local pain. It is observed clinically that loosening the "locked" muscle does relieve this pain.

The second cause is the process of central sensitization that develops within the central nervous system. People with fibromyalgia have a lower threshold for pain due to increased brain sensitivity to pain signals. Researchers believe repeated nerve stimulation causes the brains of fibromyalgia patients to change. This change involves an abnormal increase in levels of certain neurotransmitters, which are chemicals in the brain that cause nerves to communicate, and is believed to result from overwhelming the "gated" protective mechanism

DHEA

A chemical, produced only during stage 4 sleep, that initiates a cascade of events that causes proteins to repair themselves.

Protein

Complex molecules composed of amino acids that are essential to an organism structure and function.

Immune system

The body system that protects the body against invading organisms and infections.

Ligament

A tough band of tissue connecting the articular extremities of bones or supporting an organ in place.

The Basics

of afferent sensory inputs into the dorsal root ganglion of the spinal column. A "wind-up" phenomenon—repetitive stimulation of C-fibers leading to a progressive increase in electrical charges from second order neurons in the spinal cord—results in amplification of sensory impulses in the CNS, creating greater discomfort than is seen in people without fibromyalgia. **Functional MRI (FibromyalgiaRI)** testing has confirmed this process of the "wind-up" phenomenon. In the following experiment, five pounds of pressure was applied to a person's thumbnail. Pain was rated on a scale of 0 to 10. FibromyalgiaRI was performed to "map" the brain during the painful stimulus. Normal subjects reported the pain at about 3/10, and their FibromyalgiaRIs revealed two activated brain areas. Fibromyalgia patients reported the pain at about 8/10, and their FibromyalgiaRIs showed much greater activation in 13 brain areas. When the normal group's thumbnail pressure was increased to 10 pounds, they reported the pain at about 8/10, and their FibromyalgiaRIs showed many more brain areas activated. Central sensitization not only causes amplification of pain but of all sensory stimuli including sounds, visual stimuli, cold, heat, odors, and tastes as well. Consequently, relatively benign stimuli will cause marked discomfort in fibromyalgia patients with central sensitization.

Functional MRI (FibromyalgiaRI)

Functional MRI is based on the increase in blood flow to the local vasculature that accompanies neural activity in the brain.

13. Are there any inherited tendencies?

One theory suggests fibromyalgia patients have a genetic predisposition to developing an autonomic or central nervous system disorder that affects the response to severe pain. Another theory developed from the parent–child relationships that are detected in fibromyalgia. One study has demonstrated an increased prevalence of fibromyalgia in first-degree relatives of patients with fibromyalgia. Another study has shown that an autosomal dominant basis exists for fibromyalgia. Dominant inheritance means an abnormal gene from one parent is capable of causing disease, even though the matching gene from the other parent is normal. The abnormal gene "dominates" the pair of genes. If just one parent has a dominant

One theory suggests fibromyalgia patients have a genetic predisposition to developing an autonomic or central nervous system disorder that affects the response to severe pain.

gene defect, each child has a 50% chance of inheriting the disorder. Another study reports a 5% to 10% incidence of hereditary transmission and suggests that the possible gene for fibromyalgia is linked with the HLA region. Another study proposed that fibromyalgia is more common in people who have a family history of alcoholism and depression. Fibromyalgia and reduced pressure pain thresholds have been shown to aggregate strongly within families. Yet other studies have revealed specific polymorphisms in the serotonin transporter gene and the catechol-O-methyltransferase enzyme that inactivates catecholamines.

14. How is fibromyalgia diagnosed?

Currently, there is no laboratory test or imaging study that establishes the diagnosis of fibromyalgia. Doctors must rely on patient histories, self-reported symptoms, a physical examination, and an accurate manual tender point examination. In 1990 the American College of Rheumatology (ACR) developed a set of criteria to diagnose and classify fibromyalgia. Included in this description was a finding of widespread pain, present for at least 3 months, located on the right and left sides of the body as well as above and below the waist. Digital palpation with an approximately force of 4 kg (enough pressure to turn the nail bed of the thumb white) applied to at least 11 of 18 established tender points must produce pain in specific areas, including the occiput, low cervical, trapezius, supraspinatus, second rib, lateral epicondyle, gluteal, greater trochanter, and knees (see **Figure 1**). Once fibromyalgia is diagnosed, it is imperative that any underlying condition causing or perpetuating the low endurance state of the muscle be identified. These conditions include sleep disorders, endocrine problems (i.e., thyroid and parathyroid disorders), connective tissue diseases (i.e., lupus, rheumatoid arthritis, polymyalgia rheumatica), nutritional deficiencies, neurologic disorders (i.e., radiculopathy, plexopathy), myopathies, infectious diseases, and other conditions that lead to a deconditioned or debilitated state.

Currently, there is no laboratory test or imaging study that establishes the diagnosis of fibromyalgia.

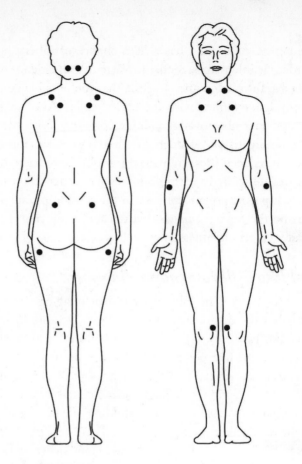

Figure 1   Tender Points Locations

15. What are trigger points?

Trigger points are discrete, focal, hyperirritable spots located in a taut band of skeletal muscle. The spots are painful on compression and can produce **referred pain**, referred tenderness, motor dysfunction, and autonomic phenomena.

Trigger points are classified as being active or latent, depending on their clinical characteristics. An active trigger point causes pain at rest. It is tender to palpation with a referred pain pattern that is similar to the patient's pain complaint. This referred pain is felt not at the site of the trigger-point origin but remote from it. The pain is often described as spreading or radiating. Referred pain is an important characteristic of

Trigger points

Places on the body where muscles and adjacent fibrous tissue (fascia) are sensitive to the touch.

Referred pain

Pain from a malfunctioning or diseased area of the body that is perceived in another area, often far from the origin.

a trigger point. It differentiates a trigger point from a tender point, which is associated with pain at the site of palpation only (see **Table 1**).

A latent trigger point does not cause spontaneous pain but may restrict movement or cause muscle weakness. The patient presenting with muscle restrictions or weakness may become aware of pain originating from a latent trigger point only when pressure is applied directly over the point.

Moreover, when firm pressure is applied over the trigger point in a snapping fashion perpendicular to the muscle, a "local twitch response" is often elicited. A local twitch response is defined as a transient visible or palpable contraction or dimpling of the muscle and skin as the tense muscle fibers (taut band) of the trigger point contract when pressure is applied. This response is elicited by a sudden change of pressure on the trigger point by needle penetration into the trigger point or by transverse snapping palpation of the trigger point across the direction of the taut band of muscle fibers. Thus, a classic trigger point is defined as the presence of discrete focal tenderness located in a palpable taut band of skeletal muscle, which produces both referred regional pain (zone of reference) and a local twitch response. Trigger points help define myofascial pain syndromes.

Table 1 Trigger Points vs Tender Points

Trigger points	Tender points
Local tenderness, taut band, local twitch response, jump sign	Local tenderness
Singular or multiple	Multiple
May occur in any skeletal muscle	Occur in specific locations that are symmetrically located
May cause a specific referred pain pattern	Do not cause referred pain, but often cause a total body increase in pain sensitivity

The Basics

Tender points, by comparison, are associated with pain at the site of palpation only, are not associated with referred pain, and occur in the insertion zone of muscles, not in taut bands in the muscle belly. Patients with fibromyalgia have tender points by definition. Concomitantly, patients may also have trigger points with myofascial pain syndrome. Thus, these two pain syndromes may overlap in symptoms and be difficult to differentiate without a thorough examination by a skilled physician.

16. What is a tender point exam?

Digital palpation with an approximately force of 4 kg (enough pressure to turn the nail bed of the thumb white) applied to at least 11 of 18 established tender points must produce pain in specific areas, including the occiput, low cervical, trapezius, supraspinatus, second rib, lateral epicondyle, gluteal, greater trochanter, and knees (see Question 14).

17. What is a trigger point injection?

Trigger point injection can effectively inactivate trigger points and provide prompt, symptomatic relief. The decision to treat trigger points by manual methods or by injection depends strongly on the training and skill of the physician as well as the nature of the trigger point itself. For trigger points in the acute stage of formation (before additional pathologic changes develop), effective treatment may be delivered through **physical therapy**. Furthermore, manual methods are indicated for patients who have an extreme fear of needles or when the trigger point is in the middle of a muscle belly not easily accessible by injection (i.e., psoas and iliacus muscles). The goal of manual therapy is to train the patient to effectively self-manage the pain and dysfunction. However, manual methods are more likely to require several treatments, and the benefits may not be as fully apparent for 1 to 2 days when compared with injection.

While relatively few controlled studies on trigger point injection have been conducted, trigger point injection and dry needling of trigger points have become widely accepted. This

Physical therapy

The treatment consisting of exercising specific parts of the body such as the legs, arms, hands, or neck in an effort to strengthen, regain range of motion, relearn movement, and/or rehabilitate the musculoskeletal system to improve function.

therapeutic approach is one of the most effective treatment options available and is cited repeatedly as a way to achieve the best results. Trigger point injection is indicated for patients who have symptomatic active trigger points that produce a twitch response to pressure and create a pattern of referred pain. In comparative studies, dry needling was found to be as effective as injecting an anesthetic solution such as Novocain® (procaine) or Xylocaine® (lidocaine). However, postinjection soreness resulting from dry needling was found to be more intense and of longer duration than the soreness experienced by patients injected with lidocaine. Studies support the opinion of most researchers that the critical therapeutic factor in both dry needling and injection is mechanical disruption of the tightened muscle fibers by the needle. Because fibromyalgia is not an inflammatory state of the muscle, cortisone preparations offer no additional benefits. Trigger point injections can be repeated several times in order to facilitate an exercise program or physical therapy.

Rob's comment:

Through my physical therapist, I found another doctor whom many of my former doctor's patients also found and migrated to. He is simply a genius in understanding fibromyalgia and the nervous system. He was so accurate with his trigger point injections that I began to get relief for months at a time. He also understood the depths of fibro and how it can eat away at every facet of your life.

18. If all other symptoms are present, but a patient presents with only seven or eight active tender points, which fail to meet the ACR criteria, do you not diagnose fibromyalgia?

The only thing this scenario implies is that the fibromyalgia patient is having a particularly good day. Tender points can come and go. Patients can have both active tender points and latent tender points. If the tender points are coming and going or if the patient is having a day where the muscle did not get overused, the patient is fortunate enough to experience a better day. In this instance, muscle will start to loosen up and there is less associated pain. That doesn't mean that patients cannot leave the office and later in the day tighten up from the drive home and then be back up to 12, 13, or 14 of the typical 18 tender point locations. The most important thing to remember is that ACR locations are only important for research study classification and are not critical for diagnostic purposes.

19. How is fibromyalgia treated?

Fibromyalgia is a heterogeneous condition comprising a range of symptoms and features.

It is important to recognize that fibromyalgia is a heterogeneous condition comprising a range of symptoms and features. Effective management must take all of these factors into account.

The successful management of fibromyalgia can be carried out utilizing a three-phased treatment approach. Any treatment used in isolation is most often doomed to fail. The initial phase should involve identification of any underlying causative factors and addressing those first (i.e., sleep, diet, connective tissue diseases, thyroid disorders, DHEA deficiency). This phase would include implementation of appropriate medication as needed to address the underlying causative factors. Another important aspect of phase one treatment is education about fibromyalgia and the causative factors. Once the particular areas of concern have been controlled or improved, phase two can begin. This phase attempts to diminish the painful tender points through the use of myofascial release, massage, physical therapy, and, when necessary, trigger point injections. The final phase attempts to improve the diminished endurance state through the use of **aerobic exercise**. However, if exercise is implemented too early as an intervention, before correcting those factors necessary to ensure muscle has an adequate opportunity to repair, further deterioration may ensue.

Aerobic exercise

Physical exercise that increases the work of the heart and lungs; examples are running, jogging, swimming, and dancing.

20. Why do some patients have more symptoms/pain than others?

The expression and response to pain is variable for all individuals. Environmental factors coupled with emotional stress, psychological factors (including anxiety and depression), degree of local trauma, genetic factors, and the body's own chemical alterations all impact the expression of pain. Further influences on the degree of pain expression derive from the extent of implementation of various management strategies/ techniques, medications, behavior modification, and exercise. Thus, recognizing those factors that help improve the pain and those that worsen the pain can have an enormous impact on how severe the pain will ultimately become.

21. Is fibromyalgia an emerging illness only in the United States?

Today it is estimated that fibromyalgia affects 7% of the world's population. Although the pain of fibromyalgia is a global experience, the approach to treatment varies greatly from country to country.

22. What is the prognosis?

Fibromyalgia is a disorder that causes enormous suffering. However, it is not life threatening. For most patients, the results are usually discouraging when using a single form of treatment in isolation. When phase two and phase three principles are utilized without first identifying and treating an underlying causative factor, results improve from direct symptomatic management. One study found that 47% of patients with fibromyalgia no longer fulfilled ACR criteria 2 years after diagnosis, and remission objectively occurred in 24.2%. When a phase one approach is also included, greater than 74% of patients will respond favorably. The mere fact that the pharmaceutical companies are now spending research and development monies on this disorder should provide increasing hope to the millions of fibromyalgia sufferers.

Jane's comment:

When I'm not feeling good, the first thing I do is review my sleep. Is it restorative? Do I have pain when I awake? To help maintain

Although the pain of fibromyalgia is a global experience, the approach to treatment varies greatly from country to country.

symptom control, I often need to rest during the day. I ask myself, "When was the last time I rested during the day?" I then rearrange my days so that I can rest. How are my pain levels? Do I need to use a Lidoderm patch to help control pain? Am I eating enough protein? Am I drinking enough water? How is my exercise going? Am I overdoing it? When was the last time my thyroid was checked? I make a point to slow down and notice that the sky is blue, and there are children playing. I remind myself how good a hot shower feels. And so on. When I slow down, I can focus again on what I need in order to be happy and to be comfortable with fibromyalgia.

I spent so many years trying to keep up with what my friends could physically do that I lost sight of the big picture: Life is to be enjoyed. I learned I had to plan a little more. I plan my days so that I can enjoy them. What things are most important to complete this week? What is most important for today? Can I hire the neighborhood teenager to help? How can my family help? Learning to ask for help and learning to say "no" can dramatically increase your enjoyment of life.

Jerry's comment:

On the same general train of thought, recognize that no matter how well you engineer your daily life to cooperate with your body, you are going to have bad days. I feel great, and I still have bad days. That's what fibromyalgia is. The trick is to have more good days than bad days, and if you do, you're already winning. Beyond that, there's not much more you can do. There is no cleansing process. You have fibromyalgia, and chances are you always will. But take it from me, someone who was completely hopeless and cynical, fibromyalgia is manageable.

Surround yourself with positive people and positive things. Nobody wants to hear how horrible it is to have fibromyalgia, and if you're anything like me, you don't want pity anyway. Focus on positive things, find funny people, and get each other laughing.

23. Who can diagnose fibromyalgia?

A rheumatologist, neurologist, primary care physician, pain specialist, and/or a **physiatrist** have all generally received some form of training in diagnosing of fibromyalgia. A physiatrist is a specialist in the diagnosis and nonsurgical treatment of pain. A physiatrist usually employs a team approach to restoring a patient's abilities (rehabilitation) through various means, such as medications, physical and occupational therapies, injections, behavioral interventions, and management of other underlying medical conditions. Therefore, it is commonplace for physiatrists to include other healthcare providers and physicians from different disciplines as part of a multidisciplinary team.

Physiatrist

A physician who specializes in physical medicine and rehabilitation.

24. What is a multidisciplinary approach to the treatment of fibromyalgia?

In the **multidisciplinary approach**, each healthcare provider (i.e., your physician, your physical therapist, your **psychologist**, your sleep physician, and so forth) treats you independently but communicates with other team members. Over time, each team member learns what the others are doing. Eventually, the team's treatments become oriented as a whole. The team is now a transdisciplinary one in which the healthcare providers' interventions overlap to fill in and reinforce the goals that characterize the team's treatment objectives.

Multidisciplinary approach

Approach that uses many experts from different disciplines working together as a team to manage and control the symptoms of fibromyalgia.

25. Should I go to a pain clinic for treatment?

Fibromyalgia sufferers should go where they can get help. If the pain specialist at a pain clinic is willing to assume the role of overseeing all aspects of fibromyalgia care, then this could be a perfect fit. Additionally, other physicians who treat fibromyalgia utilizing a multidisciplinary approach might commonly request the assistance of a pain clinic in order to provide the most complete and comprehensive care. Many treatment options provided by pain clinics are available for fibromyalgia and for many other common painful conditions that can coexist with fibromyalgia.

Psychologist

A specialist who can talk with patients and their families about emotional and personal matters and can help them make decisions.

The Basics

Mark's comment:

Never give up. That would be my most important suggestion to anyone. Do your reading. Be knowledgeable. Find out what is happening with your body and relay that to your doctor. If your doctor is not willing to listen, walk away. I've walked away from a number of doctors. If they just don't understand, they're wasting your time. When you find the right doctor, you can begin healing.

Lynn's comment:

Fibro, who? When I was first told I had fibromyalgia—actually it was written on the forms you get from the doctors as you're checking out—I never really knew what that long word meant. I thought it was just a diagnosis, and once I asked the doctor what it was, it took a while to explain it. Then you have to research it online, go to the library, learn about it, and then try to wrap your mind around it. And to modify your lifestyle to be successful, it's definitely a challenge. But a challenge that, in my opinion, you need to face head on. You can't just be totally intimidated by this work and the diagnosis. It's a challenge that you can win. It's really about wrapping your mind around fibromyalgia, getting over it, and getting on with your life.

26. Is the medical profession recognizing fibromyalgia as a medical condition?

Many physicians failed to receive any fibromyalgia education during their medical school training. As a result, many of these same physicians are uncomfortable with the diagnosis and treatment of this condition. Studies have shown between 16% and 71% of physicians are not at all comfortable in recognizing symptoms of fibromyalgia, and 25% to 73% are not at all confident in differentiating symptoms of fibromyalgia from other conditions. Education is the key, and as the healthcare community becomes better educated and as better treatment options become available, fibromyalgia will be acknowledged and accepted.

27. How do I find a physician who understands and treats fibromyalgia?

The best option is word of mouth. Ask family and friends or speak with your primary care physician to see if any fibromyalgia specialists are in your area. Check Web sites for local and national fibromyalgia organizations as these will oftentimes list physicians who treat fibromyalgia patients. Realize that while many rheumatologists, neurologists, and physiatrists are knowledgeable about fibromyalgia, not all are willing to put forth the inordinate amount of time necessary to treat this condition. Many physicians find these patients too demanding, too anxious, too depressed, or simply too difficult to treat. Find an empathetic and caring physician, one who has taken an interest in you, "the person." If you find a physician who cares about you and is willing to partner with you in your battle against pain and suffering, that's about 80% or 90% of the battle.

Sharon's comment:

In my search for answers to the pain I did not yet understand, and which assaulted me as though I had aroused a dormant live thing inside me, I consulted many top orthopedic specialists. It did not take someone with my background in science to realize that something very real was very wrong with me: the pain was too severe to be incidental or random. As unbelievable as it may sound, one orthopedic physician told me he did not know what could be wrong with me because he could see no abnormalities on the X-rays he had ordered. This son of Hippocrates actually told me that I must have bad karma.

Having given me that "diagnosis," he referred me to his partner who confirmed that no abnormalities were visible on the X-rays—and therefore did not exist. When, 3 weeks later, I was foolish enough to return for a further consultation, this dedicated physician said, "Why are you here? I told you there was nothing wrong." Unmoved by my persistence, he gave me a prescription

If you find a physician who cares about you and is willing to partner with you in your battle against pain and suffering, that's about 80% or 90% of the battle.

for an anti-inflammatory before he told me, quite plainly, not to come back.

*During the next 8 years, I traveled through many physicians' offices—MDs, DOs, alternative medical specialists, and even a shaman—looking for the cause of my pain. From every one, I heard the song familiar to fibromyalgia patients: You need to see a psychologist. Your hormones are out of balance. Your stress levels are high. You should learn to live with the pain. You just need more sleep, and you'll feel better in the mornings. If the verses varied, the refrain was the same: **There is nothing wrong with you.***

*My persistence cost me several friends who couldn't understand that living with chronic pain has everyday effects. But I developed relationships with new acquaintances who did understand chronic pain because they too suffered from it. We spoke the same language. We could share—and compare—our reactions to treatments, physicians, **alternative medicine**, physical therapists, **massage therapy**, SSRIs, tricylic antidepressants, sleeping pills, support groups, work issues, pain clinics, trigger point injections, and cognitive difficulties. We most gratefully shared the loss of our old lives. It helped immeasurably to know others who also had to adjust to a whole new world.*

My frame of mind improved, and I gained perspective. I returned to work part-time, working now through pain and exhaustion that required longer recuperation time. Finally, one physician, in an effort to dismiss me from his practice because my chronic condition was frustrating, referred me to a specialist for an EMG (a nerve conduction test). It was this specialist, a physiatrist, who began to turn my life right-side-up.

He discussed my symptoms with attention and patience. I was impressed by both the breadth of his knowledge and his openness. From the results of the EMG, he gave me a physical diagnosis; he said I had sacroiliitis. But he continued investigating my pain and, a few months later, told me there was an additional diagnosis: fibromyalgia.

Alternative medicine

A broad category of treatment systems such as chiropractic, herbal medicine, acupuncture, homeopathy, naturopathy, and spiritual devotions.

Massage therapy

Manipulation of tissues (as by rubbing, kneading, or tapping) with the hand or an instrument for therapeutic purposes.

For the next few months, during my visits and in between them with phone calls, I bombarded this physician with questions. He always took the time to answer me. And while the answer might be conditional, it was never dismissive. To this day, I am grateful for the understanding, empathy, knowledge, and time this physician gave and continues to give me. Any way he could, he helped me.

Renae's comment:

In my long and rough journey with fibromyalgia as my companion, I found nothing more important than finding professionals (including allopathic and allied healthcare practitioners) who are familiar with the disease and have an understanding temperament. I was fortunate to find an excellent physician, physical therapist, chronic pain psychologist, endocrinologist, and massage therapist. My good fortune was at least partly due to my persistence. Working with these practitioners has helped me enormously, helped me survive and even thrive along my journey in the world of chronic pain.

Lynn's comment:

Finding a physician who listens and understands is a key component to managing your fibromyalgia. If your doctor doesn't first accept and understand that fibromyalgia is truly something that needs to be treated, if your doctor is not listening to what your complaints are, what your ailments are, you're not going to be successful at all. So, finding a doctor who validates what you're saying is crucial.

28. How do I go about educating my physician about fibromyalgia?

Very gently. Most physicians subconsciously don't like patients assuming the role of medical educators. Most physicians prefer to get their information from scientific journals. Therefore, the very best thing that a patient can do is print off a brief article about fibromyalgia that another physician has written. Do not provide physicians with Web sites or patient advocacy articles. Physicians should be educated by peer-reviewed scientific information, especially when there's a question about the credibility of the disease in their own mind. The last thing that physicians want to do is look at what a patient advocacy group has written about the disorder or how it should be treated. Don't take in masses of information that might consume a lot of the physician's time. A single review article highlighting some of the recent findings will result in the most effective use of the patient visit, prevent resentment or hatred of the patient, and ultimately lead to the best care for the fibromyalgia sufferer.

29. Is it normal to have memory loss?

Altered thought processing and memory loss, or "Fibro Fog" as it is commonly known, is one of the most common complaints voiced by fibromyalgia patients.

Altered thought processing and memory loss, or "**Fibro Fog**" as it is commonly known, is one of the most common complaints voiced by fibromyalgia patients. More specifically, patients complain that they experience difficulty remembering new information or details (short-term memory loss) and feel that their mind is in a fog. Fibro Fog not only encompasses memory loss and cognitive impairment but difficulties with language and learning as well. This symptom is most likely a result of chronic **sleep deprivation**. During a normal 8-hour night of sleep, the body will undergo the majority of its physical repair and restoration during the first 4 hours when the bulk of stage 4 sleep occurs. It's during the second half of sleep that the body repairs and restores the mind. When an individual fails to get adequate amounts of both the first and second halves of sleep (i.e., those with fibromyalgia, the elderly, and hospitalized patients, especially those in intensive care units), the result most commonly observed is altered thought processing and memory loss. . . or in this case, Fibro Fog.

Fibro Fog

The cognitive dysfunction experienced by many fibromyalgia patients.

Sleep deprivation

A shortage of quality, undisturbed sleep that results in detrimental effects on physical and mental well-being.

Mark's comment:

Fibro Fog is like opening a file cabinet to locate information, only to find the folders not in any familiar order. You attempt to organize the folders alphabetically. After checking how you've done, you notice the folders are still in disarray. Repeatedly you try to reorganize until you're tired of trying. If you're disgusted with yourself you may stop and leave it for another day or try to continue. When opening the folders you find that many are missing the contents. The folders that have their contents seem to be in the wrong folder. Confused, you aimlessly search through folders and begin mixing their contents with other folders in an attempt to classify the contents in their proper folder. You do this over and over, back and forth, to no avail. At some point you ask yourself, what was I looking for? No matter how hard you try, you just don't remember.

When I'm in this Fog, it's hard to communicate with others. Finding the proper words is difficult, to say the least. And forming interesting conversation is practically unattainable. What I've learned is to set daily goals. Write them down, starting with the easiest to the more challenging. The key is to keep your expectations pushing the edge just short of failure. Then, as time goes on, I build on my successes. Eventually I find my way through the Fog.

30. Does fibromyalgia cause depression?

Fibromyalgia doesn't necessarily cause depression, but fibromyalgia and depression can be very highly associated with one another. Common sense tells us that if a person has had chronic pain for months on end and has lost his or her ability to function in the real world, then, as a reaction to those unfortunate events, depression is not unlikely. In addition, depression and fibromyalgia share a common chemical basis—serotonin. Serotonin is a chemical that has about 18 different functions in the body. Some of the these functions include the preservation of pain inhibition, the ability to get into deep stage 4 sleep, and the ability to keep the mind on an even keel, thereby preventing anxiety and depression. Serotonin levels drop precipitously in chronic pain states like fibromyalgia. The deficiency in serotonin is, therefore, responsible in part for the anxiety, altered sleep, depression, and pain of fibromyalgia.

31. How will pregnancy affect my fibromyalgia?

During pregnancy, the hormonal influences seemingly have a protective effect on the mother's body in order to protect the baby's environment. Many women report that they get a reprieve from their fibromyalgia symptoms during pregnancy, and some women even resort to multiple pregnancies in order to feel better. This finding clearly suggests that there is some hormonal level or combination of hormones that improves fibromyalgia. Doctors believe this could be due to the ovarian hormone relaxin. During pregnancy, the amount of relaxin in a woman's body increases up to tenfold. Studies show that relaxin supplements help ease symptoms in many women with fibromyalgia. Unfortunately the postpartum state results in an entirely different scenario. During this time the hormonal influence is lost. The baby's needs during the night result in fractionated, poor-quality sleep for the mother. This can be a very difficult time for mothers with fibromyalgia as they can experience significant **flare-ups**. As the baby begins sleeping through the night, mothers with fibromyalgia typically return to their original baseline condition.

In 1997, a Norwegian study was conducted on fibromyalgia and pregnancy. The study confirmed many of the previously noted observations but found that the third trimester was by far the most challenging part of a pregnancy. Fibromyalgia symptoms increased in frequency during the third trimester. This increase in symptoms could be attributed to deterioration in sleep, as an altered body contour makes sleep difficult or nearly impossible in some instances. Most of the women in the study reported that their symptoms remained more intense than normal until about 3 months after they had delivered. They also had a greater incidence of postpartum depression. However, the babies born were all healthy, full-term, and of a good birth weight.

Many women report that they get a reprieve from their fibromyalgia symptoms during pregnancy, and some women even resort to multiple pregnancies in order to feel better.

Flare-up

A period of time when symptoms reappear, becoming worse and then improving again.

Gina's comment:

Looking back, I realize that during pregnancy I felt mostly the same as before I became pregnant, and at times I even felt better. Now I'm picking up where I left off before the pregnancy began.

I treasure the lessons I learned. I learned that if I have another child, I won't be afraid or feel helpless. I'll know that any difficulties won't be worse than I can handle; I can and will cope. My advice to anyone with fibromyalgia who wants to become pregnant—or may be already pregnant and worried—is to take control, to ask for whatever help you need, and to keep asking until someone listens. Yet, even as you look for answers from professionals, never forget that you are the primary expert on your body. Stretch, exercise, take a pregnancy yoga class, eat well, and relax. You may find, as I did, that pregnancy can actually make you feel better for the duration. Your reward for doing all those exercises and asking all those questions is your wonderful baby.

When I was pregnant with our second child, Jake, I experienced similar pains/challenges as with our first child. Throughout the pregnancy I maintained a comfort level by utilizing hot and cold therapy (ice packs and heating pads) along with stretching. My physician suggested water physical therapy, and I found it to be quite relaxing.

I had an easier and quicker recovery with this birth, and in the months that followed I adjusted to having two children and the challenges of living with fibromyalgia.

My second pregnancy, as with my first, was a constant learning experience. I have found that having fibromyalgia requires a constant and ongoing search for what can help me to feel better, and I expect that my journey has just begun.

32. How does acute pain turn into chronic pain?

During an acute injury an inflammatory reaction occurs in the sensory input zone of the spinal cord corresponding to that region of the body that was injured. Over time this reaction can result in permanent scarring of this sensory zone and permanent chronic pain. Even after the body part has healed, the scarred sensory input zone of the spinal cord can still generate impulses that the brain perceives as pain. Additionally, evidence suggests that patients with fibromyalgia experience abnormal pain amplification at the level of the spine, although the specific abnormalities leading to amplification have not been completely elucidated. A "wind-up" phenomenon—repetitive stimulation of C-fibers leading to a progressive increase in electrical charges from second order neurons in the spinal cord—results in amplification of sensory impulses in the CNS, and contributes to the phenomenon of central sensitization.

Even after the body part has healed, the scarred sensory input zone of the spinal cord can still generate impulses that the brain perceives as pain.

Rob's comment:

I never told anybody I had fibromyalgia. As a guy I still thought it wasn't cool. If anyone asked, I alluded to my car accident, some falls I'd had, scoliosis—but not fibromyalgia. The only people I could share the secret name with were two coworkers. One was my own assistant, and she had it very bad. She said I was a good boss because I understood her bad days. We laughed with dark humor at how pathetic we were when we both were having a "Fibro day." However, if I hadn't had this condition myself, as a manager, I wouldn't have had the compassion to understand my coworker's pain and dilemma.

33. I have constant headaches. Is this common for someone with fibromyalgia?

It is important to realize that virtually every muscle in the body can be affected by fibromyalgia. In essence, that means that every muscle and, for that matter, every location through-out the body can hurt. The head is no exception. Two of the 18 tender points identified in the ACR diagnostic criteria are located at the right and left occiput (back of the head). When these tender points are present, they produce pain in the back of the head. In addition, tension headaches brought about from stress may be caused by the development of widespread active trigger points found scattered throughout the muscles of the head and neck.

The Basics

PART TWO

Sleep

Why is sleep important to patients with fibromyalgia?

How can you tell if you are getting into stage 4 sleep?

How can I improve my sleep?

More…

Sleep is a natural, periodic, and reversible behavioral state. While asleep, we are perceptually disengaged from the environment and unresponsive to it. Overwhelming evidence shows that sleep is essential to life. The defining features of sleep include minimal movement, stereotypic posture, reduced responsiveness to stimulation, and reversibility (the ability to awaken).

FIBROMYALGIA AND SLEEP

34. Why do we sleep?

Sleep is vital to the restoration and recovery of physiological processes degraded by continued wakefulness.

Several hypotheses exist to answer this question. First, sleep is vital to the restoration and recovery of physiological processes degraded by continued wakefulness. Second, sleep reduces metabolic rate and body temperature resulting in energy conservation. Third, a more basic biologic theory suggests that sleep reduces motor activity, thereby decreasing the likelihood of attracting predators during the hours of the day that an animal need not spend actively feeding or in pursuit of food.

Sleep is not the passive experience of withdrawing from wakefulness. It's an active progression generated by specific chemical reactions in the brain. Unlike many other neurologic functions, there is no single unique "sleep center" in the brain. Instead, sleep is a complex process that occurs in several specific regions of the brain. Three basic mechanisms coordinate and govern the processes of sleep and wakefulness: (1) autonomic nervous system balance, (2) homeostatic sleep drive, and (3) **circadian rhythms**. These mechanisms maintain sleep and wakefulness in a dynamic balance but also allow for adaptation to sudden shifts in the time and duration of sleep.

Circadian rhythm

A metabolic or behavior pattern that repeats in cycles of about 24 hours.

Rapid eye movement (REM)

A light sleep when dreams occur and the eyes move rapidly back and forth.

Non-rapid eye movement (NREM)

A recurring sleep state during which rapid eye movements do not occur and dreaming does not occur; accounts for about 75% of normal sleep time.

35. What are the stages of sleep?

There are two distinct states of sleep: **rapid eye movement (REM)** sleep and **non-rapid eye movement (NREM)** sleep. NREM is further subdivided into sleep stages 1 through 4. REM, or stage 5, is not subdivided. These stages are classified due to distinct physiologic and electroencephalographic characteristics seen in each stage (see **Table 2**). Sleep stages do not occur randomly but in cycles with each stage of the cycle progressing "deeper" into NREM sleep and ending with REM sleep (see **Figure 2**).

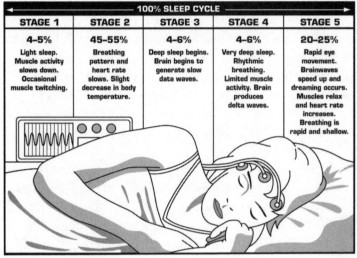

◄─────────── 100% SLEEP CYCLE ───────────►				
STAGE 1	**STAGE 2**	**STAGE 3**	**STAGE 4**	**STAGE 5**
4–5%	**45–55%**	**4–6%**	**4–6%**	**20–25%**
Light sleep. Muscle activity slows down. Occasional muscle twitching.	Breathing pattern and heart rate slows. Slight decrease in body temperature.	Deep sleep begins. Brain begins to generate slow data waves.	Very deep sleep. Rhythmic breathing. Limited muscle activity. Brain produces delta waves.	Rapid eye movement. Brainwaves speed up and dreaming occurs. Muscles relax and heart rate increases. Breathing is rapid and shallow.

Figure 2   Sleep Cycles

Table 2   NREM vs. REM Sleep

NREM	REM
4 Stages	1 Stage
Usually little or no eye movement	Rapid eye movement
Dreaming is rare	Dreaming is common
Brain activity decreases	Brain activity increases
Heart rate and blood pressure decreases	Heart rate and blood pressure increases and varies
Sympathetic nerve activity decreases	Sympathetic nerve activity increases significantly
Blood flow to the brain decreases	Blood flow to the brain increases and varies
Respiration decreases	Respiration increases and becomes more erratic
Muscles are not paralyzed	Muscles are paralyzed

Non-Rapid Eye Movement (NREM) Sleep

This stage is subdivided into several stages that distinguish the transitions from wakefulness to deeper sleep:

- Stage 1 occurs in the beginning of sleep and is the lightest stage of sleep associated with slow eye movements. People aroused from this stage often believe that they remained fully awake. During the transition into stage 1 sleep, it is common to experience muscle jerks.
- Stage 2 sleep typically accounts for 40% to 50% of sleep. It is an unconscious state from which one is easily awakened. No eye movements occur, and dreaming is very rare.
- Stage 3 is the transition stage where delta waves begin to occur, and these waves signal the start of deep sleep.
- Stage 4 is slow-wave sleep (SWS), the "deepest" stage of sleep in which there is a continuation of the delta wave. The basis for all sleep is to ultimately get into this stage of restorative sleep.

Stage 3 and stage 4 sleep are frequently combined and referred to as slow-wave sleep, accounting for about 20% of total sleep time in adults (most of which occurs in the first half of a night's sleep). The highest arousal thresholds (i.e., difficulty awakening, such as by a sound of a particular volume) are observed in stages 4 and 3, respectively. A person will typically feel more "groggy" when awoken from these stages, and indeed, cognitive tests administered after awakening from stages 3 and 4 indicate that mental performance is somewhat impaired for periods up to 30 minutes, relative to awakenings from other stages.

Rapid Eye Movement (REM) Sleep

REM sleep is also known as paradoxical sleep during which periods of fast EEG activity occur. Although dreaming can occur during both REM and NREM sleep, REM dreams are more vivid. The function of REM sleep remains uncertain, although some data suggest an important role for REM sleep in memory consolidation.

36. When is the best time to awake?

The five sleep stages combine to form one sleep cycle. Sleep cycles generally last 90 to 100 minutes. Individuals generally feel rested and refreshed only when awaking at the conclusion of a sleep cycle. Therefore, most individuals will find it easiest to awaken and feel most refreshed after 3, 4.5, 6, 7.5, 9, and 10.5 hours of sleep.

37. Why is sleep important to patients with fibromyalgia?

Many different factors can cause a decrease in the endurance of muscle, but the most common cause is the absence of restful or restorative sleep (seen in as many as 70% to 90% of fibromyalgia patients). During the course of the day's activities, microscopic damage occurs to various parts of the body, especially muscle. Sleep is necessary to repair this damage. Failure to repair the damage results in accumulated damage. Muscle that has accumulated damage protects itself from developing large tears by tightening down into trigger points. It is during deep stage 4 sleep that a cascade of events takes place resulting in protein repair. The proteins that are manufactured or repaired include muscle, immunologic proteins (infection fighting proteins), and enzymes (chemicals necessary not only for digestion but also for various cell processes). Disturbance or absence of stage 4 sleep has been shown to induce signs and symptoms of fibromyalgia. Additionally, if the sleep disorder is allowed to persist, the symptoms of fibromyalgia generally worsen.

Many different factors can cause a decrease in the endurance of muscle, but the most common cause is the absence of restful or restorative sleep (seen in as many as 70% to 90% of fibromyalgia patients).

Lucy's comment:

I experienced 4 years of numerous doctor visits, months of physical therapy, along with the probing and prodding of every part of my body and brain. There were days I honestly thought I was on the verge of insanity because nothing was permanently eradicating the excruciating pain, and no one could tell me what was happening to my body. I would lie awake at night wondering if my legs would move and allow me to walk or if my shoulders would function so that I could brush my hair, let alone take care of my family and remain employed. The physical and emotional anguish was causing a major disruption in my daily lifestyle.

Then my personal miracle took place, and I discovered that I had fibromyalgia. Finally, a name had been given to the mysterious, inconsistent symptoms that had been causing my body to throb with pain and feel like it was slowly deteriorating. More importantly, I discovered the importance of quality, restorative sleep, which resulted in a "rebirth" of my life and a deterrent to the advancement of my disorder. The regenerative power of proper sleep can never be underestimated. With the use of a prescription sleep aid, I immediately began to experience restful, complete sleep. Within a matter of days, the simple act of superior sleep resulted in comprehensive physical and mental effects. I no longer experienced the daily throbbing and searing pain at my pressure points. My muscles and joints finally responded to my conscious requests. I could even dance again! My anticipation of bodily functions dissipated, which further increased the quality of my sleep. With less pain there was a decrease of pain medication. Lastly, my memory and thought process improved dramatically. I might get an occasional stiff leg or arm, especially if I have had a stressful day in the classroom, but with a warm shower, gentle stretching, and a good night's sleep, I am revitalized and ready to experience this awesome world.

Sharon's comment:

The first step in my treatment was improving my sleep with medication. I consider this the first step in my recovery because sleeping more made me feel alert during the day. I also noticed in the months to come my good days started to outnumber the bad, and that is the first step to managing fibromyalgia.

38. How can you tell if you are getting into stage 4 sleep?

An individual who gets into deep stage 4 sleep should feel rested, refreshed, and energetic upon awakening in the morning.

An individual who gets into deep stage 4 sleep should feel rested, refreshed, and energetic upon awakening in the morning.

This is the individual who easily awakens the next morning bright and alert, ready to jump out of bed with energy to tackle the day. This is actually normal! Out of 7 days in a week, a person getting enough stage 4 sleep will feel revitalized all 7 days, not only 1 or 2 days.

39. What hormones are affected by the sleep–wake cycle?

Many hormones are directly influenced by the sleep–wake cycle. Growth hormone, insulin-like growth hormone-1 (ILGF-1), DHEA, prolactin, and parathyroid hormone levels all increase during sleep, with growth hormone, ILGF-1, and DHEA release occurring primarily during deep stage 4 slow-wave sleep. **Thyroid stimulating hormone (TSH)** secretion is suppressed during sleep.

There is one hormone that directly affects the sleep–wake cycle. The pineal hormone, **melatonin**, promotes sleep and contributes to the regulation of the sleep–wake rhythm. Melatonin is secreted primarily during darkness and is suppressed by light. Administration of exogenous melatonin in the early evening hours serves to advance the circadian clock (facilitates earlier sleep). Melatonin is widely available and has gained popularity as a sleep-promoting agent. Some studies suggest that melatonin may be useful in the treatment of delayed sleep phase syndrome, jet lag, work shifts, and **insomnia** in older people with low endogenous melatonin levels.

40. My physician uses the terms "sleep latency," "maintenance of sleep," "sleep architecture, and "sleep onset insomnia" in reference to insomnia. Could you explain each of these?

- Sleep latency is the time it takes for a person to fall asleep. The time period measured from "lights out," or bedtime, to the beginning of sleep.

Thyroid stimulating hormone (THS)

Released by the pituitary gland to increase thyroid hormone production.

Melatonin

Pineal hormone (a hormone secreted from the pineal gland) secreted primarily during the hours of darkness.

Insomnia

Inadequate quality or quantity of sleep, with difficulty initiating or maintaining sleep.

Sleep

43

- Sleep maintenance refers to maintaining undisturbed sleep free of awakenings. Sleep maintenance can be interrupted by environmental causes such as noise, a child, or a bed partner. Internal causes can include pain, anxiety, and bathroom breaks.
- Sleep architecture refers to the NREM/REM stage and cycle infrastructure of sleep. More simply stated, sleep architecture is the five stages of sleep.
- Sleep onset insomnia refers to difficulty initiating or getting to sleep. Sleep maintenance insomnia is the inability to stay asleep after sleep was initiated and is manifest by waking up too early and not being able to fall back asleep.

41. What is a sleep diary?

A sleep diary is a daily written record of an individual's sleep–wake pattern containing such information as time of retiring and arising, time in bed, estimated total sleep period, and sleep interruptions, characterized by number, duration, and causes. Additional information that the diary might include is naps (number and duration), stresses during the day, rating daily daytime sleepiness, rating daily irritability, and listing medication changes and effect. Sleep is a habit, and determining good and bad tendencies requires detailing all the happenings that transpire over a 2- to 4-week period of time. A detailed diary is indispensable for formulating a differential diagnosis and, ultimately, a treatment plan.

42. Is an overnight sleep study always necessary to determine a cause of insomnia?

Most causes of insomnia can be readily identified by a physician through a careful history and physical examination. However, relying on the observations of bed partners or other household members can often reveal additional causes such as obstructive **sleep apnea** or movement disorders that might otherwise be missed. An overnight sleep study, also known as a **polysomnogram** (see **Figure 3**), is generally reserved for

Sleep apnea

Cessation of breathing that occurs during sleep. Usually due to obstruction of the airway, it can also be due to inability of the brain to initiate respiration.

Polysomnogram

A technical term for a sleep study that involves recording brain waves for assessing the quality of sleep and airflow at the nose and mouth.

conclusively identifying these later two conditions and for guiding their treatment. Once it is deemed appropriate to perform for the care and management of insomnia, the test involves placing electrodes over the body and scalp while an individual sleeps in order to monitor brainwave activity, respirations, and body movement. The study measures:

- Sleep cycles and stages
- Electrical activity of muscles
- Eye movement
- Breathing rate
- Blood pressure
- Blood oxygen saturation
- Heart rhythm
- Leg movements
- Body position and movement

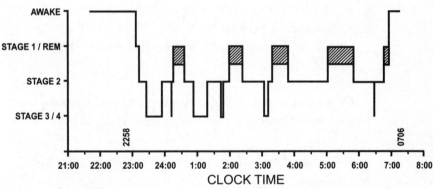

NORMAL SLEEP ARCHITECTURE FOR A HEALTHY FEMALE

Figure 3   Sleep Study Slide

Dr. Tamler's comment:

It wasn't until months later that the real cause of insomnia was revealed. The patient's husband accompanied her to her office visit for the very first time. After listening to a lengthy discussion with the physician about her insomnia, he interrupted. "Has she ever explained to you why she really has insomnia? Has she ever told you about the two elderly Rottweiler dogs that sleep with her? Has she ever told you that they are incontinent each night and at least twice a night she has to get up and change the bed sheets?"

43. How can I improve my sleep?

There are two principle forms of treatment for insomnia: conservative therapy and pharmacologic therapy.

There are two principle forms of treatment for insomnia: conservative therapy and pharmacologic therapy. Nonpharmacologic, conservative therapy focuses on both sleep hygiene and cognitive behavioral therapy (CBT), a set of behavioral techniques implemented by a psychologist or sleep specialist. The elements of sleep hygiene include:

Stimulants

Drugs that increase the activity of the sympathetic nervous system and produce a sense of euphoria or awakeness.

- Limit use of **stimulants** before bedtime.
- Do not use alcohol as a sleep aid.
- Do not exercise 3 hours before bedtime.
- Establish a conducive sleep environment (dark, cool room).
- Use the bed only for sex and sleep. No reading or TV, which stimulate the brain to remain awake.
- Reduce or, preferably, eliminate naps.
- Go to sleep and awake at the same time each day (including weekends).

Biofeedback

The use of electronic instruments to measure muscle tension in any muscle group.

Other techniques to improve sleep include relaxation techniques, **biofeedback**, hypnosis, meditation, and yoga.

44. What role does stress have on sleep and fibromyalgia?

When a person is stressed, they are anxious. When a person tries to go to sleep at night with a racing mind, worried about the previous day's events and the day's events to come, the mind cannot relax, and the individual cannot get to sleep. Subconsciously, the stress continues to be disruptive throughout the entire night causing frequent awakenings. This prevents restorative stage 4 sleep from occurring, and muscles cannot repair the previous day's damage. Moreover, the stress continues to have an impact throughout the next day. When a caricature is drawn of an individual who is stressed or anxious, the individual is portrayed with little squiggle lines by the shoulder, signifying some kind of vibration taking place in that region and suggesting that the muscles are tight and tensed with some quivering taking place. In essence, this is what really occurs. Furthermore, if the postural muscles around the head and neck are maintained in a very tight and rigid fashion, the body can't tell whether those muscles are contracting due to heavy exertion, such as carrying bales of lumber, or if the body is just keeping its muscles tight from stress. The net result is overuse of those muscles, and it has a wear-and-tear effect, ultimately producing the same painful response as vigorous labor.

45. What over-the-counter pharmacologic interventions are available for treating insomnia, and do they work?

Despite the fact that pharmacologic therapy has become increasingly available, many patients resort to using over-the-counter medications or alcohol in a desperate attempt to get sleep. Commonly used nonprescription medications include antihistamines, cough syrups, aspirin, and several unregulated dietary **supplements**. There is no evidence to support the use of such agents in the treatment of insomnia. Many of these medications, including antihistamines, are used for their drowsiness side effect but do nothing to maintain sleep or promote deep sleep. Likewise, some physicians treat insomnia with sedating prescription antidepressants and other medications that sedate as a side effect, but these fail for the same reasons. Furthermore, alcohol actually disrupts sleep, suggesting that the use of alcohol may exacerbate, rather than alleviate, insomnia.

Supplements

The addition of vitamins and minerals, in a pill form, to a person's diet.

46. What is the best class or type of drugs to use for insomnia?

Currently physicians use both prescription drugs not indicated for insomnia (i.e., sedating antidepressants, sedating antipsychotics) and prescription drugs indicated for insomnia (i.e., benzodiazepines, nonbenzodiazepines receptor agonists, melatonin receptor agonists). Of all these available choices, nonbenzodiazepines receptor agonists provide the best option for successful treatment. Because sleep is a habit, it is likely that the drug chosen will need to be used for an extended period of time until a good sleep habit is developed. Two drugs in this category, Ambien CR® and Lunesta®, have been found in double-blind, placebo-controlled clinical trials to be relatively safe for chronic use. Additionally, they maintain normal sleep architecture, suggesting that patients using them can get into stage 4 sleep. Conversely, benzodiazepines (i.e., Valium®, Xanax®, Ativan®, Restoril®, Halcion®) actually prevent stage 4 sleep and are addictive when used chronically. Rozerem® is FDA approved for patients with sleep onset insomnia. Rozerem is a melatonin receptor agonist promoting sleep induction but does nothing for sleep maintenance. It, however, has been used when necessary in combination with the nonbenzodiazepines receptor agonists. Another agent seeking FDA approval for treating fibromyalgia-associated insomnia is Xyrem®. Xyrem is a metabolite of GABA (Gamma-aminobutyric acid) and its precise mechanism of action is unknown.

Elaine's comment:

Although I knew as a healthcare professional that sleep was very important for the mind and the body, I had no idea how much sleep impacted my fibromyalgia. I also was very unaware that I was not getting restorative sleep.

I can see now very clearly that interrupted sleep, or not enough sleep, directly causes my pain levels to rise, and I am also aware that my mind/brain does not function as well when I don't get enough sleep or quality sleep. My physiatrist explained about the impact sleep has on the symptoms of fibromyalgia and prescribed medications to assist me in obtaining quality sleep and sufficient length of sleep. I noticed that this made significant differences not only in improving my pain symptoms but also my mental outlook and cognitive abilities. I find proper dosing of medication(s) essential. I also find that regular and consistent exercise, both aerobic and nonaerobic, has great positive bearing on the length and the quality of my sleep. If I do not get "the sleep that I need," I experience both physical and mental/cognitive symptoms that negatively impact my daily functioning.

Recent articles demonstrate that lack of sleep or interrupted sleep (poor sleep) causes persons to have higher anxiety levels and less ability to think and problem solve. While these articles were not specifically addressing fibromyalgia patients, they were very helpful for me because as a fibromyalgia patient I do know that anxiety causes me to physically hold tension in my muscles. When this happens, it only makes sense that my pain levels will increase.

*In the past I was not consciously aware of how much holding I did. I also wasn't aware of the effects that sleep played in this whole picture. As a result of visits to my **psychiatrist**, my physical therapy, and my psychological treatment, I learned to become attuned to my muscle tension, and what to do and how to release this. Now, I check my body frequently for muscle tension throughout the day. Noticing this provides me with much more choice because I can engage in breathing exercises and thought changing that can discharge muscle tension. There is no question to me that sleep plays a major and significant role in fibromyalgia.*

Psychiatrist

A medical doctor who specializes in the treatment and prevention of mental and emotional disorders.

47. What is restless leg syndrome?

Restless leg syndrome is characterized by an unpleasant, uncomfortable creeping, crawling, tingling, pulling, twitching, tearing, aching, throbbing, prickling, or grabbing sensation in the legs that produces an uncontrollable urge to relieve these

Sleep

sensations by moving the legs frequently. This symptom typically occurs at rest or before sleep and is alleviated by activity. Studies show that symptoms of restless leg syndrome and leg cramps are significantly more prevalent in patients with fibromyalgia and in those with rheumatoid arthritis.

Studies show that symptoms of restless leg syndrome and leg cramps are significantly more prevalent in patients with fibromyalgia and in those with rheumatoid arthritis.

48. What is a sleep specialist?

A sleep specialist is a physician certified in the subspecialty of sleep medicine who specializes in the clinical assessment, physiologic testing, diagnosis, management, and prevention of sleep and circadian rhythm disorders. Sleep specialists treat patients of any age and use multidisciplinary approaches. Disorders managed by sleep specialists include, but are not limited to, sleep-related breathing disorders, insomnia, hypersomnia, circadian rhythm sleep disorders, parasomnias, and sleep-related movement disorders.

49. Is it safe to use herbal products for insomnia?

Many patients experiment with or use herbal products such as valerian root, ginkgo biloba, skull cap, and passion flower. Herbal products have a tranquilizing and sedating effect, but may also cause daytime sedation. These products pose several potential problems including drug interactions with other herbals or with prescription products. Predicting drug interactions with herbal products is problematic for two reasons. First, herbal products aren't regulated by the Food and Drug Administration. Second, there is no quality control in the manufacturing process, so every ingredient in the herbal products isn't always known and listed on the label. Therefore, the amounts of the substances present in each tablet can vary widely from batch to batch. For these reasons, always check with your pharmacist or physician before using prescription and herbal medications together.

PART THREE

Associated Pain Conditions

What causes facial pain?

Is there a connection between interstitial cystitis and fibromyalgia?

What is irritable bowel syndrome (IBS)?

More...

Fibromyalgia patients most often have associated fatigue, sleep disorders, irritable bowel syndrome, migraine headaches, immune system or endocrine system disorders, tension headaches, periodic limb movement disorder, restless leg syndrome, temporomandibular pain syndrome, interstitial cystitis, and vulvodynia.

50. What causes facial pain?

Temporomandibular dysfunction (TMD) causes pain and dysfunction in the head, neck, face, and jaw. These symptoms are often multiple and varied. TMD is a musculoskeletal disorder, which means that it affects muscles and bones. Sometimes people refer to TMD as TMJ. The correct term, as recommended by the American Dental Association, is TMD, or temporomandibular disorders. Both TMD and fibromyalgia affect the muscles of the face, jaw, head, neck, shoulders, and back. Unfortunately, both TMD and fibromyalgia often go undiagnosed. Eighty-five percent of people who suffer from fibromyalgia also suffer from TMD. We see the disorder most frequently in women between the ages of 20 and 50. Emotion and stress play an important role in TMD. TMD may be a sign that the patient is under stress. Anything that relieves stress is helpful, such as reading, exercising, listening to music, and the like. If the stress is getting to be a bit much, counseling may help you learn how to manage it. It is almost impossible to get relief from TMD if the underlying emotional issues are not addressed. Biofeedback is often used to gradually learn how to reduce muscle contractions.

51. Who should I see for facial pain—my physician or a dentist?

Keep in mind that, for most people, discomfort from TMD eventually goes away whether treated or not. Simple self-care practices are often effective in easing the symptoms. If you need more treatment, seek the advice of a dentist and aim for treatment that is conservative and reversible. If possible, avoid treatments that make permanent changes in the bite or jaw.

Temporomandibular disfunction (TMD)

Conditions characterized by facial pain and restricted ability to open/move the jaw.

Both TMD and fibromyalgia affect the muscles of the face, jaw, head, neck, shoulders, and back.

Here are some tips:

- Avoid chewing gum and clenching your teeth.
- Eat soft foods.
- Eat small bites of food and control yawns to avoid opening your mouth wide.
- Maintain good posture and eat nutritious foods to promote joint and muscle healing.
- Hold the telephone, instead of cradling it against your shoulder.
- Eliminate spasms and pain by using mouth guards, moist heat, and medicines.
- Get counseling, stress reduction, or biofeedback/relaxation training.
- Have misalignment of your teeth corrected and, in severe cases, consider surgery.

If irreversible treatments are recommended, be sure to get a reliable second opinion. Many practitioners, especially dentists, are familiar with the conservative treatment of TMD. Because TMD is usually painful, pain clinics in hospitals and universities are also a good source of advice and second opinions. Specially trained facial-pain experts can often be helpful in diagnosing and treating TMD.

52. What is interstitial cystitis (IC)?

Interstitial cystitis/painful bladder syndrome (IC/PBS) defined by the International Continence Society (ICS) as "complaint of suprapubic pain, related to bladder filling, accompanied by other symptoms such as increased daytime and nighttime frequency, in the absence of proven urinary infection or other obvious pathology." Despite a century of study, the etiology of IC has been elusive. IC is a syndrome of urinary urgency, frequency, and pelvic pain but is often associated with other chronic conditions such as irritable bowel syndrome, chronic fatigue, fibromyalgia, migraine headaches, and pelvic floor dysfunction. It is unclear if the bladder is a primary pain generator or an "innocent bystander" in a more

Associated Pain Conditions

diffuse process. More research is needed to characterize patients with symptoms of IC to determine who would benefit from different treatment targets.

53. Is there a connection between interstitial cystitis and fibromyalgia?

Many patients diagnosed with IC/PBS also have symptoms consistent with fibromyalgia.

Many patients diagnosed with IC/PBS also have symptoms consistent with fibromyalgia. In 2008, a survey performed by Dr. Kenneth Peters, Chief of Urology at William Beaumont Hospital in Royal Oak, Michigan, demonstrated that 21% of the IC population at the hospital had symptoms of fibromyalgia. More research is needed to understand this association, including what percentage of those with IC have fibromyalgia.

Renae comments:

There are many similarities between fibromyalgia and IC. I have found that just like fibromyalgia, IC is not well recognized within the medical community or the general public. Not many people know what the condition is and look quite perplexed when I state the name of the condition. I have to admit it is a cumbersome word to just pronounce! And, like fibromyalgia, IC often goes undiagnosed or misdiagnosed, and it takes a diligent patient to search out physicians who understand and are able to run the appropriate tests to make the diagnoses. Once again, it is important to note that, just like fibromyalgia, IC is not a psychosomatic disorder nor is it caused by stress. Another point is that diet is very important to help control the symptoms but does not cause the conditions.

Vulvodynia

According to the International Society for the Study of Vulvovaginal Disease (ISSVD), vulvar discomfort, most often described as burning pain, occurring in the absence of relevant visible findings or a specific, clinically identifiable neurologic disorder.

54. What causes pelvic pain (vulvodynia)?

The exact cause of **vulvodynia** is not known. Vulvar vestibulitis syndrome (now called vestibulodynia) has been reported in 11% of women with IC in surveyed populations. Vestibulodynia is characterized as severe pain upon touch of the vulvar vestibule which is located posterior to the glans clitoris, between the labia minora, containing the urethral and vaginal openings and Bartholin's ducts.

Vestibulodynia is often considered a subtype of vulvodynia; however, in vulvodynia the pain is present even without sensory stimulation, and the location of pain may include the vulva, perineum, and inner thighs in addition to the vestibulum. The International Society for the Study of Vulvovaginal Disease (ISSVD) defines vulvodynia as "vulvar discomfort, most often described as burning pain, occurring in the absence of relevant visible findings or a specific, clinically identifiable neurologic disorder." The cause is unknown. It is diagnosed by touching the area with a cotton swab and noting any pain (mild, moderate, or severe, or score from 0 to 10 on the visual analog scale [VAS]). This "burning" pain is suggestive of a neuropathic pain response. There may be pain fiber proliferation, erythema of the tissues, and hypertonicity of the levator muscles.

The vulvar pain must be present for at least 3 months and infections, dermatologic, neoplastic, and neurologic conditions ruled out. Clinically, there is not a more widely used standardized test than the cotton swab (Q-Tip) test for vulvodynia and its subtypes at this time. Vulvodynia was found to be the fourth most common IC-associated symptom affecting 25% of women with IC. Extrapolations based on three studies examining the prevalence of vulvodynia in the United States suggest that more than 2.4 million women have vulvodynia.

55. Is vulvodynia related to fibromyalgia?

There is strong evidence of interrelated pain disorders including vulvodynia, fibromyalgia, interstitial cystitis, and irritable bowel syndrome. The exact cause is not known yet. There are a variety of medications and therapies used to treat both IC and vulvodynia. Antihistamines, antidepressants, anti-inflammatories, and physical therapy have been used to minimize symptoms of both. In addition, other therapies used for IC such as transcutaneous electrical nerve stimulation (TENS) and InterStim should be explored for their effect on vulvodynia as well as their urinary symptoms. Other useful therapies for vulvodynia include topical agents (lidocaine

There is strong evidence of interrelated pain disorders including vulvodynia, fibromyalgia, interstitial cystitis, and irritable bowel syndrome.

or compounded medications such as baclofen, gabapentin, and amitriptyline), oral medications (gabapentin, pregabalin, and calcium citrate), complementary therapies (yoga, guided imagery, and cognitive behavioral therapy) or a low-oxalate diet. Surgery for vulvodynia may be helpful in the recalcitrant cases but is utilized as a last resort since symptoms may be transient in many women.

56. What is Raynaud's phenomenon? Is this part of fibromyalgia?

Raynaud's disorder causes painful coldness and color changes in the fingers and toes. Many people with fibromyalgia also suffer from Raynaud's attacks.

Fibromyalgia patients suffer from chronic excessive sympathetic activation. One effect is cold hands and feet due to constriction of blood vessels in the fingers and toes. Research shows that this constriction is greater in females than in males. This suggests that the sympathetic fight-or-flight response has a greater effect in females and explains the higher rate of fibromyalgia in females.

57. What is irritable bowel syndrome (IBS)?

Irritable bowel syndrome (IBS)

A chronic functional gastrointestinal disorder primarily characterized by abdominal pain and disturbed bowel functioning (diarrhea and/or constipation). It is present in 33% to 77% of individuals with fibromyalgia.

Irritable bowel syndrome (IBS) is a gastrointestinal disorder present in 33% to 77% of individuals with fibromyalgia. This prevalence rate is far higher than the 10% to 15% rate of IBS in the general population. IBS is one of several "functional" gastrointestinal disorders. A functional disorder is one in which no structural abnormality can be found, but function is disturbed.

The diagnosis of IBS is based on a specific cluster of bowel symptoms, primarily recurrent or persistent abdominal pain associated with diarrhea, constipation, or both. Secondary symptoms, such as bloating or the sudden urge to defecate, are also associated with the disorder.

Scientific study of IBS now examines its **overlapping conditions** with other medical conditions. Researchers have discovered that IBS not only co-occurs at high rates with some other digestive tract disorders, such as functional dyspepsia (stomach distress and indigestion), but also co-occurs at much higher rates than expected with four chronic health problems that have little to do with the intestinal tract: fibromyalgia, chronic fatigue syndrome, temporomandibular joint disorder (TMJ or TMD), and chronic pelvic pain.

58. Do fibromyalgia patients have signs and symptoms that overlap with hypothyroidism and adrenal insufficiency?

There is a significant controversy in the fibromyalgia literature as to whether fibromyalgia is caused by unrecognized **hypothyroidism**. Patients with fibromyalgia have clinical signs and symptoms that overlap with both hypothyroidism and adrenal insufficiency. It is therefore imperative to rule out these two endocrine disorders.

To treat a fibromyalgia patient with hypothyroidism, I prescribe a branded, synthetic T4 and adjust the dosage to attain a TSH level of 0.5–2.0 mU/L. My experience with patients who have both fibromyalgia and hypothyroidism is that attaining this goal often fails to produce a normal sense of well-being. This may be due to the overlap of symptoms between the two diseases or to unrealistic expectations of the treatment's benefits.

There is also significant controversy in fibromyalgia literature as to whether fibromyalgia is caused by unrecognized adrenal insufficiency. One hypothesis is that fibromyalgia patients have altered brain function that alters pain processing by the hypothalamic–pituitary–adrenal axis and the autonomic nervous system. The fatigue, sleep disturbances, myalgias, gastrointestinal complaints, and impaired cognitive function may be due to misalignment of the internal biological clock with abnormal sleep–wake cycles.

Associated Pain Conditions

Overlapping conditions

A secondary illness that accompanies the primary illness affecting an individual. Patients with fibromyalgia are often affected by one or more overlapping illnesses, such as restless leg, interstitial cystitis, or tension headaches.

Hypothyroidism

Underactivity of the thyroid gland, causing tiredness, cramps, a slowed heart rate, and possibly weight gain.

There is significant controversy in fibromyalgia literature as to whether fibromyalgia is caused by unrecognized adrenal insufficiency.

57

Clinical studies of fibromyalgia patients show normal circadian rhythms and normal diurnal cortisol and melatonin levels during the day and night. In addition, the hypothalamic–pituitary–adrenal axis of fibromyalgia patients has been tested by inducing **hypoglycemia** through insulin injection. Hypoglycemia creates severe physiological stress, which activates the axis. Fibromyalgia patients respond with slightly lower ACTH levels than others do, but their cortisol response to stress is normal. Treating fibromyalgia requires a combination of pharmacologic and nonpharmacologic therapies. Although eliminating all the pain isn't possible in most fibromyalgia patients, partial relief can provide significant improvement in psychological distress, cognitive ability, sleep, and physical ability. The most effective treatment plan should not rely on pain medication exclusively but combine the use of exercise, physical therapy, psychological support, and patient education.

Hypoglycemia
An abnormally low level of glucose in the blood.

Renae's comment:

Hypothyroidism, manifested by profound fatigue, muscle weakness, and generalized malaise, closely resembles fibromyalgia. A few years after being diagnosed with fibromyalgia, I was diagnosed with Hashimoto's Thyroiditis — an autoimmune disease in which the immune system attacks the thyroid gland. I was now hypothyroid, for which the standard treatment is Synthroid®, a synthetic replacement for thyroid hormones T3 and T4 that restores normal levels of them in the body. The medication ordinarily works like a charm, but did not for me.

I was eager to start treatment, but after six weeks, the medication did not seem to be helping. My endocrinologist suggested I try Nature Thyroid®, a natural thyroid medication made from a pig's thyroid. (Unlike Armour®, another medication made by harvesting pig thyroid, Nature Thyroid has no inert ingredients added to it.) After 6 weeks it did help with my fatigue levels. By no means was it the answer to the pain and fatigue I live with, but there was an improvement.

I feel very fortunate because my physician was willing to work with the natural medication. In fact, now when his fibromyalgia patients report sensitivities to medications or hormones, he will even suggest the use of a natural replacement.

We, as patients, need to feel comfortable discussing the need to try alternate types of medications, and hopefully your physician is willing to "think outside the box" and find whatever it takes to help control your pain and fatigue.

PART FOUR

Pharmacologic Management

What medications are prescribed for the treatment of fibromyalgia?

Which drugs are currently FDA approved for the treatment of fibromyalgia?

Why are fibromyalgia patients so sensitive to medications?

More...

59. What medications are prescribed for the treatment of fibromyalgia?

Drug therapy clearly plays a role in the treatment of pain. However, no single drug or class of drugs has proven to be the best choice for fibromyalgia pain. Therefore, the physician is left to sort out which of the many options may offer the greatest benefit to his or her patients. Only by taking the medications as prescribed and not skipping or omitting doses can a reliable and optimal result be attained. This is because some medications must be taken on a regular schedule, whereas others may be taken as needed to achieve the desired effect.

Medications that have been tried, with varying degrees of success, in fibromyalgia include:

- Nonnarcotic **analgesics** (i.e., Tylenol, **tramadol**)
- **Nonsteroidal anti-inflammatory drugs (NSAIDs)**
- Muscle relaxants
- Tricyclic antidepressants
- Select serotonin reuptake inhibitors (SSRIs)
- **Serotonin and norepinephrine reuptake inhibitors (SNRIs)**
- **Anticonvulsants**
- Stimulants
- Hypnotics/sleep aids
- Dehydroepiandrosterone (DHEA)

60. Do NSAIDs help in the treatment of fibromyalgia?

While NSAIDs are commonly used in the treatment of fibromyalgia, most patients find little benefit or effectiveness when these medications are used alone. However, this class of drugs may be useful analgesia adjuncts when combined with antidepressants. Furthermore, fibromyalgia patients may have other conditions that do respond to NSAIDs, such as acute and chronic inflammatory musculoskeletal disorders, headache, and fever.

Analgesic

A medication or agent that reduces pain.

Tramadol

A centrally acting analgesic for the treatment of pain in fibromyalgia. Also know as Ultram.

Nonsteroidal anti-inflammatory drugs (NSAIDs)

Drugs that act against inflammation, reduce fever, relieve muscle pain, and prevent blood clots.

Serotonin and norepinephrine reuptake inhibitors (SNRIs)

A type of antidepressant medication that increases the levels of both serotonin and norepinephrine by inhibiting their reabsorption into cells in the brain.

Anticonvulsants

Drugs given to prevent seizures.

61. What are SSRIs?

Select Serotonin Reuptake Inhibitors (SSRIs) are a class of antidepressants that selectively block the reabsorption (break-down) of serotonin, a neurotransmitter that dampens pain responses and triggers stage 4 sleep. Therefore, despite their typical use to treat mood disorders such as depression and anxiety, SSRIs have also been proven to be beneficial in reliev-ing pain and fatigue as well as improving the sleep disorders of fibromyalgia. Medications in this group include Prozac® (fluoxetine), Zoloft® (sertraline), Paxil® (paroxetine), Celexa® (citalopram), and Lexapro® (escitalopram). The best studied SSRI, Prozac, was found to decrease pain and fatigue while improving ability to function. There is some evidence to also indicate that other SSRIs may be just as helpful in treating fibromyalgia. Treatment with SSRIs is not always successful and even when the treatment does work, some people may find the side effects of these medicines unacceptable.

Side effects of SSRIs include:

- GI complaints including nausea, loss of appetite, diarrhea
- Mood complaints including irritability, anxiety, or dulled sensorium
- Sleep complaints including insomnia or drowsiness
- Sex complaints including loss of libido, sexual desire, or ability
- Constitutional complaints including weight gain, headaches, orthostatic hypotension, or dizziness

Many of these side effects generally improved after a few days of continuous use.

Other considerations:

- Using an antidepressant medicine to treat fibromyalgia does not mean that the condition is "all in your head."

Using an antidepressant medicine to treat fibromyalgia does not mean that the condition is "all in your head."

- The dose of an SSRI used to treat fibromyalgia is usually the same as that needed to treat depression.
- Studies suggest that using an SSRI and a tricyclic antidepressant together may be more successful at breaking the cycle of pain and sleep problems caused by fibromyalgia than using either of these medications alone.
- Studies have found that daily use of SSRIs may increase the risk of bone fracture in adults over the age of 50.
- SSRIs may cause drug interactions because they inhibit enzyme systems in the liver that break down other medications. These medications accumulate faster than the body can dispose of them. This can lead to higher drug concentrations and potentially increased pharmacological effects as well as increased adverse side effects. SSRI drug interactions have been reported with Xanax (alprazolam), tricyclic antidepressants, Coumadin® (warfarin), MAO inhibitors, Dilantin® (phenytoin), Tegretol® (carbamazepine), and theophylline.
- While unlikely, taking SSRIs and triptans (a class of medicines used to treat migraine headaches) together can cause a very rare but serious condition called **serotonin syndrome**.

Serotonin syndrome

A hyperserotonergic state that is a very dangerous and potentially fatal side effect of serotonergic enhancing drugs; it can have multiple psychiatric and nonpsychiatric symptoms.

62. How do the SSRIs raise serotonin levels?

SSRIs actually block the degradation or breakdown of serotonin. This maintains the serotonin in the brain for a longer period of time increasing the serotonin effect. The best analogy to use to demonstrate how this works is a bathtub. If water is flowing from the faucet into the bathtub but the drain is wide open, then the water empties right down the drain and nothing accumulates. An SSRI is equivalent to a drain plug. As soon as a drain plug is fitted into place, the level of water starts to accumulate in the bathtub. Now the water levels rise and water is available for a bath.

63. What are SNRIs?

Another group of antidepressants are the selective serotonin/norepinephrine reuptake inhibitors (SNRIs). They selectively block the reabsorption of both serotonin and norepinephrine. Thus, they are also known as dual reuptake inhibitors. Medications in this group include Cymbalta (duloxetine), Effexor® (venlafaxine), and Savella™ (milnacipran). Two small studies found that patients who completed 8 weeks of Effexor (venlafaxine) therapy experienced at least a 50% reduction in fibromyalgia symptoms including significantly improved pain, less fatigue, better sleep, less morning stiffness, less depression and anxiety, and improvements in the disability caused by fibromyalgia. Cymbalta and Savella demonstrated efficacy in a number of outcome variables independent of its effect on mood in two high-quality multicenter studies conducted over a 3-month period of time.

Side effects of SNRIs include:

- GI complaints including nausea, indigestion, constipation, or loss of appetite
- Mood complaints including irritability, depression, or dulled sensorium
- Sleep complaints including insomnia, lethargy, or drowsiness
- Sex complaints including loss of libido, sexual desire, or ability
- Constitutional complaints including weight gain, dry mouth, headaches, elevated blood pressure, sweating, hot flashes, loss of balance, orthostatic hypotension, or dizziness

Cymbalta (duloxetine) is FDA approved for the treatment of fibromyalgia.

Other considerations:

- Cymbalta (duloxetine) is FDA approved for the treatment of fibromyalgia.
- Savella (milnacipran) is FDA approved for the treatment of fibromyalgia.
- SNRIs are sometimes prescribed instead of tricyclic antidepressants because they tend to work faster and cause fewer side effects.

Savella (milnacipran) is FDA approved for the treatment of fibromyalgia.

- SNRIs are not recommended for people with heart conditions because of the norepinephrine effect.
- Similar to SSRIs, taking SNRIs and triptans together can cause a very rare but serious condition called serotonin syndrome.

64. What are anticonvulsants?

Anticonvulsants are a class of drugs designed to prevent seizure activity. They are also useful in neuropathic pain (pain that originates within nerves). Medications in this group include Neurontin® (gabapentin), Lyrica (pregabalin), Topamax® (topiramate), and Keppra® (levetiracetam). Both Neurontin and Lyrica reduce the calcium-dependent release of several neurotransmitters, resulting in a diminished number of electrical signals passing between nerves in the central nervous system. Neurontin is the best studied and best tolerated anticonvulsant for treatment of neuropathic pain associated with diabetic neuropathy, postherpetic neuralgia, mixed neuropathic pain syndromes, phantom limb pain, Guillain-Barré syndrome, and the acute and chronic pain from spinal cord injuries. In a 12-week study, researchers found that fibromyalgia participants who were treated with Neurontin displayed significantly less pain, better sleep, and less fatigue compared with participants who received a placebo. Multiple studies, lasting as long as 1 year, have been carried out using Lyrica. These studies reveal that patients with fibromyalgia experience not only a significant reduction in pain, but also improvements in the areas of sleep quality, fatigue, global function, and quality of life.

Side effects of anticonvulsants include:

- GI complaints including nausea, constipation, or upset stomach
- Cognitive complaints including depression, amnesia, decreased thought processing, or dulled sensorium

- Sleep complaints including sedation, somnolence, fatigue, lethargy, or drowsiness
- Neurologic complaints including double vision, blurred vision, involuntary eye movements, tremor, or ataxia
- Constitutional complaints including weight gain, dry mouth, lower extremity swelling, or dizziness

Other considerations:

- Lyrica (pregabalin) is FDA approved for the treatment of fibromyalgia.
- There are no significant drug interactions with Neurontin.
- Added sedation may occur when using anticonvulsants with other medications that depress the central nervous system.
- Antacids given concurrently with Neurontin reduce its absorption by 20%. If antacids are taken, Neurontin should be taken 2 hours later.

Lyrica (pregabalin) is FDA approved for the treatment of fibromyalgia.

65. What are tricyclic antidepressants, and are they still used for the treatment of fibromyalgia?

Tricyclic antidepressants are yet another class of antidepressant medications used in the treatment of fibromyalgia. This class includes the first available antidepressant medications and, logically, the first studied for fibromyalgia. Tricyclic antidepressants generally function as norepinephrine reuptake inhibitors; however, two (Elavil® and Tofranil®) also have weak serotonin reuptake inhibition. Researchers believe that this gives tricyclic antidepressants their analgesic effect. Medications in this group include Elavil (amitriptyline), Sinequan® (doxepin), Pamelor® (nortriptyline), Tofranil (imipramine), and Flexeril® (cyclobenzaprine). Randomized, controlled trials show that 10 to 50 mg of amitriptyline at bedtime is effective. Flexeril is marketed as a muscle relaxant, but structurally it is a tricyclic. In randomized, controlled trials lasting 6 to 12 weeks, patients given 10 to 40 mg per day also found it effective.

Side effects of tricyclic antidepressants include:

- GI complaints including constipation
- Sleep complaints including sedation, somnolence, fatigue, lethargy, or drowsiness
- Neurologic complaints including blurred vision, impaired balance, impaired gait, or impaired attention levels
- Constitutional complaints including weight gain or dry mouth
- Additional complaints including skin rashes, jaundice, sexual dysfunction, decreased tear flow, urinary retention, arrhythmias, or abnormalities that prevent the muscle cells of the heart from contracting in an efficient, synchronized pattern

There are other considerations:

- Doses recommended for fibromyalgia are much smaller than the doses used to treat depression.
- For patients who need to be slowly titrated on the medication, doxepin (10 mg/ml) is available as a liquid.
- Tricyclics depress activity in the brain and spinal cord. Accumulative depressant effects may occur if they are taken along with other medications that depress the central nervous system, such as antihistamines, tranquilizers, sleep medications, narcotics, muscle relaxants, and alcohol.
- Expect to wait 1 to 3 weeks for maximum sleep modification and analgesic effect.

66. I use Elavil for sleep. Is this an effective drug?

Elavil and Desyrel® (trazodone), two first generation drugs, have significant anticholinergic side effects including dry mouth, heart problems, and sedation. It is because of their sedative side effect that these medications were typically chosen to treat fibromyalgia. However, if a patient is put to sleep with

Elavil but then is kept up all night with a dry cotton-mouth, the medication is a poor choice due to the disruptive nature to deep stage 4 sleep. Until 1992, tricyclic antidepressants were all that were available and thus the best choice at the time. They were also viewed as ideal medications because of their antidepressant properties (it was believed that all fibromyalgia patients were depressed). However, studies now show that the doses that are used for sleep in fibromyalgia are incapable of providing antidepressant characteristics. In addition, while strong evidence exists to demonstrate Elavil's effectiveness in helping sleep and overall well-being, better medications have been developed as alternatives with less concerning side effects and better targeting of specific neurotransmitters.

Jane's comment:

I did not like the Elavil. Though it helped me sleep, I awoke feeling drugged. In addition, I started craving sugar. Never in my life had I wanted straight sugar on a spoon. Needless to say, I started to gain weight. I took the Elavil for a while and started feeling a little better, but I gained 25 pounds. So I stopped the Elavil and lost 20 pounds. Then the pain and fatigue increased, so I went back on the Elavil. This started a vicious cycle.

67. Why is it sometimes necessary to try many different drugs to treat my symptom?

The World Health Organization recommends a stepped approach to managing pain. During initial treatment, the lowest dose of a single agent is used. The dose is titrated to determine the effectiveness of the medication. If a single medication doesn't control the pain, then an additional medication from another class is added. This method incorporates all the different types of medications to maximize pain control. During each step, the patient is assessed to determine his or her response to the treatment. Fibromyalgia patients present with different symptoms and severity of symptoms. As a result, it is common for physicians to try different drugs in various combinations.

The World Health Organization recommends a stepped approach to managing pain

68. Which drugs are currently FDA approved for the treatment of fibromyalgia?

There are three medications currently approved by the U.S. Food and Drug Administration (FDA) for the treatment of fibromyalgia. Lyrica (pregabalin), manufactured by Pfizer, was the first to receive approval in June 2007; Cymbalta (duloxetine), manufactured by Eli Lilly, received approval in June 2008; and Savella (milnacipran), manufactured by Cypress Bioscience, Inc., received approval in January 2009.

Fibromyalgia Impact Questionnaire (FIQ)

The FIQ is an assessment and evaluation instrument developed to measure fibromyalgia patient status, progress, and outcomes. It has been designed to measure the components of health status that are believed to be most affected by fibromyalgia.

Cymbalta was found to be effective in treating fibromyalgia in a 12-week randomized, double-blind placebo-controlled trial.

Lyrica was found to be effective in treating fibromyalgia in an 8-week randomized, double-blind placebo-controlled trial. The study compared various doses of pregabalin in 529 patients. The study reported that Lyrica at 450 mg/day significantly reduced the average severity of pain in the study compared with placebo (-0.93 on a 0 to 10 scale; $P \le 0.001$), and significantly more patients in this group had $\ge 50\%$ improvement in pain at the end point (29%, versus 13% in the placebo group; $P = 0.003$). Lyrica at 300 and 450 mg/day was associated with significant improvements in sleep quality, fatigue, and global measures of change. Lyrica, at 450 mg/day, improved several domains of health-related quality of life. Dizziness and somnolence were the most frequent adverse events. Rates of discontinuation due to adverse events were similar across all four treatment groups. The authors concluded that Lyrica at 450 mg/day was efficacious for the treatment of fibromyalgia, reducing symptoms of pain, disturbed sleep, and fatigue compared with placebo. Lyrica was well tolerated and improved global measures and health-related quality of life.

Cymbalta was found to be effective in treating fibromyalgia in a 12-week randomized, double-blind placebo-controlled trial. The study compared a 60-mg dose of Cymbalta to a placebo in 207 patients. The study reported that Cymbalta-treated subjects improved significantly more ($P = 0.027$) on the **Fibromyalgia Impact Questionnaire (FIQ)** total score, with a treatment difference of -5.53 (95% confidence interval -10.43, -0.63), but not significantly more on the FIQ pain score (P = 0.130). Compared with placebo-treated subjects, Cymbalta-treated subjects had significantly greater reductions in Brief Pain Inventory average pain severity score (P = 0.008), Brief Pain Inventory average interference from pain score (P = 0.004), number of tender points (P = 0.002), and FIQ stiffness score (P = 0.048), and had significantly greater improvement in mean tender point pain threshold (P = 0.002), CGI-Severity (P = 0.048), PGI-Improvement (P = 0.033), and several quality-of-life measures. Cymbalta treatment improved fibromyalgia symptoms and pain severity regardless of baseline status of major depressive disorder. The authors concluded that Cymbalta was an effective and safe treatment for many of the symptoms associated with fibromyalgia in subjects with or without major depressive disorder.

Savella was found to be effective in treating fibromyalgia in a 12-week randomized, double-blind, placebo-controlled, flexible dose escalation monotherapy trial. The study compared milnacipran twice daily, milnacipran once daily, and placebo in 125 patients. Eighty-four percent of all milnacipran patients escalated to the target dose of 200 mg with no tolerability issues. Of the milnacipran-treated patients, 37% reported at least a 50% reduction in the intensity of their pain, compared to just 14% of placebo patients (P = 0.0395). Milnacipran twice daily was also statistically superior to placebo treatment on the FIQ, the McGill pain questionnaire, and a 24-hour recall visual analogue pain scale. Furthermore, milnacipran patients reported significant improvement in fatigue on the FIQ fatigue scale and 75% of all milnacipran-treated patients reported overall global improvement, compared to 38% in the placebo group (P = 0.004). The results of the study revealed that both the once- and twice-daily groups showed statistically significant improvements in pain, as well as improvements in global well being and fatigue, and the drug was generally well tolerated.

Another drug actively seeking FDA approval is Xyrem (sodium oxybate), a GABA agonist and neuroprotective nutrient that is classified as an orphan drug. In one study, Xyrem effectively reduced the symptoms of pain and fatigue in patients with fibromyalgia and dramatically reduced the sleep abnormalities (alpha intrusion and decreased slow-wave sleep) associated with the nonrestorative sleep characteristic of this disorder.

69. Should I be concerned with the side effects of the medications I am taking?

Acetaminophen
The generic name for Tylenol.

All medications have side effects, including Tylenol (**acetaminophen**), and all have the potential to make an individual feel worse. Manufactures are required to list all potential side effects, although this does not mean that every patient will experience all of these reactions. In fact, the FDA requires the manufacturers to list all patient complaints experienced while taking a medication during the drug's FDA-approval process. Therefore, antidepressants will have depression listed as a side effect and hypnotics will have drowsiness listed. True side effects of a medication are the ones that occur at a frequency significantly different than those experienced while taking a placebo. If a concern develops about a medication's side effect, the prescribing physician should be notified as soon as possible to determine the best course of action.

If you have a complaint about a product regulated by the FDA, they would like to hear about it. Two reporting systems are available:

1. Consumer Complaint Coordinators (CCC): Located in FDA offices throughout the United States and Puerto Rico, they will listen, document your complaint about an FDA-regulated product, and follow up as necessary. Consumers should report problems to the CCC for their geographic region. (http://www.fda.gov/opacom/backgrounders/complain.html)

MedWatch
The Food and Drug Administration's reporting system for adverse events.

2. **MedWatch**: Used for reporting any adverse events (unexpected side effects) that occur while using human healthcare products and FDA-regulated products such as medicines, over-the-counter products, supplements,

cosmetics, and medical equipment. (https://www.access
data.fda.gov/scripts/medwatch)

70. What is the role of a compounding pharmacy?

For patients with fibromyalgia, **compounding pharmacies**
play a completely different role than conventional pharmacies.
They offer medications in different forms and different dosages than those available and supplied by commercial pharmaceutical manufacturers. They also offer unique medications
and combinations not produced for nationwide distribution.
Compound pharmacists typically have more training, equipment, and knowledge in the area of compounding than traditional pharmacists. A compound pharmacy has thousands of
dollars invested in special equipment such as capsule-making
machines, sensitive scales to measure accurate doses, ventilat-
ing hoods for safety, mills to reduce particle size, and various
mixing devices. As a result of this equipment and their expertise, compound pharmacists will typically prepare unique
dosage forms of capsules, creams, suppositories, and liquids
on a daily basis.

Examples of medications that can be obtained through a
compounding pharmacy are:

- Liquid forms of medications supplied in various con-
  centrations
- Transdermal gels
- Capsules (in both immediate- and sustained-release
  versions)
- Suppositories
- Oral troches

There are different reasons for using each delivery method and
each one effectively dispenses the correct dose of medication
to the patient.

For patients with fibromyalgia, compounding pharmacies play a completely different role than conventional pharmacies.

Compounding pharmacy

A facility that both makes and sells prescription drugs. A compounding pharmacy can often prepare drug formulas that are specially tailored to patients.

71. *Are there any concerns with the use of herbs and supplements?*

The use of herbs and supplements can pose several problems. First, these products aren't regulated by the FDA. Therefore, they can make unsubstantiated claims of safety and effectiveness. Realizing that fibromyalgia patients will do almost anything to relieve pain, fatigue, and suffering, many of these unregulated companies prey on fibromyalgia patients, attempting to convince them that a particular herb or supplement is necessary to resolve the syndrome. Second, there is no quality control or accountability during the manufacturing process. Therefore, every ingredient in the herbal products is not always identified or listed on the label. Additionally, the relative amounts of the substances contained in each pill can vary widely from batch to batch. Finally, there can be very serious drug interactions with these over-the-counter products and traditionally prescribed medications. Thus, it is imperative that fibromyalgia patients always check with their pharmacist or physician before using prescription and herbal medications together.

Dr. Tamler's comment:

*I noticed some extra containers in the bagful of medications brought in by the patient. They happened to be the nonprescribed supplements that she was taking. Her son living out West was an herbalist and had told her he wanted her to take these products. Of course he had his mother's best interest in mind. One of the herbs was Arnica Montana, used in liniment and ointment preparations for strains, sprains, and bruises. Arnica preparations used topically have been demonstrated to have anti-inflammatory properties and assist normal healing processes. However, if ingested internally, this herb not only produces severe gastroenteritis and internal bleeding of the digestive tract, but **heart muscle paralysis** as well. After I had voiced my concerns, the patient later found out that her son neglected to tell her that the product was suppose to be used topically. She stopped using herbs and supplements altogether.*

72. What are some of the visual side effects that occur with medications used to treat fibromyalgia?

There are several visual complications that can occur with prescription and over-the-counter medications, although most of them are temporary and reversible. These side effects include:

- **Dry eye disease (DED)**: A condition in which the clear front surface of the eye, the cornea, no longer remains moist
- Accommodative spasms: Cause blurred vision, which is the second most common visual complaint of patients with fibromyalgia
- Binocular dysfunction

Dry eye disease (DED)

Decreased tear production or increased tear film evaporation.

73. Why are fibromyalgia patients so sensitive to medications?

With fibromyalgia, it is as if someone has turned up an amplifier within the body. Every response is amplified: sounds, smells, sensitivity to touch and pain. All of these are overly exaggerated due to an overly sensitive central nervous system. As a result, all body systems have the potential to overrespond to any stimulus presented to the body, such as medications, chemical additives, perfumes, etc.

74. Does one drug work better than the others?

There currently is no single drug to cure fibromyalgia, and no drug is clearly superior to another. The best regimen is usually established through closely coordinated care with a physician interested in treating fibromyalgia and its associated conditions. Oftentimes by simply listening to the patient, the most effective medication regimen can be instituted.

There currently is no single drug to cure fibromyalgia, and no drug is clearly superior to another.

PART FIVE

Complementary Approach

How can I avoid a flare up?

What are self-management skills?

What nutritional therapy/recommendations would you suggest for fibromyalgia?

More...

Fibromyalgia treatment involves the positive blending of both mainstream medicine and alternative treatments. The patient most likely to "succeed" is open-minded. Implementing self-management strategies can have rich rewards—symptom relief and the resulting ability to function at a higher level so you enjoy improved quality of life.

Because fibromyalgia is a disorder with multiple presentations, its management must take multiple approaches. There is no single "tried-and-true" recipe for treatment. Management varies according to the severity of symptoms in each patient.

The key to effective management is collaboration between knowledgeable healthcare providers and a patient's self-management techniques. Among the patient skills that matter most is a positive attitude.

75. What is cognitive behavioral therapy, and how is it helpful to those with fibromyalgia?

Cognitive behavioral therapy (CBT) is a blend of two types of psychotherapeutic techniques. The cognitive part focuses on the individual's mental environment. The therapist helps the individual identify maladaptive beliefs about their illness and reduce expectations for failure to solve problems in a more adaptive fashion. Cognitive therapy focuses on the use of rational thinking to help a person gain an accurate understanding of the nature of their condition so that the condition can be managed more effectively. The behavioral component focuses on the way the person's symptoms are affected by various factors so that the individual can develop better strategies for managing their symptoms via modifications in their behavior.

For example, patients with fibromyalgia tend to try to ignore their pain levels while performing activities for as long as they can. This strategy is commonly employed by most people without fibromyalgia while performing their activities of daily

Cognitive behavioral therapy (CBT)

A type of psychotherapy in which the therapist teaches the patient to restructure his or her cognitive beliefs (thought patterns) and hence, behavior.

living as a way of completing tasks in spite of mild discomfort or fatigue. When individual with fibromyalgia tries to ignore and push through the pain, the pain increases to very high levels and they are often unable to complete the task or, in more severe cases, end up in bed for days on end. Individuals with fibromyalgia need to learn to identify when their pain levels are increasing so they can take breaks and employ relaxation techniques to keep the pain from escalating. For example, a female executive with fibromyalgia had to walk very long distances in her job and would often miss work on Thursday or Friday because her pain and fatigue levels would build over the course of the workweek. By taking a few minutes and sitting down on benches when the pain and fatigue increased, she was able to keep the pain and fatigue levels from increasing to intolerable levels and was able to stop missing work.

76. What is involved in cognitive behavioral therapy, and who should I see for this therapy?

Cognitive behavioral therapy is generally conducted by psychologists who have been trained in these techniques. Cognitive behavioral therapy is conducted in three phases. The first phase involves education concerning the nature of fibromyalgia, self-monitoring of symptoms, and goal setting. The second phase involves acquiring the skills to accurately predict which methods (taking breaks, slowing down, reprioritizing, altering activity order, practicing relaxation, taking medication, sleep hygiene, aerobic exercise) provide the best outcome. The third phase involves employing the techniques in real life. Most CBT practitioners are psychologists, although CBT can be conducted by other types of practitioners who are trained to perform the techniques.

Cognitive behavioral therapy is conducted in three phases.

Jane's comment:

My pain management psychologist helped me learn the difference between good pain and bad pain. He helped me learn to structure my days and not overdo. He taught me that if I have five units of energy for the day, why waste four units walking the grocery store? I should use a scooter to get my groceries. By not walking, I saved that energy to spend quality time with my husband. I learned not to struggle with pain just to do the dishes. I'd fill the sink with water and dishes, then lie down. After 10 minutes, I'd wash the dishes, fill the sink again, and lie down again. I followed this process until I had the strength to wash all the dishes. My pain management psychologist also taught me how to recognize my fatigue signals. I had ignored them for so long that I had to relearn them. One of the most crucial elements of this healing process was recognizing the anger I had because I was sick. I felt that I had no control over my life and that my body had betrayed me. My pain management psychologist's help was very important. Through biofeedback I learned to recognize that I was contracting muscles I wasn't using. Doing so adds to muscle pain and fatigue. I learned how to relax those muscles. I learned that I put way too much stress on myself. Because I felt tired and unable to do things like clean or see friends, I would obsess over not having vacuumed or dwell on the thought that going out to dinner and dancing with friends was too much and life was so unfair. Over time I learned a new outlook: Do I really need to vacuum? Will it make that much difference if I don't do it until Saturday? Why don't I meet friends for dinner and then come home? They are my friends; they will understand or they should.

Jenny's comment:

The doctors at the pain clinic soon referred me to a chronic pain psychologist who works with fibromyalgia patients and specializes in treating people living in chronic pain. It was wonderful to talk to someone who had studied fibromyalgia. He could finish my sentences about the pain. His face showed not only that he was listening, but that he really cared. He helped me manage the pain and find ways to relax. Equally important, he taught me ways to say "No." All my life, I've tried to do everything for everyone all the time. It has been hard for me to accept that I can no longer do that, and it's been hard for others to understand. I see this wonderful psychologist regularly.

77. What are behavioral pain management techniques?

Certain activities can reduce sympathetic and central nervous system activation. Play quiet, calming music; avoid noisy environments; wear ear plugs; dress warmly in cold temperatures; shop when stores aren't crowded; avoid loud people; soak in a hot tub or whirlpool; use heating pads; and so forth.

Slow down. Hurrying activates the sympathetic nervous system. It causes your muscles to contract more. Understand that slowing down is hard to do. Initially, your psyche will rebel, because it associates hurrying with goal achievement. The faster I go, the more tasks I can complete per unit time. When I slow down, I feel like I'm not getting anything done. Slowing down is hard because it reduces short-term feelings of accomplishment. This can arouse feelings of inadequacy, laziness, and guilt.

Learn to conserve. If you have moderate to severe fibromyalgia and you want to attend a wedding on Saturday, get plenty of rest on Thursday and Friday. Get your clothing ready several days in advance. On the day of the wedding, get some rest after the ceremony and before the reception. Make sure you have a comfortable chair (bring a pillow if necessary). Try to find a comfortable seating position, and take breaks in the lounge or sit in your car when you need to. Don't plan much for the next day, so you can give your body a chance to recover.

Prioritize. If you want to give your child the quality time he or she needs, don't try to keep an immaculate house. Your children aren't going to remember that the house was clean. But they may remember that you preferred to do housework rather than spend time playing with them. The same goes for your partner. When your partner returns from work, he or she may be more pleased if the house is a little messy but you are feeling good, are in a good mood, and can be up and around.

Complementary Approach

Figure out how to move/position your body without increasing the pain. This may sound easy, but it can be difficult. Severe pain is so traumatizing to the psyche that, once it subsides, the psyche tries to forget how bad it was. Therefore, it's hard to remember what movements you should avoid. In addition, patterns of body movement are overlearned habits that we do automatically. For years, a fellow with severe lower back pain bent at the waist to brush his two dogs every day. One day he tried sitting on a footstool and was amazed at how much less pain he experienced when he brushed his dogs in this new position.

78. What is catastrophizing?

Catastrophizing

Occurs when a person ruminates about all the terrible things that are probably going to happen.

Catastrophizing occurs when a person ruminates about all the terrible things that are probably going to happen. It is an ineffective cognitive method of coping. When you are faced with a threat, such as being in pain for a long period of time, focusing on all the terrible things that could happen generates increased anxiety, dread, and hopelessness about the future. In addition, research using function **magnetic resonance imaging (MRI)** indicates that catastrophizing is associated with increased activation of brain regions involved in cognitive and emotional activation. Finally, catastrophizing is also associated with increased pain sensitivity in fibromyalgia patients.

Magnetic resonance imaging (MRI)

A noninvasive, non-X-ray diagnostic technique based on the magnetic fields of hydrogen atoms in the body. MRI provides computer-generated images of the body's internal tissues and organs.

79. What is mindfulness, and how is it used to counteract the tendency to catastrophize?

Mindfulness is a form of deep relaxation that involves focusing on being "in the moment." This involves learning how to stop the "mental chatter" that mirrors everyday concerns, past hurts inflicted by others, reasons why one is angry, etc. Coupled with learning how to stop the mental chatter is learning to focus internal bodily sensations that occur during deep relaxation and enhanced experiences of various sensory phenomena.

Mindfulness

A form of deep relaxation that involves focusing on being "in the moment."

Practice mindfulness. Try to enjoy your surroundings (air, plants, people, music, etc.) to their fullest. This requires mental discipline and a refocus on the quality of your experiences as opposed to the quantity of them. What we really desire is contentment with what we have, which requires that we stop focusing on what we don't have. It is human nature to take what we have for granted, and it is important to work on not doing so. In addition, practice deep relaxation techniques. Biofeedback training can also help you in this situation, so that you can learn how to relax muscles and reduce nervous system activation.

Relaxation skills can moderate fibromyalgia pain and often moderate other features of the disorder, such as sleep disorder, tender point sensitivity, and overall feelings of well-being. Relaxation, assisted by biofeedback training, raises the trainee's sense of self-efficacy—the confidence that he or she can do something to improve his or her condition.

80. What is biofeedback?

Biofeedback involves using various sensors to record bodily functions and simultaneously present visual and auditory information in order to allow a person to gain voluntary control over functions that are normally involuntary.

Mark's comment:

Biofeedback made me aware of how much stress has to do with your condition. There were many types of stress I was undergoing at the time, and through biofeedback you can actually look at a monitor as it shows you how tense your muscles actually are and that you have the ability to actually lower some of the tension in your body.

81. How is biofeedback used in the treatment of fibromyalgia?

The greatest controlled research support for biofeedback in the treatment of fibromyalgia is surface **electromyogram (sEMG) biofeedback**. In sEMG biofeedback of fibromyalgia, the therapist attaches sensors that record the electrical activity of muscles. Research has shown that fibromyalgia patients tend to have resting sEMG levels an average of 4 to 5

Biofeedback involves using various sensors to record bodily functions and simultaneously present visual and auditory information in order to allow a person to gain voluntary control over functions that are normally involuntary.

Electromyogram (sEMG) biofeedback

Surface EMG biofeedback allows therapists to record the electrical activity of muscles through sensors attached to the skin.

times the resting activity of normal control subjects. The therapist guides the patient through the process of learning how to develop voluntary control over these resting muscle contractions. It is important for the therapist to be familiar with common pitfalls that interfere with learning deep muscle relaxation such as trying too hard, becoming competitive with the devices, focusing excessive attention on the feedback signals, not repositioning often enough, etc.

82. What other forms of biofeedback are being used in treating fibromyalgia?

Some therapists are performing EEG (brain rhythm) biofeedback to try to reduce the central sensitization that characterizes fibromyalgia. Some therapist are also using heart rate and respiration biofeedback to train a deep relaxation response. Finger temperature biofeedback has a long research record of being effective in treating the Raynaud's Phenomenon (cold hand attacks) that is experienced by many fibromyalgia patients.

83. What other behavioral techniques are being used in treating fibromyalgia?

Hypnosis is sometimes helpful in pain management. In addition, some therapists are reporting some symptom reduction using audiovisual entrainment, a treatment that consists of flashing lights and rhythmic auditory sounds that are designed to alter brain rhythms.

84. How can I find a biofeedback therapist in my area?

Biofeedback therapists obtain certification from the Biofeedback Certification Institute of America (BCIA). In addition to written and oral exams, they must undergo supervised internship training and, after being certified, are required to obtain 20 hours of continuing education credit per year.

85. Do fibromyalgia patients experience the stages of grieving?

Yes, allow yourself to grieve your reduced functional capacities. Each activity you're no longer able to engage in causes a grief reaction. Grief is the feeling of loss, such as in the loss of a loved one. Mourning a loss is a process with five stages:

1. Denial
2. Anger
3. Bargaining with God (when applicable)
4. Sadness/depression
5. Acceptance

When you become unable to engage in activities that give you a sense of accomplishment, you lose the joy those activities brought you. So, it is important to find new activities that restore that sense of accomplishment without increasing the pain.

Think outside the box. Try container vegetable or herb gardening, talking to support group comembers, listening to books on tape, cooking for scout groups, volunteering, and so on. If the sadness becomes overwhelming and you feel hopeless, talk to someone you trust (such as a minister or health professional) about what you should do. Reaching acceptance means that you aren't denying your limitations, and you feel less sad and angry.

Mark's comment:

Probably my biggest hurdle was to accept the fact that I had something that I couldn't control. I lived most of my working and private life being a leader by example, the person who could overcome and adapt to any situation, the man who could get the job done, and being the provider, supporter, and role model to my family. I then found myself in a position where I didn't have control over the way I felt anymore and it just devastated me—literally devastated me.

Complementary Approach

86. How does physical therapy help patients with fibromyalgia syndrome?

Physical therapy utilizes four types of interventions that benefit fibromyalgia patients:

- Exercise: includes stretching, strengthening, aerobics, coordination exercises, and balance training
- Therapeutic modalities: **ultrasound**, electrical stimulation, low-level light therapy, heat, and cold
- Manual therapy: includes soft tissue mobilization, massage, myofascial release (type of massage), spray/stretch, manual stretching, joint mobilization, and proprioceptive neuromuscular facilitation
- Patient education: consisting of instruction in proper posture, body mechanics, ergonomics, and self care

All four of these interventions help the two main problems associated with fibromyalgia—central nervous system hypersensitivity and muscle dysfunction.

Exercise improves flexibility, coordination, and muscle strength. It increases endurance and tolerance to activity. Stretching stimulates circulation to the muscles—relaxing them and facilitating the removal of waste products (lactic acid). Aerobic exercise, along with the well known benefits to the circulatory system, increases the release of **endorphins** (hormones) that decrease pain signals in the brain. Exercise is movement, and most fibromyalgia patients are afraid of moving because it is painful. If we do not move we "rust." Our muscles stiffen and weaken leading to pain and discouragement.

Fibromyalgia patients have trouble with balance for several reasons. They frequently have pain in the legs and the lower back—areas that help send feedback to the brain (**proprioception**) to tell us where our body is in space, which is important in balancing. Pain disrupts the proprioceptive feedback to the brain, leading to loss of balance and coordination. Tightness and

Ultrasound

An electrical modality that transmits a sound wave through an applicator into the skin to the soft tissue in order to heat the local area; for relaxing the injured tissue and/or dispersing edema.

Exercise improves flexibility, coordination, and muscle strength.

Endorphins

Any of a group of proteins with potent analgesic properties that occur naturally in the brain.

Proprioception

The ability to sense the location, position, orientation, and movement of the body and its parts.

weakness in the legs and trunk further contribute to poor balance. Standing on one leg, within easy reach of something to hold onto to steady yourself (kitchen sink), for a goal of 2 minutes is the most helpful exercise to regain your sense of balance.

Therapeutic modalities such as ultrasound, electrical stimulation, light therapy, heat, and cold block pain signals from the muscles to the brain, breaking the pain cycle associated with central nervous system hypersensitivity. These modalities help by increasing blood flow, which helps to heal tight and damaged muscles. Ultrasound and electrical stimulation vibrate muscle tissue, breaking up the "knots" frequently found in tight fibromyalgic muscles.

Manual therapy, especially massage, is frequently the only treatment that can loosen the tightness in fibromyalgic muscles. Skilled hands can feel how much pressure to apply and in what direction to get the muscles to relax and the tissue restrictions to release. Manual therapy gives instant feedback to the patient and practitioner to whether the muscles are relaxing. Manual stretching by the physical therapist teaches the patient what proper stretching should feel like and what muscles are most problematic. PNF (proprioceptive neuromuscular facilitation) is hands-on treatment that involves manual techniques to facilitate stretching or retrain (strengthen) weak muscles.

Instructing the patient in how to take care for themselves with proper posture and body mechanics is crucial to maintain the benefits received in physical therapy treatment. The patient going home and sitting awkwardly at his computer for several hours just negates all the positive effects of treatment.

The patient going home and sitting awkwardly at his computer for several hours just negates all the positive effects of treatment.

Sharon's comment:

Physical therapy was also suggested to help control my pain. But finding a physical therapist who understood fibromyalgia was as challenging as finding an understanding physician had been. For one thing, I found most physical therapy sites too eager to start exercises that included free weights and machines, which always made me worse. For another, I found few places where patients were given time to talk to a therapist before starting treatment. I never felt comfortable putting my questions to the aides who actually performed the therapy, so I was constantly changing sites, searching for a center that offered the all-around therapy situation I felt I needed. Finally, one of my new friends recommended a therapist at a center near my home. Eighteen years later, this therapist continues to treat me.

The problem with physical therapy, as with other fibromyalgia treatments, is that it isn't designed specifically for treating fibromyalgia. Therefore, some ways of administering it can make fibromyalgia worse. That's why it's crucial to find a therapist who understands fibromyalgia. My experience taught me that, when considering a therapy site, that's the time to ask the therapist whether they've worked with the disorder and what success he or she's had.

Jane's comment:

On the medical side, I had a lot of physical therapy, some of it in water. Finally, I started getting better. I started walking on my treadmill 1 minute a day. After a week, I moved up to 2 minutes. Although I could have walked longer, I knew when to stop so that I didn't overdo. So I started slow and listened to my body for signals. As I got better, I was taken off Zoloft. I also cut back, then eliminated, the Vicodin, then the Ultram. It is amazing to think that at one time I was taking eight Vicodin and eight Ultram a day and still having pain.

87. Why do many patients feel worse with physical therapy treatment?

Many physical therapists do not understand the underlying problems with fibromyalgia, in particular central nervous system hypersensitivity. Fibromyalgia patients' brains have a lower threshold to pain so they do not tolerate the same stretching and strengthening exercises normally given to other patients. They also have tight and knotted muscles, further lowering their pain threshold. Interrupting the pain cycle must be done before attempting exercise.

There is a three-step protocol to treating fibromyalgia patients:

- Phase one consists of relaxing the muscles utilizing modalities such as heat and ultrasound. Manual therapy of massage and soft tissue mobilization breaks up restrictions in the muscles, decreasing muscle guarding and tightness. This leads to less pain and prepares the muscles for stretching and strengthening exercises. Phase one lasts about 1 to 2 weeks with a frequency of three treatments per week.
- Phase two involves the same treatments, but stretching and low-intensity aerobic exercise is begun. Patient education in proper postures, body mechanics, and ergonomics is done throughout all the phases. During these first two phases the brain begins to learn not to overreact to the pain, and the muscles begin to repair themselves. The patient is able to relax, which helps break up the pain cycle. Now that the patient is feeling better and his or her muscles have more flexibility, he or she can begin to tolerate strengthening exercises. At home, heat is used to relax the muscles and block pain. Gentle stretching exercises are also done.
- Phase three begins with strengthening exercises as well as other exercises that target the patient's unique and specific problems, such as loss of balance or coordination. Muscles that were found weak in the initial evaluation are targeted.

Most patients even in a moderate amount of pain are able to tolerate 4 to 5 minutes each on an exercise bicycle, walking on a treadmill, and an upper body bicycle. By using several different machines, one area of the body is not overworked.

Complementary Approach

Throughout the course of treatment, aerobic exercise is increased by a couple minutes until 30 minutes of steady exercise is achieved at a low intensity. Movement is the most important aspect of the treatment. It increases circulation as well as gets the body moving, which has a positive psychological effect on patients when they realize they are able to move without pain. Movement also modulates (decreases) pain by blocking pain signals.

Movement is the most important aspect of the treatment.

Key points to remember with physical therapy treatment are:

- Soft tissue mobilization (massage) is done gently, slowly working deeper as muscles relax and loosen. Massaging perpendicular to the muscle fibers is better tolerated and should be done first. Pushing directly down onto trigger points (tender areas of muscle restriction) usually aggravates fibromyalgia patients' pain.
- Manual therapy is applied to only a few areas of the body per treatment to lessen posttherapy soreness. Since fibromyalgic muscles are tighter and have more knots, extra muscle waste products (lactic acid) are released with massage. Most fibromyalgia patients do not tolerate a 1-hour full body massage because of this.
- Stretching is done slowly, gently, and to just the muscles that are the tightest and, whenever possible, should be done after warming up with hot packs or low intensity aerobic exercise.
- Strengthening is tolerated best with low weight and 20 to 30 repetitions maximum. Weight is only increased when 30 repetitions are done easily and without pain. Distribute strengthening exercises to several different muscle groups usually focusing on the postural muscles.

88. How can I avoid a flare-up?

Fibromyalgia patients have less strength, less endurance, and more tightness, so flare-ups are somewhat inevitable.

Fibromyalgia patients have less strength, less endurance, and more tightness, so flare-ups are somewhat inevitable. There are many things you can do to decrease the pain intensity and frequency. Using ice, heat, and balms to block pain signals gives short-term relief. Getting regular massages helps lessen the accumulation of restrictions in muscles. It is important to stretch the tightest muscles daily to maintain flexibility and prevent knots from returning. A physical therapist can show you the best stretches for your problem areas. Regular aerobic exercise (three to four times a week) helps maintain and increase endurance while benefiting the cardiovascular system. Aerobic exercise improves endorphin release, which mellows the nervous system and blocks pain. Movement of the body involved in aerobic exercise helps coordination and balance and lubricates your joints. Most patients have trouble when they stop doing their home program and become sedentary, stiff, and weak, leading to a return to a cycle of pain. Practicing good ergonomics and body mechanics prevents injury and aggravation of hypersensitive muscles.

89. What should I expect at my first physical therapy visit?

A physical therapist does an initial evaluation on the first visit. The evaluation consists of taking a medical history, including a history of your current problem, and getting to know what makes your pain worse and better. Also noted on the first visit is what other medical conditions you have and how they might influence how your fibromyalgia manifests itself. Next, the therapist does an objective exam that consists of testing your flexibility and strength, as well as feeling and palpating the muscles for trigger points or tightness. Physical therapists experienced in treating fibromyalgia can usually tell the difference between patients with fibromyalgia and how their muscles feel compared to those who do not have it. Fibromyalgic muscles tend to be tighter, feel "gunky," and have more knots and trigger points. After the initial evaluation, the therapist will make a list of your problems and come up with a plan of care that targets your specific areas of pain and dysfunction. There is usually time to answer your questions and give you an idea of what to expect with treatment.

Complementary Approach

Sometimes you will get treatment such as heat and electrical stimulation that can help begin to relax your muscles and block pain. You may also have a short massage. The initial visit usually lasts about 90 minutes.

90. How do I find a physical therapist who understands fibromyalgia?

The American Physical Therapy Association (www.apta.org) has a list of physical therapists in your area. You want to pick a therapist who specializes in orthopedic and manual therapy. Call the clinic and find out if they schedule enough time for patients (two patients per hour) and whether they do hands-on treatment. Ideally and most importantly, you should ask them what fibromyalgia is. They should be able to answer that it is a central nervous system hypersensitivity syndrome as well as a muscle dysfunction problem. Many healthcare professionals, including physical therapists, do not yet understand these important aspects of fibromyalgia. Some schools still teach that fibromyalgia is mostly a psychological problem.

91. Does yoga help relieve the pain and discomfort of fibromyalgia?

Leading medical authorities now recognize fibromyalgia pain as involving central sensitization, a malfunction of the pain-processing centers in the brain and spinal cord. Unfortunately, this not only causes pain, but also limits the brain from having normal sensations.

Repetitive movements and exercise in poor alignment cause pain, which leads to exercise-related flares (sudden worsening of fibromyalgia symptoms). So we become afraid to move and exercise. Then we ache, because the tissues are deprived of oxygen by low muscle tone and immobility. All this pain makes us afraid to use our bodies. We become tense and anxious, so we move clumsily and reinjure ourselves. We curl up in a protective fetal position to sleep or support ourselves with numerous pillows, never lying flat to fully open the chest. Doing this contributes to shallow breathing, which in turn contributes to **hypoxic** muscle pain and aching. All this leads to poor circulation, which causes tossing and turning to get blood to all areas. This unconscious shifting deprives us of deep sleep. Fatigue contributes to pain, clumsiness, and brain fog, which contribute to more injuries and even more pain—a vicious cycle.

Yoga can help with all these problems. Breathing practices increase the oxygen supply to the tissues, reducing aching. Increased oxygen to the brain can help clear brain fog. An exercise done slowly with meticulous attention to posture and alignment, yoga postures allow us to exercise without microinjuries, thus reducing the chances of exercise-related flares. By constantly varying your yoga practice (which is easy to do because there are many yoga poses), you avoid the hyperpathic pain triggered by repetitive motions. By learning new postures and movements, you provide new sensory input to the brain, thus bypassing the learned pain patterns of allodynia and learning new ways to feel your body. By learning deep relaxation skills, you improve your sleep. Also, by exercising regularly, you improve your muscle tone and circulation, providing adequate blood supply to all your muscles so you can sleep better.

92. How does acupuncture help those with chronic pain?

Pain is one of the great remaining mysteries of medical science. But we are getting ever closer to answers. We do know that many sets of nerve-cell fibers are involved, each secreting their own neurotransmitter to communicate with the nerve cells they connect to. Some of these neurotransmitters make it easier for the pain-sensing nerve fibers to fire, which increases our sensitivity to pain. Other neurotransmitters make it harder for the nerve fibers to fire, thus decreasing our sensitivity to pain. In other words, some act as an accelerator, and others act as a brake. Morphine, for example, is of the latter type. It kills pain because it is a neurotransmitter that inhibits

Fatigue contributes to pain, clumsiness, and brain fog, which contribute to more injuries and even more pain—a vicious cycle.

Hypoxic
Deficient in oxygen.

Yoga
A system of exercises that help your control of the body and mind. It also improves your breathing and focuses the alignment of your body.

Complementary Approach

the transmission of pain stimuli. The brain naturally produces it when we are in pain—though not in the massive amounts that a physician can prescribe. Normally, the brain increases production of opiates and other pain-killing neurotransmitters to desensitize us to pain that doesn't go away.

Chronic pain represents a hyperactive state of the central (brain and spinal cord) and peripheral (outside the brain and spinal cord) nervous systems in which both systems become sensitized to pain. Over time, the nervous systems begin to overrespond to pain stimuli. This means that it takes less stimulation to cause pain and that pain is felt for a much longer period of time following the stimulus.

Moreover, in chronic pain, the sympathetic nervous system is often in a heightened state of arousal. The sympathetic nervous system is a massive network of nerves throughout the brain, spinal cord, and body that causes the familiar "fight-or-flight" response, in which the body is almost instantly prepared for a dangerous emergency. Heart rate increases, breathing rate increases, blood pressure rises, emotions flare, adrenalin flows. Needless to say, it's unhealthy to be in this aroused state more or less permanently. It leads to high blood pressure, irritable bowel symptoms, anxiety, and despair.

Acupuncture acts on pain-sensing nerve-fiber transmission in two ways. One way is by increasing the strength of inhibitory (pain-blocking) circuits in the brainstem. The brainstem circuits at the top of the spinal cord act as pain gates that are closed by acupuncture. The other way is by reducing the excitability of pain circuits in the spinal cord and brain. These acupuncture-induced alterations reduce the hypersensitivity of the nervous system that develops in chronic pain. It also works by calming the chronically hyperaroused sympathetic nervous system, which reduces the muscle contractions present in fibromyalgia.

Acupuncture

The practice of piercing specific sites on the body, called pathways or meridians, with thin needles in an attempt to relieve pain associated with some chronic disorders.

Acupuncture-induced alterations reduce the hypersensitivity of the nervous system that develops in chronic pain.

In all these systems, the treatment improves circulation of **Qi**, blood, and fluids. Treatment also helps the body's mechanisms for maintaining a steady state, thus moving you toward better balance and better health.

Qi
Energy flow.

93. How does massage benefit those with fibromyalgia?

Fibromyalgia patients experience an abnormal level of muscle tension caused by shortened and tight muscles tissue. Chronic muscle tension of a lasting nature gradually increases in intensity and pain. The effectiveness of massage therapy is that it directly affects the muscles, fascia, and circulatory system. When deep pressure is applied to this tightened muscle tissue and then released, it releases the blood and lymph flow to make its way into the tissue, providing it with nourishment (oxygen). This increased flow will also carry waste products, such as lactic acid, out of the muscle and fascia and into the bloodstream. Deep pressure massage also elongates muscles and tendons and softens fascia, allowing circulation and relief from tension.

The fascia in the body plays an important part in the pain of fibromyalgia patients; myofascial release helps dampen the pain. Its focus is the package that we're wrapped in, the connective tissue and every muscle and muscle fiber. The fascia gets restrictions in it; it tightens down and sticks to itself. It has an elastic quality, so as you work with it, you warm it up and it starts smoothing with you, independent of the muscle and the tissue (the skin).

As with all types of body work, it is essential that the therapist has experience working with fibromyalgia patients and understands the disorder. When patients follow a maintenance program once a week or bimonthly, massage has been found to work better than other therapies in providing relief.

Mark's comment:

Deep myofascial release is very important. When my muscles become stuck I experience overall muscle pain, muscle spasms, restless legs, head and neck pain, muscle stiffness, limited motion, muscle loss and constant aching pain in those muscles in addition to other muscles groups. Left untreated, trigger points develop and spread, causing more stuck muscles, more pain, more sleepless nights, more anxiety, more dysfunction, and the feeling your body is a toxic. Having deep myofascial release in conjunction with trigger point injection gave me relief from pain, a greater range of motion, offered more freedom of motion, and allowed more blood flow, which promoted more healing to happen. Deep myofascial release helps sleeping. Proper sleep reduces pain and stiffness in the muscles and helps clear the mind. When you're in constant pain your body and mind actually forget what it's like not to feel pain and tends to remain guarded. I stretch every morning in a hot tub, and as needed, which increases range of motion and releases toxins from the stuck muscles. It also prepares my muscles for activity and reduces the incidents of injury. I learned to balance my activity with rest, being aware not to overwork my muscles. This is still the most difficult to do because of my nature to be productive and never give up.

Denise's comment:

Massage has been a lifesaver for me. I was diagnosed with fibromyalgia in 1983 and have tried many different remedies for the pain over the years. Massage has been the most beneficial in my experience. Discovered to be helpful during early physical therapy sessions, massage has relaxed my muscles and eased my pain and stress like nothing else. A wonderful massage therapist works on me for an hour a week and I would see her more often if I could! She is not a luxury in my life—she is a necessity. I also use a shiatsu massager first thing every morning to loosen my muscles in order to function during the day. This is the only thing that keeps me going! I find it very difficult to exercise, and I feel with massage at least my tissues are being moved regularly. And it feels fantastic, too.

94. What can patients do at home to reduce symptoms?

One very common treatment is to use items that are soft and round, such as a tennis ball or some other kind of firm ball, in order to apply acupressure (a direct pressure to the painful area or tender point for 20 to 60 minutes in order to break up the tightened, restricted fibers). The rationale for this form of treatment comes from the following analogy: When an individual suddenly develops a charley horse in the middle of the night, the natural inclination is to grab at the muscle, start to massage it, and then stretch it out. This is a reflexive, instinctive action. On the other hand, when a partial area of muscle tightens producing the same painful phenomenon, the body has no reflex to address the problem. Despite this fact, when the same treatment technique is used—massaging out the muscle knot, stretching out the fibers, and then bringing them back to their normal resting length—the exact same results can be achieved. The result is successful pain relief!

95. What are self-management skills?

There is no known cure for fibromyalgia, but the symptoms can be managed. This is a process that involves making wise choices and changes that will positively affect your overall health. The optimum treatment of fibromyalgia is, therefore, a classic blend of the efforts of the patient and the doctor. **Self-management skills** are vital to avoiding flare-ups and living without pain. Whether the issue is pain, fatigue, or cognitive difficulties, patients must listen to their body and adjust daily activities depending on what each day is like.

How you manage fibromyalgia varies, depending largely on how severe your symptoms are. They can range from very mild and occasional to severe and persistent, so there's considerable variance in the appropriate level of management. Self-management requires not only self-awareness, but also diligence—active participation on the patient's part.

The optimum treatment of fibromyalgia is a classic blend of the efforts of the patient and the doctor.

Self-management skills

A process that involves making wise choices and changes that will positively affect your overall health.

With a positive attitude, self-awareness, and diligence, the resulting decrease of pain and tenderness, plus the increase of strength and energy, markedly improve our lives.

The saying "knowledge is power" applies strongly to fibromyalgia. Educating ourselves about the disorder is the first step to wellness. It's enormously empowering to know what we're dealing with. With fibromyalgia, we must have faith in the body's ability to heal and be proactive about our treatment. The first step to feeling better is to feel capable of taking control of our healing. Understanding the battlefield is often half the battle. As we who have fibromyalgia develop a better understanding of our condition, it becomes far easier to recognize both our limitations and our capabilities. As we empower ourselves with knowledge, our journey becomes much easier to travel.

Pacing and moving is essential to all of us because it allows the blood to move freely. In most individuals, movement is pleasurable; stretching feels wonderful, and moderate exercise makes us feel stronger and free of pain. The person with fibromyalgia feels little of this.

Everyone—from doctors to chiropractors to physical therapists—encourages patients to stretch. Few tell their patients how tricky it can be to find the right stretching program because it is not their area of expertise. So doctors send patients to a gym where someone puts a pair of weights in their hands and says "Your muscles are weak. You will feel better if you lift weights, and you will get stronger over time." This works in theory only and is the worst thing you could do.

When the skin under the skin (fascia) is too tight and full of knots, it can't strengthen. It will just rip more and hurt more. I always use the analogy of the clothesline. If your clothesline of muscles is ripped, old, and shrunk, it may be able to handle a blouse, but it can't sustain the weight of a winter coat. Trainers who ask you to lift weights but don't provide you with an alternative have little experience with individuals with chronic pain. Ask your physical therapist (or doctor) about gentle strengthening exercises to make your muscles more resilient.

Journaling can be a key to discovering triggers. This doesn't have to be a time-consuming process; jotting down what occurs to you is all that's necessary. The more informal you are, the more likely you are to be honest about your feelings. Journaling is also a useful tool for recording any changes in your medications or dosages, or keeping track of dietary changes and their effect.

Journaling
The process of recording information about your daily life.

Journaling also helps us communicate more productively with our physician. No one can recall accurately specific reactions to medications, dates new symptoms started, and so on. Referring to our daily notes makes any doctor's visit more productive.

One of the most important techniques for managing fibromyalgia is to prioritize activities. Most patients find their energy levels highest in the morning and lowest in the afternoon. So it stands to reason that we should try, whenever possible, to accomplish our most important, energy-consuming tasks in the morning. "First things first" is one of the most useful axioms anyone ever came up with.

One of the most important techniques for managing fibromyalgia is to prioritize activities.

Overexertion always exacts a price. When tempted, remind yourself that this is one of the bad things about fibromyalgia you can control. Whenever we think it's safe to increase our activities, the only responsible way is to take baby steps in that direction. If we don't, chances are we'll end up taking a giant step backwards. By going forward at a strictly measured pace, we can avoid a flare-up of symptoms.

Renae's comment:

It is important for patients to understand their limitations are different from other fibromyalgia patients. We must learn not to overstress with things we cannot change. My journey is ongoing;

I realize what will make me feel worse and what will assist me in feeling better.

Margo's comment:

Once I accepted this, that it wasn't going away, and I learned to move slower, then I could do more things. If I tried to move fast and do everything I could do before, I wasn't going to get anything done because I would be hurting so badly that I would end up lying on the couch the rest of the day. But if I would just do a little bit, lie down and take a break, then feel better, get up and do a little bit more, eventually I would get more things done.

96. Does stress increase my pain levels?

The number one cause of flare-ups is stress.

The number one cause of flare-ups is stress. We sometimes forget that stress is a natural, normal force that's part of everyone's life. However, it affects people differently, and the range of effects even on the healthiest folks is very broad. For anyone with fibromyalgia, stress is always a serious issue. The only way to manage our condition effectively is to find and keep a balance between work, rest, and play.

Although stress is a normal part of life, for us it is likely to arise from the simplest daily routines. Merely living with chronic pain is in itself a constant source of stress.

It's also natural for anyone with a chronic condition to have some negative thoughts. And these thoughts bring additional stress. Because negative thinking increases pain, we need to replace any negative thoughts with pleasant, positive affirmations.

Sometimes, changes in environmental factors (such as noise, temperature, and weather exposure) can cause stress and exacerbate the symptoms of fibromyalgia, and these factors need to be modified. Many patients report that sticking to a schedule is beneficial—that is one reason why vacations are difficult for many of us—making it all the more urgent to develop everyday tools for dealing with ongoing stress.

Probably the best tool is taking time out of each day to let go of the demands of that day. There are numerous ways to do this: biofeedback, yoga, meditation, tai chi, and reading are all techniques that may help you relax.

97. What nutritional therapy/recommendations would you suggest for fibromyalgia?

There is no single food that can cure fibromyalgia, but there is no question that what we eat can ease the symptoms of this challenging condition. I have seen patients experience improved energy and concentration and endure less Fibro Fog and fatigue by following **nutritional therapy/recommendations** and improving their nutritional intake.

Most fibromyalgia patients have what are known as **perpetuating factors**. These are biochemical imbalances that make muscles more vulnerable to trigger points and render some therapies less effective or lasting. (These imbalances are one reason why many patients don't respond to physical therapy.) A major example of a perpetuating factor is a diet with nutritional inadequacies. Think of these inadequacies as potholes that pose a continual threat to the machine that is your body.

Fibromyalgia patients typically eat diets high in **carbohydrates** and extremely low in protein. The basic components of muscle are proteins and minerals. Yet the typical fibromyalgia patient's diet is low in protein, so he or she lacks the material to repair and maintain healthy muscle. When protein is supplied to the body in an insufficient amount, protein synthesis can be inadequate or fail to take place. For this reason high levels of protein in the diet are required.

Typically, a 40-30-30 diet, in which 40% of the diet is made up of carbohydrates, 30% protein, and 30% fat, is adequate to supply the protein requirements, providing kidney function is not compromised. The higher levels of protein provide an intermediate fuel source that can control the hypoglycemia often seen in fibromyalgia patients.

Complementary Approach

Nutritional therapy/ recommendations
Using food and supplements to encourage the body's natural healing.

There is no single food that can cure fibromyalgia, but there is no question that what we eat can ease the symptoms of this challenging condition.

Perpetuating factors
Factors that interfere with healing or enhance the progression of myofascial pain.

Carbohydrates
One of the three main classes of food and a source of energy. Carbohydrates are the sugars and starches found in breads, cereals, fruits, and vegetables.

Renae's comment:

Nutrition

The process by which an individual takes in and utilizes food material.

Nutrition plays a very important role. My doctor always reminds me I need to eat better. Because of fibromyalgia we suffer from fatigue and depression and eating comfort foods helps lift our spirits. And eating nutritiously is a daily goal. It's a challenge I am working on with a nutritionist.

Mark's comment:

Nutrition is a real important part of my program. Because my muscles don't tolerate the level of exercise I should be getting, other factors become involved, like being overweight, low endurance, lack of energy, diabetes, high cholesterol, excessive yeast in the blood, shallow breathing, slow heart rate, and lack of mental sharpness. I have learned that I need to eat to live, not live to eat. It was easy to use food as a source of comfort as to how I was feeling. What I eat is as important as how much. In order to get back the energy I was lacking and reduce more pain, I eliminated processed foods and refined carbohydrates from my diet. My body did not process them very well and they made me feel lethargic. I select what type of protein I eat and monitor the types of fat. I eat fruits and vegetables that are low in sugar, dark leafy greens, legumes, beans, whole grains, almonds, and walnuts. If I can't make it I don't eat it. In addition, I drink lots of water and take dietary supplements that give me more energy and boost my immune system. Getting nutrients to your cells seems to be the key to vitality and healing.

And they're all things you need to work at on a daily basis, so it's a very hard challenge from day to day.

98. How do I find a support group in my area?

The National Fibromyalgia Association has a network of support groups across the United States and encourages participation within the fibromyalgia community. Participation in support groups can provide an opportunity to reach out to others who have had similar challenges and foster an improved understanding of lifestyle management.

Perhaps one of the most important benefits of participating in a support group is a decreased sense of isolation so many people feel when they are experiencing chronic pain. In a support group environment, feelings of anger, depression, guilt, and anxiety can be expressed, validated by others, and accepted as a normal response to living with chronic pain. Having the freedom to express negative feelings and to identify with one another helps participants to realize they are not alone in their struggle. They can experience a sense of emotional relief from the support of others.

Perhaps one of the most important benefits of participating in a support group is a decreased sense of isolation.

Keep in mind that if one group doesn't work for you, it's worth going a little out of your way to find another. In the long run, participating in a fibromyalgia group that works well can be enormously helpful and therapeutic. Also, you will have an opportunity to share what your own experience has taught you, and helping others is among the best therapies there is.

Rob's comment:

It's funny in an odd way that I could tell one friend that another friend has cancer but cannot talk about fibromyalgia. Why, after all this time? Maybe because few people realize how bad it can be and don't care or understand the disease and its devastating tentacles into your life. Or maybe because it isn't mainstream enough to be acceptable and good lunch talk? When I finally made the decision to attend a fibromyalgia support group, it was a sense of relief to see other men in the auditorium. Men tend to be very stoic, but as our comfort levels increased I found I was not the only "man" trying to present a macho image but suffering with pain under my mask. The group is now a part of my life as are my physical therapy, physicians', and psychologist appointments.

99. How can I help to bring about fibromyalgia awareness?

Participating in awareness day activities and advocacy efforts have paid off. Doctors are beginning to recognize that fibromyalgia is real and more physician education programs on the condition are readily available.

In 1993, not a single project on fibromyalgia was funded by the National Institutes of Health (NIH), the branch of the US government that oversees awards for biomedical research. The number of studies funded on fibromyalgia has slowly increased. Today, an estimated $10 million is spent on fibromyalgia by the NIH each year. Many of the fibromyalgia projects funded by the NIH are making a true difference in determining the physiological mechanisms responsible for the many symptoms of this condition, but not all of them are patient-relevant. For a current list of projects being funded through your tax dollars, visit the government's "Estimates of Funding for Various Diseases, Conditions, Research Areas" at www.nih.gov/news/fundingresearchareas.htm.

Inroads have been made, but there is still a great deal of work to be done. While you may think you are just one person and your voice is too small to be heard, this is just not the case. In fact, it is essential that you write to your elected officials and to the NIH. That's how grassroots lobbying exerts its impact. The greater number of people who write (snail mail and e-mail) and call, the more impact we have. First, you should be aware of many important facts about fibromyalgia. There are a multitude of people, associations, and agencies dedicated to helping people, including the American Pain Foundation and the National Fibromyalgia Partnership. It's not necessary to make a trip to Washington, DC, to become an advocate for fibromyalgia awareness. Writing letters to your local elected officials is a start and a way for you as a patient and citizen to make your voice heard!

Today, an estimated $10 million is spent on fibromyalgia by the NIH each year.

100. Where can I find information about fibromyalgia?

Educating oneself about fibromyalgia, or any other disease, is synonymous with empowerment. Fibromyalgia is not only an enigma to patients and families, but also to the medical community. As patients we must be open to discussing questions and concerns with our healthcare providers. We have included a list of fibromyalgia-related and other professional Web sites that patients have found very helpful (see Appendix). Google Scholar is another valuable resource for journal articles published by medical journals.

Complementary Approach

Appendix

Web sites

American Academy of Craniofacial Pain
520 West Pipeline Road
Hurst, TX 76053
www.aacfp.org

American Academy of Medical Acupuncture
4929 Wilshire Boulevard, Suite 428
Los Angeles, CA 90010
(323) 937-5514
www.medicalacupuncture.org

American Academy of Neurology
www.aan.com

American Academy of Pain Medicine
13947 Mono Way #A
Sonora, CA 95370
(209) 533-9744
www.painmed.org

American Academy of Physical Medicine and Rehabilitation
One IBM Plaza, Suite 2500
Chicago, IL 60611
(312) 464-9700
www.aapmr.org

American Academy of Sleep Medicine
One Westbrook Corporate Center, Suite 920
Westchester, IL 60154
(708) 492-0930
www.aasmnet.org

American Chronic Pain Association
P.O. Box 850
Rocklin, CA 95677
(800) 533-3231
www.theacpa.org

American College of Rheumatology
1800 Century Place, Suite 250
Atlanta, GA 30345-4300
(404) 633-3777
www.rheumatology.org

American Fibromyalgia Syndrome Association
P.O. Box 32698
Tucson, AZ 85715
(520) 733-1570
www.afsafund.org

American Massage Therapy Association
500 Davis Street, Suite 900
Evanston, IL 60201
(847) 864-0123
www.amtamassage.org

American Pain Foundation
201 N. Charles Street, Suite 710
Baltimore, MD 21201-4111
www.painfoundation.org

American Pain Society
4700 W. Lake Avenue
Glenview, IL 60025
(847) 375-4715
www.ampainsoc.org

American Physical Therapy Association
1111 N. Fairfax Street
Alexandria, VA 22314
(800) 999-2782
www.apta.org

Arthritis Foundation
P.O. Box 7669
Atlanta, GA 30357-0669
(800) 687-2277
www.arthritis.org

Association for Applied Psychophysiology and Biofeedback
10200 W. 44th Avenue, Suite 304
Wheat Ridge, CO 80033-2840
(303) 422-8436
www.aapb.org

Centers for Disease Control and Prevention
1600 Clifton Road
Atlanta, GA 30333
(800) 232-4636
www.cdc.gov

Chronic Pain and Fatigue Research Center
www.med.umich.edu/painresearch

Division of Rheumatology at the University of Michigan
www.med.umich.edu/intmed/rheumatology

CO-Cure
A fibromyalgia/chronic fatigue database with resources, articles,
and clinical updates
www.co-cure.org

Fibromyalgia Network
P.O. Box 31750
Tucson, AZ 85715
(800) 853-2929
www.fmnetnews.com

FM-CFS
Support groups throughout Canada
http://www.fm-cfs.ca

Food and Drug Administration
www.fda.gov

HealthFinder
A gateway consumer health Web site with access to innumerable publications and other resources
www.healthfinder.gov

Helping Our Pain and Exhaustion
23915 Forest Park
Novi, MI 48374
(248) 344-0896
www.hffcf.org

House and US Representatives
House of Representatives: www.house.gov
United States Senate: www.senate.gov

Immune Support and ProHealth
Web site with medical articles, advice from leading physicians, a support community, and up-to-date news on nutrition and wellness
www.immunesupport.com
www.prohealth.com

Interstitial Cystitis Association
www.ichelp.org

International Academy for Compounding Pharmacists
www.iacprx.org

International Association for Chronic Fatigue Syndrome
27 N. Wacker Drive, Suite 416
Chicago, IL 60606
www.iacfsme.org

Job Accommodation Network
www.jan.wvu.edu

Lupus Foundation
www.lupus.org

Massage Finder Information
www.massagetherapy.com/home/index.php

Medline Plus
www.nlm.nih.gov/medlineplus/fibromyalgia.html

Medline Plus Drug Information Website
www.nlm.nih.gov/medlineplus/druginformation.html

Men with Fibromyalgia
www.menwithfibro.com/home.html

National Center for Complementary and Alternative Medicine
NCCAM Clearinghouse
P.O. Box 7923
Gaithersburg, MD 20898
(888) 644-6226
www.nccam.nih.gov

National Fibromyalgia Partnership
www.fmpartnership.org

National Fibromyalgia Research Association
www.nfra.net

National Headache Foundation
820 N. Orleans, Suite 217
Chicago, IL 60610
(888) NHF-5552
www.headaches.org

National Library of Medicine
Represents every significant library program, from medical history
to biotechnology
www.nlm.nih.gov

National Women's Health Resource Center
157 Broad Street, Suite 106
Red Bank, NJ 07701
(877) 986-9742
www.healthywomen.org

NIH Office of Dietary Supplements
ods.od.nih.gov

Partnership for Prescription Assistance
www.pparx.org

Appendix

PubMed
The US National Library of Medicine's huge online medical database
www.ncbi.nlm.nih.gov/pubmed/

Restless Legs Syndrome Foundation
1610 14th Street, Suite 300
Rochester, MN 55901
(507) 287-6465
www.rls.org

The TMJ Association
P.O. Box 27660
Milwaukee, WI 53226
(262) 432-0350
www.tmj.org

Vulvar Pain Foundation
203 N. Main Street, Suite 203
Graham, NC 27253
(336) 226-0704
www.vulvarpainfoundation.org

Womenshealth.gov
(800) 994-9662
www.4woman.gov

Books

Fibromyalgia and Chronic Myofascial Pain Syndrome: A Survival Manual.
Starlanyl, D., Copeland, M. E.
Oakland: New Harbinger Publications, 1996.

Myofascial Pain and Dysfunction: The Trigger Point Manual. 2nd ed.
Simons, D. C., Travell, J. C., Simons, L. S.
Baltimore: Lippincott Williams & Wilkins, 1999.

Orthopaedic Physical Therapy Secrets. 2nd ed.
Placzek, J. D., Boyce, D. A.
Philadelphia, PA: Hanley & Belfus, Inc., 2001.

Fibromyalgia: The Complete Guide From Medical Experts and Patients
Ostalecki, S.
Sudbury, MA: Jones & Bartlett Publishers, 2008.

Papers

The American College of Rheumatology 1990 criteria for the classification of
    fibromyalgia: report of the multicenter criteria committee.
Wolfe, F., Smythe, H. A., Yunus, M. B., et al.
Arthritis Rheum 1990;33:106–172.

Fibromyalgia: An "Invisible" Disability
Barrett, D. A.
www.quackwatch.org/03HealthPromotion/fibromyalgia/fms03.html. Accessed
    February 14, 2000.

Documentary

Fibromyalgia: Fitting the Pieces Together
www.hffcf.org
www.mccicorp.com
248-358-4700

Magazines

Massage Magazine
www.massagemag.com

Yoga Journal
www.yogajournal.com

Journals

American Family Physician
www.aafp.org/online/en/home/publications/journals/afp.html

American Journal of Physical Medicine and Rehabilitation
www.amjphysmedrehab.com

Archives of Physical Medicine and Rehabilitation
www.archives-pmr.org

Johns Hopkins White Papers
www.johnshopkinshealthalerts.com/bookstore/index.html

Journal of Arthritis & Rheumatism
www.rheumatology.org/publications/ar/index.asp

Journal of Chronic Fatigue Syndrome
www.cfs-news.org/jcfs.htm

Journal of Rheumatology
www.jrheum.com

Journal of Musculoskeletal Pain
www.haworthpress.com/journals

Journal of the American Medical Association
jama.ama-assn.org

Physical Medicine and Rehabilitation Clinics of North America
www.pmr.theclinics.com

Rheumatology International
www.springer.com/medicine/rheumatology/journal/296

Glossary

A

Acetaminophen: The generic name for Tylenol.

Acupuncture: The practice of piercing specific sites on the body, called pathways or meridians, with thin needles in an attempt to relieve pain associated with some chronic disorders.

Acute: Condition of short duration that starts quickly and has severe symptoms.

Adjuvant: Drugs that augment the effects of analgesics. They include antidepressants and anticonvulsants.

Aerobic exercise: Physical exercise that increases the work of the heart and lungs; examples are running, jogging, swimming, and dancing.

Allodynia: An altered sensation in which normally nonpainful events are felt as pain.

Alternative medicine: A broad category of treatment systems such as chiropractic, herbal medicine, acupuncture, homeopathy, naturopathy, and spiritual devotions. Alternative medicine is also referred to as "complementary medicine." The designation "alternative medicine" is not equivalent to holistic medicine, which is a narrower term.

Analgesic: A medication or agent that reduces pain.

Anticonvulsants: Drugs given to prevent seizures.

Autonomic nervous system: System of the brain that controls key bodily functions not under conscious control, such as heartbeat, breathing, and sweating. The autonomic nervous system has two divisions: the sympathetic nervous system and the parasympathetic nervous system. The sympathetic nervous system accelerates heart rate, constricts blood vessels, and raises blood pressure. The parasympathetic nervous system slows heart rate, increases intestinal and gland activity, and relaxes sphincter muscles.

B

Biofeedback: The use of electronic instruments to measure muscle tension in any muscle group.

C

Carbohydrates: One of the three main classes of food and a source of energy. Carbohydrates are the sugars and starches found in breads, cereals, fruits, and vegetables. During digestion, carbohydrates are changed into a simple sugar called glucose.

Catastrophizing: Occurs when a person ruminates about all the terrible things that are probably going to happen.

Central nervous system: The brain and spinal cord.

Central sensitization: A malfunction in the brain's pain recognition centers that causes people with fibromyalgia to experience pain instead of normal sensations.

Chronic disease: A disease showing little changes or of slow progression; the opposite of acute.

Chronic fatigue syndrome: A condition of excessive fatigue, cognitive impairment, and other varied symptoms. Classified by the World Health Organization (WHO) as a disease of the nervous system, it is of unknown etiology and could last months or years, causing severe disability.

Circadian rhythm: A metabolic or behavior pattern that repeats in cycles of about 24 hours.

Cognitive behavioral therapy (CBT): A type of psychotherapy in which the therapist teaches the patient to restructure his or her cognitive beliefs (thought patterns) and hence, behavior.

Complementary approach: A group of diverse medical and healthcare systems, practices, and products that are not presently considered to be part of conventional medicine.

Compounding pharmacy: A facility that both makes and sells prescription drugs. A compounding pharmacy can often prepare drug formulas that are specially tailored to patients; for example, a compounding pharmacy could create liquid versions of medications normally available only in pill form for patients who cannot swallow pills.

Craniosacral therapy: A gentle form of manipulation. Craniosacral therapists manipulate the craniosacral system, which includes the soft tissue and bones of the head (cranium), the spine down to its tail end (the sacral area), and the pelvis. This manipulation also works with the membranes that surround these bones and the cerebrospinal fluid that bathes the brain and spinal cord.

D

Degenerative joint disease: Osteoarthritis or rheumatoid arthritis.

DHEA: A chemical, produced only during stage 4 sleep, that initiates a cascade of events that causes proteins to repair themselves.

Dolorimeter: A device for quantifying the threshold of pain.

Dry eye disease (DED): Decreased tear production or increased tear film evaporation.

E

Electromyogram (sEMG) biofeedback: Surface EMG biofeedback allows therapists to record the electrical activity of muscles through sensors attached to the skin.

Endorphins: Any of a group of proteins with potent analgesic properties that occur naturally in the brain.

F

Fascia: A fibrous membrane covering, supporting, and separating muscle and some organs of the body. Also known as soft tissue.

Fibro Fog: The cognitive dysfunction experienced by many fibromyalgia patients.

Fibromyalgia: A chronic disorder characterized by widespread musculoskeletal pain, fatigue, and multiple tender points that occur in precise, localized areas, particularly in the neck, spine, shoulders, and hips. It also may cause sleep disturbances, morning stiffness, irritable bowel syndrome, anxiety, and other symptoms.

Fibromyalgia Impact Questionnaire (FIQ): The FIQ is an assessment and evaluation instrument developed to measure fibromyalgia patient status, progress, and outcomes. It has been designed to measure the components of health status that are believed to be most affected by fibromyalgia.

Flare-up: A period of time when symptoms reappear, becoming worse and then improving again.

Flexibility: The ability of muscle to relax and yield to stretch forces.

Food and Drug Administration: The FDA is responsible for protecting the public health by assuring the safety, efficacy, and security of human and veterinary drugs, biological products, medical devices, our nation's food supply, cosmetics, and products that emit radiation.

Functional MRI (FibromyalgiaRI): Functional MRI is based on the increase in blood flow to the local vasculature that accompanies neural activity in the brain.

H

Hyperalgesia: An extreme reaction to a stimulus that is normally painful.

Hypermobile: Abnormally flexible.

Hyperpathia: Abnormally severe pain from a stimulus that normally is slightly painful.

Hyperthyroid: Excessive functionality of the thyroid gland marked by increased metabolic rate, enlargement of the thyroid gland, rapid heart rate, high blood pressure, and various secondary symptoms.

Hypoglycemia: An abnormally low level of glucose in the blood.

Hypothyroidism: Underactivity of the thyroid gland, causing tiredness, cramps, a slowed heart rate, and possibly weight gain.

Hypoxic: Deficient in oxygen.

I

Immune system: The body system that protects the body against invading organisms and infections.

Initiating factors: Factors that cause the onset of myofascial pain.

Insomnia: Inadequate quality or quantity of sleep, with difficulty initiating or maintaining sleep.

Irritable bowel syndrome (IBS): A chronic functional gastrointestinal disorder primarily characterized by abdominal pain and disturbed bowel functioning (diarrhea and/or constipation). It is present in 33% to 77% of individuals with fibromyalgia.

Ischemia: Lack of blood flow to a body part, often caused by constriction or obstruction of a blood vessel.

J

Joint: The point of connection between two bones or elements of a skeleton (especially if the articulation allows motion).

Journaling: The process of recording information about your daily life.

L

Ligament: A tough band of tissue connecting the articular extremities of bones or supporting an organ in place.

M

Magnetic resonance imaging (MRI): A noninvasive, non-X-ray diagnostic technique based on the magnetic fields of hydrogen atoms in the body. MRI provides computer-generated images of the body's internal tissues and organs.

Massage therapy: Manipulation of tissues (as by rubbing, kneading, or tapping) with the hand or an instrument for therapeutic purposes.

MedWatch: The Food and Drug Administration's reporting system for adverse events.

Melatonin: Pineal hormone (a hormone secreted from the pineal gland) secreted primarily during the hours of darkness.

Mindfulness: A form of deep relaxation that involves focusing on being "in the moment."

Multidisciplinary approach: Approach that uses many experts from different disciplines working together as a team to manage and control the symptoms of fibromyalgia.

Muscle: A body tissue consisting of long cells that contract when stimulated and produce motion.

Myofascial pain: Pain and tenderness in the muscles and adjacent fibrous tissues (fascia).

N

Neurotransmitters: Chemicals in the brain, such as acetylcholine, serotonin, and norepinephrine, that facilitate communication between nerve cells (neurons).

Non-rapid eye movement (NREM): A recurring sleep state during which rapid eye movements do not occur and dreaming does not occur; accounts for about 75% of normal sleep time.

Nonsteroidal anti-inflammatory drugs (NSAIDs): Drugs that act against inflammation, reduce fever, relieve muscle pain, and prevent blood clots.

Norepinephrine: A neurotransmitter found mainly in areas of the brain that are involved in governing autonomic nervous system activity, especially blood pressure and heart rate.

Nutrition: The process by which an individual takes in and utilizes food material.

Nutritional therapy/recommendations: Using food and supplements to encourage the body's natural healing.

O

Overlapping conditions: A secondary illness that accompanies the primary illness affecting an individual. Patients with fibromyalgia are often affected by one or more overlapping illnesses, such as restless leg, interstitial cystitis, or tension headaches.

P

Palpate: To touch or feel.

Perpetuating factors: Factors that interfere with healing or enhance the progression of myofascial pain.

Physiatrist: A physician who specializes in physical medicine and rehabilitation.

Physical therapy: The treatment consisting of exercising specific parts of the body such as the legs, arms, hands, or neck in an effort to strengthen, regain range of motion, relearn movement, and/or rehabilitate the musculoskeletal system to improve function.

Polysomnogram: A technical term for a sleep study that involves recording brain waves for assessing the quality of sleep and airflow at the nose and mouth.

Predispose: Having factors that increase the risk of myofascial pain.

Proprioception: The ability to sense the location, position, orientation, and movement of the body and its parts.

Protein: Complex molecules composed of amino acids that are essential to an organism structure and function. Meats, eggs, and dairy products are significant sources of protein. You can also get protein from a variety of grains, legumes, nuts, and seeds. Proteins are the "building blocks" of the human body.

Psychiatrist: A medical doctor who specializes in the treatment and prevention of mental and emotional disorders.

Psychologist: A specialist who can talk with patients and their families about emotional and personal matters and can help them make decisions.

Q

Qi: Energy flow.

R

Rapid eye movement (REM): A light sleep when dreams occur and the eyes move rapidly back and forth.

Raynaud's phenomenon: Discoloration of the fingers or toes due to emotion or cold in a characteristic pattern over time: white, blue, and red.

Referred pain: Pain from a malfunctioning or diseased area of the body that is perceived in another area, often far from the origin.

Rheumatoid arthritis (RA): A chronic disease characterized by stiffness and inflammation of the joints, loss of mobility, weakness, and deformity.

ROM: Range of motion. The amount of movement at one joint or multiple joints of the body.

S

Select serotonin reuptake inhibitor (SSRI): A type of drug that is used to treat depression. SSRIs slow the process by which serotonin (a substance that nerves use to send messages to one another) is reused by nerve cells that make it. This increases the amount of serotonin available for stimulating other nerves.

Self-management skills: A process that involves making wise choices and changes that will positively affect your overall health.

Serotonin: A neurotransmitter within the central nervous system.

Serotonin and norepinephrine reuptake inhibitors (SNRIs): A type of antidepressant medication that increases the levels of both serotonin and norepinephrine by inhibiting their reabsorption into cells in the brain.

Serotonin syndrome: A hyperserotonergic state that is a very dangerous and potentially fatal side effect of serotonergic enhancing drugs; it can have multiple psychiatric and non-psychiatric symptoms.

Sleep apnea: Cessation of breathing that occurs during sleep. Usually due to obstruction of the airway, it can also be due to inability of the brain to initiate respiration.

Sleep deprivation: A shortage of quality, undisturbed sleep that results in detrimental effects on physical and mental well-being.

Soft tissue: The ligaments, tendons, and muscles in the musculoskeletal system.

Somatic: Pertaining to the body.

Stimulants: Drugs that increase the activity of the sympathetic nervous system and produce a sense of euphoria or awakeness.

Substance P: A protein substance that stimulates nerve endings at an injury site and within the spinal cord, increasing pain messages.

Supplements: The addition of vitamins and minerals, in a pill form, to a person's diet.

Sympathetic nervous system: The part of the autonomic nervous system that raises blood pressure and heart rate in response to stress.

Syndrome: A group of symptoms as reported by the patient and signs as detected in an examination that together are characteristic of a specific condition.

T

Temporomandibular disfunction (TMD): Conditions characterized by facial pain and restricted ability to open/move the jaw.

Temporomandibular joint (TMJ): The connecting hinge mechanism between the base of the skull (temporal bone) and the lower jaw (mandible).

Tender points: Sites where the interdigitating fibers of the muscle become mechanically locked into a position that produces pain.

Thyroid: A gland located beneath the voice box (larynx) that produces thyroid hormone. The thyroid helps regulate growth and metabolism.

Thyroid stimulating hormone (THS): Released by the pituitary gland to increase thyroid hormone production.

Tramadol: A centrally acting analgesic for the treatment of pain in fibromyalgia. Also know as Ultram.

Tricyclic antidepressants: A group of drugs used to relieve symptoms of depression. These drugs may also help relieve pain.

Trigger points: Places on the body where muscles and adjacent fibrous tissue (fascia) are sensitive to the touch. These areas are generally in the upper and lower back muscles, but they may occur elsewhere. Also, an area of low neurological activity that when stimulated or stressed transforms into an area of high neurological activity with referred sensations to other parts of the body.

U

Ultram (tramadol): A (synthetic) analgesic (pain reliever).

Ultrasound: An electrical modality that transmits a sound wave through an applicator into the skin to the soft tissue in order to heat the local area; for relaxing the injured tissue and/or dispersing edema.

V

Vulvodynia: According to the International Society for the Study of Vulvovaginal Disease (ISSVD), vulvar discomfort, most often described as burning pain, occurring in the absence of relevant visible findings or a specific, clinically identifiable neurologic disorder.

W

Wax and wane: Refers to symptoms that come and go without definitive cause.

World Health Organization: The directing and coordinating authority for health within the United Nations' system. It is responsible for providing leadership on global health matters, shaping the health research agenda, setting norms and standards, articulating evidence-based policy options, providing technical support to countries, and monitoring and assessing health trends.

Y

Yoga: A system of exercises that help your control of the body and mind. It also improves your breathing and focuses the alignment of your body.

INDEX

Index

Index

W9-AJZ-810

Adventure Guide to

SICILY

Joanne Lane

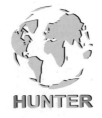

HUNTER

HUNTER PUBLISHING, INC.
130 Campus Drive, Edison, NJ 08818-7816
☎ *732-225-1900 / 800-255-0343 / fax 732-417-1744*
www.hunterpublishing.com; e-mail comments@hunterpublishing.com

IN CANADA:
Ulysses Travel Publications
4176 Saint-Denis, Montréal, Québec, Canada H2W 2M5
☎ *514-843-9882 ext. 2232 / fax 514-843-9448*

IN THE UNITED KINGDOM:
Windsor Books International
The Boundary, Wheatley Road, Garsington
Oxford, OX44 9EJ England; ☎ *01865-361122 / fax 01865-361133*

ISBN 978-1-58843-627-6
© 2007 Hunter Publishing, Inc.

For complete information about the hundreds of other travel guides offered by Hunter Publishing, visit us at www.hunterpublishing.com

All rights reserved. No part of this publication may be reproduced, stored in a retrieval system, or transmitted in any form, or by any means, electronic, mechanical, photocopying, recording, or otherwise, without the written permission of the publisher.

This guide focuses on recreational activities. As all such activities contain elements of risk, the publisher, author, affiliated individuals and companies disclaim any responsibility for any injury, harm, or illness that may occur to anyone through, or by use of, the information in this book. Every effort was made to insure the accuracy of information in this book, but the publisher and author do not assume, and hereby disclaim, any liability for loss or damage caused by errors, omissions, misleading information or potential travel problems caused by this guide, even if such errors or omissions result from negligence, accident or any other cause.

Cover photo: Harbor at Castellammare del Golfo (Steve Geer)

Maps © 2007 Hunter Publishing, Inc.
Index by Inge Wiesen

4   3   2   1

Contents

THE STAR SYSTEM

Adventure Travel Guides cover all the sights and attractions. But, vacation time is limited and precious, so we steer you to the best and the not-to-be-missed with a star system. Attractions that earn one star (★) are worth a visit. Two stars (★★) mean you should exert a bit of effort to go there. When you see three stars (★★★), just do it. You won't be sorry.

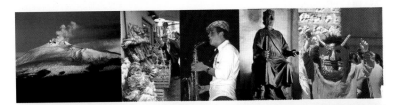

Introduction

"L'Italia senza Sicilia non lascia immagine nello spirito: qui è la chiave di tutto." (To see Italy without Sicily is not to see Italy at all, for Sicily is the key to everything.) Wolfgang Goethe

Sicily has long been regarded as Italy's ball to kick. Its position at the toe of the mainland's boot has inspired many jokes at its expense. But Sicily actually has a lot to throw back. There aren't many places in the world where you can ski and then hit the beach afterwards for a refreshing dip; enjoy temperate climates year-round; go to markets with the most astounding array of seafood; see Greek,

Roman, Etruscan, medieval and Arabic architecture all in one town as you meet some of the friendliest people in the world. The island of Sicily is like another world compared to the rest of Italy – only three km away over the Messina Straits. And in fact the people proclaim themselves Sicilians first, with distinct differences in language, culture, food and day-to-day living. Many visitors find this surprising but refreshing. The richness in culture is seen in the architecture, theater, cinema and art found everywhere. Despite the poverty, unemployment and much-publicized Mafia control, it's a vibrant and volatile place but far safer than tourists expect.

Sicilians have a strong sense of community, the pace of life is slow, schedules seem to have no importance and it can be simultaneously frustrating, entertaining and totally memo-

rable. But, whether you come here to fish, dive, hike, ski, play golf or trace your family origins, there is plenty that is appealing to visitors.

History

 Sicily has a diverse history which has left it with an abundance of archaeological remains, architectural marvels and an eventful past. It was a constant pawn for marauding forces in the Mediterranean for over 6,000 years because of its strategic location. Each has contributed in some way to the richness of Sicilian culture but often at a cost as inhabitants bore the weight of one colonizer after another.

Prehistory/Ancient Civilizations

The Italian peninsula has supported human life for thousands of years. Cave paintings in Addaura on Monte Pellegrino confirm the presence of a Paleolithic culture in Sicily between 20,000 and 10,000 BC.

The Carthaginians & Greeks (750-215 BC)

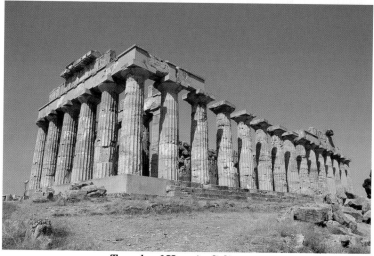

Temple of Hera in Selinunte

After 900 BC Mycenean and Aegean trading contacts were replaced by Carthaginian ones from North Africa, particu-

larly in western Sicily. The Carthaginians were originally Phoenicians from the eastern Mediterranean and they settled at Palermo, Solunto and Mozia in the eighth and seventh centuries BC – at the same time the Greeks were establishing colonies on the eastern coast of Sicily in Siracusa and Gela. The Greeks challenged the Carthaginians for control of Sicily and pushed them back to the western part of the island. The island was in a constant state of civil war.

The scattered Greek colonies throughout Italy were known as Magna Graecia or Greater Greece, and their populations and wealth eventually overtook that of Greece itself. Under their rule Siracusa grew to become the rival of Athens. As a result, in 415 BC Athens dispatched an armada to help Segesta in their war with Siracusa-supported Selinus. Siracusa itself came under siege in 413 BC, but easily repelled its attackers.

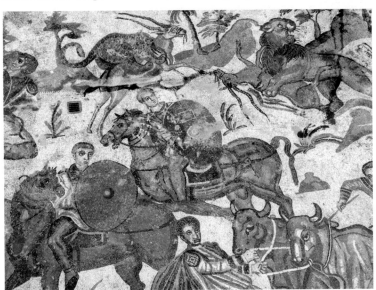

Mosaic of hunters from a Roman villa near Piazza Armerina
(Galen R Frysinger, www.galenfrysinger.com)

Romans & The Empire (218 BC-468 AD)

Roman rule began when Siracusa fell in 211 BC. It became Rome's first province outside of the Italian peninsula. For 700 years Sicily was a province of Rome and became Rome's granary. Huge tracts of forests were cut for grain cultivation, Sicily's temples were stripped of their treasures, while the popu-

lation was denied Roman citizenship and treated almost as slaves. As a result there were two major slave revolts. The Romans did not establish new settlements but Romanized the existing Greek ones, creating a Greco-Roman society. When the Republic finally began to decline, some peace and prosperity returned to the island. Sicilians were finally granted citizenship in the third century AD and it once again became an important center for trade.

Barbarians, Byzantines & Arabs (468-1061)

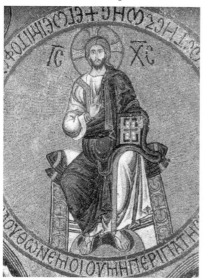

Mosaic in Palermo's Byzantine St. Mary's of the Admiral church

The centralized power of Rome over Sicily evaporated in 410 AD and a period of foreign rule by Vandals and Ostrogoths from North Africa ensued from AD 468 until 535. However, Barbarian rule was short and ended when the Byzantine general Belisarius took the island in 535. Sicily was then annexed to the Byzantine Empire, a medieval state ruled from Constantinople.

The island enjoyed a few centuries of Byzantine rule that were largely peaceful and prosperous, although taxation was high. The Byzantine cultural influence lasted well into the Arab and Norman eras in Sicily. Under the Byzantines, Greek remained the culture and language of the majority. But Constantinople was never able to give much attention to Sicily and Muslim-Arab piratical attacks were common from North Africa as the Moors gained power in the Mediterranean. The Sicilians traded with the Arabs but nonetheless coastal raids became commonplace.

In 700 the island of Pantelleria was taken and it was only due to internal struggles among the Arabs that they did not invade Sicily. By 800 many Arab merchants lived in Sicilian cities and trade agreements were signed. But in 827 a fully fledged Arab invasion took place. Thousands of Arabs,

Berbers and Spanish Muslims, known collectively as Saracens, landed at Marzara del Vallo and took Palermo in 831. Palermo became the capital of the Arabs in Sicily and one of the world's greatest cities, with gardens, mosques and palaces. The Arabs brought with them other benefits: they resettled rural areas, renovated and extended irrigation, introduced new crops, developed mining, a salt industry, commerce and extended religious tolerance.

However the Arabs were prone to divisive feuding. Sicily lost its central position in the Arab Mediterranean empire and became vulnerable again. The Byzantines attempted to retake the island but it was the Normans who eventually conquered.

The Norman Conquest (1060-1194)

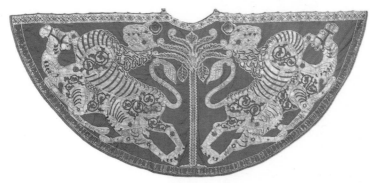

Robe of the Norman king of Sicily, Roger II, made in 1133

The most brilliant age of Sicily's history of occupation belongs to the Normans who seized Messina from the Arabs in 1061 and captured Palermo 11 years later. It took them almost three more decades of bloody fighting to take the entire island. Their reign was brief but they managed to bring a lasting legacy of art and architecture in just over a century of rule. In that time five Norman kings ruled in Sicily.

The Normans had a policy of acceptance and integration, using the existing frameworks available to form a governmental class. They introduced a Latinized aristocracy and superseded the Arabic language with French and Italian. The fine mosaics at Monreale, outside Palermo, attest to the Norman's brilliant architectural abilities.

However, the death of William II in 1189 created a crisis in Norman Sicily. Henry the Hohenstaufen (or Swabian) arrived with a fleet to take over. There was little opposition and he crowned himself King of Sicily.

The Swabian Dynasty (1194-1266)

When Henry V died, the throne passed to his son Frederick II. Frederick imposed an authorative stamp on society and

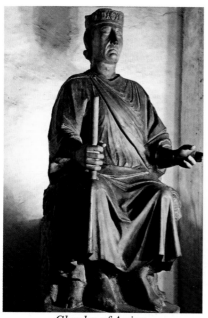

Charles of Anjou,
by Arnolfo Di Cambio

attempted to restore the broad framework of the Norman state. He encouraged the arts, science, law, medicine and Sicilian vernacular poetry. There was some measure of peace in Sicily during his half-century of rule until he died. The pope wanted to deprive the Swabians of their possession of Sicily and sold the throne to the king of England. Ten years later a new French pope deposed the English king and gave Sicily to the brother of the French king, Charles of Anjou. Charles immediately embarked on a campaign against the Sicilian population who had supported the Swabians. He plundered land and gave it to his followers, heavily taxing the population to cover the costs of recent wars. His punitive actions caused the nobility to turn against him, which began the Sicilian Vespers in 1282, a revolt against the French. Power passed to the Aragon dynasty and five centuries of Spanish rule followed.

The Spanish (1282-1713)

Because of its domination by Spain during this period, the Renaissance had little impact on Sicily. Feudal bonds continued with the granting of large portions of land to the Spanish

aristocracy in return for military service. During the centuries of Spanish rule, feuding, economic stagnation, corruption, increased taxes, plague and earthquakes burdened the people. The Catholic Church also rose to power under the Spanish. It was during this period that brigandry developed, with small gangs of armed peasants robbing large estates and causing mayhem, burning crops, killing livestock and the bailiffs whom the Spanish nobility had left in charge to collect rent when they moved to the cities. These bands were both feared and admired by the peasantry and were referred to as "*mafia*."

The 17th & 18th Centuries

This period saw continued unrest as short-term rulers controlled the island while it also suffered from natural disasters – an eruption of Mt Etna in 1669 and an earthquake in 1693. Austria was given the island in 1707 but ruled for just four years until a Spaniard, Charles of Bourbon, arrived to claim the throne of the Two Sicilies (Sicily and Naples). Following his death, Sicily passed under the control of the House of Savoy, an Italian family from southeast France. Again this was short-term and it was traded to the Austrians in 1720. In 1734 the Spanish again reclaimed the island.

During the Napoleonic Wars, Sicily was one of the few places in Italy left unconquered by Napoleon. However, when he took Naples (part of the Two Sicilies) the King fled to Palermo under the protection of the British. When the tax demands on the Sicilan peasantry led to open revolt, the British intervened and persuaded King Ferdinand IV to summon a new parliament and adopt a constitution where Sicilian independence was guaranteed and feudalism abolished. When the British left after Napoleon's defeat, Ferdinand revoked the move.

Unification

Uprisings were common during this period and reached the ears of Giuseppe Garibaldi, who decided it was time to begin his war for the unification of Italy. In 1860 he arrived in Marsala with 1,000 men to liberate the island from Bourbon rule and Sicily became free of Spain for the first time since 1282. A 99½% majority voted in favor of a union with the new kingdom of Italy under Vittorio Emanuele II. However, within a

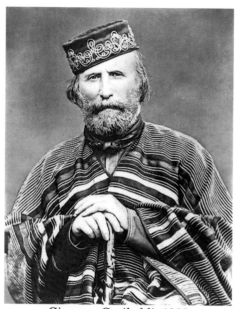
Giuseppe Garibaldi, 1866

few years Sicilians began to question whether the change of ruler had achieved anything. The populace was dissatisfied and in the years leading up to 1914 one and a half million Sicilians left their land for North and South America.

During this period the power of the Mafia grew. In the vacuum of power that existed between the people and the state, gangs drawn up along family lines took on the role of intermediaries between tenants and owners of land, sorting out disputes and regulating affairs in the absence of an effective judicial system.

By the 20th century, the island was suffering from emigration losses and from the effects of another earthquake in Messina.

The World Wars

The onset of World War I was a further blow to the Sicilian economy. In 1922, when Mussolini gained power, he sent Cesare Mori to Sicily to put an end to the Mafia. Thousands of suspected Mafiosi were imprisoned, but it simply drove the criminal class further underground or abroad, where it flourished. In the 1930s Mussolini encouraged wheat production in Sicily to give his nation more economic and agricultural self-sufficiency. However, the increase in wheat production was at the cost of the diversity of crops Sicily required and caused soil exhaustion and erosion.

In exchange for the wheat production, Mussolini promised to return land to its rightful owners and introduce reform, but WWII put an end to that. During the war Sicily was occupied by the Germans and suffered heavily. The Allied invasions were successful in liberating the island from German rule but

at the cost of heavy bombing and the return to power of the Mafia. Few Sicilian towns escaped aerial bombardment in a month of heavy fighting before the Germans abandoned the island. Messina in the island's east was the most heavily bombed of all Italian cities. The Mafia had played a key role in the Allied landings and subsequent success and, in return, those who had been imprisoned under Fascism were freed.

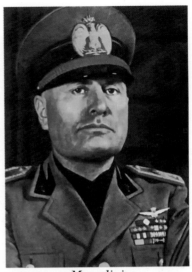

Mussolini

The Republic

After WWII radical changes occurred in Sicily. Anarchy, hunger, banditry and crime were widespread. The Mafia returned to their seats of power and a separatist movement pushed for independence from the mainland. In response to this, Sicily was granted regional autonomy in 1946, with its own assembly and president. In the same year Italy was declared a republic. During the latter half of the 20th century the Democrazia Cristiana (DC or Christian Democrats) became powerful, promising reforms and appealing to traditional values. The center-right Catholic party was aided by the Mafia, ensuring they came out at the top of the polls. In return, the Mafia received favorable contracts in the 1950s building period. In 1992 Sicily returned to the headlines when two anti-Mafia magistrates, Giovanni Falcone and Paolo Borsellino, were assassinated. The events triggered a general upheaval in Italian political life. Today Sicily is probably better off than at any oter point in its changeable history, but it still faces many economic, social and political problems.

Geography/the Land

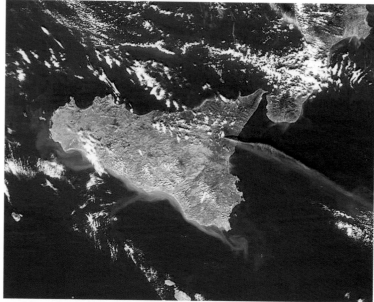

Sicily from space

Sicily is the largest of the Mediterranean islands, with an area of 10,023 sq. miles. It is surrounded by two parts of the Mediterranean Sea, the Ionian and Tyrrhenian. Around it lie a number of smaller islands: the Aeolians and Ustica in the north, the Egadi to the west and the Pelagie islands and Pantelleria in the south.

Sicily was probably once connected to mainland Italy, just three km as it is from Calabria, and also to Africa, 160 km away. The island is triangular in shape and was name Trinacria (three points) by the Greeks.

THE TRISKELE

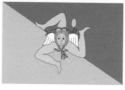

The Triskele or Trinacria is the ancient symbol of Sicily – the image of a woman with three running legs. When the Greeks circumnavigated the island they noted the three capes – Capo Peloro, Capo Pachino and Capo Lilbeo

– that formed a triangle and called the island Trinakrias, meaning three promonotories. The Romans called it Trinacrium, meaning "star with three points." It is thought that the symbol originated during the Greek occupation as Greek coins have been found bearing the symbol. The original face on the symbol was that of Medusa, whose gaze had the power of petrifying anyone who looked at her. She had snakes upon her head instead of hair and the three legs symbolized the three corners of the island. Medusa's face has now been replaced by the friendlier image of an agrarian goddess with wheat stalks coming out of her hair, symbolizing Sicily's fertility.

Terrain

Some 83% of Sicily's surface area is mountainous or hilly, especially in inland regions. The remaining area includes level coastal areas and a large expanse of plains near Catania. The most extensive mountain areas are in the north and east. In the east is Mount Etna, the highest point on the island at 3,340 m (10,958 ft) and Europe's largest active volcano. Sicily actually has two of Italy's 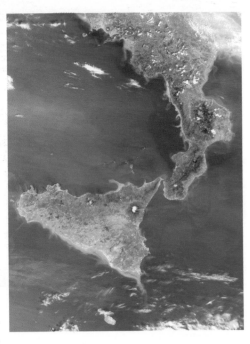 three active volcanoes, the other located on Stromboli in the Aeolian Islands.

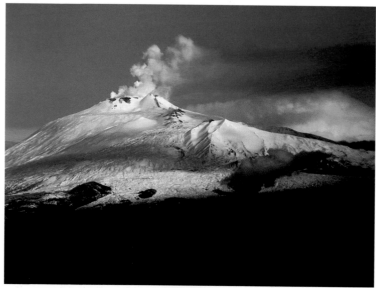

Mt. Etna

Sicily's precarious position over two continental plates makes it prone to earthquakes. A 1693 quake damaged many towns in the southwest. In 1908 Messina was almost destroyed and in 1968 the western part of the island was badly affected. The seismic activity, however, has also created tourist the attractions of Mt Etna, Stromboli and Volcano, where you can climb the volcanoes and bathe in thermal mud.

Regions

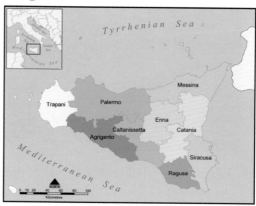

There are nine provinces in Sicily that take the name of their capital town or city – hence the Agrigento province also includes the city of Agrigento. The provinces have an associated two letter code –

Agrigento which includes the Pelagic Islands (AG), Caltanisetta (CL), Catania (CT), Enna (EN), Messina, which includes the Aeolian Islands, (ME), Palermo, including Ustica, (PA), Ragusa (RG), Siracusa (SR) and Trapani, including the Egadi Islands and Pantelleria, (TP).

Climate

 Sicily's mild Mediterranean climate of hot, dry summers and short, mild winters makes it one of the most agreeable in Europe and perfect for travelers in every season. The intermediate seasons are short and more an extension of summer than of winter. They can also be warm enough for swimming in if the sirocco winds from Africa are blowing. There's also plenty of sun to be had (see the table below), with the average number of hours of sun per year at 2,500, compared to 2,000 on the Italian peninsula and 1,800 in southern France.

In July and August the temperatures rise and the hot, dusty African sirocco winds blow. Space is at a premium on the coast, with jostling crowds from Italy and Europe. You will also find hotel prices higher and availability reduced. Temperatures usually hover in the high 80s to low 90s F but it can be hotter on the southern and western coasts than elsewhere in Sicily as these areas are most affected by the Saharan sand carried on sirocco winds. The cities are also oppressive during the summer. At this time of year the best places to be are on the coast or in the interior where the upper reaches are cool and green.

The coldest months of the year are December and February when day temperatures are around 50°F and night time temperatures fall to about 32°, but rarely below. Winter is the wettest time of year and the highest rainfall occurs in November. During the winter the interior sections of the island are wet and windy and the upper reaches can even be bitterly cold, especially after dark. Inland, around Enna, it can get snowed under, but this then allows for skiing at Piano Battaglia (Madonie mountains) or Mount Etna. The most snow tends to fall in January.

May and June or September and October are the best options for vacationers. You can still swim and there are fewer crowds. Autumn months are pleasant, with good food harvests.

Rainfall

Sicily's climate is subtropical, tending to desert, with rainfall typical of similar regions on the northern coasts of Africa. Most rainfall, if any, occurs in November and three-fourths of the annual total falls between October and March. June, July and August are the driest months of the year. Winter rains are scarce in the interior and heavier in the west and north of the island. Sunny Palermo has typically less rainfall annually than any other large city in Italy at about 19 unches per year.

Water shortages are common in Sicily. Not only has Sicily recorded a diminishing annual rainfall and has the lowest annual records in the country at 15 inches but there are also no major rivers and lakes in the country to sustain the needs of the population. Some areas like the offshore islands have no fresh water at all due to low rainfall or high evapotranspiration.

Italy as a whole has the highest water consumption per capita in Europe and the third-highest in the world. In Sicily population demands on water resources are also high. Leakages from reservoirs and badly maintained distribution networks also cause significant water losses, as does outright theft. In summer water restrictions are evident in major Sicilian cities.

Flora & Fauna

 The differences in geology and climate around the island encourage a rich range of plant life, with everything from subtropical species to flora more typical of Northern Europe. Much of the plant life was

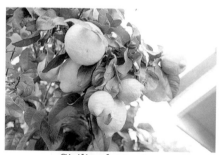
Sicilian lemon tree

brought in by various invading powers such as the Greeks and Phoenicians, who introduced vines, olives, figs and pomegranates. The Arabs planted dates, lemons, almonds and bitter orange used for marmalade, candied fruit and essence. Sweet oranges arrived in the 16th century via the Portuguese

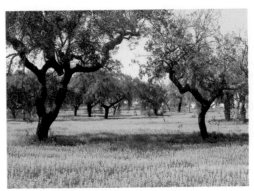
Cork oaks in a field of lupins

and tomatoes and prickly pears arrived about the same time. The mandarin was imported at the beginning of the 19th century and eucalyptus was also introduced to combat malarial marshlands. Sicily has also been noted as a grain-producing territory since the Romans first cultivated the terrain to send back produce to Rome.

Today Sicily's coastal areas feature citrus orchards, olive trees and vineyards. Mountain slopes are typically covered with broom, lavender, rosemary, wild olives, dwarf palms, lentisk, cork

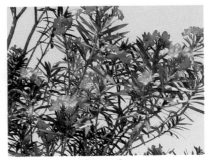
Oleander

oaks, oleanders, carob trees and tamarisks. The great forests that once covered the island remain mostly in the Nebrodi,

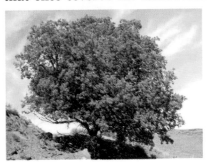
Olive tree

Madonie, Peloritani and on the Etna slopes. These woodlands comprise oak trees, holm oaks, cork oaks, chestnut trees and beech trees. Other plants include agaves, palms, plane trees, ficus, cedar, mulberry and eucalyptus.

The slopes of Mt Etna are particularly fertile and cultivation of olives, grapes, citrus and other fruits is very successful in the lower

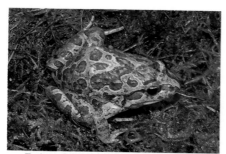
Painted frog or Disglossus pictus
(Fabrizio Li Vigni)

areas. On the higher slopes there are pistachio plantations, walnuts, almond, chestnut, pine, birch and oak trees.

Sicily's changes in climate and environment over the centuries, compounded by man's influence, have changed its wildlife as well. Birds of prey and big mammals have largely disappeared, including the near-extinct wolf and long-extinct Sicilian deer. Wildcats, martens, dormice (rare), hedgehogs, wild rabbits, weasels, beavers, squirrels and wild boar are among those that remain. Bird species include the falcon, pilgrim hawk, windhover, kite, eagle, rock partridge and imperial crow. Migratory birds such as the common

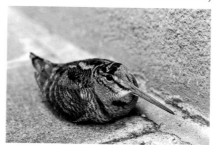
Eurasian woodcock (Mark Schröder)

wader, pink seagull, greater sea swallow and the spoonbill still stop off in Sicily. The island also has a large number of insects and invertebrates, including the spotted grass snake. There is a local species of toad that grows almost eight inches long, as well as several varieties of frog and gecko lizard. Freshwater fish were found in the island's rivers until the end of the 19th century until they were fished out, but eels can still be found.

The seas around Sicily are home to large numbers of blue-fin tuna and swordfish, which are also popular delicacies (see the *Cuisine* section later in this chapter). The great white shark exists in the southern waters of the Mediterranean but attacks are very rare.

Ecology & Environment

Sicily is an incredibly beautiful country and steps are now being taken to protect its fauna and flora through the recent

creation of parks and nature reserves. However, the numerous foreign rulers over the centuries all took their toll on the environment. For example, woods and forests covered Sicily before the Romans arrived and cultivated the terrain to grow wheat, which they sent to Rome. Later the Arabs reduced the forest sizes even more as Sicilian wood came into great demand for use in ship building. They did introduce citrus fruits and install irrigation systems. However, by the 16th century the island's interior was largely deforested and today the remnants of Sicily's woods and forests can be found only in the three national parks and 90 natural reserves. The primary tracts of forest are in the Nebrodi Mountains near Messina, the Madonie Mountains closer to Palermo and areas such as the woods of Ficuzza.

In more recent times environmental damage has continued. In the 1930s Mussolini exploited Sicily for wheat production, resulting in soil exhaustion and erosion. And all throughout the 20th century industrialization and urbanization have created pollution problems – smog is a common problem in big cities and some of the island's more beautiful areas have been fouled. You'd be advised not to swim in industrial areas around Gela, Porto Empedocle, Augusta and Trapani.

Illegal construction is another problem in Sicily. The Mafia launder money in many construction projects and residents have often built illegally, creating ugly suburbs in previously pristine garden areas and houses that are unfinished to avoid taxes.

Sicily has been a little slow introducing laws to protect its natural treasures and in fact a Ministry for the Environment was only created in 1986. Recycling is still disappointingly uncommon and littering too common.

National Parks

Sicily's forests are confined largely to the 86 parks and natural reserves around the island. Of these, four are regional parks of significance. The **Parco Fluviale dell'Alcantara** is a 30-mile-lomg reserve with spectacular natural sculptures along the River Alcantara near Catania. The **Parco dell'Etna** was established in the late 1980s to protect the slopes of the volcano from further development. The region is divided into four areas with different levels of protection and includes the towns around the volcano. **Parco dei Nebrodi**

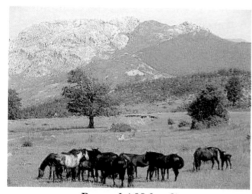

Parco dei Nebrodi

was established in 1993 and comprises some of the most important and largest wooded areas of Sicily (about 140,000 acres). The park has a lot of arboreal species and wildlife, including San Fratello horses (unique to Sicily), sheep, pigs and cattle that can be found everywhere – including the middle of the misty mountain roads. The **Parco delle Madonie** is a mountainous woodland east of the capital. It was set up in 1989 to protect the region, the only reserve where people live.

The island groups form most of the marine protected areas and a variety of mountains, caves, lakes, rivers and other islands are protected by the remaining reserves. Two of the more beautiful coastal reserves include the stunning

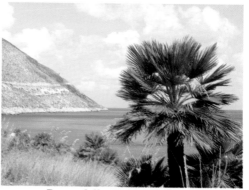

Parco dello Zingaro (Stefan C)

Parco dello Zingaro to the northwest of Palermo and **Vendicari** on the southern coast. Historically significant areas include **Bagni di Cefala** (Arab baths) and **Pantalica** (cliff-side tombs). Visit www.parks.it for more information.

Government

Sicily became a self-governing region in 1946 with Palermo as its capital. It has had its own parliament and president since 1947. This means Sicily has a wider range of economic and administrative powers than

other regions of Italy but it has limited legislative powers in such areas as tourism, transport, industry and the environment.

But the real driving power behind Sicily's political system since autonomy was granted has been the Mafia. Mafia influence in the national legislature has long been suspected, but never proven outright and any new authority's willingness to curb it usually fades quickly.

The Economy

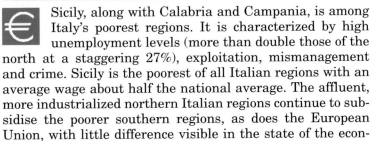 Sicily, along with Calabria and Campania, is among Italy's poorest regions. It is characterized by high unemployment levels (more than double those of the north at a staggering 27%), exploitation, mismanagement and crime. Sicily is the poorest of all Italian regions with an average wage about half the national average. The affluent, more industrialized northern Italian regions continue to subsidise the poorer southern regions, as does the European Union, with little difference visible in the state of the economy.

Some believe Sicily's problems are centuries in the making. Certainly foreign domination in Sicily has left its mark on the economy. Many of these occupying powers neglected the economy or some, like the Normans, left fine monuments but little economic independence. Vegetation and forests were cleared, the locals heavily taxed and the island prevented from developing and making the most of its potential. Little changed for Sicilians after unification and what was modernized brought associated ills. Pockets of the island were ruined by construction and industry and yet little has been done to tackle the real problems such as emigration, poverty and unemployment.

The Italian government set up the Cassa del Mezzogiorno in 1950 to rebuild the economy. European aid poured in with it through subsidies, grants, loans and tax incentives. However, much of the aid was siphoned off by organized crime and the government finally scrapped the scheme in 1992, responding to frustration expressed by northern states. The EU however continues to subsidize the Sicilian economy.

After these state-supported industrial ventures failed there were hopes for private investment. But so far investors have

been difficult to attract. The protection money and payoffs to politicians required for building permits and business operating licenses have discouraged northern and foreign firms.

Money laundering in Sicily is almost a way of life. Business people often request false or inflated receipts for outsourced services. Corruption exists at all levels. Public building contracts are assigned based on bribery and kickbacks. Anti-Mafia certificates were introduced for business registrations and public contracts but have done nothing to change the situation. While the Mafia are often behind shady transactions, it's now a new Mafia of white collar professionals who work together collaboratively in a new underworld of "respectable" deals.

The proposed closures of the Fiat factory in Termini Imerese over the past few years has been an ongoing source of concern for the Sicilian economy, with many job losses. The company is launching new models and eliminating top-of-the-range car production as part of its latest market strategy to return the company to full production by 2008.

Sicily's economy still relies on agriculture, although there are other strong industries, including sulphur production, fishing and petrochemicals. All are challenged by outside competition. Tourism is probably the most hopeful of all the industries but the road to recovery will not be easy.

Employment

Every year about 10,000 Sicilians leave home to search for work (see *Population* later in this chapter) and those that stay behind usually move to the cities for better opportunities. Unemployment is currently estimated at about 27% (over 35% for women and over 50% for those under 25). Unemployment peaks in the province of Enna and the cities of Catania, Palermo and Messina. Employment in Sicily is generally divided into the agricultural sector (12%), industry (20%) and tourism/commerce (68%). The monthly income per inhabitant is estimated at half that of a Milanese resident. Sicilian families living at the country's poverty level are about 31%. Real GDP growth has been negative on three occasions since 1992 and on average remains below the national average.

Sicily has a limited industrial base and even most university graduates are fortunate if they find jobs in Sicily. Those that do find work are often poorly paid. There is no minimum wage

law in Italy and employers can exploit the unemployment conditions by grossly underpaying their staff or even hiring illegally. The best job options for young people are in family-run businesses.

The government is working hard to create thousands of low-paying jobs with programs like Articolisti and LSU (Lavoro Socialmente Utile). However professionalism is often secondary to the social prestige of a job title and people sometimes seem to work only between frequent coffee breaks. Obviously there are exceptions like Sicily's world-class orchestras and highly developed archaeology and history fields. But women remain seriously under-represented in important positions, are underpaid and sexual harassment is not unusual.

Bribes or political favors are used to obtain positions and personal recommendations are important. This means one must be personally known to establish a business relationship or obtain employment. Even if you're only marginally competent, a good recommendation can get you a good job.

Education

In Sicily value for education has not been a strong point. Compulsory education has helped when it is enforced but in many poorer districts of Sicily children can be found not attending school. In Palermo one in six children aged 12 to 14 chooses not to go to school. Italy's minimum school-leaving age is 16, raised from 14 years just a few years ago and may soon rise to 18 years. Figures from 2005 show that 9% of Italians are functionally illiterate and this figure may be higher in Sicily.

Customs & Lifestyle

The long domination of foreign powers in Sicily left its imprint on the people and their culture. The separation from the Italian mainland has also created a separate mentality in the people, who see themselves as Sicilians first and Italians a distinct second.

In Sicily, parental, familial and peer influences are strong and the mother is the center of it all. Family events such as first communions and weddings take on a momentous importance. Sicilian children live with their parents into their adulthood, usually until they marry. This is partly because it is hard to find a job that pays well enough to permit a young person to

be more independent. Even young mothers seem very dependent on their own mothers. The family bonds are something foreigners often cite as a virtue, but it can also be limiting. Foreigners staying with Sicilian families may find them unusually protective

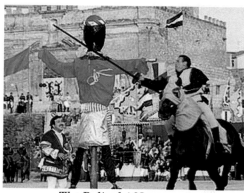

The Palio dei Normanni

tive – in itself an endearing quality. However, for those used to more freedom within their own family contexts, it can seem confining.

Religious events in Sicily are still celebrated with gusto, despite a decreasing number of churchgoers. Other local festivals range from aristocratic to popular and from medieval to folk festivals, and are the best places to see many of the traditional styles of dress and transport which have largely disappeared from day-to-day life. Some

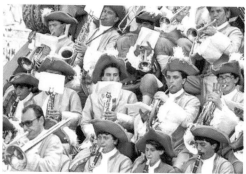

At the Festino di Santa Rosalia

festival highlights include the **Palio dei Normanni** in Piazza Armerina (12-14 August), **Festino di Santa Rosalia** (10-15 July), celebrating their patron saint, the **Misteri of Trapani** (Easter) and **La Scala** (24-25 July), illuminating the ceramic stairs of Caltagirone. At the "**Ballu di li Diavuli**" (Devil's Dance) participants wearing devil masks and with goatskins over their shoulders make fun of bystanders, accompanied by the sound of bugles. Religious icons are carried in a procession and the devils try to prevent the Virgin from meeting her dead Son. In the end, they are defeated by two warrior angels.

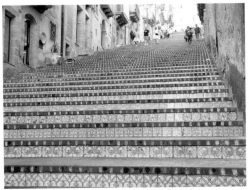

The ceramic stairs of Caltagirone

Sicilian society is still largely socialist and you may notice that employees of public services are sometimes careless about the way they treat customers. For example, post office officials and bus ticket inspectors tend to presume that everyone is dishonest. Be prepared for similar treatment, although they can be more lenient with tourists. Be positively assertive wherever possible.

Another notable characteristic is a seeming reluctance to stand in

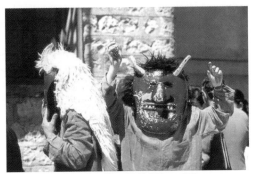

The "Ballu di li Diavuli"

line. Expect people to crowd bank tellers, ticket booths, food stands and cashiers, disregarding whoever may have arrived first. The best solution is to put out your elbows and join in.

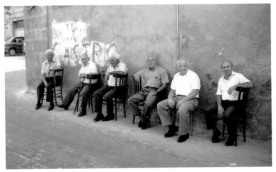

Sicilian men (Joanne Lane)

For visitors Sicilians also seem to have a rather unorthodox sense of time and priorities, reflected especially in the long closure of stores and business from

1 to 4 pm. Around 5 pm, activity increases again in the main piazzas and streets as people take a *passeggiata* (stroll) to socialize or do their shopping.

Legally, Sicilian women have the same rights as men but, socially, many also conform to traditional roles in society. For example, Sicilian women are often reserved with men they don't know, even in a business situation. Sexual harassment can be common in the workplace and young men will call out "*ciao bella*" to women they don't know. Expect a lot of tooting and whistling.

The vast majority of working Sicilian women are employed in lower-paying professions, such as secretaries and sales clerks. Few are real entrepreneurs, physicians or lawyers and they also receive lower salaries than men for comparable work. ARCI Donna (Via Alessio di Giovanni 14, Palermo, ☎ 091-345-799, www.arcidonna.org) is a national association working to promote equal opportunities for women. They list women's representation in government as 0% nationally, 3.8% regionally and 5½% in local politics. The overall representation of women in Sicilian government is 11.8%, notably less than the national level of 15.9% for Italy as a whole

As regards marital and sexual laws, Italy has been somewhat slow to establish a legal position. Divorce was legalized in Italy only in the 1970s, rape became a serious crime (a violent felony) only in the late 1990s, and "private" prostitution is actually legal under most conditions. However, brothels and related activities are not.

Dress & Fashion

On average Italians dress better than Americans. The *bella figura* is an important part of Italian life and there is some shame felt in making a *brutta figura* or bad impression. Good shoes are an important part of the equation and often the first thing new acquaintances may notice. American visitors are often identifiable by the large white sneakers they wear – not something Italians wear outside the gym. Smart dressing for dinner is also important. You may not be able to match the heel sizes and sweeping coats of the local women, but dressing well will help you fit in.

While Italian women dress well, they do not wear skimpy or see-through clothing. In churches make sure you dress modestly or you may be refused entry. This means no shorts or short skirts, and shoulders should be covered.

Love & Relationships

Sicilian men are possibly even more forward with women than their north Italian counterparts. Certainly as a whole Sicilians tend to be more expressive. Young people in Sicily are usually forced, for economic and social reasons, to live at home with their parents. They often lack privacy at home and may appear more reserved as couples within the family context. However, courting couples meet in city parks and squares where they can be more affectionate.

Population

Sicily is one of the most densely populated islands in the Mediterranean and has a higher percentage of births to deaths than the mainland. The population is something over five million, mainly concentrated in the two large cities of **Palermo** (750,000) and **Catania** (376,000) on the northern and eastern coasts. Development of industry has also favored migration from high altitude zones and the interior to the coasts, although historically the coasts were also important for maritime trade. **Caltanisetta** is the most populated inland city, with a population of 61,300.

The Sicilian population has been drained somewhat by mass emigration. Between 1880 and 1910, 1½ million Sicilians left Sicily for the United States. Now it is estimated that about 10,000 people leave the island every year for work opportunities in Northern Italy or abroad in Canada, the United States and Australia. These people are usually younger, leaving an ageing populace behind.

Taormina shopper (Galen R Frysinger, www. galenfrysinger.com)

Ironically, immigrants from outside the EU have flooded into Sicily in search of the same opportunities and there are large populations of Tunisians, Africans, Pakistanis, Bangladeshis and Chinese in the cities.

Sicily has always been a melting pot of cultures and peoples. Today's inhabitants are descended from Greeks, Italians, Phoenicians, and the pre-colonial indigenous peoples known as Sicans, Elymi, and Sicels. There is also some Norman and Spanish blood still present due to their respective conquests of the island. Today, Sicilians residing in the east, southeast, and northeast portions of the island are considered primarily of Greek and Sicel descent. Cities like Syracuse, Messina, Agrigento and Taormina were originally Greek settlements; and the southwest, west and northwest had Phoenician/Arab and Sican inhabitants. Trapani and Palermo were also Phoenician settlements. Those with Norman or Spanish blood are found mostly in the large northern cities such as Palermo and Cefalù.

Religion

The earlier inhabitants of Sicily like the Sicans, Sicels, Elami, Phoenicians, Carthaginians and ancient Greeks were polytheistic and created their own Gods. Later, the Romans also adopted the Greek gods as their own. Judaism was the first monotheistic faith in the Mediterranean region. Christianity built upon Judaism and was then followed by Islam during the Norman era (1070-1200). Sicily's Muslims gradually converted to Christianity, and over time the remaining Byzantine (Orthodox) clergy were replaced by Latin (Catholic) priests. The Jewish population emigrated or converted to Christianity after an infamous Spanish decree in 1492. By 1500 Sicily was Roman Catholic, except for a few Albanian Orthodox communities whose churches soon affiliated themselves with Rome.

In Italy today 85% of people are Catholics but only 25% attend mass regularly and many children are never baptized. In Sicily religion has remained an important part of life. Most of the island are still practicing Roman Catholics although the most devout are now ageing. But young people still attend mass once a week, and Catholic traditions, religious processions and ceremonies are still celebrated with gusto. Feast days are often also holidays.

Sexual Attitudes

Nudity

There does seem to be some tolerance for and even obses- sion with naked- ness, especially in advertising, within the Italian culture. However, see- through or skimpy clothing is not toler- ated and people wearing them can expect to be harassed. Take your

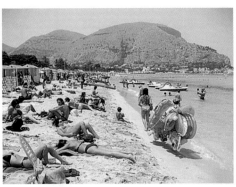

On the beach, Palermo

cues from locals in regards your dress. Topless sunbathing is another area in which cues should be taken from others on the beach. It is legally tolerated but not always acceptable. Beach attire is also usually confined to the sand and not appropriate for walking back to hotels or restaurants.

Gay Life

Attitudes towards homosexuality in Sicily are generally less tolerant than in the north of Italy and the more religious southern society influences this to a considerable degree. In Sicily gay couples may still find it hard to get a *matrimoniale* or double bed. However, as long as one doesn't make a *brutta figura* (bad show), some tolerance prevails. There is no legis- lation in Sicily discriminating against the lifestyle.

The gay scene in Sicily has been expanding, with popular institutions including Palermo's Pietro Montana Gay Culture and Art Center, the Sauna Mykonos in Catania (the first gay sauna in Sicily) and accommodation such as the B&B Casa Gaya in Siracusa. See www.gaysicilia.org and www.gay.it for helpful news and listings of gay-friendly businesses. Arci Gay (www.arcigay.it/eng/) is the main association operating in Italy for rights of homosexual people.

The Outside World

Sicilians have traveled overseas for much of the last century, particularly in periods of economic difficulty before and after

the World Wars. One and a half million Sicilians left their homeland in the years leading up to 1914. The outside world is thus very familiar with the Sicilian way of life, in some ways far more so than that of Northern Italy. In fact the prototypical Italian in many countries is thought of as a short, stocky, dark-haired Sicilian, and Italian restaurants world-wide often serve Sicilian cuisine – cannoli desserts, olive oil and the crushed-ice drink granita.

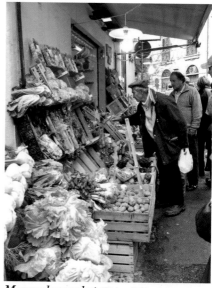

Monreale market (Galen R Frysinger, www. galenfrysinger.com)

Sicilians are generally a welcoming people and enjoy interacting with other nationalities. Their friendly, chatty good will is quite a contrast to images tourists have of the Mafia.

While a lot of Sicilians have left the country to search for greater economic or professional opportunities, ironically many also come into Sicily in search of the same. In Sicily today immigrants have worked hard to open businesses and you're likely to see Internet cafés and call centers operated by Indians or Pakistanis, Chinese shops and restaurants, Nigerians harvesting grapes and olives, Tunisians with shops selling North African carpets and other products and Romanians or Russians employed as live-in housekeepers or nurses to assist an aging parent. Gypsy populations in Palermo live in camps at the edge of the city. Most have a Muslim Balkan origin and arrived in the 1960s.

Politics

Sicily is semi-autonomous, with special powers granted under the constitution, as well as its own parliament and president. This means it has a wider range of economic and administrative powers than other regions of Italy but it has limited legis-

lative powers in such areas as tourism, transport, industry and the environment.

However, a century of indoctrination through Fascist and Communist governments has left Sicilians somewhat ignorant of their national history. Communists and Neo-Fascists are now a minority of the population but they continue to affect society with their squabbles, strikes and corruption. High schools and universities are still highly politicized and professors are often hired based on their political leanings.

Sports

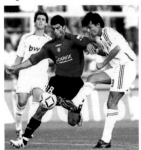

Italian sports are similar to those of other European countries. Football (soccer), rugby, basketball, skiing, archery, race car driving and skating are popular and are followed by keen fans. Chess, cards and bocce are also commonly played, usually by the older population. Messina has made it to the *Serie A* national soccer league and has done much to lift the game on the island. As a culture, however, few Italians exercise regularly, particularly those over 35. Men seem obsessed with football, but few play and sports are not encouraged in high school programs.

PUMPING IRON

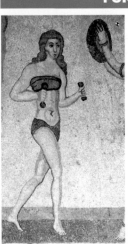

A mosaic in the ancient Roman villa in Piazza Armerina shows women working out with barbells and dumbbells. The mosaic is almost 2,000 years old, indicating that possibly women's bodybuilding could have been invented here. The image of Sicilian women pumping iron does not quite fit today in a society where negotiating pavements in high heels is almost the only exercise women get and the average diet consists of coffee, pastries and pasta.

Music

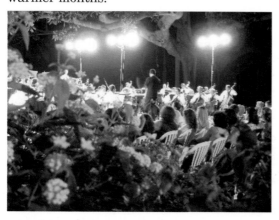

Sicily does not have its own rock music scene and its airways are usually saturated with Italian, British and American mainstream chart music. Occasionally big international bands make it here in the summer. Local councils in big cities such as Palermo, Messina and Catania also sponsor open-air concerts in public areas during the warmer months.

Traditional music still has a following, if somewhat more more modest. There is a great variety of Christian music including a cappella devotional songs from Montedoro and many brass bands, such as Banda Ionica, was founded in 1997 and consisting of 20 young musicians who play traditional songs. Harvest songs and work songs are also indigenous to this agricultural island. Sicilian flute music, called *friscaletto*, is popular among traditionalist Sicilians, as are Messina's male choirs.

Sicily's most famous musician was the great composer **Vincenzo Bellini** (1801-1835), who died at the age of 34. He wrote 10 operas that were not truly recognized until after his death. The current music star is teenager saxophonist **Francesco Cafiso** (www.francescocafiso.it) from Vittoria, who plays regularly in Sicily and at European, American and even Australian concerts.

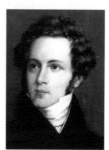

Vincenzo Bellini

Sicily's Greek and Roman theaters in Taormina, Segesta, Siracusa and Tindari often host classical music concerts and visiting international orchestras,

although Sicily's orchestras are also world-class. (The view of Mt Etna from the Taormina stage is unforgettable.) The opera season runs from October to June. The **Teatro Massimo** in Palermo (www.teatromassimo.it) and the **Teatro Bellini** in Catania are the best places to view a performance. Many smaller theaters throughout Sicily have their own music programs too.

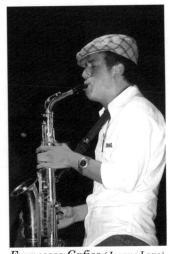

Francesco Cafiso (Joanne Lane)

Popular music festivals/concerts include **Musicale Trapanese** (Trapani, July), **Sciacca Jazz** (Sciacca, July), the **Renaissance Music Festival** (Erice, August), and the **Festival of Holy Music**, including chants and hymns performed traditionally (Monreale, October/November).

Film & Television

Most towns have a movie theater but English-language films are always dubbed into Italian, frustrating for tourists, although it is amusing to hear Bruce Willis or Arnold Schwarzenegger speaking in sexy Italian accents. In summer, many tourist resorts and towns show open-air films in the piazzas. In July an international film festival is held in Taormina with screenings in the picturesque Greek theater. Portopallo in the island's far south also has a film festival in August.

DID YOU KNOW THEY WERE SICILIAN?

Many Sicilians have made their move on the world stage in sport, politics, film, music and other fields. Take a look:

Sicilian-American

Charles Atlas (1892-1972), body builder
Joe DiMaggio (1914-1999), baseball player
Mario Puzo (1920-1999), author
Tony Bennett (born 1926), singer, painter
Al Pacino (born 1940), actor

Martin Scorsese (born 1942), film director
Tony Danza (born 1951), actor
Marisa Tomei (born 1964), actress

Part Sicilians

Frank Sinatra (1915-1998), singer, actor
Frank Zappa (1940-1993), musician
Robert De Niro (born 1943), actor
Sylvester Stallone (born 1946), actor, filmmaker
Cyndi Lauper (born 1953), pop singer
Natalie Imbruglia (born 1975), pop singer

On Location

The glorious Sicilian landscape has long been used effectively for film locations. Among them are Roberto Rossellini's *Stromboli: Terra di Dio* (1949) with Ingrid Bergman, and Francis Ford Coppola's *Godfather* trilogy. Scenes for Part II (1974) were filmed in Savoca near Taormina and Ficuzza. Scenes for part III (1990) used locations in Palermo. The epic *Nuovo Cinema Paradiso* (1989) filmed by Giuseppe Tornatore makes use of the island's interior, particularly the splendid piazza in Palazzo Adriano, while Michael Radford used locations on offshore islands Salina and Pantelleria for *Il Postino* (1994).

Theater

 Sicilians are fond of their theater and you can find small theaters in all main towns and cities which have music programs and dramatic arts, particularly in the summer months. Palermo alone has 13 theaters and Catania marginally fewer. In Siracusa, Tindari and

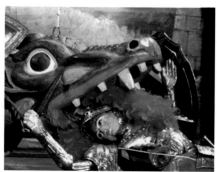
Puppet show

Taormina the Greek and Roman theaters provide dramatic settings. The biggest and most famous classical dramas on the island take place in May and June in Siracusa and during Pirandello week in Agrigento in July. Unfortunately for visitors, all performances are in Italian.

Puppet theater has been popular in Sicily since the 14th century and is still followed by vocal audiences, who know the stories backwards and forwards. Puppets or marionettes are used to unfurl the tales, usually in unintelligible Sicilian dialect, about the Paladins, the 12 peers of Charlemagne's court. There is often a lot of fighting, battles, love interests and activity – the perfect recipe to keep the audience entertained. To see the puppets, stage sets and related gimmicks go to the Museo delle Marionette or Museo Etnograifco Pitre in Palermo or Museo Vagliasindi in Randazzo.

Language

 Most Sicilians are bilingual in Italian and Sicilian, although regional dialects can vary. English speakers are only to be found in cities, hotels, airports and restaurants. Therefore it is recommended that you learn at least a few words and phrases in Italian before you arrive (see the language section at the back of the book). This is particularly handy in remote parts of Sicily, although in these regions you will not understand local dialects spoken by older people.

Sicilian is often referred to as a dialect of standard Italian when it is really a separate Romance language descended from Vulgar Latin – a unique blend of Greek, Latin, Aragonese, Arabic, Longobardic and Norman-French elements.

The Sicilian language has an extensive vocabulary of 250,000 or more words. Sicilian is also spoken around Reggio di Calabria and in southern Puglia in Italy. It had a significant influence on the Maltese language, with Malta a part of the Kingdom of Sicily until the late 18th century.

Sicilian has always been a largely unwritten language and was discarded by aristocrats and literate classes for Tuscan by the 17th century. Thus the language came to be considered as vulgar and was spoken only by the masses. A brand of Tuscan became the official written language around 1700, before which most documents were recorded in Latin. In Norman times, official documents were issued in Greek, Latin, Arabic and sometimes Norman French.

The national government tried to suppress Sicilian after 1860, but it remained the native language until the 20th century. Today Italian appears to have supplanted Sicilian as the spoken language of today's Sicilians. Wider literacy through media like television and the Internet have further dimin-

ished the use of Sicilian. However, there are still probably more speakers of Sicilian than of any other Italic language, except standard Italian. Regional dialects still exist and differ greatly from region to region. Many young people from country and inner city areas do not always speak, read or write standard Italian proficiently.

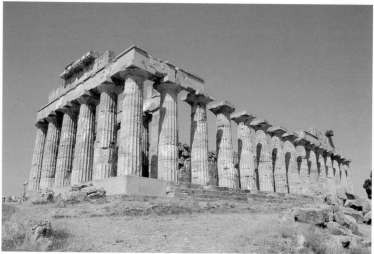

Temple of Hera, Selinunte

Arts & Architecture

Sicily's numerous invaders left a rich legacy of architecture and art bringing craftsmen, traders and artists to the island. Combined with local styles, that created an unusual hybrid. The Hellenistic age is most visible in the Doric temples at Selinunte, Segesta, Syracuse and Agrigento. There are also the rock tombs at Sant'Angelo Muxaro and pottery remnants like the beautiful black and red kraters (vases). The Romans left theaters, aqueducts and

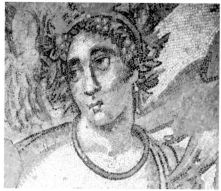

Mosaic from Roman villa at Piazza Armerina (Galen R Frysinger, www. galenfrysinger.com)

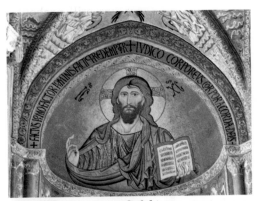

Norman mosaics at Cefalú (Galen R Frysinger)

the fantastic Roman villa outside Piazza Armerina with its beautiful mosaics. The Byzantines converted a lot of the Doric temples to Christian basilicas. It was the Normans who left the most evidence of their rule in Sicily, with strongholds, churches, cathedrals, extensive mosaics, palaces, chapels and much more. The mosaics at Monreale are probably the main feature of this period. The Renaissance brought medieval styles popular on the Italian mainland to Sicily. The Baroque age settled into Sicily following an earthquake in 1693 when many towns in the south were rebuilt in this style. In the 19th and 20th centuries Art Nouveau was the predominant style, especially in Palermo.

Today a decorative ceramics trade continues to flourish in Caltagirone and Santo Stefano di Camastra. Sicily is also home to two prominent folk art traditions, both drawing heavily on the island's Norman influence. Donkey

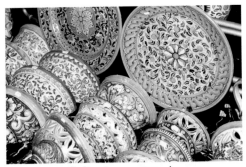

Caltagirone ceramics

carts are painted with intricate scenes from the Norman romantic poems. The same tales are told in traditional puppet theaters which feature handmade wooden marionettes (see *Theater* earlier in this chapter).

Literature

Sicilian literature first flourished in the 13th century when the Sicilian School of poetry began in Frederick II's court. The School produced poems of courtly love and inspired much subsequent Italian poetry.

There was then a gap until the 19th century, when more successful authors emerged. Giovanni Verga from Catania helped bring Sicilian literature into the 20th century with his novels and short stories. Luigi Pirandello (1867-1936) emerged as a Nobel Prize winner for his play, *Six Characters in Search of an Author*, as did the poet Salvatore Quasimodo. Few modern playwrights have escaped his influence. Giuseppe Tomasi di Lampedusa (1896-1957) wrote the famous novel,

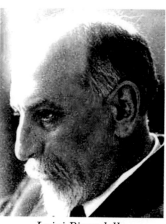

Luigi Pirandello

The Leopard, about the decline of the Sicilian aristocracy. It is considered one of the masterpieces of 20th-century Italian and European literature.

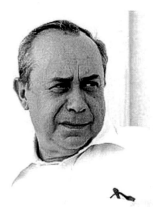

Leonardo Sciascia

Today a handful of authors continue to be acclaimed. Natalia Ginzburg from Palermo writes semi-autobiographical pieces that capture the essence of gestures and everyday life. Leonardo Sciascia from Agrigento attacks the past and present of Sicily in his novels and essays. His successes include *Il Giorno della Civetta* (*The Day of the Owl*) about the Mafia. Other noteworthy 20th-century writers include Ellio Vittorini and Gesualdo Bufalino. Andrea Cammilieri's book series about

Inspector Montalbano (see *Films & Television* earlier in this chapter) has also made him a popular author.

Sicily continues to be included in literature written primarily for foreign audiences. The most famous 20th-century novel of this type is probably Mario Puzo's *The Godfather*, which portrays Sicilian life. It also made it to the silver screen in three epic films.

Myths & Legends

The Mafia

It is hardly possible to write about Sicily without giving the Mafia due mention, though its important to note that organized crime doesn't pose a threat to visitors. Mafia shootings are rare and you are unlikely to witness one firsthand or come into contact with Mafia activity. There are seedy types and quiet streets best left alone, but the Mafia are not concerned with tourists. Even if you pick out a potential Mafia type, it is more likely to be somone who had too much wine at lunch, woke up cranky from siesta or is just your average Sicilian grand-

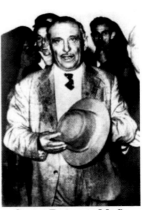

Genco Russo, a Mafia boss in the 1960s

father; all of whom on closer acquaintance are the friendliest people you might want to know.

It's also important to highlight the distinction between mafia and "the Mafia." Mafia refers to a criminal mentality; the Mafia, to a specific criminal organization. Sicily is the home of the original Sicilian Mafia, or *Cosa Nostra*, which claims a history dating back to the 13th century and feudal times, when they defended the poor against the tyranny of Sicily's rulers.

In the original Palermo dialect the word *mafioso* once meant beautiful, bold or self-confident. So anyone called a *mafioso* had an intangible attribute probably closest to the English word "cool." It was actually the Italian government that attached criminal connotations to the word in 1865 and it then entered general usage.

The Mafia's complex system of justice is based on the code of silence known as *omerta*. The system worked so well that many doubted its very existence until 1982, when a high-ranking member, Tommasso Buscetta, was arrested in Brazil and agreed to incriminate other members.

Mussolini made many anti-Mafia purges to establish a Fascist structure in Sicily and largely succeeded. Many *mafiosi* fled abroad to risk being jailed and those that escaped to the United States developed the Mafia there. The Mafia did not become powerful in Italy again until after WWII, when it developed into an organization more ruthless and stronger than ever before. At a 1989 meeting in Nice, the Sicilian Mafia and the Calabrian and Neapolitana Mafia met representatives of the Colombian and Venezuelan drug cartels and carved up the world's heroin and cocaine markets. The Sicilians retained the heroin trade. Not only are they involved in drug-trafficking, but also arms deals, finance, construction, tourist development, public sector projects and Italian politics.

In the 1990s there was a lot of Mafia violence in Sicily as the *Cosa Nostra* tried to eliminate opposition. They assassinated two anti-Mafia judges in Palermo with separate bomb blasts. However, as a result, the Italian government finally took action and the Sicil-

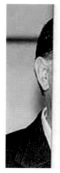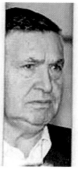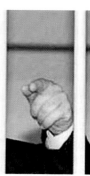

Salvatore Riina

ian godfather, Salvatore "Toto" Riina, was arrested. He was head of the powerful Corleone clan and the world's most wanted man since 1969.

It is alleged that *Cosa Nostra* had direct contact with representatives of Silvio Berlusconi when he was planning the birth of his political party, Forza Italia.The deal that was alleged was for the repeal of Law 41 bis and other anti-Mafia laws in return for electoral deliverances in Sicily. Indeed the party has a stronghold in Sicily, holding all 61 Sicilian seats in

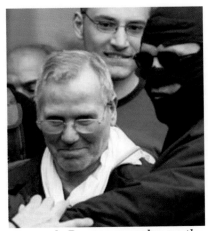

Bernardo Provenzano, who ran the Mafia after Salvatore Riina's arrest, was himself arrested in 2006

Parliament but no one has suggested a link between Berlusconi and *Cosa Nostra* directly.

What has become more common in Sicily now is the development of a "mafia culture." This is an essentially white collar element of professionals who collaborate to control building contracts, politics and power.

Media portrayal of the Mafia has been extensive, with novels like *The Godfather* by Mario Puzo later made into films by Francis Ford Coppola. Other films include *Goodfellas*, directed by Martin Scorsese, *Bugsy* starring Warren Beatty, *Donnie Brasco* about the first FBI agent to infiltrate the Mafia, *The Untouchables* about Eliot Ness and his law enforcers in the USA fighting Al Capone and *Casino*, starring Robert De Niro.

Regional Food & Wine

 Be prepared to give your taste buds some serious exercise in Sicily. The food and wine here is among its greatest attractions and its fame and accessibility worldwide means you will probably have tasted it long before you arrive. The real thing is only better. Sicilian chefs

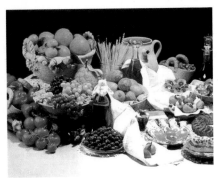

Sicilian buffet

have been sought after since the fifth century BC and in medieval times they were used in foreign courts, much like French chefs today.

Endless invaders all made an impact on Sicilian cuisine and you can find Greek, Arab, Norman, Spanish and English elements in the food. This means that the cuisine has a lot more to offer than just pasta and pizza. It still uses a staple of pasta, tomato sauces and fresh vegetables, but also local supplies like chilies, tuna, sardines, swordfish, olives, pine nuts and capers. Mild winters and long summers also mean fruits and vegetables are available during more of the year and tend to be a lot larger. Browsing local markets should be a daily pastime for any visitor so you can simply admire the array of produce. The best news for travelers is that eating well should not blow your budget. A full meal with local wine generally costs about €20 a head.

Tipping, Service Charges & the Bill

Most restaurants charge a *coperto*, or cover charge, for each person seated – to "cover" the table with a table cloth and serve bread. The *coperto* has persisted because Italians are traditionally cheap tippers. Tipping is not expected, particularly if a service charge is already included, but if you do feel inclined, 10% is acceptable. In some bars and cafés you may have to pay first before you take your receipt to the bar staff to procure drinks and food. In restaurants and trattorias you ask or are given *il conto* (the bill) at the end of the meal.

Restaurants

Restaurants like pizzerias, open in the evenings generally from 8 pm Tuesday through Saturday, and are usually closed on Sundays and Mondays. Some restaurants will also open for lunch about 12:30 pm, but most serve pizza only in the evening. On public holidays and weekends it is a good idea to reserve a table. Once you are seated, the bread will arrive on the table and you can help yourself – don't worry about getting crumbs on the tablecloth! Overcharging is uncommon in Sicily, but, where possible, order from a written menu with prices indicated. To find cheaper restaurants, avoid those located near hotels or on main streets, especially those that offer "tourist menus." Try a local hangout on a side street.

Sicilian Cuisine

Breakfasts, Snacks, Sweets

In Sicily people start the day with milky coffee (*cappuccino*) and a pastry or *cornetto* filled with jam, custard or chocolate.

Another common breakfast is *granita* (lemon flavored crushed ice) inside *brioche* (sweet bread). Street food in Sicily usually consists of rice balls, potato croquettes, fritters and mini-pizzas. It is tasty and easily portable. *Arancine* are a particular favorite, fried rice balls stuffed with meat or cheese. *Panini* (sandwiches) are available almost anywhere in

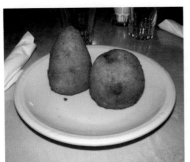

Rice balls (Galen R Frysinger, www.galenfrysinger.com)

bars and *alimentaris* (grocers). A *tavola calda* is a good place to pick up hot snack foods like *arancine* and *patatine fritte* (chips) or even a hot meal. They are usually found in bigger towns and around train stations. A *rosticceria* serves spit-roast chicken, hamburgers or hot dogs.

Sicilian sweets are unparalleled and deservedly famous. Popular dishes include *cassata* – a rich, sugary cake filled with ricotta and sugar. *Cannoli* are tubular fried pastries stuffed with ricotta and rolled in chocolate. These dishes may taste different here than in other parts of Italy because the ricotta in Sicily is made from sheep's milk. Some north Italian pasticcerias will import Sicilian ricotta for their own *cannoli*. Arab influences are particularly prevalent in Sicilian sweets. Marzipan is used extensively. A well-known Sicilian dessert is *frutta di martorana*, an almond marzipan pastry colored and shaped to resemble real fruit.

In much of Sicily events are celebrated with traditional sweets. For example *cassata* is typically made to celebrate Easter.

Gelato (ice cream) in Sicily is also particularly good, as is *granita*, a sweetened crushed ice flavored with lemons or strawberries served mainly in summer from street carts and bars/cafés. For the best gelato head to a popular *gelateria* (easy to pick by the crowds waiting outside), rather than a restaurant or supermarket. Most bars have a good selection of ice cream but do look for those that make it on the premises.

There is some evidence to suggest ice cream was created in Italy or, if not, at least perfected when Marco Polo observed the Chinese practice of pouring syrup onto snow. In any case, the manufacture of ice cream in many countries has been the re-

sult of Italian migration and Sicily is generally credited with being the home of such ices in the Western world. In Sicily the Greeks and Romans employed lumps of Etna's snow to chill their wine, while the Arabs used it to chill their *sarbat*. The Italian word for sorbetto and the English word sherbert come from these sweet fruit syrups the Arabs drank diluted with ice water. Granita is a development of this.

GRANITA

To make your own you will need:

■ one cup chopped and crushed fruit (including juice)
■ one cup of white granulated refined sugar
■ four cups of water

Preparation: Chop and crush the fruit. Heat the sugar in two cups of water until it dissolves. Remove and allow to cool. Add the remaining water and crushed fruit. Freeze for 40 minutes, then remove and mix thoroughly to granulate it before putting it back in the freezer for another 20 minutes. The texture should resemble grains or flakes.

Pizzas

Pizza in Sicily is second only to that of Naples in quality. Here it is flat and not deep-pan, and usually cooked in wood-fired ovens (*forno a legna*). *Sfincione* is a local form of pizza prepared on thick bread with tomatoes, onions and anchovies. It is found more in bakeries than in pizzerias.

Vegetarians

Vegetarians will find ample food fare to keep them happy. Many pasta sauces are based on tomato and dairy products and non-meat pizzas are easy to find. There are also plenty of delicious salads to sample. *Caponata* is a tasty salad made with eggplant, olives, capers and celery. There is also an artichoke (*carciofi*) version. *Panella* is a thin paste made of crushed or powdered *ceci* beans and served fried. *Maccu* is a creamy soup made from the same bean. *Croquet* are fried potato dumplings made with cheese, parsley and eggs.

Meat Dishes

Most traditional Sicilian meat dishes are made with lamb or goat. The most famous is probably *vitello alla marsala* (veal marsala) cooked in the sweet marsala wine. Chicken *alla marsala* can be prepared using a similar recipe and method. *Milza* (veal spleen) sandwiches are a local delicacy but not necessarily to everyone's taste.

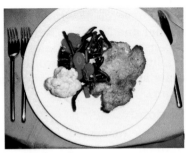

Veal cutlet (Galen R Frysinger)

Drinks

Café (coffee) is popular in Sicily, as in all of Italy, with the usual varieties such as *cappuccino, macchiato, café latte* and so on. Try *café corretto* for something different – coffee served with a drop of alcohol. Iced tea mixed with lemon (*té freddo*) is a common drink in summer and excellent for taking the heat off. Juices and water are commonly available but make sure you try the Sicilian specialty *granita*, a crushed ice-drink that comes in several flavors. *Frullato* is a fresh fruit shake. Ask for *aqua* (water) or *aqua minerale* (mineral water), which are usually provided free of charge with another purchase at a bar. *Latte di Mandorla* is another Sicilian specialty. The drink is basically almond pulp and water and is best served fresh at a bar.

Alcohol

The drinking culture in Sicily is very different to Britain and America. At just about every meal you will be offered *vino* (wine) in either *bianco* (white) or *rosso* (red), and Sicilian children are brought up on it from an early age. Local wine is a lot cheaper, usually unlabelled and may surprise for its quality (ask for *vino della casa)*. Sicily has a name for its quality everyday wines like *Corvo* and *Regaleali*, which are also found in other parts of Italy. *Marsala* is a particularly famous Sicilian dessert wine, which is sometimes sweetened and mixed with eggs.

The Aeolian Islands produce their own specialties and in Taormina they serve an ice cold almond wine. Sicilians also like their liqueurs and offer the same ones as on mainland Italy, such as *amaro* and *grappa*. But on the east coast you can

find *Fuoco dell'Etna* which is, as its name suggests, a volcanic experience. *Birra* (beer) drinkers may find the Italian and Sicilian versions, *birra nazionale*, a little weak (Peroni, Dreher and Messina). Imported beers tend to be a little more expensive. Beer is usually served in bottles as *piccolo* (a third of a litre) or *grande* (two-thirds). In some bars, bigger restaurants and all *birrerias* you can get draught lager (*birra alla spina*).

Seafood

Sicily is renowned for its seafood. Anchovies, sardines, tuna and swordfish are abundant and combined with pasta like *spaghetti con le sarde* (spaghetti with sardines), *finnochio con sarde* (fennel with sardines) and *seppia* (cuttlefish) served in its own black sauce with pasta. Swordfish is normally grilled, and smaller

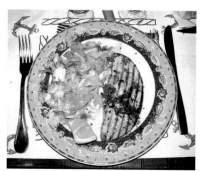
Swordfish (Galen R Frysinger)

fish, like snapper, are sometimes prepared in a vinegar and sugar sauce. Most menus allow you to choose from a base of seafood (*pesce*) or meat (*carne*).

Cheeses

Pecorino, provolone, canestrato, piacentinu, provola, tuma, primo sale, maiorchino, ragusano, ricotta salata, caciocavallo, and sheep's-milk ricotta are some of the main cheeses to try in Sicily, made from cows or goats milk. Ricotta is used in many sweet dishes.

Sicilian Olives

Local Sicilian olive oil is fragrant and appetizing due to its fertile soil. The ancient Athenians actually preferred Sicilian olive oil to their own, even though they grew some of the same varieties. Olive oil is perfect for pouring on fresh salads and is used liberally in cooking.

■ Just the Facts

Passport

European Union (EU) citizens plus those from Switzerland, Slovenia, Croatia, Malta and Turkey can travel to Sicily with their national identity cards alone. All non-EU nationals must have a passport that is valid until after you return home. People from the United States, Canada, Australia, Japan, Switzerland, Israel and New Zealand may enter the country for stays of three months with a valid passport; other nationals should consult their embassies about visa requirements. Citizens of the United Kingdom need only a valid passport to enter Italy for an unlimited stay.

If you lose your passport or it is stolen in Sicily, notify the police, obtain a statement and then contact your embassy or consulate as soon as possible. Make two photocopies of your passport's data page in advance, one to be kept by someone at home and another to carry with you, but separate from your original passport.

You must register with the police within three days of entering Italy. If you are staying in a hotel, this will be done for you; otherwise you should register at the local police station or *Questura*.

Visas

All non-EU nationals entering Italy for reasons other than tourism (eg. study or work) will need to contact an Italian consulate, as they may require a specific visa. A **Schengen visa** is valid for up to 90 days allowing travel in all Schengen countries (Austria, Belgium, Denmark, Finland, France, Germany, Iceland, Italy, Greece, Luxembourg, Netherlands, Norway, Portugal, Spain and Sweden). But check to make sure Italy has no restrictions on certain nationalities. You must apply for a visa in your country of residence and you can apply for no more than two Schengen visas in any 12 month period. They can not be renewed in Italy.

Study visas are required for non-EU citizens to attend a university or language school.

Non-EU citizens need a **work permit** (*permesso di lavoro*) to work in Sicily.

To get a *permesso di soggiorno*, allowing you to study, work legally or live in Sicily, is fairly straightforward for EU citizens. For other nationalities it can be more involved. Usually you need a valid passport with a visa stamp to indicate your date of entry into Italy, a special visa issued in your own country if you are planning to study, four passport photographs and proof you can support yourself financially.

Travel Insurance

It is wise to take out a travel insurance policy to cover any medical problems and theft, loss or damage to your personal items while you are in Sicily. Italy has free reciprocal health agreements with other member states of the EU. Travel agents or specialist travel insurance companies will give you the best advice on choosing an insurance policy. In any case, always read the policies and fine print carefully.

Emergency Numbers

These are the national emergency telephone numbers:
- Military Police (*Carabinieri*) ☎ 112
- Emergency services/Police (*Polizia*) ☎ 113
- Fire Brigade (*Vigili del Fuoco*) ☎ 115
- Road assistance (*Soccorso Stradale*) ☎ 116
- Road service ACI (*ACI Soccorso Stradale*) ☎ 803-116
- Sea Rescue (*Soccorso in Mare*) ☎ 1530
- Ambulance (*Ambulanza*) ☎ 118
- Medical Emergencies Catania (Guardia Medica) ☎ 095-377-122
- Medical Emergencies Palermo (Pronto Soccorso) ☎ 091-702-0347, after 8 pm ☎ 091-591-647

Telephones

Orange public telephones are operated by Telecom Italia and come with clear instructions printed on them (also in English). These are generally found in the street, train stations, some big stores, some bars and unstaffed Telecom centers. These phones generally accept only telephone cards (*carte/schede telefoniche*) but you may find some still accept both cards and coins and even commercial credit cards. For calling within Italy, phone cards are avail-

able in various denominations from *tabacchi* or newsstands. Make sure you break off the perforated corner before trying to use them. Local calls cost €.31 per unit (about five minutes).

The peak time for domestic calls is 8 am-6:30 pm Monday to Friday and 8 am-1 pm Saturday. Cheaper rates apply 6:30 pm-8 am, on Saturday afternoons and all day Sunday.

Different peak times apply for international calls. Cheap rates to the UK are 10 pm to 8 am Monday to Saturday and all day Sunday; to the USA and Canada from 7 pm to 2 pm Monday to Friday and all day Saturday and Sunday; and to Australia from 11 pm to 8 am Monday to Saturday and all day Sunday.

The cheapest options for international calls are either a telephone charge card where you can use access codes and a PIN number to make calls that are charged to your own domestic account; or, better still, an international phone card. This card is known locally as *carta telefonica internazionale* and is available at *tabacchi*. To make a call, follow the instructions on the back of the card. If you want to make a reversed charge/ collect international call *(carico al destinatario)* dial ☎ 170 from a public telephone.

International Phone Codes

- Australia ☎ 61
- Ireland ☎ 353
- New Zealand ☎ 64
- UK ☎ 44
- USA and Canada ☎ 1
- France ☎ 33
- Germany ☎ 49
- Greece ☎ 30
- Spain ☎ 34

Other codes are listed in Italian phone books.

Calling Sicily

The country code for Italy is 39. Italian telephone numbers can have varying numbers of digits, so don't assume they're wrong because of that.

Sicily City Codes

Since July 1998, area codes have been included in all phone numbers within Sicily even when dialing locally in the same city. This is a list of the major city codes in Sicily:

- Agrigento ☎ 0922
- Catania ☎ 095
- Cefalù ☎ 0921
- Enna ☎ 0935
- Messina ☎ 090
- Palermo ☎ 091
- Siracusa ☎ 0931
- Taormina ☎ 0942
- Trapani ☎ 0923

Helpful Numbers

- ☎ 176 – general information in English
- ☎ 170 – to place international calls with operator assistance
- ☎ 12 – directory enquiries

Toll-free numbers (*numeri verdi*) all begin with the prefix ☎ 800. The prefix ☎ 848 indicates a national number charged at a local rate.

- **Italian white pages** – www.paginebianche.virgilio.it/index.html
- **Italian yellow pages** – www.paginegiallo.virgilio.it

Time Zones

Sicily is an hour ahead of GMT/UTC in winter and two hours ahead in the daylight saving season (last Sunday in March to last Sunday in October). This operational time is the same as most West European countries, except for Britain, Ireland and Portugal, which are one hour behind. However, Italy makes the changeover to daylight saving a little differently. See www.timeanddate.com if you're not sure.

Language

If you don't speak Italian and plan on traveling without an Italian speaker it would be wise to learn at least a few words and phrases. English is not widely spoken even in cities and it will help if you know some basics. See our language glossary at the end of the guide for common words and phrases.

Taxes

% A value-added tax (IVA or VAT) of 20% is added to clothing, wine and luxury goods sold in Italy. On consumer goods it's already included in the price tag, but it may not be on services. To reclaim your tax see the *Reclaiming Vat* section later in this chapter.

Expect a service charge and 9% IVA or VAT tax to be included in hotel rates. In luxury or five-star hotels it can be 12%. Restaurants do not add tax to the bills, though a service charge of approximately 15% may be included. Check restaurant menus first; sometimes it may already be included in the prices.

Opening Hours

Shops in Sicily usually open from 9 am to 1 pm and 4 to 8 pm, Monday to Friday. However, many restaurants and some other shops stay closed on Mondays. Major tourist offices and large supermarkets may open continuously even on weekends, including Sundays. Smaller shops generally close on Saturdays at 1 pm and are closed all day Sunday.

Banks tend to open from 8:30 am to 1:30 pm and 2:45-3:45 pm Monday to Friday (times may vary slightly across the island). They are closed on weekends. Pharmacies open 9 am-12:30 pm and 3:30-7:30 pm. They close Saturday afternoon and all day Sunday. When closed, they will list other pharmacies that are open. In big cities there are 24-hour pharmacies. Most churches open from early morning until noon or 12:30 pm, and again from 3 or 4 pm, closing at 6 pm or after the last mass.

Sicilian bars and cafés are open from 7 am to 8 pm continuously and may go much later. Discos and clubs usually open at about 10 pm but don't fill until midnight. Restaurants are open from approximately 12 pm to 3 pm and 7:30 to 11 pm. Restaurants and bars are required to close one day each week; it's usually a Monday.

Museum and gallery opening hours tend to be 9:30 am-8 pm, sometimes with a midday break. Most are closed on Monday. Archaeological sites open 9 am-12 pm and 4-7 pm Monday to Friday and 9 am-12 pm Saturday; summer hours may be longer.

Post offices open Monday to Saturday 9 am-2 pm. Central and main district post offices may stay open until 6:30 or 7 pm on weekdays. On the last day of the month all post offices close at midday.

In August many stores close in the afternoons or may stay closed altogether for at least two weeks.

When to Go

 The best months for sightseeing in Sicily are April, May, June, September and October when the weather is mild. The Easter period attracts floods of visitors and is probably best avoided. July and August are the hottest months and rather uncomfortable for traveling. Not only can it be stifling hot in the cities, but even the beaches are not a respite from the heat and you'll be sharing the sands with thousands of others. Prices go up during this period, although most of the action culminates around Ferragosto, the August 15 holiday.

You can swim in Sicily into November. September and October are particularly pleasant months. September is the time for harvests of wine, olives, figs, hazel nuts, and the accompanying celebrations. Autumn months are beautiful in the vineyards when the leaves turn to red and orange, mushrooms are plentiful and temperatures are still pleasant. Winters can be mild in Sicily, although there are rainy periods. Do note that Christmas and New Year attract a lot of visitors and reservations can be difficult and expensive. At all times of the year local festivities and events can also put prices up or make availability scarce.

Immigration & Customs

Documents

Driving Licenses & Permits: Foreign driving licenses are usually honored by car rental agencies but you should obtain an international driving permit if your license is not issued by an EC nation or if you plan to use private cars. Permits usually cost about $10-$15 and are easily available from the American or Canadian Automobile Association. In the United Kingdom see the Automobile Association or Royal Automobile Club and in Australia the RACQ, VIC or your state road association. Requirements are to hold a valid driver's license in

your country and be at least 18 years of age. You must carry your driver's license along with your international driving permit.

Hostel Cards: Hostel cards can save you money on accommodation in Italy but, due to the limited number of hostels in Sicily, they would not be worth purchasing for use here alone. Some of the cards that do function in Sicily include the VIP Backpackers network card (www.vipbackpackers.com) for independent hostels and YHA or HI (www.ostellionline.org or www.hihostels.com). Both offer about 5% discounts to members for accommodation, tours, car rental and other travel.

Student & Youth Cards: If you are a student or under 26 years old you also qualify for travel concessions. Always take your school or university institutional card along, but you may also need an internationally recognized card like the ISIC (International Student Identity Card) or ISE (International Student Exchange, www.isecards.com). Other card options include the ISTC (International Student Travel Confederation) for students of any age, faculty/teacher members and youths aged 12 to 26 years. There's also the IYTC (International Youth Travel Card) if you're over 26 years and the ITIC (International Teacher Identity Card) for full-time teachers. Student travel organizations such as STA (Australia, UK, USA), Council Travel (USA) and Travel CUTS (Canada) can issue these cards. The Euro <26 card (www.euro26.org) is another option. It is available in 37 countries in Europe and you don't need to be a student or European citizen. In Italy the card costs €11. Go to Associazione Carta Giovani, Via Albalonga 3, Rome (☎ 06-6496-0345, www.cartagiovani.it).

A European Passport is also useful to gain access to museums for discounted prices if you're under 26 or over 65.

The International Student Exchange (ISE card) is one option that offers discounts for travel. It is not quite as established as the ISIC but many of the establishments that discount ISIC also give discounts to ISE holders. The card costs $25 and can be ordered online from www.isecards.com.

In Sicily you can go to the branch of Centro Turistico Studentesco e Giovanile (CTS, ☎ 199-501-150 or ☎ 06-441-1166 in Rome, www.cts.it) to obtain ISIC, ITIC and Euro<26 cards. You have to join the CTS first for €28. See the website for all Sicily offices. Here is a list of those in Palermo and Catania:

Just the Facts

- Via Nicolo Garzili 28/g, Palermo, ☎ 091-332-209
- Via Danimarca 44/b, Palermo, ☎ 091-670-3634
- Via Etna 11, Catania, ☎ 095-250-0391
- Via Ventimiglia 153, Catania, ☎ 095-530-223

Senior Cards: Senior Citizens can use their national pensioner cards to get discounts on rail and other travel, accommodation packages, tours and even museum entry. European passport holders who are over 65 often receive discounted or even free entry to museums.

Copies: You should make two copies of your most important personal and travel documents before you leave home. Take one with you and leave the other with someone back home. These documents should include passport data and visa pages, credit cards, travel insurance policy, important transport tickets, driving license, travel itinerary and any other useful information.

Customs Procedures

In July 1999 duty-free sales within the EU were abolished. This means travelers within the EU can no longer purchase goods free of excise tax and VAT. However, duty-free sales continue for those traveling to destinations outside the EU. If you're entering Italy from outside the EU you may bring in the following items duty-free: 200 cigarettes, 1 litre of spirits, 2 litres of wine, 60 mls of perfume, 250 mls of toilet water and other goods to a total value of €175. If you have anything over this limit you should declare it on arrival and pay the duty. Carry the receipts with you at all times.

Reclaiming VAT: Tourists who are residents of countries outside the EU may claim a refund on the tax added to purchased items if the item was purchased for personal use and cost more than €154.94 and if the retail outlet is an affiliate of the system. Look for signs saying "Tax-free for tourists," or ask the shopkeeper. You must fill out a form at the point of purchase and have it stamped and checked by Italian customs when you leave the country (if you are visiting several European Union countries be ready to show officials what you've bought when you leave the EU and keep the receipt). Return the form by mail within 60 days to the vendor who will make the refund either by check or to your credit card. Sometimes this can be done immediately at major airports. Global Refund (☎ 0331-283-555, www.globalrefund.com) offers this service in major airports and border crossings for a processing fee.

In Italy receipts must be retained for all goods and services. The person at the cash register should hand one to you automatically. You can be fined if you don't have one. This is a new law aimed at tightening controls on the payment of taxes in Italy.

Costs

Sicily is probably not as cheap as you might hope but neither is it as expensive as mainland Italy. August is the most expensive time on the island and all resort areas put their prices up during this period. However, it is still a cheaper option than northern Italy even during this time and outside of peak periods prices drop dramatically. The less-visited areas offer better deals than tourist Meccas like Erice, Cefalù, Siracusa, Taormina, the Aeolian Islands and Pantelleria. However, because they are little-visited there may also be only a few options for places to stay and eat. Campsites are unfortunately rather expensive in Sicily and youth hostels are few and far between. Gas is expensive at €1.20 per litre but public transportation is less expensive than in places like Germany, the UK and USA.

A prudent traveler could scrape by on €40 per day by staying in a youth hostel or campsite, eating one simple meal per day, buying a sandwich for lunch and traveling slowly. For €60 per day you could stay in cheaper guesthouses or small hotels, with one sit-down meal and museum visit per day. For a single traveler, however, this may be hard to manage as hotel rooms are usually cheaper per person for a double. For mid-range hotels, two meals, a drink or two and other comforts should be possible on €100 per day. If you're renting a car add another €50 per day to cover rental, gas and parking costs.

This table shows how daily costs might break down:

Campsite/hostel/budget accommodation	€15
Breakfast (coffee + pastry)	€2.50
Snack lunch	€5
Sit-down lunch	€10
Coffee	€1
Sit-down dinner	€10-20
Transport for inner city or small distances	€5-10
Metro ticket inner city	€0.90

Just the Facts

Transport over longer distance €10-15
Medium-range hotel €30-50
Museums €5-10

HOTEL PRICE CHART	
€	Up to €25 per day
€€	€26-€55
€€€	€56-€85
€€€€	Over €85

All accommodation prices given represent the cheapest available double room in high season. These rooms may or may not have an en-suite bathroom or shower. Out of season you may be able to negotiate a lower price than those suggested here. In campsites and hostels the prices listed are per-person.

To save money while you travel you could avoid staying in places that include breakfast, as most consist of coffee and pastry only. Unless it's an upmarket place, you'll probably get a better tasting and cheaper breakfast in a café. If you're staying anywhere long-term, ask for available discounts. Places that allow you to cook your own food are a good option as there are plenty of markets around to pick up produce.

The key shown here indicates the cost of meals. The pricing scale is for a typical Sicilian meal, including the purchase of house wine, water and a first and second plate.

If you're eating out, make sure you check the fine print on menus before you sit

DINING PRICE CHART	
Price per person for an entrée, including house wine.	
€	Up to €12
€€	€13-€25
€€€	€26-€35
€€€€	Over €35

down. Most restaurants charge a *coperto* (cover charge) or *servizio* (service fee), which can be very high in touristy places. Restaurants on the main *corso* (street) are usually more expensive. Local haunts down side-streets or alleyways are usually a better bet. Check the prices first, of course. In a bar or café, if you stand at the bar to drink your coffee or eat a sandwich, the price may be half what it would be if you sat at a table.

Currency

Since January 2002 the euro (€)has been the unit of currency for all transactions in Italy and the EU. All receipts still have the lira (L) value marked on them and you may hear older people still discussing amounts in *vecchia lire* (old lira). The conversion rate has been set at €1 = 1936.27L.

The euro is divided into 100 cents. Coin denominations are one, two, five, 10, 20 and 50 cents, €1 and €2. Notes are €5, €10, €20, €50, €100, €200 and €500. The notes and coins are legal tender across the euro zone and you don't need to change money in these member states. For more information on the euro go to www.europa.eu.int/euro.

Banks, ATMs & Currency Exchange: Most Sicilian banks open Monday to Friday 8:30 am-1:20 pm and 3-4 pm. The main banks you will see are the Banco di Sicilia, the Banca Populare Sant'Angelo, the Cassa di Risparmio and the Banca Nazionale di Lavoro.

You can exchange money in banks, post offices and currency exchange booths (bureaux de change or *cambios*). Check the rate and commission charge before proceeding with the transaction. Banks usually offer a better exchange rate, but they may charge €1.29 or more in commission. ATMs normally set their rates by those of major banks, though you pay more on the transaction. Post offices have a flat commission rate of €.52 and charge a maximum of €2.60 per transaction. Traveler's checks always attract higher fees.

Large hotels, airports and main train stations can also handle traveler's checks and cash exchanges.

Exchange rates at the time of writing were:

Australia . . . . A$1 . . . . €0.60245
Canada . . . . C$1 . . . . €0.71393
New Zealand . . . . NZ$1 . . . . €0.50568
UK . . . . £1 . . . . €1.45250
USA . . . . US$1 . . . . €0.79339

For help finding exchange rates for your local currency go to www.oanda.com.

Don't count on finding an ATM in smaller towns, particularly in rural areas. The word for ATM in Italian is *bancomat*.

Cash: Pickpockets and bag snatchers are a problem in some tourist areas so it's best not to carry around more cash than what you need for one or two days. Keep an emergency stash separate from other valuables in case you lose your travelers' checks or credit cards. Cash is still the only form of purchase in markets, small guesthouses and shops, so you will need it for many transactions.

 You should be able to order some euro notes from your bank before setting out or from branches of Thomas Cook or American Express. Alternatively, there are ATMs at both arrival airports in Sicily where you can get ready cash. Most ATMs take international cards wherever the Maestro or Cirrus symbol is displayed. There is usually a small charge for this transaction.

Travelers' Checks: Travelers' checks are a safe way of carrying your money around as they are replaceable if lost or stolen. Make sure you keep a list of the checks in a separate location from the notes so you can make a claim. If they are stolen, report the loss immediately to their nearest office.

Travelers' checks are available from most banks or from Thomas Cook (www.thomascook.co.uk or www.us. thomascook.com) and American Express (www. americanexpress.co.uk or www.americanexpress.com). It's best to get your checks made out in a selection of denominations and in euros, but checks in sterling or dollars are widely accepted in Sicily too.

Credit & Debit Cards: Cards are the simplest and safest way to carry money around. They give you access to ATMs (*bancomats*). Make sure you have a pin number that will work overseas. If for some reason the ATM rejects your card, try another or several before ringing internationally. There are ATMs all over Sicily, although few in small towns.

Visa, MasterCard, Eurocard, Cirrus and Eurocheque are accepted throughout Sicily. These cards are preferred over American Express, although in tourist areas American Express is usually accepted.

Credit cards are increasingly common in Sicily, but not accepted everywhere. It is a good idea to make sure you can use your card first before trying to pay for a meal, hotel or other purchase with it. Some places may require a minimum expenditure.

Going Metric

To make your travels in this region easier, we have provided the following chart that shows metric equivalents for the measurements you are familiar with.

GENERAL MEASUREMENTS

1 kilometer = .6124 miles

1 mile = 1.6093 kilometers

1 foot = .304 meters

1 inch = 2.54 centimeters

1 square mile = 2.59 square kilometers

1 pound = .4536 kilograms

1 ounce = 28.35 grams

1 imperial gallon = 4.5459 liters

1 US gallon = 3.7854 liters

1 quart = .94635 liters

TEMPERATURES

For Fahrenheit: Multiply Centigrade figure by 1.8 and add 32.

For Centigrade: Subtract 32 from Fahrenheit figure and divide by 1.8.

Centigrade	Fahrenheit
40°	104°
35°	95°
30°	86°
25°	77°
20°	64°
15°	59°
10°	50°

Debit cards are available from outlets like Thomas Cook and you can deposit an amount of money onto the card that can be withdrawn by using a pin code (*codice segreto*) from ATMs. Divide your money among the cards and use them until your credit expires. You will pay a transaction fee to use the ATM.

The MasterCard number in Italy is ☎ 800-870-866; for Visa, it's ☎ 800-819-014. American Express is ☎ 800-874-333. Diners Club is ☎ 800-864-064.

Money Wiring/International Transfers: For emergency money in Sicily you can use a money wiring service through the foreign office of a large Italian bank or through major banks in your own country to a nominated bank in Sicily.

However, the speediest option is to send money through an agent like Thomas Cook (www.thomascook.co.uk, www.thomascook.com), MoneyGram (www.moneygram.com) or Western Union (www.westernunion.com). All have agents in Sicily. The procedure is for the sender and receiver to turn up at an outlet with a passport or ID.

Post Offices

Post offices normally open Monday to Saturday from 8:30 am to 6:30 pm. In smaller towns the post office may not be open on Saturdays and usually everywhere else they close at noon on the last Saturday of the month. However, you can buy *francobolli* (stamps) at a *tabacchi* and sometimes in other shops. This is advisable if you know the value required as post office lines can be long and service slow. The delivery service is not much better. Sicilian mail is notoriously slow and may need up to two weeks to reach destinations like the United States, Canada, Australia and New Zealand. Use *posta prioritaria* to express an item within Italy. *Posta celere* is for urgent mail within Italy or abroad but has a maximum up to 20 kg/44 lbs. for international destinations and up to 3 kg/6.6 lbs. for Italian destinations. Both services guarantee delivery within 24 hours in Italy and three to five days abroad.

■ Holidays

Sicilians take their annual holidays in August and generally head to the seaside or into the mountains. Many businesses close during August, especially

around the Feast of the Assumption or *Ferragosto* on August15th. The Easter Break or *Settimana Santa* is another busy holiday period.

Major Public Holidays in Sicily:

- January 1 - New Year's Day (*Anno Nuovo*) celebrations take place on New Year's Eve (*capodanno*)
- January 6 - Ephiphany (*Befana)*
- March/April - Good Friday (*Vernerdi Santo*), Easter Monday (*Pasquetta*)
- April 25 - Liberation Day (*Giorno della Liberazione*). Marks the end of the German presence and Mussolini with the Allied victory in Italy
- May 1 - Labor Day (*Giorno del Lavoro*)
- June 2 - Festival of the Republic
- August 15 - Feast of the Assumption (*Ferragosto*)
- November 1 - All Saints' Day (*Ognissanti*)
- December 8 - Feast of the Immaculate Conception (*Concezione Immaculata*)
- December 25 - Christmas Day (*Natale*)
- December 26 - St Stephen's Day (Boxing Day, *Festa di Santo Stefano*)

Feast days of patron saints are observed locally and you may find businesses and shops closed on these days.

Major Festivals & Pilgrimages

- *January*

Epiphany (*Befana*): This festival is celebrated around Sicily but is particularly colorful in Piana degli Albanesi (near Palermo) with a parade and fireworks display.

- *February*

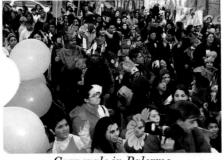

Carnevale in Palermo

Carnevale: This holiday takes place the last week before Ash Wednesday when towns stage carnivals to enjoy themselves in the last let-your-hair-down opportunity before the sacrificial period of Lent. Sciacca's festivities

Just the Facts

are renowned in Sicily, as are those of Taormina, Acireale and other places on the Ionian coast.

Feast of Saint Agatha (*Festa di Sant'Agata*): Catania celebrates this feast of its patron saint from the 3rd to the 5th of the month. The saint's relics are paraded through town amidst food stalls and fireworks.

Sagra del Mandorlo in Fiore: This festival during the second week of February celebrates the almond blossom in Agrigento.

■ *April*

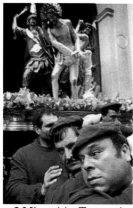

Easter (*Pasqua*): An important festival in Sicily, celebrated by solemn processions and passion plays. Trapani's procession of *I Misteri* is famed, as are similar processions in Marsala, Enna and Piana degli Albanesi. But every town in Sicily will have some procession and celebration. You may also want to look at the celebrations at Prizzi in the western interior and San Fratello on the Tyrrhenian coast.

I Misteri in Trapani

Motor Racing (*Corsa Automobilistica*): The start of the racing season begins the last week in April at Lago di Pergusa near Enna. The season runs until the end of September.

■ *July*

Feast of St Rosalia (*Festa di Santa Rosalia*): Palermo's biggest annual party is

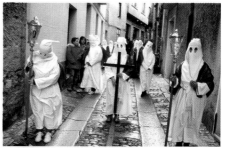

Trapani Good Friday procession

held in honour of one of its patron saints from the 11th to the 15th. The saint's relics are paraded from the city cathedral and there is music, food, dancing and partying.

Feast of St James (San Giacomo): On July 24 and 25 every year, the colorful ceramic steps in Caltagirone are lit by many colored paper lamps to celebrate this feast day.

■ *August*

Medieval Pageant (*Il Palio dei Normanni*): This two-day celebration in Piazza Armerina on the 14th and 15th commemorates Count Roger's taking of the town from the Arabs in the 13th century. There are costumed parades, town processions, jousts and general good cheer.

■ *September*

Pilgrimages (*Pelegrinaggi*): There are numerous pilgrimages that take place in Sicily, but the most interesting are to Mt Pellegrino on the 4th (near Palermo) and to the church at Gibilmanna in the Madonie and Tindari on the 8th.

■ Transportation

Getting Here

Sicily is not a major European destination and therefore direct flights to the island are limited. You can fly directly from London, New York and Paris on a charter flight in summer or scheduled services via an airport on the Italian mainland. From other countries all flights go via the mainland first, probably to Rome or Milan. It's no problem to pick up onward flights to Sicily from these two centers or Napoli. Alternatively train or bus the rest of the way. Boats are also an option from Naples, Rome, Genoa or Livorno. You probably won't want to drive to Sicily as expensive tolls and a long commute through the mainland make it expensive and time consuming.

By Air

 Sicily is not served by intercontinental flights and most likely you'll get a connecting flight or even change airlines in Rome or Milan. Palermo and Catania are served by flights from Italian destinations. **Alitalia** (www.alitalia.com) is the major carrier to Sicily (both Palermo and Catania). **Sardinia Meridiana** (www.meridiania.it) also has flights between Italy and Sicily. In summer there are charter flights from European centers like London. The highest fares are during the Easter period and between June and August. Shoulder seasons include September to October and April to May. The best prices are November to March with the exclusion of Christmas and New Year. However, accommodation packages may offer good deals for a cheap holiday at all times of the year.

Major Airports

There are two main airports in Sicily: **Aeroporto Falcone Borsellino** or **Aeroporto Punta Raisi** (☎ 091-702-0127 or toll-free 800-541-880, www.gesap.it) 32 km west of Palermo; and **Aeroporto Fontanarossa** (☎ 095-723-9111 or 095-340-505, toll free 800-605656, www.aeroporto.catania.it), seven km south of Catania. The small **Aeroporto Vincenzo Florio** at Birgi, Trapani (☎ 0923-842-502, www.airgest.com) is a military airport open also to civil traffic. Companies servicing this airport include **Air One** (www.flyairone-it) and **RyanAir** (www.ryanair.com, Trapani-Pisa) and various charter flights. Flights connect to Roma Fiumicino, Milan, Turin, Venice, Bari, Catania, Lampedusa and Pantelleria.

Booking Flights

To ensure a good deal on your ticket, compare prices from several travel agents, Internet sites and travel ads in newspapers. Start looking early as cheaper tickets usually need to be purchased well in advance.

Booking your flight online can save you money by cutting out the cost of agents or middlemen, although agents can also have better access to the cheapest deals going, find ways to avoid inconvenient layovers and get good travel insurance.

If you are working or studying in Italy for more than one year you may wish to get a one-way ticket and utilize the cheap tickets out of London to come home. Students or travelers under 26 years should always ask for youth/student fares. Children under 12 or seniors over 65 may also be able to get discounts. If you are flying from Australia or New Zealand, ask about stopovers to break the journey.

Following are some online booking sites.

www.travelocity.com: Online air travel info and reservations sites for cars, rail, hotels and other packages.

www.priceline.com: Travel deals allowing you to quote your own price from the US.

www.cheapflights.com: Air travel and latest deals from the US.

www.hotwire.com: Deals from the US and Canada and associated packages.

www.skyscanner.net: All-airline search engine.

www.expedia.co.uk and **www.expedia.com**: Discounted airfares, online travel planning.

www.flightline.co.uk: Cheap flights and holidays from the UK with UK tour operators.

www.ebookers.com: This site allows you to select your country of origin (European) and search for discounted flights.

www.travelshop.com.au: Site listing flights from Australia and good-value package deals plus last-minute offers.

www.studentflights.com.au: Cheap Australian travel offers for students and backpackers.

www.bigliettie-aerei.it: An Italian site containing a database with low cost rates.

Flights from Italy

Air New Zealand (☎ 132-476 in Australia, 0800-737-000 in New Zealand, www.airnnewzealand.com).

British Airways (☎ 1300-767-177 in Australia, 09-966-9777 in New Zealand, www.britishairways.com).

Malaysia Air (☎ 132-627 or 02-9364-3500 in Australia, 0800-777-747 in New Zealand, www.malaysiaair.com).

Qantas (☎ 13-13-13 in Australia, 0800-808-767 in New Zealand, www.qantas.com.au).

KLM (☎ 1300-303-747 in Australia, fax 1300-787-747, www.klm.com).

Thai Airlines (☎ 03-8662-2266 in Australia, 09-377-3886 in New Zealand, www.thaiair.com).

Alitalia (☎ 02-9244-2445 in Australia, 09-308-3357 in New Zealand, www.alitalia.it).

Cathay Pacific (☎ 131-747 or 02-9251-3460 in Australia or 09-379-0861 in New Zealand, www.cathaypacific.com).

Garuda (☎131-223 or 02-9334-9944 in Australia, 09-366-1862 in New Zealand, www.garuda-indonesia.com).

Japan Airlines JAL (☎ 02-9272-1111 in Australia, 09-379-9906 in New Zealand, www.japanair.com).

Singapore Airlines (☎ 131-011 or 02-9350-0100 in Australia, 09-373-7731 or 0800-808-909 in New Zealand, www.singaporeair.com).

Agents & Packages

Flight Center (☎ 133-133 in Australia, 800-243-544 in New Zealand, www.flightcenter.com.au, www.flightcenter.co.nz).

STA Travel (☎ 1300-733-035 or 03-9207-5900 in Australia, 0508-782-872 in New Zealand, www.statravel.com.au, www.statravel.co.nz).

Thomas Cook (☎ 131-771 or 800-801-002 in Australia, 0508-782-872, 09-379-3920 in New Zealand, www.thomascook.com.au).

Trailfinders (☎ 1300-780-212 or 02-9247-7666, www.trailfinders.com.au).

Specialist Tour Operators

CIT (☎ 02-9267-1255, www.cittravel.com.au). Specialist tour operator to Sicily taking in major cities and sights and the Aeolian islands.

Drive Travel (☎ 03-8781-1120, www.drivetravel.com). Driving holidays in Sicily.

Hidden Italy (☎ 02-9957-4511, www.maryrossitaravel.com). Guided walks in Sicily including Palermo, Taormina, the Madonie park and Aeolian islands.

Peregrine Adventures (☎ 03-9662-2700, www.peregrine.net.au). Walking and cycling adventures.

Intrepid Travel (☎ 1300-360-667, www.intrepidtravel.com.au).

By Sea

Unless you fly you have to take a ferry to get to Sicily until the much talked about bridge or tunnel across the straits of Messina is completed. The shortest sea crossing is from Villa San Giovanni in Calabria. You can also board a ferry in Naples, Genoa or Livorno for Palermo. In high season you should pre-book a passage, especially if you have a vehicle. At other times you can simply walk on, but check the winter schedules carefully as services are less frequent. The website www.traghetti.com (☎ 899-500-097) lists all schedules.

From Villa San Giovanni

Car ferries make the crossing to Messina frequently in about half an hour. In summer months there can be longer delays. The **Ferrovie dello Stato** or **FS Italian Railways** (☎ 892-

021, www.trenitalia.com) operates 30 car and passenger train ferries daily (one-two hourly, 40 minutes). On **Caronte** ferries (☎ 090-641-6352, www.carontetourist.it) foot passengers travel for free (€19 for small cars, departures every 10 minutes).

From Reggio di Calabria

For a quicker passage try the passenger-only *aliscafi* (hydrofoils) from Reggio di Calabria to Messina, 15 minutes farther south of Villa San Giovanni. FS operates 18 hydrofoils daily Monday to Saturday and 12 times on Sunday (about once hourly, 25 minutes).

Meridiano (www.meridianolines.it) operates 21 times daily Monday to Friday (departing hourly, nine services for commercial vehicles only, one hour), 12 times on Saturday (every two hours), and once on Sunday evening. Foot passengers €1. 50, cars €10.

From Naples

Tirrenia (☎ 050-754-492 for English, ☎ 081-317-2999 call center, www.tirrenia.it) operates two overnight car ferries daily all year between Naples and Palermo (10 hours, from €36.04 in low season). A day service operates in summer months only (eight hours, from €36.04 in low season).

SNAV (☎ 091-611-4211, www.snavali.it) has a fast once-daily service linking Naples to the Aeolian Islands from June to mid-September (5½ hours, €77). Another once-daily service runs overnight from Naples to Palermo (10½ hours, from €15) with two extra Saturday services in summer (daily and overnight, 10½ hours). The boats also carry vehicles.

Ustica Lines (☎ 0923-873-813, www.usticalines.it) also uses Naples on the mainland to Trapani (via Ustica, Favignana and Levanzo) on Monday, Thursday, Friday and Saturday from June to September (seven hours, €85). The Friday service is July and August only. Another service runs to Milazzo in summer only (seven hours, €88.20).

Siremar (☎ 091-749-3111, www.siremar.it) runs from Naples to Milazzo via the Aeolian Islands (twice weekly, 15-20 hours). Prices start from €36.80 in low season.

From Cagliari

A weekly Tirrenia service operates between Palermo and Cagliari in Sardinia (13½ hours, from €26.14 in low season) and from Cagliari to Trapani once weekly all year with an extra service in summer (10 hours, from €21.49 in low season).

From Rome

SNAV has overnight car ferries from Rome Civitavecchia to Palermo on Tuesday, Thursday and Saturday from April 29 to October 31 (13 hours, from €38). Another service runs on Sunday in the summer months. Ferries depart from Porto Civitavecchia about one hour from Rome by train.

Grandi Navi Veloci or **Grimaldi** (☎ 899-199-069, www1. gnv.it) links Roma Civitavecchia to Palermo (daily departures, 12 hours, from €40).

From Genoa

Grandi Navi Veloci has daily departures for Genoa (20 hours, from €59) from Terminal Traghetti at Via Milano 51 in Genoa.

From Malta

Virtu Ferries (☎ 095-535-711, www.virtuferries.com) runs between Malta and Pozzallo and Catania from March to October (€28 single passenger). Cars can be transported on some services. Services run at least three days weekly with numerous services on some days (1½ hours to Pozzallo, three hours to Catania).

From Tunisia

Grandi Navi Veloci has a service from Palermo to Tunis twice weekly overnight (10 hours, € 60).

Ustica Lines has a new service from 2006 that runs from Trapani to Tunisia to Tunis (from €42.50) and Sousse (from €52.50).

FERRY SCHEDULE FROM ITALY TO SICILY	
Company	**Frequency & duration**
Villa San Giovanni - Messina	
FS car ferries	1-2 hourly, 40 mins

Caronte car ferries	every 10 minutes, 20 mins
Reggio di Calabria – Messina	
FS ferries	hourly, 20 mins
Meridiano car ferries	21 daily Mon-Fri, 12 Sat, 1 Sun; 60 mins
Genova - Palermo	
Grandi Navi Veloci/Grimaldi	daily departures, 20 hours
Rome – Palermo	
Grandi Navi Veloci/Grimaldi	daily departures, 12 hours
Snav	3 times weekly April-October, on Sundays in summer, 13 hours
Naples - Aeolian Islands	
Siremar	2 weekly, 15-20 hours
Snav	1 daily (June-mid September), 5½ hours
Naples - Palermo	
Tirrenia	2 overnight car ferries daily, 1 day service in summer only, 8-10 hours
Snav	1 service overnight daily (mid April to early Oct), 2 additional Saturday services in summer, 10½ hours
Naples - Milazzo	
Ustica Lines	1 daily, summer only, 7 hours
Naples - Trapani via Ustica, Favignana and Levanzo	
Ustica Lines	3 weekly, summer only, 7 hours
Cagliari - Palermo	
Tirrenia	1 weekly, 13½ hours
Cagliari - Trapani	
Tirrenia	1 weekly, extra services in summer; 10 hours
Tunisia - Trapani	
Grandi Navi Veloci	2 weekly, 10 hours
Malta - Pozzallo	
Virtu Ferries	minimum 3 days weekly (increasing in summer), March to October, 1½ hours

Malta - Catania	
Virtu Ferries	minimum 2 days weekly, 3 hours

By Train

 If time is on your side, you may want to go to Sicily by train. For information on Italian trains call ☎ 848-888-088 in Italy or visit the Italian train sites www.trenitalia.com. Direct express trains run from Milan and Rome to Palermo, Catania and Siracusa. Rome-Palermo and Rome-Siracusa takes at least 10 hours.

Timetables

Train timetables in the station are available at the end of the platforms, with the *arrivi* (arrivals) on a white background and the *partenze* (departures) in yellow. The station of origin and terminating station are listed, along with major intermediate stops and arrival times. The electronic boards on the station wall are for imminent arrivals and departures and will list current information about delays and platform numbers. Sometimes the platform number is not displayed until moments before the train arrives, so stay alert! The other place to get timetable information is the automated touch-screen machines located in major stations. You can also purchase tickets in these machines (see *Tickets* below). A complete schedule of all trains in the country and fares can be bought at most newsstands or check it on-line at www.trenitalia.it

Train Types

There are several different types of trains in Italy. *Locali* are the slow all-stops kind and generally travel locally only. *Regionali* are marginally faster and travel farther beyond their originating region. *Interregionali* and *espresso* trains cover longer distances and are not necessarily all-stops. The InterCity trains are faster long-distance trains. **Eurostar Italia** (ES) trains are the top of the range – air-conditioned trains that require a seat booking.

Tickets

Ticket prices are based either on the type of train or the class you travel. On *locali* and *regionali* only second-class seats are

available; on other trains you pay a little more for first class where it is available. Faster trains also require a supplement. The quickest way to get a train ticket is from the station's automated machines. These accept cash and credit cards. They may not always have change available but will give a credit slip that can be used towards your next ticket. If you do queue up at the windows you can be in for a long wait. Major stations now offer a line for trains that are departing in the next few minutes. Look out for windows that display the Eurostar sign as they only sell tickets on ES trains. If you are traveling short distances only, go to a *tabacchi* or *cafe* at the station to get 20-km, 40-km or 60-km tickets. They will usually have a sign saying *biglietti in vendita* (tickets for sale).

Whatever ticket you buy, it must be stamped in one of the yellow machines around the station displaying the sign *convalida* before boarding the train. If it's a round-trip ticket make sure you stamp it each way. Tickets are valid for two months until they are stamped. Once you stamp them they are valid for 24 hours. Tickets are only valid for six hours after they are stamped for travel on distances of less than 200 km. See the details on the back of the ticket for more information.

Long-distance trains must generally be booked in advance.

Rail Passes

Many rail tickets are valid in Italy, including Eurail, InterRail, Europass and Flexipass tickets. Some of these include:

The **FS Cartaverde Pass** for travelers under 26. It is valid for one year and reduces train fares by 20%. If you're over 60, you can purchase the **Carta d'Argento** (Silver Card), which allows a 40% discount on first-class rail travel and a 20% discount on second-class travel.

The **Trenitalia Pass** is available for adults, small groups and youth for three to 10 days of travel within two months. It is for non-Italian residents only.

For extended travel, ask about the *biglietto chilometrico*, valid for travelers of all ages, that entitles you to 3,000 km with a maximum of 20 trips.

The **Eurail Pass** is considered by many as the best option for traveling through Europe, and Italy is one of the 18 countries where you can use it. A variety of passes are available for different times and classes.

Rail Ticket Agencies

- www.eurostar.com. Eurostar reservations.
- www.raileurope.com. Rail passes in Europe, regional passes, tickets and schedules.
- www.railconnection.com. Online rail passes with Rail Connection.
- www.trenitalia.com. The official Italian rail site for Italian rail passes and timetables.
- www.inter-rail.net. Information about travel in Italy, train passes and timetables.
- www.eurorail.com. Agent selling the Eurorail pass.
- www.railplus.com.au. Australian site selling European packages.
- www.cittravel.com.au. CIT World Travel Australia.

By Bus

 Traveling to Sicily by bus is a long haul and not necessarily cheaper than trains or even flights. There is also no direct service to Sicily from outside Italy. Eurolines goes as far as Rome; from there you will have to change carriers to get to Sicily.

Ticket Agencies

European

Eurolines offices (www.eurolines.com, ☎ 055-357-110) cover all of Europe. Check the website for a full list. The Rome office is at Circonvallazione Nomentana 574, Lato Stazione Tiburtina, ☎ 064-440-4009. **UK Eurolines** runs to Rome in 32 hours at 7:30 am on Monday, Wednesday and Friday for £74. No services run direct to Sicily; the closest stop is Naples.

Italian

Segesta/Interbus (☎ 091-342-525, www.interbus.it) has one daily departure that leaves Rome from Piazzale Tiburtina to Messina (€31, nine hours), two for Palermo (€35,65, 12 hours) and Syracuse (€34,60, 12 hours). The office is at Saistours, Piazza della Repubblica 42, ☎ 064-819-676.

Interbus (☎ 0935-565-111) and **Etna Trasporti** (☎ 095-348-131) connect Sicily with Puglia, Milan and Turin.

Segesta Internazionale connects Sicily with Germany, Belgium, France and Luxembourg (☎ 091-342-525).

SAIS Autolinee (☎ 091-616-6028, www.saisautolinee.it) buses can be taken from Venice to Sicily.

By Car & Motorcyle

Unless you're already journeying around mainland Italy by car or motorcycle, it's not the best way to reach the island. Air, train or ferry are definitely preferred. If you do have a car, you must take a car ferry across the strait.

Rental Agencies

Cars can be rented at airports and major cities. See *Getting Around* below.

Getting Around

Getting around in Sicily by public transport is not difficult, although services may not always seem very efficient. Trains link the major cities and connect most of the coastline, while buses go to most other places. Without a doubt having your own car is the best way of getting around if you can cope with the traffic and the parking.

By Car & Motorcycle

A car is the best way to move around in Sicily as public transportation can be unreliable. Major highways provide good access to the coast and through the interior. The A20 connects Messina and Palermo, while the A18 links Messina and Catania. Through the center from Catania to west of

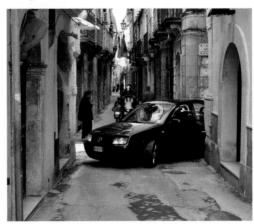
A difficult turn in Taormina
(Galen R Frysinger, www.galenfrysinger.com)

Cefalù is A19; farther west of Palermo the A29 runs to Trapani and the airport and south to Mazara del Vallo. The *superstrada* S115 is another major road running along the southern coast. Other *superstrade* bisect the island.

Driving in Sicily's big cities can leave you a sweaty, shaking mess and squeezing into small parking spaces is definitely not for the faint-hearted; unless you're well accustomed to the roads. The worst times are usually 8 to 9 am on weekdays and from 1 to 2 pm. Saturday evenings are also busy between 7 and 9 pm. The best way to tackle the cities is to leave your car somewhere safe and head out on foot. Outside of built-up areas you'll find well maintained roads with few vehicles (except for the busy coastal routes).

Parking is restricted in the narrow streets of historic centers (*centri storici*) and usually limited to local vehicles. The best place to park is in a guarded lot. Areas that are signposted *Zona Disco* (disk zone) allows free parking for limited periods but you must display your time of arrival. If you can't get a cardboard disk, use a piece of paper. The *parcometro* is also common now in some cities. You put coins in a machine for a stamped ticket and leave it on the dashboard.

For safety while driving, carry a good map, flashlight and mobile phone. If you break down, call the **Automobile Club d'Italia** or ACI dispatchers (☎ 803-116) who should have English-speaking operators. Another good number is the **CAT Phone Service Center** (☎ 06-4477), also provided by ACI, who have multilingual staff that can tell you about road and weather conditions, highway tolls, ferries, mileage distance and automotive procedures.

Gas stations open Monday to Saturday 7 am-7 pm, with a break at lunchtime. Some have automatic self-service pumps that accept only bills and/or credit cards. At the time of writing, *benzina senza piombo* (unleaded gas) cost about €1.25 per litre. The stations on the *autostrade* are open 24 hours. Gasoline is called *benzina* and diesel is *gasolio*.

Driving in Sicily is on the right and road rules are the same as on the mainland. Sicilian drivers can be aggressive. Speed limits are 130 kph (80 mph) on *autostrade,* 110 kph (70 mph) on state and provincial roads, 90 kph (56 mph) on secondary and local roads and 50 kph (31 mph) in urban areas. Drink driving is fined heavily, as is speeding where it is enforced. Police can levy on-the-spot fines in Italy. Seat belts and children's car seats are compulsory.

Car Rentals

Cars can be rented at airports and key locations in major cities like the central railway station and ports. Rates start from €35 a day for an economy car like a Fiat with unlimited mileage. If you want an automatic you must specify when you reserve the car, and higher rates will apply. Tax can come to an additional 20% and if you rent from the airport there's an associated 14% fee. Always check what insurance cover you get before you rent.

In Italy you must be 21 years of age to rent a car and a credit card is required as a warranty. If you need a child car seat, request one in advance. A further cost is usually applicable for the rental. Your country's driver's license is acceptable to rent a car; if you want to get an international driver's license, see the *Documents* section. For contact details of all rental car offices in Sicily go to the websites below.

- **Avis** (www.avis.com or www.avisautonoleggio.it)
- **Hertz** (www.hertz.com)
- **Maggiore** (www.maggiore.it)
- **National Car Rental** (www.nationalcar.com)
- **Budget** (www.budget.com)

By Bus

 Buses are generally considered more reliable and faster than trains; they are also air-conditioned and connect major and minor cities. They can be slightly more expensive than trains. You should be able to get bus timetables from local tourist offices or they may be posted at the bus stop (usually the central square) in smaller towns. In larger cities the main intercity bus companies have ticket offices or use travel agencies. For overnight transport you should book ahead – for example if you are leaving Sicily for the Italian mainland. Otherwise, it is fine to just turn up and grab a seat on board when the bus comes. Various companies serve the different routes.

Useful Phone Numbers

SAIS (☎ 091-616-6028 Palermo, ☎ 095-536-168 or 095-536-201 Catania, www.saisautolinee.it) connects Palermo, Catania, Messina and Siracusa from the train stations. SAIS also operates on the south and east coasts and in the interior, including the towns of Catania, Agrigento, Enna, Taormina

and Siracusa. **Cuffaro** (☎ 091-616-1510, www.cuffaro.info/index.htm) connects Palermo with centers like Agrigento, Racalmuto, Favara, Canicatti, Grotte, Comitini and Castrofilippo. **Etna Trasporti** (☎ 095-530-396, www.etnatrasporti.it) operates between Catania, Caltagirone, Piazza Armerina and Taormina. **Interbus** (☎ 095-532-716, www.interbus.it) operates between Messina, Taormina, Catania and Siracusa.

See individual chapters below for detailed information on bus transport.

By Train

 The train lines in Sicily connect Messina, Taormina, Siracusa and Palermo and are run by the state railway **Ferrovie Dello Stato** (www.trenitalia.com, ☎ 848-888-088 or 892-021). There is one private line, the **Ferrovia Circumetnea** which does a circuit of Mt Etna (see the Mt Etna chapter later in the guide).

Train delays in Sicily are common and journeys can be notoriously slow and frustrating. Some Sicilians advise that you travel by bus where possible. There are *metropolitana* (metro) systems in Catania and Palermo. See individual chapters below for more information.

By Boat

 The only places where you will rely on boats for getting around in Sicily are on the islands. Generally, services for the Aeolians run from Milazzo but you can also get there from Palermo and Messina. To get to the Egadi Islands use Trapani as the departure base, to the Pelagic Islands from Porto Empedocle near Agrigento, Ustica from Palermo and Pantelleria from Milazzo and Trapani. See more details below.

These companies service the offshore islands:

SNAV (☎ 091-611-8525, www.snavali.com). Hydrofoils from: Milazzo to the Aeolians.

Ustica Lines (☎ 0923-873-813, www.usticalines.it). Hydrofoils from Trapani to the Egadi Islands, Lampedusa to Linosa, Pantelleria to Trapani.

Siremar (☎ 091-749-3111, www.siremar.it). Ferry and hydrofoil from Palermo to Ustica, Trapani to the Egadi Islands,

Porto Empedocle to Lampedusa/Linosa, Milazzo to the Aeolian Islands.

By Air

 Flying within Sicily is expensive but, if your time is limited, you may want to fly to the more distant islands such as Pantelleria and the Pelagic Islands. Otherwise, it is far more cost effective to get a boat (see the previous section). You can book flights at the airports, online or at travel agencies. See the listings abve in this chapter.

To Lampedusa Airport

(☎ 0922-971-548)

Alitalia (☎ 06-2222, www.alitalia.it) flies twice daily to Lampedusa from Palermo, as does **Air Sicilia** (☎ 091-702-0310, www.airsicilia.it). Air Sicilia also has a flight from Catania to Lampedusa. **Air One** (☎ 091-70201, www.flyair-one.it) flies from Palermo to Lampedusa.

To Pantelleria Airport

(☎ 0923-911-398, www.pantelleriairport.it)

Air One flies to Pantelleria from Rome, Milan, Venice, Bari and Trapani. Also from Bologna in summer. **Meridiana** flies from Palermo. Alitalia has direct charter flights from Rome, Milan, Venice and Bologna.

Cycling

 Biking in Sicily is a good way to get around, although you can't really talk about cycle-tourism as there are not a lot of established cycle tracks. But there is a good road network for quiet passages and magnificent scenery. Bikes are generally available for rent in most towns although it may be harder to get good mountain bikes. See the regional sections below for local information. If you're planning long-term rental you may want to consider buying a bike. Bikes can be taken on trains for a small additional supplement and are free on ferries. Make sure you bring your own tools, spare parts, inner tube repair kit, helmet and a good lock to safeguard against theft.

We have listed numerous itineraries in this guide, but many travel companies offer both group and self-guided excursions, where they provide detailed route information. See the travel agents mentioned earlier in this chapter and the following list

Just the Facts

of mountain bike clubs and associations. Unfortunately, much of the website information is in Italian only.

Ragusani Volanti (www.ragusanivolanti.it) is a group of passionate cyclists from Ragusa. The website lists their trips and mountain bike routes around Ragusa.

Sole & Bike (www.solebike.it), operating from Acireale, presents various itineraries in the area and also organizes tours and accommodation for cyclists. Routes include Mt Etna, the Lemon Coat and historic sites.

Ciclo Turismo (www.cicloneb.it) operates in the Parco Regionale dei Monti Nebrodi.

Nebrodi Cycling Tours (☎ 0941-438-730, www.nebrotours. com) offers a range of itineraries in the Nebrodi Mountain Park, including other walking and gastronomic tours.

Lo Zoccolo duro Bike (http://web.tiscali.it/lozoccoloduro_bike/) is dedicated to mountain biking in Sicily. Itineraries are listed for the Aeolian Islands, Mt Etna and other national parks in Sicily.

Club Green Bike (☎ 338-749-6406, fax 178-226-0815, www. ragusa.net/mtb/). The Green Bikes Club in Ragusa lists all their club news online, plus itineraries in the Ragusa area including Modica, Chiaramonte Gulfi and Monti Iblei.

Acquaterra Mountainbike (Piazza Cavour 14, Catania, ☎ 095-438-954, http://web.tiscali.it/acquaterrabike) meets every Thursday evening from October to June at their office. They do mountain bike trips every three weeks for eight months of the year. There are more regular summer programs and tours of national parks in Sicily. They also have night tours of Catania's monuments. There is a membership fee to join in any trips.

Palermo Bike Affair (www.bokos.it/bikeaffair) is a group of Palermo-based bikers. They do regular rides of Palermo and surrounding areas and even as far as Etna and Ficuzza. In 2004 they did a complete circuit of the island. See the website for useful route information.

Bikes on the Road (www.bikesontheroad.it) has monthly excursions from Agira taking in surrounding areas.

Montainbike Sicilia (☎ 095-434-859, Via Napoli 45, Catania, www.montainbikesicilia.it) promotes both city, off-road and children's riding through a number of excursions and activities.

Rent Bike (☎ 346-231-7451, www.rentbike.it) in Acireale rents city and mountain bicycles for use all over Sicily and can provide transport to/from arrival points in Sicily. Bikes start at €13/day, €63/week, €126/two weeks.

Siciclando (☎ 091-754-1626, Via P.pe di Pantelleria 37, Palermo, www.siciclando.com) is a group of people keen on biking and walking, offering tours and producing publications with itineraries. They have three major routes through Western and Eastern Sicily.

Acquaterra (Via Antonino Longo 74, ☎ 095-503-020, www.acquaterra.it) is based in Catania but does cycling just above everywhere Sicily on the disused railroads and through all the nature reserves.

The Sicilian Regional Ministry for Tourism, Communication and Transport, in conjunction with Siciclando, has published a guide, *Sicily by Bike*, that you can request by emailing urp.dipturismo@regione.sicilia.it. It contains nine itineraries, one for each province of Sicily. Siciclando worked in conjunction with Palermo Tourism to produce a similar book of cycle itineraries in the Province of Palermo. Email editorial@palermotourism.com for details.

■ *Italian Bike Associations*

Federazione Ciclistica Italiana (Stadio Olimpico, Curva Nord, Roma, ☎ 06-36851, www.federciclismo.it) hosts events and can provide bike information for all Italy.

Federazione Italiana Amici della Bicicletta or **FIAB** (☎ 041-921-515, www.fiab-onlus.it) has publications, itinerary suggestions, events, and help for families with children. In English, Italian and German. They have subsidiary sites – www.bicitalia.org, which is seeking to creating a national highway of cycling routes, and www.bimbimbici.org, with information on traveling with children by bicycle.

Albergabici (www.albergabici.it) is a useful organization listing cyclist-friendly accommodation around Italy, including 52 locations in Sicily.

BicItalia and FIAB together have produced a map of the national cycling route that extends throughout all of Italy. The route in Sicily loops around the island from Messina, following the coast to Catania and down to Siracusa as part of the Number 1 Ciclopista del Sole and EuroVelo's Middle Europe route (www.ecf.com). At Siracusa the Number 1 route

culminates, but the EuroVelo continues to the ferry at Pozzallo for Malta. Another route from here continues to Gela, Agrigento, Marsala, Trapani and Palermo. Detailed itineraries are available on the websites and through organization publications.

■ Special Concerns

Safety

You're unlikely to become a victim of the Mafia in Sicily, but there are some elementary rules worth observing for hassle-free holidays. It's definitely not a good idea to wander the city streets alone after dark, especially in Palermo or Catania. Do not wear expensive jewelry, watches or flaunt other possessions. Avoid quiet areas and keep your bags either on you or in sight at all times. Internal money belts are the safest defense against pick-pockets; external waist packs not only peg you as a tourist but are easy prey in crowds. Any bags should be slung across your body rather than loosely off a shoulder. Only take money with you for one day's purchases and distribute the rest through your luggage.

REPORT ANY LOSS

Dealing with local police can be a headache but is a must if you wish to claim any insurance on lost or stolen items. See the emergency numbers at the beginning of this chapter.

Sickness or Injury

EU citizens may use Italy's health services under the same terms as Italian residents. Get form E111 from main post offices. The Australian Medicare system also has a reciprocal healthcare arrangement with Italy. However, it's always best to travel with your own travel insurance (see *Travel Insurance* earlier in this chapter).

Sicily does not present too many health concerns. Vaccinations are not required unless you plan to continue on to North Africa. The most common complaints in Sicily are the heat in summer and upset stomachs. Water is generally safe to drink,

although it may taste funny. Fountains are available in all towns but watch out for signs saying *aqua non potabile*, meaning the water is not safe to drink.

Farmacie (pharmacies) dispense prescriptions and should be able to give you advice on minor ailments. In bigger towns and cities there's usually one all-night pharmacy. When they close they are required to list those currently open.

Every town has a *medico* (doctor) whom you may visit. The pharmacy can point you in the right direction or you can consult the *Pagine Gialle* (Yellow Pages). Take your E111 form to the doctor with you to get free treatment and prescriptions for medicines at the local rate. Brand names can differ so take any empty medication bottles in with you. Dentists are not covered under the E111 and can be expensive.

Travel with medicines you are familiar with and may need, but general medicines like *l'aspirina* (aspirin) are commonly available. If you are seriously ill go to the *Pronto Soccorso* (emergency section) at the hospital or phone ☎ 113 and ask for *ospedale* or *ambulanza*.

People with Disabilities

There are services for disabled travelers in Sicily but it would be wise to check where they are available before setting out. The Italian State Tourist offices in your country (listed later in this chapter) may be able to give you a list of Italian associations for the disabled and what help is available in Sicily. **CIT** offices (listed later in this chapter) should also be able to help with hotels that have facilities for the disabled.

The Italian Railway, **Ferrovie dello Stato (FS)**, does have trains with carriages for passengers in wheelchairs. 1,200 trains run daily with disabled access and there is a nationwide reservations number, ☎ 199-30-30-60, to facilitate booking services for disabled passengers. Two hundred stations provide a disabled customer assistance service and you can also click the wheelchair icon on the **TrenItalia** (www.trenitalia.com) website for a list of towns that have wheelchair access in the train stations. TrenItalia also prints special timetables that detail services and fares for the disabled. It is also available in Braille and on audiocassette.

Some useful organizations to contact in Italy include the **Italia Per Tutti** website (www.italiapertutti.it) where you can choose the location you are going to and the kind of disabled services you need. *Turismo per tutti* is a quarterly magazine published by the Cooperative Integrate (☎ 800-271-027, www.coinsociale.it) for disabled tourists. They also have mobility and tourism services and can help you with guided tours and transport for disabled passengers. **Anthai** (www.anthai.org), **AIAS** (www.aiasmilano.it), and **Accessible Italy** (www.accessibleitaly.com) are some other useful groups.

Senior Travelers

Seniors receive discounts on public transport and on admission to some museums so always ask if you qualify. The minimum age is generally 60 years. For those over 65, many entrance fees are waived. Travel packages may also be available for seniors through senior organizations and travel agencies. Ask at home before you leave.

Families

 Traveling with children of any age in Sicily should not present difficulties. There are plenty of activities to keep them interested, travel is safe and hygienic and Italians love children and will do their best to spoil them. There are discounts for children on public transport and on admission to museums, galleries and other sites. Get into the habit of asking for a *sconto bambino* (child's discount) before you purchase tickets. Restaurants may be able to provide high chairs or cushions and offer half-portions (*mezza porzione*) or children's portions (*porzione da bambino*).

Most hotels will have a different fee structure for children, although some simply charge them as adults. If you need additional services such as cribs or high chairs, ask about these when you reserve.

■ Information Sources

Embassies & Consulates

 See www.esteri.it for a full list of embassies and consulates.

Canada
Embassy – Level 21, 275 Slater St, Ottawa, ON K1P 5H9, ☎ 613-232-2401, fax 613-233-1484, ambasciata.ottawa@esteri.it.

USA
Embassy – 3000 Whitehaven St NW, Washington, DC 20008, ☎ 202-612-4400, fax 202-518-2154, www.italyemb.org.

Britain
Embassy – 14 Three Kings Yard, London W1Y 4EH, ☎ 020-731-2200, fax 020-731-2230, ambasciata.londra@esteri.it.

Australia
Embassy – 12 Grey St, Deakin, Canberra, ACT, ☎ 02-6273-3333, fax 02-6273-4223, ambasciata.canberra@esteri.it.

New Zealand
Embassy – 34-38 Grant Rd, Thorndon, Wellington, ☎ 04-4735-339, fax 04-4727-255, ambwell@xtra.co.nz.

Italy
Consulates in Palermo
UK: Via Cavour 121, 90133, ☎ 091-326-412, fax 091-584-240.
In Catania: Via Verdi 53, 95100 Catania, ☎ 095-741-0330.
USA: Via Vaccarini 1 Palermo, ☎ 091-305-857, fax 091-343-546.

Embassies in Rome
Australia: Via Alessandria 215, 00198, ☎ 068-527-21.
Canada: Via Zara 30, 00198, ☎ 064-459-81.
New Zealand: Via Zara 28, 00198, ☎ 064-417-171.
UK: Via XX Settembre 80a, 00187, ☎ 064-220-0001.
USA: Via Veneto 119a, 00187, ☎ 064-674-1.

Tourist Offices

Sicilian tourist offices consist of the regional offices, APT (Azienda Promozione Turistica), and local offices known as AST (Azienda di Soggiorno e Turismo). In many small towns and villages the local tourist office is also called a Pro Loco. The APTs usually have both local and regional information and are located in the capital towns of the provinces. The other offices tend to have local information only and may be little more than a small room, though they can provide a lot of useful information.

Just the Facts

CHANGES TO APT

It was rumored that Sicily's APT offices were due for a structural change and/or closure at the time of publication. But the new structure of tourism offices in Sicily is still unknown (or undecided) as of now. Do be aware that the APT details listed in the guide may change in the future.

The quality of tourism offices can vary a lot outside of major cities and tourist areas. It is unlikely they will speak English in smaller towns and they may have run out of printed information by the end of the tourist season. However, generally most will be helpful and they should be able to give you a list of hotels, a map and information on major sights.

The APT produces the helpful accommodation guide *Guida dell'Ospitalita nella Provincia*, which contains up-to-date information on camp sites, hostels, hotels and other accommodation.

Most offices are open 9 am-12:30 or 1 pm and 4-8 pm Monday to Friday. Hours are often extended during summer and popular destinations are open all or part of Saturday and Sunday. Most tourist offices are conveniently located in the main piazza, the corso or at the railway station. Ask for the *ufficio del turismo* or *l'ufficio di informazione*.

For a full list of Italian state tourist offices operating in Italy see the Italian State Tourism Board (ENIT) website, www.enit.it. For offices abroad, see www.italiantourism.com and these in the list below:

■ **Australia** – Level 4, 46 Market Street, Sydney, NSW 2000, ☎ 02-9262-1666, fax 02-9262-1677, italia@italiantourism.com.au.

■ **Canada** – Suite 907, South Tower, 175 Bloor St East, Toronto M4W 3R8, ☎ 416-925-4882, fax 416-925-4799, enit.canada@on.aibn.com.

■ **New Zealand** – c/o Level 4, 46 Market Street, Sydney, NSW 2000, Australia, ☎ 02-9262-1666, fax 02-9262-1677, italia@italiantourism.com.au.

■ **UK** – 1 Princes St, London W1R 9AY, ☎ 020-7408-1254, fax 020-7399-3567, www.italiantouristboard.co.uk, italy@italiantouristboard.co.uk.

■ **USA** – Italian Government Tourist Board (www.italiantourism.com).

- **Chicago**: Suite 2240, 500 North Michigan Avenue, Chicago, IL 60611, ☎ 312-644-9335, fax 312-644-3019, enitch@italiantourism.com.
- **Los Angeles**: Suite 550, 12400 Wilshire Blvd, Los Angeles, CA 90025, ☎ 310-820-1898, fax 310-820-6357, enitla@italiantourism.com.
- **New York**: Suite 1565, 630 Fifth Avenue, New York, NY 10111, ☎ 212-245-5618, fax 212-586-9249, enitny@italiantourism.com.

Other sources for information include Italy's national travel agency known as CIT or Citalia outside Italy. Sestante CIT (Compagnia Italiana di Turismo) offices have extensive information on Sicily, can organize tours, book hotels, make train reservations, sell Eurail and train passes. Their offices include:

- **Australia** – Sydney: Level 2, 263 Clarence Street, NSW, 2000, ☎ 02-9267-1255, fax 02-9261-4664. Melbourne: Level 4, 227 Collins Street, VIC 3000, ☎ 03-9650-5510, fax 03-9654-2490.
- **Canada** – 7007 Islington Avenue, Suite 205, Woodbridge, Ontario L4L 4T5, ☎ 905-264-0158, cittours@cittours-canada.com.
- **UK and Ireland** – Marco Polo House, 3-5 Lansdowne Road, Croydon, Surrey CR9 1LL, ☎ 020-8686-0677, 8686-5533.
- **USA** – Level 10, 15 West 44th Street, New York, NY 10036, ☎ 212-730-2121.

Maps

The best map of Sicily is published by the Touring Club Italiano (www.touringclub.it, *Sicilia*, 1:200,000). It costs €7 and can be found in bookshops, airports and tourist outlets in Sicily or at Amazon.com. A legend explains the symbols in Italian, English, German, Spanish and French. Likewise, the Touring Club produces maps to Mt Etna (*Parco dell'Etna*, 1:50,000), the Nebrodi and Madonie parks.

Other maps include the *Sicily International Road* (Hammond International) with city and regional insets, the Michelin *Sicily Map No. 432* and other maps by Rough Guides and Insight Guides. The AA produces the *Road Atlas Italy* and Michelin also has a *Road Atlas* at a scale of 1: 300,000 and a *Motoring Atlas*.

Local tourist offices can also hand out reasonable town plans and regional maps and you'll find the maps in this guide should be fine for most purposes. You can also purchase maps on www.amazon.com.

Useful Websites

General Sites

- **www.bestofsicily.com** – Comprehensive website with everything from nature, history and politics to sights, tours, eating, shopping and accommodation.

- **www.initaly.com** – Thousands of pages written by Italians and travelers, recognized by the Italian Government Tourist Board.

- **www.siciliaonline.it** – Italian language site with daily weather news, travel information, school and work information.

- **www.backpackitaly.com** – City guides to Catania and Palermo plus all-around travel advice about Italy for independent travelers.

- **www.cts.it** – CTS (Centro Turistico Studentesco e Giovanile) is a student travel organization. The site is mostly in Italian, listing special offers and travel information.

- **www.sicilianculture.com** – Details cultural aspects of Sicilian life including food and drink, people, history, language, music, dance and other traditions.

- **www.parks.it** – Sicily's national and regional parks, protected areas and more.

- **www.emmeti.it/welcome/sicilia/index.uk.html** – Accommodation, restaurants, cooking and tourist information on Sicily and Italy.

Regional Information

- **www.regionesicilia.it** – Regione Sicilia provides information about offices and government on the island and tourism. Mostly in Italian.

- **www.aaptit.pa.it** and **www.palermotourism.com** – Official website of the AAPIT in Palermo with city news, time tables and events. In English, French, German and Italian.

- **www.apt.catania.it** or **www.provincia.catania.it** – Information on the province of Catania.

- **www.apt-siracusa.it** or **www.provincia.siracusa.it** – Hospitality, transport, itineraries and maps for the province of Siracusa.

- **www.apt.trapani.it** or **www.provincia.trapani.it** – Official website of the APT Trapani.

- **www.provincia.agrigento.it** – Official site of the province of Agrigento.

- **www.provincia.enna.it** or **www.apt-enna.com** – Sites about Enna and the region.

- **www.provincia.messina.it** – Messina.

- **www.provincia.ragusa.it** or **www.ragusaturismo.com** – Information on the province of Ragusa.
- **www.provincia.cl.it** or **www.aapit.cl.it** – Information on the province of Caltanisetta.
- **www.isole-sicilia.it** – Information on all the Sicilian islands including the Aeolians, Egadi, Pelagian, Pantelleria, Ustica and Mozia.

Transport

- **www.alitalia.it** – Italian national air carrier.
- **www.trenitalia.com** – Train website for Italy in Italian and English. Check times and prices and Italian rail passes.
- **www.traghetti.com** – Links to all ferries servicing Sicily.
- **www.saisautolinee.it** – Sicilian bus service details online including time tables and prices.
- **www.interbus.it** – Sicilian bus carrier. Timetables and prices listed online.
- **www.aziendasicilianatrasporti.it** – Hours and routes of the AST (Azienda Siciliana Trasporti) buses that service major cities in Sicily.

Accommodation

- **www.camping.it/sicilia** – Italian campsite and tourist resort web site in English, French, German and Italian.
- **www.ostellionline.org** – Listing of hostels in Italy.
- **www.thinksicily.com** – Apartments and flats for rent around the island.
- **www.specialplacestostay.com** – English travel guide with online listings of quality farm stays, bed and breakfasts and hotels all personally inspected.
- **www.hostelworld.com** – Online booking engine to secure accommodation in a range of categories.

Other

- **www.paginegialle.it** – Italian yellow pages online.
- **www.paginebianche.it** – Italian white pages online.
- **www.enit.it** – Italian State Tourist Office site.

Useful Books

Walking in Sicily by Gillian Price (2002, www.cicerone-guides.co.uk) has excellent walking itineraries around the island with helpful transport and accommodation information. Regione Sicilia produces ***The Archipelago of the Sun*** (2002) with information covering all of Sicily and the islands. Each of the nine provincial tourism

offices (APT) produce their own material, including a guide to accommodation in the region. The Palermo tourist office in particular has an amazing array of literature. The Touring Club Italiano (www.touringclub.it) not only produces maps but also guides to the regions and provinces. Their red hard-back *Sicily* (€46.50) is considered by many the definitive guide to visiting the island. *The Madonie Park* by Francesco Alaimo lists excursions and information about the Parco Madonie. It sells for €10 in tourist and park offices. For specific dining information you'd want to consider *Gambero Rosso* (www.gamberorosso.it) selections on wines and food. *Jamie's Italy* by famed English chef Jamie Oliver (2005) is also a good look at eating in Italy with some detail on Sicily locations.

Newspapers & Magazines

The Sicilian daily is *Il Giornale di Sicilia* and you should find this everywhere. The *Gazzetta dello Sport* is also commonly found, recognizable for its pink color and sport news. Each city has its own press (see sections of this guide for details). These are useful for transport timetables, concerts, film listings and local news. For example in Catania there is *La Sicilia* and in Messina *La Gazzetta del Sud*. National papers like Milan's *Corriere della Sera* (authoritative, right-wing), Turin's *La Stampa* and Rome's *La Repubblica* (middle to left wing) each publish a Sicilian edition. Other papers include *L'Unita*, a former Communist Party organ and *Il Manifesto*, a more radical and readable left-wing daily.

If you're looking for English-language newspapers, these are usually found in big cities like Palermo, Catania, Messina, Taormina and Cefalù. Check shops in the train station and the main piazza or corso. They are usually a few days late.

TV & Radio

Italian television may not be your bag but it's worth a look to see what the locals watch. Television in Italy is deregulated. The three state-run channels are RAI 1, 2 and 3 and face tough competition from independent operators headed by former Prime Minister Silvio Berlusconi, who owns Canale 5, Italia 1 and Rete 4. Most television output includes an endless array of Italian cabaret shows, game shows and variety programs that are all equally appalling. The RAI channels tend

to have some more serious reporting and news, RAI 3 in particular has some interesting programs.

As with television there are three state-owned radio stations (RAI-I 1332 AM or 89.7 FM), RAI-2 (846 AM or 91.7 AM) and RAI-3 (93.7 FM) which have classical and light music with news broadcasts and discussion programs. Most of the other programs feature nonstop dance music and lots of advertising.

Sicilian radio stations include RGS (Radio Giornale di Sicilia) available at 102.7 in Palermo, 107.9 in Messina and 100.6 in Catania. See www.rgs.fm for more information. The station features sports news and all the usual popular music.

■ Top 20 Things to Do

There's so much to see and do, eat and drink, snorkel and hike, and celebrate in Sicily and you can't do it all in one trip! So here's a look at 20 highlights of a visit to the island.

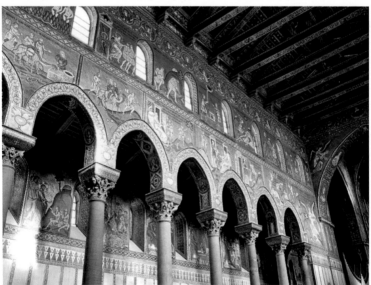

The church in Monreale (Galen R Frysinger, www.galenfrysinger.com)

1. **Monreale** – The breathtaking mosaics in the church at Monreale near Palermo are among the most important in the Christian world. Their vibrant colors and detail are a tribute to their medieval craftsmen.

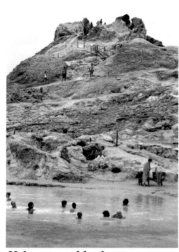

Volcano mud baths (Joanne Lane)

2. **Thermal Bathing** – The *fangi* or thermal baths on Volcano in the Aeolian Islands are a surreal experience for images of wallowing mud-smeared tourists, the aromas of the foul-smelling sulphur, and the fantastic benefits for skin and arthritic complaints. It's a perfect way to recover from long travel days.

3. **Mount Etna** – The slopes of the slumbering giant volcano are a fantastic place to hike, mountain bike, ski, 4WD and explore. The volcano dominates much of the eastern side of the island and its formidable presence is everywhere in the lava buildings and volcanic ash that covers all the surrounding towns with a thin layer of dust.

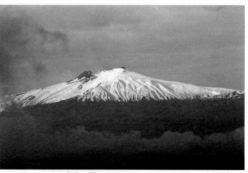

Mt. Etna (Joanne Lane)

4. **Granita** – This refreshing ice drink is commonly drunk in the summer months with the crushed ice topped by fresh lemon or other fruit juices and sometimes topped by fresh whipped cream *(panna)*. It's a real thirst quencher with a zip. Locals will recommend where you might find vendors for the best *granite*.

5. **Parco dello Zingaro** – Picture delightful swimming coves, gravel beaches, unspoiled country and pristine blue ocean. That's what you'll find at Parco dello Zingaro. The park is accessible only by foot. This is one of Sicily's most beautiful coastal regions, stretching seven km from near Scopello to just south of San Vito Lo Capo.

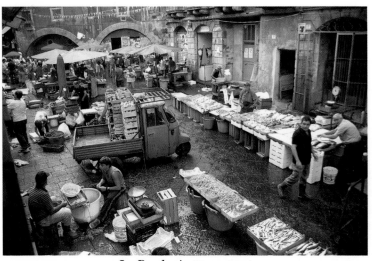

La Pescheria (Joanne Lane)

6. **La Pescheria** – Catania's fishermen's market comes alive every morning with the cries of salesmen, the hustle of shoppers and every type of seafood imaginable.

7. **Palio dei Normanni** – This annual August festival in Piazza Armerina is a colorful pageant of medieval costumes, re-enacted battles, and horsemanship as the four districts of the town compete for the coveted Palio banner.

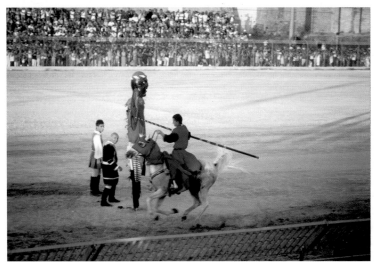

Palio, Piazza Armerina (Joanne Lane)

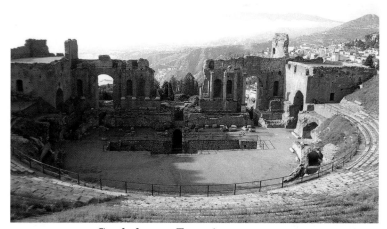

Greek theater, Taormina (Joanne Lane)

8. Greek Theater – Taormina's Greek theater has one of the most stunning locations in the world, with views of both Mt Etna and the jeweled sea below. It is still used frequently for concerts and theater.

9. Parco Regionale delle Madonie and **Parco dei Nebrodi** – It's impossible to list one of these fabulous woodlands without mentioning the other, even though they are remarkably different. Nebrodi has 140,000 acres of woodland and is home to much wildlife, including the beautiful San Fratello horses as well as many wild pigs and goats that like crossing the road. The Monti Madonie on the other hand is

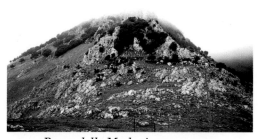

Parco delle Madonie (Joanne Lane)

the place to ski during the winter months from Piano Battaglia. It is equally popular in summer for picnicking and hiking.

10. **La Scala, Caltagirone** – The 142 stairs decorated with hand-painted designs are a testament to the skills of Sicily's ceramic artists. During the annual Festival of St James on July 24 and 25 every

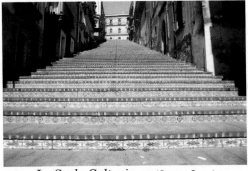

La Scala Caltagirone (Joanne Lane)

year, the stairs are lit by thousands of colored paper lamps.

11. **Ginostra** – This tiny hamlet on Stromboli is a world removed from the bustle of crowds that come to the island to do the night ascent of the active volcano. Ginostra seems almost forgotten by the modern world with donkeys tethered outside houses, craggy-bearded men, white terraced houses, limited electricity and services. The perfect hideaway.

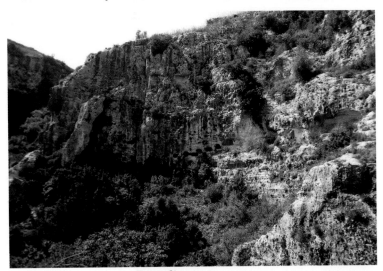

Pantalica (Joanne Lane)

12. **Pantalica** – This high ravine is spectacular enough on its own but has the added attraction of prehistoric tombs that litter the sheer walls. Trails follow the valley floor between refreshing swimming holes and up to the higher reaches of the ravine.

13. Snorkeling at Isola Bella – This tiny isle is one of the most photographed spots on the eastern coast and is a fantastic snorkeling location that can be easily reached from Taormina or Catania. The water here is remarkably clear and you can explore the grottoes in a pedal boat or by swimming.

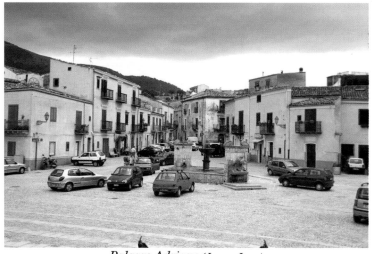

Palazzo Adriano (Joanne Lane)

14. Palazzo Adriano – The delightful medieval square of Palazzo Adriano was made famous by Giuseppe Tornatore's 1989 classic *Cinema Paradiso*. It must be Sicily's largest town square. Its cobbled stone pavement is lined with churches.

15. Tempi di Agrigento – One of the world's most important archaeological sites is a feast of columns, altars, statues and stone amidst a countryside of blooming almond trees.

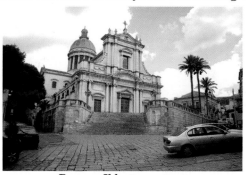

Ragusa Ibla (Joanne Lane)

16. Ragusa Ibla – In the heart of Baroque country, Ragusa Ibla is a delightful maze of narrow streets, steep inclines and houses stacked one on top of the other. It's also the filming location for one of

Sicily's popular television series, *Inspector Montalbano.*

17. **Capo Passero** – The southernmost tip of Sicily is more Arab than European in appearance, with dome-shaped houses, swirling Saharan sirocco winds and archetypal fishing villages, such as Portopalo di Capo Passero. The local tuna fishery flourished here for most of the last century. It is owned by the Baron of Belmonte and is open to the public.

18. **Birdwatching at Vendicari Riserva** – This narrow strip of marshy coastline provides a rare and protected habitat for migratory species, including flamingos, grey herons, little egrets, white and black storks and ducks. There's also pleasant walking, beaches and an old tuna fishery, *la tonnara.*

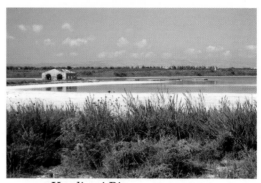

Vendicari Riserva (Joanne Lane)

19. **Gola di Alcantara** – This deep gorge invites a picnic, a swim if you can bear the freezing water, or even a hike past the boulders and waterfalls.

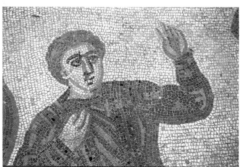

Mosaic at Villa del Casale (Joanne Lane)

20. **Villa Romana del Casale** – The mosaics discovered at this Roman villa near Piazza Armerina date from the fourth century AD and are unrivaled for their quality and extent.

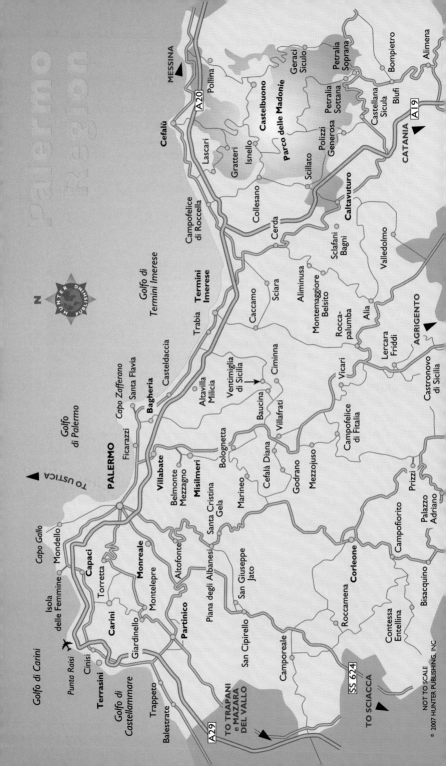

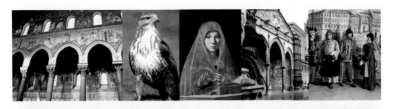

Palermo

The capital of Sicily is immediately enticing despite its frenetic traffic, pollution and heady markets. It's an exciting, in-your-face and up-your-nose kind of city that's brash, fast and loveable – one of those places that is both loathed and loved in almost the

same heartbeat. Jamie Oliver accurately described it as "modern-day anarchy" when he toured in 2005 writing and filming *Jamie's Italy* (BBC). There is crumbling architectural wealth, the diversity of multi-ethnic communities, an energetic population, tantalizing markets and wonderful coastlines, with the island of Ustica lying just off the coast. You can also retreat to the heights of Monte Pellegrino to the north or to the fine beach of Mondello.

However, don't be fooled by the romantic side of the island capital. The pleasant squares with kids playing soccer during school hours usually signal that it's a low-income area. In the city center there are crime problems and even acts of terrorism. A bomb exploded near the APT in 2005. It's not the safest place in the world.

Palermo began in the eighth century BC when Phoenicians established a trading post here and it became the Carthaginian center of Sicily. In 254 BC the Romans arrived and power shifted to Syracuse as Palermo fell into a decline. Throughout the centuries Palermo has hosted the Vandals, the Ostrogoths and the Arabs, who built the beautiful mosques and palaces. When the Arabs retreated in the 11th century the Norman period began – possibly Palermo's finest era. In 1208 Palermo became the capital of the Holy Roman Empire – the highest pinnacle in the ancient world. Then the French Angevins came to the throne, followed by the Spanish

Aragonese, and Palermo lost its power and prestige. During WWII the city was targeted by the Allies stationed in North Africa and many neighborhoods still retain the bombing damage. The postwar years were marred by Mafia corruption, although officials are now trying to fight their insidious influence and regain some of the city's architectural heritage with restoration works on Teatro Massimo and the Kalsa district, among the most recent projects.

The famed German poet Johann Wolfgang Goethe came to Palermo in 1768 and wrote that the city was "easy to grasp in its overall plan, but difficult to get to know in detail." His description wouldn't be too far off today but we hope our guide will help you discover some of the city's intricacies.

PALERMO HIGHLIGHTS

■ **Monreale** – The ceiling of the church at Monreale in the heights above the city is a stunning example of medieval workmanship, with some of the most important of Christian mosaics in the world.

■ **Vucciria Market** – The heady delights of Palermo are best experienced on foot in this bustling age-old market. Let your feet do the walking past stalls selling everything from film, batteries and electrical cord to mouth-watering delicacies like sun-dried tomatoes, eggplant and home-made pasta.

■ **Mondello** – The pleasant beachfront, with fine seafood dining on ceramic plates, is a good excursion from the capital.

■ **Monte Pellegrino** – Escape from the hustle and bustle of Palermo into the pleasant park area to the sanctuary on top. Bus it or walk to stretch your legs.

■ **Ustica** – The turtle-shaped island off the coast is a pleasant day-escape from the busy capital. Its sparkling clear waters are perfect for scuba-diving.

■ **Monte Iato** – This small mountain 30 km west of Palermo is a rocky slope littered with the remains of ancient cities in one of the region's most beautiful areas.

■ **Getting Here**

By Air

 There are no direct intercontinental flights to Palermo but you can get a connecting flight in Rome or Milan via Alitalia (www.alitalia.com) or Sardinia Meridiana (www.meridiania.it). In summer there are charter flights from European centers like London, although Ryan Air now offers regular services from London Stansted to Palermo. Flights to/from mainland Italy connect with Ancona, Bergamo, Bologna, Florence, Forli, Gennova, Lampedusa, Milan, Naples, Pantelleria, Pisa, Rome, Turin, Venice and Verona. There are also regular flights to Cologne, Hannover, London Stansted, Madrid, Monaco, Paris, Stockholm, Tunis and Zurich. For more information, see the *Getting There* section at the beginning of the guide.

The **Aeroporto Falcone Borsellino** or **Punta Raisi** (☎ 091-702-0127, toll-free 800-541-880, www.gesap.it) is 30 km from the center of Palermo on the *autostrada* A29 Trapani-Mazara del Vallo. Airlines serving the airport include:

- Alitalia (☎ 848-865-649, www.alitalia.com)
- Alpi Eagles (☎ 899-500-058, www.alpieagles.com)
- Air Malta (☎ 091-625-5848, www.airmalta.com)
- Air-One (☎ 091-702-0368, www.flyairone.it)
- Meridiana (☎ 091-652-5020, www.meridiana.it)
- Ryan Air (☎ 899-899-844, www.ryanair.com)
- Tunis air (☎ 091-611-1845)
- Volare – AirEurope (☎ 800-454-000)
- Wind Jet (☎ 095-723-458)
- Gruppo Volare (☎ 091-702-0294)
- Mistral Air (☎ 06-790-451)
- Spanair (www.spanair.com)
- eVOLAvia (☎ 899-000-929, www.eVOLAvia.com)
- Hapag-Lloyd (☎ 199-192-692)
- Helvetic (☎ 02-6968-2684, www.helvetic.com)
- MyAir (☎ 899-500-060, www.myair.com)

Buses and trains operate to and from the airport; see the sections below.

By Bus

 The main intercity bus station is east of the train station on Via Paolo Balsamo. Most of the bus companies have offices in this area. For a full list of their addresses and telephone numbers see the Palermo Tourism website (www.palermoturismo.com) or their booklet, *Agenda Turismo*.

Autolinea Prestia e Comande (☎ 091-580-457) blue buses connect the airport with the Stazione Centrale FS in 50 minutes. The stop is outside on your right as you leave the station. The route runs from Hotel Elena in Piazza Giulio Cesare outside the station to the airport with one stop at Hotel Politeama on Via Lazio angolo Via Liberta-Via Belgio. Departures are every 30 minutes at 5 am-11 pm from the city and 6:30 am-12 pm midnight from the airport. Allow an hour to reach the airport.

The **Autolinea S.A.L.** (Via 25 Aprile, Agrigento, ☎ 0922-401-360) links the airport with Agrigento and Porto Empedocle. The service runs at 12:45 pm and 7:30 pm from the Palermo airport (daily, 2½ hrs, €8.60).

Segesta (Viale dei Picciotti, ☎ 091-616-7919) links the airport to Trapani once daily at 12:45 pm (70 mins, €6.40) and also has a daily service direct to Rome.

Autolinee Gallo (☎ 091-617-1141, www.saistrasporti.it) runs from the airport to Sciacca and Ribera at 2:55 pm daily (1½-two hrs; €7.25 to Ribera; €6.40 to Sciacca).

Bus Salemi (☎ 0923-981-1120, www.autoservizisalemi.it) has a service from the airport to Castelvetrano (12 daily, 50 mins, €5.80), Mazara del Valo (two hrs five mins, €6.95) and Marsala (two hrs 35 mins, €7.50).

Cuffaro (Via Balsamo, ☎ 091-616-1510) has services to Agrigento (seven daily, two hours), while **Camilleri** (Via R. Gregorio, ☎ 091-617-1861) operates four daily services.

Salemi (Via R Gregorio, ☎ 091-617-5411) operates to Marsala (16 daily, two hours).

SAIS (Via Balsamo, ☎ 091-616-6028) goes to Piazza Armerina (five daily, two hours 20 mins, €10.30) and Catania departing every hour from 5 am-10 pm. Connections from Catania can take you on to Taormina.

Tarantola (Stazione Centrale, ☎ 0924-31020) runs to Segesta (three daily).

Interbus (Via Balsamo, ☎ 091-616-9039) goes to Siracusa (three hrs 15 mins, three daily).

AST (☎ 0931-462-711, www.aziendasicilianatrasporti.it) operates to Catania (14 daily), Ragusa (five daily), Corleone (nine daily), Cefalù, Palazzo Adriano (two daily) and Montelepre (seven daily).

By Train

 All trains arrive and leave from Stazione Centrale (☎ 892-021, www.trenitalia.com) in Piazza Giulio Cesare at the southern end of Via Roma. There is left luggage, railway police and also tourist information services (see *Information Sources* below) at the station. Some trains do stop at Stazione Notarbartolo in the northwest of the city, but if you want the central station stay on the train. Trains arrive and depart to/from Reggio di Calabria, Naples and Rome and for destinations around Sicily such as Messina, Catania, Siracusa and Agrigento.

The **Trinacria Express** (☎ 091-704-4007) operates to and from the airport and Stazione Centrale FS in 45 minutes (hourly, €5). It runs at 4:45 am-9:40 pm from the central station; and at 5:32 am-10:55 pm from the airport.

By Ferry/Hydrofoil

 All ferry services dock at Stazione Marittima off Via Francesco Crispi, about a 10-minute walk to/from the city center. Services connect Palermo to Naples, Livorno, Genoa, Rome, Cagliari and Salerno. There is a baggage deposit in operation here from 7 am-8 pm daily and an Internet point and phone center (9 am-1 pm, 4-7 pm).

Grandi Navi Veloci (☎ 091-587-801, www.gnv.it) operates from Palermo to Genoa (daily except Monday) and Livorno (Tues, Thurs and Sat night). **Grimaldi GNV** (☎ 091-611-3691, www.grimaldi.it) has services between Palermo and Civitavecchia (near Rome), Salerno and Genoa. **Tirrenia** (☎ 091-602-1235, www.tirrenia.it) runs between Palermo and Naples and Cagliari. **SNAV** (☎ 091-631-7900, www.snav.it) operates ships to Naples.

Palermo is also linked to the Aeolian Islands (**Ustica Lines**, ☎ 0923-873-813, www.usticalines.it) and Ustica (**Siremar**, ☎ 199-123-199, www.gruppotirrenia.it/siremar) in Sicily.

See the *Getting There* section at the beginning of the Guide for more details on services from Palermo to destinations outside Sicily.

Palermo

Car & Motorcycle

Driving into Palermo is traumatic at best and not recommended. Not only are the roads busy and fast but the directional signs are confusing. The city is accessible via the A20 from Messina and the A19 from Catania (208 km). The A29 runs from Palermo to Trapani and Mazara del Vallo (also for the Birgi airport). Agrigento and Palermo are linked by the SS121 through the interior of the island. Look for signs saying *centro* or *stazione centrale* to get to the inner city.

Car rental agencies available at the airport include:

- **Avis**, ☎ 091-591-684
- **Hertz**, ☎ 091-213-112
- **Maggiore**, ☎ 091-591-681
- **Auto Europe**, ☎ 091-591-250

There are Avis, Only Rent, Italy by Car and Maggiore offices at the port. At Notarbartolo train station you can find Europcar and Maggiore offices. A local rental car agency is **Alfa Car Rental** which rents cars and scooters (Via Emerico Amari 91, ☎ 091-602-3455, www.alfacarrental.com).

■ Getting Around

By Air

You can actually rent helicopters and planes in Palermo, with the correct documents, of course. Go to **Aeroambulanza**, Via Marchese di Roccaforte (☎ 091-586-031, 091-6257-575).

By Train

Palermo has a *metropolitana* (metro) system that runs from 6:10 am-10:35 pm about every 25 minutes. A single fare of 120 minutes travel time is €1. For more information call FS ☎ 848-888-088. You can also contact the Stazione Centrale for information (☎ 091-603-1111, www.palermocentrale.it).

By Bus

AMAT (☎ 091-690-2690, www.amat.pa.it) operates the city buses. AMAT booths can sell tickets, provide a small book of routes and parking tickets.

Centro Storico (historic center). . . . . €.52
120-minute ticket . . . . €1 (can be used on the metro)
One-day ticket. €3.35
20 x 120-minute tickets. €18.10
20 x one-day tickets €43.60

Key bus routes include Catacombe Cappucini (327) and Monreale (389) from Piazza Indipendeza; Mondello (806) and Monte Pellegrino (812) from Piazza Sturzo; Sferracavallo (628) from Piazzale De Gasperi; and the Circolare servizio (101) from Stazione Centrale. This latter service does not run between midnight and 4 am.

Other buses operating in the city include the **Circolare Minibus** (one-day tickets €.52), the **Linea Rossa** (every 10 mins) from S. Domenico to Croci and Stazione FS; and **Linea Gialla** (every 15 mins) from Stazione FS to Oreto, Policlinico, Ballaro, Piazza Pretoria, Via Alloro, Kalsa and Orto Botanico.

City Sightseeing Worldwide (☎ 091-589-429, Piazza Castelnuovo 6, www.palermo.city-sightseeing.it) operates two tours in Palermo in their distinctive red open-top buses. The first is the Historical Town Tour (Red Line) from Piazza Politeama to Teatro Massimo, Quattro Canti, botanical gardens, Royal Palace, Cathedral, Vucciria market and the port (every 30-60 minutes). The second route is the Villas & Zisa Castle (Blue Line) from Politeama Theater to the English Garden, Villa Malfitano, Zisa Castle, Mercato del Capo, Teatro Massimo and the port (every 60 minutes). Buy your tickets on board, in hotels or authorized agencies (€20 for adults, €10 for children age five-15).

By Taxi

Taxi ranks are available at the airport (☎ 091-591-662), Stazione Centrale (☎ 091-616-001) and Notarbartolo Station (☎ 091-343-506).

Palermo

By Car & Motorcycle

 Driving around Palermo is not advised unless you've survived other Italian cities like Rome or Naples. There's an incredible labyrinth of one-way streets, with fast-moving traffic, and Palermitans do not seem to respect road rules. Theft of and from vehicles is a big problem, as is parking. You should use an attended car park if your hotel has no parking space. It costs from €1/hr. Street parking in Palermo is €.75/hr, 8 am-10 pm.

There are some paid parking places at Stazione Centrale, Piazza G. Cesare 43 and at L'Oasis Verde, Corso Tukory 207. You can also find places near the port in Via Guardione 81 and Via Stabile 10. In the town center, options include Via Abela 13, Via Agrigento 42, Via Belmonte 18 and Piazzetta Parlatoio 6 (Corso Emanuele).

If you're in a camper and need a spot to pull up, there are two major spots: **Camper Service** (Piazza Giotto, ☎ 091-7291-111) costs €18.59 for daily parking, electricity and a daily bus ticket. Water supplements are €4.13. **Area Attrezzata Parcheggio Camper Custodito** (Via dell'Osa Maggiore 11, ☎ 380-3577-231) costs €7 daily for water, lights and battery. You can pay also by the hour or monthly.

Motorbikes can be rented from any of the following companies:

- **Motorent**, Via E. Amari (☎ 091-602-3455)
- **Rent a Scooter**, Via S. Meccio 10 (☎ 091-336-804)
- **Sicily By Car**, Via M. Stabile 6/a (☎ 091-581-045)

By Bike

 You can rent bikes from:
   - **Toto Cannatella**, Via Papireto 14 (☎ 091-322-425)
   - **Kursaal Kalhesa**, Foro Umberto I 21 (☎ 091-616-2828)
- **Bio Eco Ambiente**, Via Marchese Ugo (in front of Giardino Inglese)
- **Bici Rent**, with three locations in Giardino Inglese, Via Magliocco and Piazza Unita d'Italia (9 am-7 pm)
- **Western Union office**, cruise terminal, €6/day
- **Hotel Letizia**, Via dei Botai 30 (☎ 091-589-110)

■ Information Sources

 AAPIT Palermo (Piazza Castelnuovo 35, ☎ 091-7020-289, www.palermotourism.com, Mon-Fri 8 am-midnight, Sat and Sun 8 am-10 pm) is the most efficient tourist office in all of Sicily. Their staff can and will help you with just about anything. The **APT** office at Stazione Centrale is open Mon-Fri 8:30 am-2 pm, 2:30-6 pm (☎ 091-616-5914). The **Assessorato Turismo Comune di Palermo** (Mon-Sat, 9 am-1 pm, 3-7 pm, closed Sun and holidays) has a kiosk in Piazza Politeama for concert, museum, map, hotel and transport information.

If you want any Palermo publications, have a look for any of the following: *Agenda*, *Un Ospite a Palermo* (listing events, museums, taxi, flight timetable and more free in hotels), *Lapis* (free biweekly street press listing cultural events, live music, cinema, bars and clubs; www.lapisnet.it) or *Il Giornale di Sicilia* (daily newspaper of Sicily). These publications are available from tourist information points or newsagents.

■ Events

Palermo's Biggest Party

How many saints can a city have? Well, in Palermo there are 20 "ordinary" saints, 15 "principal" saints, four female "patron saints" (see the *Quattro Canti*) and the one that watches over them all – Santa Rosalia. Santa Rosalia is believed to have saved the people of Palermo from the plague in 1624. And from July 11th to 15th each year in sweltering heat the people of the city celebrate the Festa di Santa Rosalia. The saint's relics are paraded through the city for four days along with fireworks, partying and general pandemonium. It's a good time to visit if you can find a bed and join in the music, food and general fun. A note for the curious – Sicily has almost 700 saints for its 389 towns.

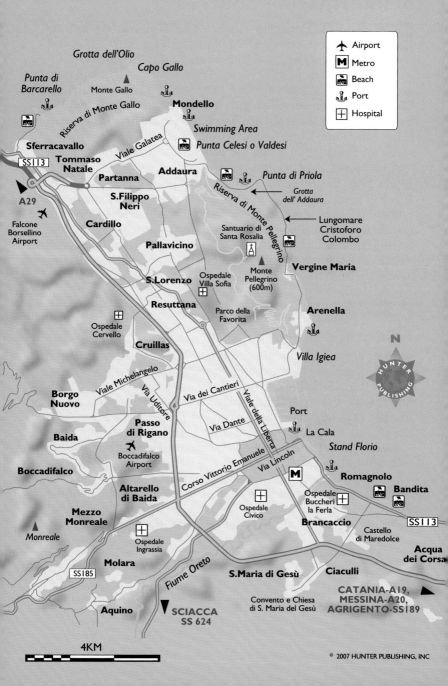

Palermo

Grotta dell'Olio

Capo Gallo

Punta di Barcarello

Monte Gallo

Riserva di Monte Gallo

Mondello

Swimming Area

Sferracavallo

Viale Galatea

Punta Celesi o Valdesi

SS113

Tommaso Natale

Addaura

Punta di Priola

Partanna

Riserva di Monte Pellegrino

Grotta dell' Addaura

A29

S.Filippo Neri

Santuario di Santa Rosalia

Lungomare Cristoforo Colombo

Falcone Borsellino Airport

Cardillo

Pallavicino

Monte Pellegrino (600m)

Vergine Maria

Ospedale Villa Sofia

S.Lorenzo

Resuttana

Parco della Favorita

Arenella

Ospedale Cervello

Cruillas

Villa Igiea

N

HUNTER PUBLISHING

Viale Michelangelo

Via Uditore

Via dei Cantieri

Viale della Libertà

Borgo Nuovo

Port

Passo di Rigano

Via Dante

La Cala

Baida

Boccadifalco Airport

Stand Florio

Boccadifalco

Corso Vittorio Emanuele

Via Lincoln

M

Romagnolo

Bandita

Altarello di Baida

Ospedale Civico

Ospedale Buccheri la Ferla

Mezzo Monreale

Brancaccio

SS113

Monreale

Ospedale Ingrassia

Castello di Maredolce

Acqua dei Corsa

Molara

Fiume Oreto

S.Maria di Gesù

Ciaculli

SS185

CATANIA-A19, MESSINA-A20, AGRIGENTO-SS189

Aquino

SCIACCA SS 624

Convento e Chiesa di S. Maria del Gesù

4KM

© 2007 HUNTER PUBLISHING, INC

Legend:
✈ Airport
M Metro
Beach
⚓ Port
⊞ Hospital

■ Sightseeing

COMMON PALERMO SIGHTS

- An entire family on one scooter with mum, dad, kids and shopping bags.
- Kids playing soccer in the street.
- Traffic jams.
- Bustling markets.
- Fresh octopus or sea urchins sliced and doused in lemon.
- Granite drink stalls in summer.
- Dog poo on the pavements!
- Three-wheelers laden with things to sell.

Walking the Historical Center

Historic Palermo sits compactly around the central crossroads, the Quattro Canti, which neatly divides the core into four quarters: the Albergheria and Capo, which lie west of Via Maqueda, and the Vucciria and La Kalsa to the east. In the past each quarter was almost a separate entity with its own dialect, trade, palace and market. Today the quarters still retain their medieval character, web-like streets, outstanding art work in hideaway churches and traffic-free alleys. The best way to explore these little streets is on a bicycle or on foot, but

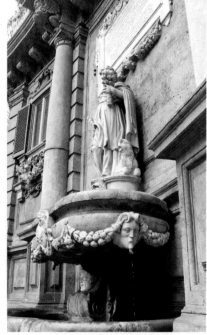

One of the Quattro Canti, detail
(Galen R Frysinger, www.galenfrysinger.com)

Palermo

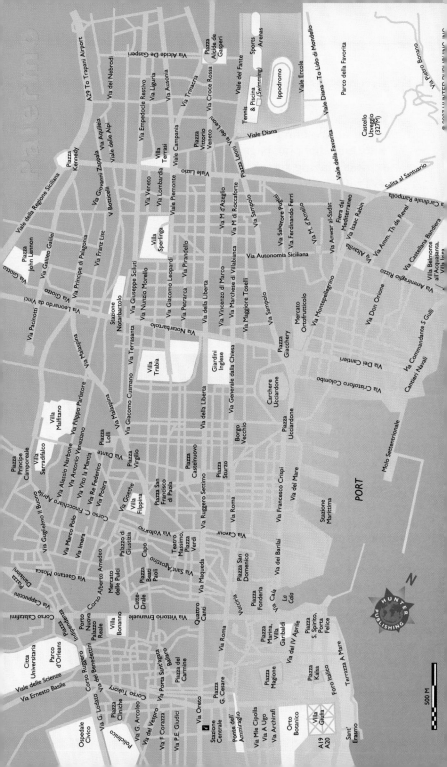

Palermo

A29 To Trapani Airport

Via Alcide De Gasperi

Piazza Alcide de Gasperi

Sports Arenas

Parco della Favoria

Via Piero Bonanno

Via dei Nebrodi

Via Liguria

Via Ausonia

Viale del Fante

Ippodromo

Tennis & Piscina (Swimming)

Castello Utveggio (327h)

Salita al Santuario

Viale Diana - To Lido di Mondello

Viale Ercole

Viale della Favorita

Via Empedocle Restivo

Via Aquileia

Via Trinacria

Via Croce Rossa

Piazza Vittorio Veneto

Viale Diana

Via Giovanni Zappala

Viale delle Alpi

Villa Terrasi

Viale Campania

Via Leoni

Viale della Regione Siciliana

Piazza Kennedy

Via Botticelli

Via Principe di Palagonia

Via Franz List

Via Veneto

Via Lombardia

Viale Piemonte

Via M. d'Azeglio

Via M di Roccaforte

Viale Lazio

Piazza Leoni

'a Cardinale Rampolla

Via Galileo Galilei

Piazza John Lennon

Via Giotto

Villa Sperlinga

Via Giuseppe Scilurt

Via Nunzio Morello

Via Giacomo Leopardi

Via Pirandello

Via Petrarca

Via della Liberta

Via Vincenzo di Marco

Via Marchese di Villabianca

Via Maggiore Toselli

Via Sampolo

Via Salvatore Puo

Via Ferdinando Ferri

Via M. d'Amelio

Via Anwar al-Sadat

Via Isaac Rabin

Fiera del Mediterraneo

Via Amm. Th. De Revel

Via Castellana Bandiera

Villa Belmonte all'Acquasanta

Villa Igiea

Via Leonardo da Vinci

Via Pacinotti

Stazione Notarbartolo

Via Terrasanta

Via Notarbartolo

Villa Trabia

Giardini Inglese

Piazza Giacchery

Mercato Ortofrutticolo

Via Montepellegrino

Via Don Orione

Via Commandante S Gulli

Via Ammiraglio Rizzo

Via Malaspina

Via Giacomo Cusmano

Via Generale dalla Chiesa

Carcere Ucciardone

Via Del Cantieri

Cantieri Navali

Villa Malfitano

Via Filippo Parlatore

Piazza Lolli

Via Dante

Via Virgilio

Piazza Castelnuovo

Via della Liberta

Borgo Vecchio

Piazza Ucciardone

Via Cristoforo Colombo

Molo Settentrionale

Piazza Principe Camporeale

Villa Serradifalco

Via Alessio Narbone

Via Antonio Veneziano

Via Vito la Mantia

Via Re Federico

Via Polara

Via Goethe

Villa Filippina

Piazza San Francisco di Paola

Piazza Sturzo

PORT

Via Gugliemo II Buono

Finocchiaro Aprile

Corso Finocchiaro Aprile

Via Imera

Via Marco Polo

Palazzo di Giustizia

Teatro Massimo, Piazza Verdi

Via Volturno

Via Ruggero Settimo

Via Roma

Via Francesco Crispi

Via del Mare

Stazione Marittima

Piazza Dinshoni

Piazza Cappuccini

Via Gaetano Mosca

Corso Alberto Amedeo

Mercato delle Pulci

Capo

Piazza Beati Paoli

Via Sant'Agostino

Via Maqueda

Piazza San Domenico

Via Cavour

Piazza Fonderia

Via dei Bartiai

'a Cala

La Cala

Corso Calatafimi

Citta Universitaria

Parco d'Orleans

Porta Nuova Palazzo Reale

Piazza Indipendenza

Villa Bonanno

Cattedrale

Via Vittorio Emanuele

Quattro Canti

Via Roma

Vuccirie

Piazza Marina, Villa Garibaldi

Piazza S. Spirito, Porta Felice

Viale delle Scienze

Via Ernesto Basile

Corso Ruggero

Via G. Lodato

Via Benedettini

Corso Tukory

Via Porta Sant'agata

Ballaro

Piazza del Carmine

Piazza Sant'agata

Via del IV Aprile

Piazza Magione

Piazza Kalsa

Foro Italico

Ospedale Civico

Policlinico

Piazza Cliniche

Via G. Arcoleo

Via del Vespro

Via F Corazza

Via P.E. Giudici

Via A Ugo

Stazione Centrale

Ponte dell'Ammiraglio

Via Oreto

Piazza G. Cesare

Via Mle Cipolla

Via Archirafi

Orto Botanico

Villa Giulia

Terrazza A Mare

Sant'Erasmo

A19 A20

N

HUNTER PUBLISHING

500 M

© 2007 HUNTER PUBLISHING, INC.

once you hit the main thoroughfares you'll want to consider some form of transport.

Quattro Canti & Around

The busy intersection of Corso Vittorio Emanuele and Via Maqueda is known as ★Quattro Canti or four corners. It was first laid out in 1608 and finished in 1620 with a Spanish Baroque façade in each corner and three tiers, including a fountain at the bottom. Statues above represent the

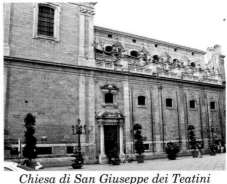

Chiesa di San Giuseppe dei Teatini
(Galen R Frysinger)

four seasons, four Spanish viceroys and the patron saints of the city's four areas. On one of the corners sits the Baroque **Chiesa di San Giuseppe dei Teatini** (Mon-Sat 7:30 am-12 pm, 5:30-8 pm; free) with its elaborate columns, paintings and stuccos, marble floors and domes.

In the nearby **Piazza Pretoria**, a short walk away, you'll see white nude figures in the central fountain that shocked the populace when they were first unveiled in

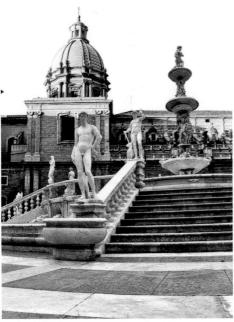

Piazza Pretoria (Galen R Frysinger)

Palermo

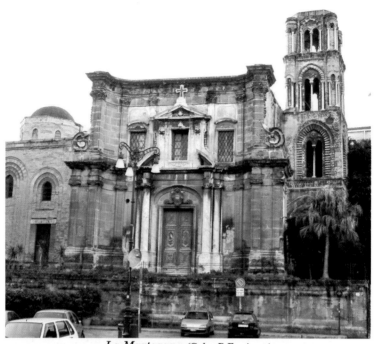

La Martarana (Galen R Frysinger)

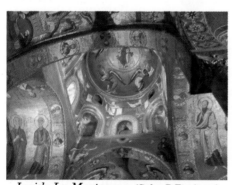

Inside La Martarana (Galen R Frysinger)

1554. They earned the nickname *fontana di vergogna* (Fountain of Shame) and ladies passing by used to cover their eyes. Turning down Via Maqueda you'll come to Piazza Bellini, more like a car park, and the splendid **La Martarana** church (Mon-Sat 8:30 am-1 pm, 3:30-5:30 pm; free). It is next to the **Cheisa di San Cataldo**, named *Martarana* after the famed Palermo sweet (see *Where to Eat*). And once you've seen the interiors you'll see the association with sweets. If you haven't yet been to **Monreale** you'll defi-

nitely find the splen-
did mosaic interior
impressionante. The
architecture is a mix
of Byzantine, Norman
and Baroque. The
beautiful setting is no-
tably popular for wed-
dings and baptisms
when it is closed for
tourists. Along with
mass, these are times
best avoided.

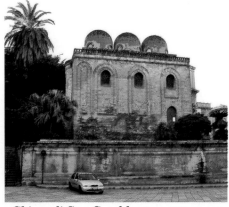

Chiesa di San Cataldo (Galen R Frysinger)

The Albergheria

This district is borded by Via Maqueda and Corso Vittorio
Emanuele northwest of Stazione Centrale and it once housed
the barons and the employees of the Norman court. Most of it
is a warren of streets dominated by a busy street market. In
this tangle of streets are some fine churches and the remnants of World War II bombing that have never been put
right. The shells of buildings are particularly noticeable in
Via Ponticello. Farther up this road is the imposing **Chiesa
del Gesu** or **Casa Professa** (Piazza Casa Professa; Mon-Sat
7-11:30 am, 5-6:30 pm; Sun 7 am-12:30 pm). It was built by
the Jesuit Fathers with the support of the Spanish Viceroy;
the interiors are richly decorated with stucco and inlaid marble.

Farther down Via Ponticello is **Piazza Ballaro** where a lively
fruit and vegetable market fills the streets all the way down
to Piazza del Carmine, past huge, slightly shabby edifices.
This is one of Palermo's best daily markets, known as Ballaro
(7 am-8 pm, Wed 7 am-12 pm), with the cries of street vendors
creating a chatter of noise, great bargains on fresh produce,
and, if you're hungry, it's a good place to sample some local
cuisine, such as *arancini*, fresh octopus or marinated eggplant. In this area the Arab influence is apparent, with street
and café signs written in Italian and Arabic. You may also
hear Arabic spoken in the streets.

From here, head away from Via Maqueda up any of the main
roads to **Via dei Benedittini**, where the other two notable

Palermo

structures in this area can be found. **San Giovanni degli Eremiti** or St John of the Hermits (Mon-Sat 9 am-7 pm, Sun 9 am-1 pm, €4.20) was built in 1132 and today is surrounded by a peaceful garden. It is one of Palermo's most famous Arabic-Norman relics, with five domes topping the church, which was built upon the remains of a mosque. Behind the church on Corso Re Ruggero is **Palazzo d'Orleans**, which is now the official residence of Sicily's president.

Cross the main road and you'll find yourself gaz-

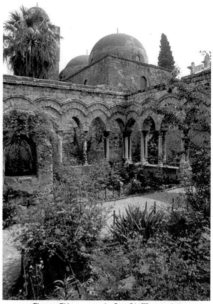

San Giovanni degli Eremiti

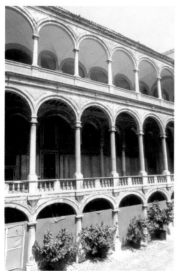

Palazzo dei Normanni

ing at the wonderously enormous **Palazzo dei Normanni** or **Palazzo Reale** (Piazza Indipendenza, ☎ 091-705-7003, Mon-Sat 8:30 am-12 pm, 2-5 pm; Sun 8:30 am-2 pm, €6). The Norman Palace is at the center of the old city and has been used as a residence by just about everyone – the emirs, the Norman kings, Spanish viceroys and, since 1947, has been the seat of the Regional Sicilian Assembly. Tight security checks the crowds of tourists coming here, so expect lines.

Inside the palace is the magnificent ★**Capella Palatina**

(Piazza Indipendenza, ☎ 091-705-6001, Mon-Sat 8:30 am-12 pm, 2-4:30 pm, €4). It's not as large as Monreale but the mosaics are stunning. This was the royal chapel of Roger II, built between 1132 and 1143. It's quite small and can feel crowded even with just one tour group, so come as early in the day as possible or you'll find yourself trying to peer over hordes of camera-touters.

To discover more about the Albergheria district, consider the "A is for Albergheria" tour in the *Adventures on Foot* section later in this chapter.

FILM LOCATIONS IN PALERMO

Palermo's brooding qualities make an excellent backdrop for both Italian and American films.

L'Avventura (1960, Michelangelo Antonioni).

Il Gattopardo (1963, Luchino Visconti) – Casa Professa, Piazza Rivoluzione, in the Kalsa in Piazza S. Giovanni Decollato, Piazza dellaVittoria and Piazza Sant'Euono. The ballroom scene was filmed in Palazzo Valguarnera Gangi.

Tanto da Morire (1997, Roberta Torre) – Vucciria market.

Cada Veri Eccelenti (1976, Francesco Rosi) – Opens in the Convento dei Cappuccini with the macabre images of mummified bodies.

The Talented Mr Ripley (1999, Anthony Minghella) – Gave audiences a brief look at the Sicilian capital when Ripley arrives in Italy at the Art Deco terminal. The "Venetian" church where Smith-Kingsley rehearses the Stabat Mater is in fact the 14th-century Chiesa Martorana in Piazza Bellini.

Jamie's Italy (2005, BBC) - used the Borgo market for the episode where Jamie Oliver learns about street food.

Godfather III (1990, Francis Ford Coppola) – Utilized the long-disused Town Hall for Michael Corleone's return to Sicily; Villa Malfitano; and the stairs of Teatro Massimo for the final scene when Al Pacino's character finally meets his waterloo.

Cattedrale & the Capo

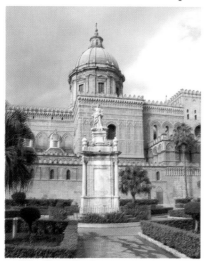

The Cattedrale (Galen R Frysinger)

The Capo area is on the southwestern part of Corso Vittorio Emanuele and if you're at the Palazzo Reale it's a short walk across the Corso. If you loop around the back of the Palazzo you can pass through the Porta Nuova, a gate erected in 1535.

Walking back towards the Quattro Canti you will pass the enormous **Cattedrale** (Corso Vittorio Emanuele, ☎ 091-334-376, 9:30 am-5:30 pm; free), which is set back in gardens on the left side of the Corso. This Norman relic was founded in 1185 but remained unfinished for centuries. Subsequent additions are slightly out of character with the original 12th-century look, creating a hybrid concoction. However, it does remain impressive, with a triple apse on the eastern end, matching towers, a Catalan-Gothic façade, arches and Norman carvings. Latice, columns, bell towers, steeples, domes and mosaics all compete for attention on the outside of the building, making

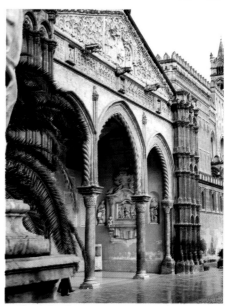

Cattedrale entrance (Galen R Frysinger)

the inside appear plainer by comparison. But there are some interesting attractions inside, including the remains of monarchs in the chapels, the tombs in the crypt and the rings and skullcap removed from the tomb of Constance of Aragon in the 18th century. Access to the tombs is along Via Bonnello.

Strolling up Via Matteo Bonello you'll come to the Mercato delle Pulci (see *Markets* later in this chapter), an open-air market selling antiques and junk in Piazza Peranni. From here,

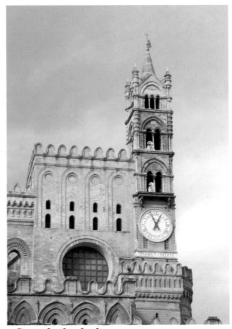

Cattedrale clock tower (Galen R Frysinger)

turn down into the Capo quarter. This is one of Palermo's oldest sections and it's a rather run-down neighborhood of battered buildings, decaying portals and decrepit medieval gates. The central focus is the market that extends on either side of Via Porta Carini and down Via Sant'Agostino. Clothes, shoes, belts, music, clothes, bags, food and the usual market goods are on sale from early morning until 7 pm daily, except on Sunday. Architectural wonders are scarce in the Capo area although you should keep an eye out for **Sant'Agostino** (☎ 091-584-632, Mon-Sat 7 am-12 pm, 4-6 pm; Sun 7 am-12 pm) on Via Raimondo. The church was built in the 13th century by the Charamonte and Sclafani families and includes some superb lattice-work, 16th-century cloisters and sculpted doorways.

The other feature in this area is the massive 19th-century **Teatro Massimo** (Piazza Verdi, ☎ 091-609-0831, Tues-Sun 10 am-3:30 pm, €3). Supposedly, this is the largest theater in Italy and it was recently restored in 1997 after being closed

for many years. Come for a performance – check the schedule online at www.teatromassimo.it for opera or ballet between October and May – or visit during opening hours when you can admire the marble, dome and columns where nobility have gathered for centu-

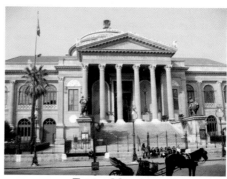

Teatro Massimo

ries. Farther away from Quattro Canti up Via Ruggero Settimo you come to Palermo's other huge theater, the 19th-century **Politeama Garibaldi** in the huge double square of Piazza Politeama (made up of Piazza Castelnuovo and Piazza Ruggero Settimo). This theater is built in Pompeiian style and houses the Galleria d'Arte Moderna (see the *Museums* section later in this chapter). It is only open for performances (☎ 091-605-3315, November-May).

THE ANTICHI MERCATI (OLD MARKETS)

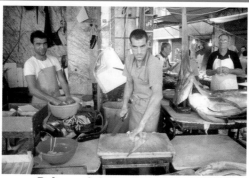

Palermo fish market (Joanne Lane)

Raucous cries of *pesce fresca* (fresh fish) or *pasta fatto a mano* (handmade pasta) ring from Palermo's daily markets – still the life blood of the old city and a huge outdoor supermarket for locals and tourists alike. The streets in this area are like Arab souks with market goods hung or displayed in stalls and stores, cheery vendors and tantalizing aromas. It's

definitely more Algeria or Tunisia than Europe. All Palermo's markets open weekdays from early morning to evening and are closed on holidays.

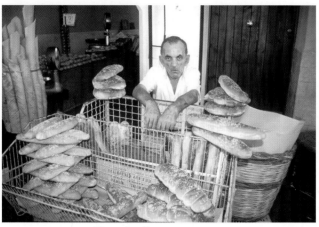

Bread seller (Joanne Lane)

Palermo

★★**La Vucciria** – In Piazza Caracciolo and the surrounding area. The origins of the name suggest it was a butcher's market but today you can find everything: fresh fish, fruit and vegetables, clothes and more. Closes midday Wednesday.

Il Capo – This market extends along Via Sant'Agostino and Via Porta Carini. This market has a bit of everything, with clothes (some second-hand), housewares, plus the usual fruits and vegetables.

Ballaro – The Ballaro market is held in the old Albergheria quarter between Piazza Carmine and Ballaro Square.

Casa Professa – New and used clothes, materials and second-hand goods are sold from near the Piazza outside the church.

I Lattarini – This market is next to Piazza Borsa (Via Roma), where you can find canvas and ropes, wholesalers of wool and cotton for embroidery, underwear, socks, handkerchiefs, hiking clothes, rubber boots, miltary boots, jumpers and knitwear.

Mercato delle Pulci – This flea market in Piazza Domencio Peranni runs weekdays from morning until afternoon selling antiques and modern objects.

Mercatino di Piazza Marina – This market at Piazza Marina is held on Saturday and Sunday selling bric-a-brac and crafts.

Mercatino Antiquariato – Held the first Sunday of the month in Piazza Unita d'Italia (Villa Sperlinga).

Borgo Vecchio – Il Borgo market between Piazza Sturzo and Piazza Ucciardone is the only one in Palermo that stays open late. It attracts a lot of younger people and it's where Jamie Oliver grilled his fish in his recent TV/book series *Jamie's Italy*.

Vucciria & Old Harbor

The Vucciria market starts near the Chiesa di Sant'Antonio on Via Roma just up from Corso Vittorio Emanuele. The winding streets leading down to the harbor are lined by fish stalls, tiny restaurants, junk stores, card players and shoppers, all trying to fight for a spot in the tiny alleyways. It's a cacophony of noise and excitement, especially first thing in the morning and at lunch time when the local restaurants become busy (see *Where to Eat* later in this chapter).

The market also extends to **San Domenico** (☎ 091-329-588, Mon-Sun 9-11:30 am, Sat and Sun 5-7 pm) in Piazza San

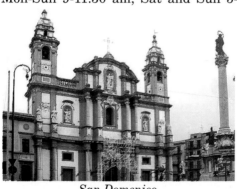

San Domenico

Domenico. The 18th-century façade is best viewed at night when its double pillars and slim towers are lit. Inside are tombs of famous Sicilian parliamentarians, poets and painters. Behind the church on Via Bambinai is the splendid **Oratory of Rosario** (☎ 091-609-0308, Mon-Fri 9 am-11 pm, May-July 9 am-1 pm, closed in August, €2.50). It was constructed in the 16th century and decorated with stuccos by Serpotta. This small chapel contains some of Palermo's best Baroque decora-

tions. Serpotta lined the walls with allegorical features and the altarpiece is by Van Dyck. In the ante-chamber is the story of the Crucifixion.

Another point of interest in this area is the **Piazza Olivella** beyond the imposing **Palazzo delle Poste** (Palermo's main post office) farther up Via Roma. The church of **Sant'Ignazio all'Olivella** displays more of Palermo's Baroque touches. Located nearby is the Museo Archaeologico Regionale (see *Museums*).

La Cala

The area between Via Roma and the waterfront was the most heavily bombed section of the city during WWII and remains one of the poorest areas, although it is now being renovated. Most likely you'll hit the waterfront after following the Vucciria markets through to Piazza Fonderia. From here you can cross Corso Via Vittorio by the church of **Santa Maria della Catena**, named after the chain that used to close the harbor in the 15th century. There are several seafood restaurants in this area (see *Where to Eat*). The Corso ends at **Porta Felice** down at the waterfront. The medieval

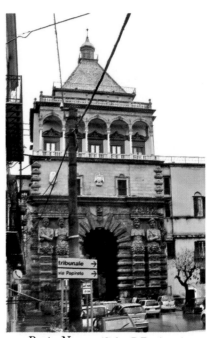

Porta Nuova (Galen R Frysinger)

city once lay between this gate and **Porta Nuova** at the other end of the Corso. As you come down the Corso toward the sea, a road on your right (Via Butera) leads to the delightful **Museo delle Marionette** (see *Museums* later in this chapter), a must for puppet lovers. The area beyond Porta Felice was flattened during the war and has since been rebuilt into a

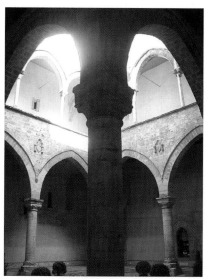

Palazzo Chiaramonte

promenade known as **Foro Italico**. On summer evenings it is particularly busy with strolling locals and *gelateria* stalls.

If you double back along the Corso you'll find the **Giardino Garibaldi** on your left, a tropical parkland once used for jousting tournaments and executions, but now for restaurants and card players. The **Palazzo Chiaramonte** lies on the east side of the square. It was built in the 14th century as a commission by the powerful Baron Manfredi Chairamonte. The family lived there for just 89 years until the last member was beheaded in the square in 1396. Since the family's demise, the Palazzo has had numerous roles. First, it was the seat of the viceroys in Sicily, then home to the Inquisition from 1685 to 1782, the city's law courts until 1972 and now it's the administrative center for the university. It's open to the public for infrequent exhibitions.

La Kalsa

The region between the waterfront and Via Roma on the other side of Corso Vittorio Emanuele is known as La Kalsa. The word Kalsa comes from the Arabic *khalisa*, meaning pure, although that's not an accurate description for this neighbourhood during the last 50 years. It was heavily bombed in WWII and was poverty-stricken. Until recently it was best avoided by tourists, but the creation of park lands on the former bomb sites has given it a face lift and an excellent program of free concerts and recitals is now held in the ruins of the Chiesa di Santa Maria dello Spasimo. You should still avoid the empty streets at night and definitely not venture out at night in this area alone.

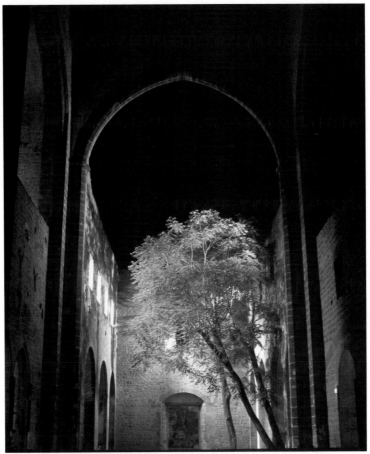

Santa Maria dello Spasimo (Sebastian Fischer)

Lo Spasimo (☎ 091-616-486, Mon-Sun 9 am-11:45 pm) is a complex of buildings south of Piazza Marina along Via della Vetreria. It includes the **Chiesa di Santa Maria dello Spasimo**, built in late Gothic style during the Renaissance. The church has been roofless for centuries and was recently restored and opened to the public as a concert and performance venue. The season runs between June and September.

Beyond the park, **Palazzo Abatellis** on Via Alloro houses Sicily's most important art gallery, **Galleria Regionale** (see *Museums* below). Next door is the 15th-century **Chiesa di Santa Maria degli Angeli** (☎ 091-616-5221, Mon-Fri 9 am-

5 pm, Sat 9 am-1 pm, Sun 10 am-12:30 pm), also known as La Gancia. The church houses an organ dating from 1620, the oldest in Palermo.

Via Alloro is bordered by numerous palazzi and squares of historical importance. **Piazza Croce dei Vespri** has a cross marking the spot where the French died in the 1282 Sicilian Vespers rebellion. On the corner with Via Aragona is the entrance to **Palazzo Valguarnera Gangi**, where the ballroom scene for *The Leopard* was filmed. Turn left into Via Aragona to get to the **Piazza della Rivoluzione**, where a fountain marks the point of the 1848 uprising's start.

Villa Giulia and the **Orto Botanico** are just a few minutes walk from here along Via Lincoln. See *Parks & Gardens* below.

PARKS & GARDENS

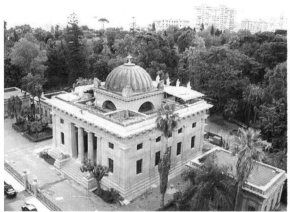

Orto Botanico

Palermo is not all decaying buildings and magnificent edifices. You won't be hard-pressed to find some delightful green areas for a picnic or a respite from the bricks and mortar. Here's a selection:

Parco della Favorita – Palermo's grandest park lies north of the city at the foot of Monte Pellegrino. There are sports grounds and stadiums at one end where Palermo's main soccer team plays and formal gardens beyond. To get here, take bus 101 from the train station to Stadio Partanna where you change for bus 614 or 645. If you want to walk, head out on Via Maqueda toward Giardino Inglese.

Orto Botanico – This botanical garden in the Kalsa area dates from 1795 and features tropical plants from all over the world. Access is on Via Lincoln, 26 (☎ 091-623-8141, Mon-Fri 9 am-8 pm, Sat 9 am-1 pm; €3.50).

Giardino Inglese – This pretty little park lies along Viale della Liberta past Piazza Crispi and is enroute to Parco della Favorita listed above. The two could be part of a combined walking itinerary (☎ 091-702-5471, 8 am-8 pm).

Villa Garibaldi – This park is also in the Kalsa area off Piazza Marina near the harbor. It dates from 1864 and has some huge shady trees.

Villa Giulia – This is another park in the Kalsa area next to the botanic gardens listed above and dates from the 18th century. The park has some deer and a children's play area (Via Lincoln, ☎ 091-740-m.4028, 8 am-8 pm, free).

For a full list of the parks, see www.palermotourism.com.

Museums & Galleries

REDUCED PRICES

European citizens under 18 or over 65 have free entry to the following museums and monuments in Palermo: Galleria Regionale Siciliana, Museo Archeologico Salinas, Palazzo Mirto, Chiostro di Monreale, Castello della Zisa, La Cuba and San Giovanni degli Eremiti. EU citizens between 18 and 25 pay a reduced price. There are also *biglietti cumulativi* (all-in-one tickets) for the following places:

1. Zisa, Cuba, Chiostro Monreale, San Giovanni Eremiti (€12 – valid for two days)
2. Museo Archeologico Regionale Salinas, Galleria Regionale della Sicilia at Palazzo Abatellis, Palazzo Mirto (€12 – valid for two days)
3. Galleria Regionale della Sicilia at Palazzo Abatellis, Palazzo Mirto (€7 – valid for one day)
4. Galleria Regionale della Sicilia in Palazzo Abatellis, Museo Archeologico Regionale A. Salinas (€10 – valid for two days)
5. Museo Salinas, Palazzo Mirto (€7)

Palermo

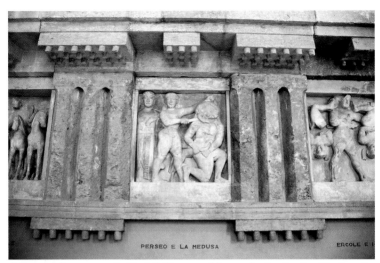

Metopes from temple C of Selinunte, Museo Archeologico Regionale
(Bernhard J. Scheuvens)

Museo Archeologico Regionale

A vast collection, including Greek stone carvings from Selinunte, original mosaic floors, the largest collection of ancient anchors in the world and finds from archaeological sites throughout the island, such as Selinunte, with its stone carvings. (Piazza Olivella 24, ☎ 091-611-805, Mon 8:30 am-1 pm, Tues-Sat 8:30 am-6:45 pm, Sun 9 am-1:30 pm; €6).

Galleria Regionale della Sicilia

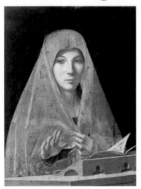

This is considered by many to be Sicily's most important art gallery and is located inside Palazzo Abatellis, with sculpture and paintings from the 14th to 16th centuries. Other rooms feature Arabic ceramics, Sicilian art and frescoes, and one is actually the palace's former chapel. (Palazzo Abatellis, Via Alloro 4, ☎ 091-623-0011; Tues and Wed-Fri 9 am-1 pm and 2:30-7 pm; Mon, Sat and Sun 9 am-1 pm; €6).

The Virgin Annunciate, ca. 1475, by Antonello da Messina

Museo Internazionale delle Marionette Antonio Pasqualino

If you only see one museum in Palermo this is probably the one you want to fit into your schedule, as it gives an excellent insight into Sicilian culture, plus the craftsmanship on display is exemplary. Puppet-lovers will enjoy the 3,500-piece collection from all over the world featuring suits of armor, plus the expressive faces and detail of the marionettes. It's good for children

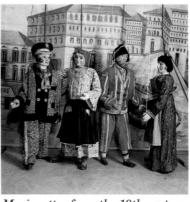

Marionettes from the 19th century

too and on Fridays in July there are puppet shows every week. (Piazzetta Niscemi 5, ☎ 091-328-060, www.museomarionettepalermo.it, Mon-Fri 10 am-1 pm, 3:30-6:30 pm; €5).

Museo Etnografico Pitre

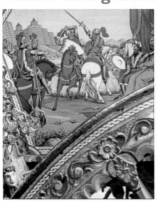

This museum provides great insight into Sicilian folklore and culture. The Sicilian puppets and painted *carretti* (carts) are a big attraction, but there are also Sicilian handicrafts and other cultural items such as 19th-century lace dresses, tapestries, tools, masks, costumes and *presepe* (nativity scenes). (Palazzina Cinese, Via Duca Abruzzi 1, ☎ 091-740-4893, Tues-Sat 9 am-7:30 pm, Sun 9 am-1 pm; €5).

Galleria d'Arte Moderna

This gallery inside the Teatro Politeama-Garibaldi features modern and contemporary Italian art. The theater itself is only open during performances. (Via F. Turati 10, ☎ 091-588-951, Tues-Fri 9 am-8 pm, Sun 9 am-1 pm; €5).

For a full list of museums, see www.palermotourism.com.

PALERMO'S PUPPET THEATERS

There has been a small resurgence of interest in traditional puppet theater. And today puppet theaters receive some funding to continue their work. The puppets, or rather marionettes, first became popular in the Middle Ages, depicting medieval charac-

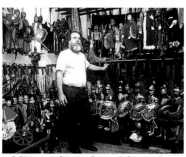

Mimmo Cuticchio of Cuticchio Puppet Theater

ters and legendary events loosely based on their historical counterparts. Characters include Orlando, one of Charlemagne's knights, the Norman knights of King Roger of Sicily and the Saracens (Moors). Most of the stories feature fighting, love and much activity, keeping both children and adults enter-

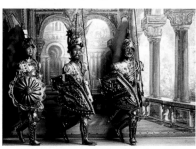

tained. The marionettes are made of wood, with cloth and metal accessories. There are still a handful of marionette makers working in Sicily, particularly in Palermo, Catania and Messina, who sell

In the Museo delle Marionette

many of their creations as souvenirs. To see a performance go to the **Museo delle Marionette**, **Museo Etnografico Pitre** (see *Museums & Galleries* for both) or **Cuticchio Puppet Theater** (Via Bara all'Olivella 95, ☎ 091-323-400, www.figlidarte-cuticchio.com). **Teatro Carlo Magno** (Borgo Vecchio, Via Collegio di Maria 17, ☎ 091-814-6971) has weekend performances at 5:30 pm. Other puppet shows may be held at Teatro Argento (Via Pietro Novelli, 1/a) or Teatro Ditirammu (Via Torremuzza 6, ☎ 091-617-7865, www.teatrinoditirammu.it).

Other Sights

Castello della Zisa

The squat, solid and square 12th-century castle was a palace begun by William I in 1160 and finished by his son William II. Its name comes from the Arabic *el aziz*, meaning magnificent.

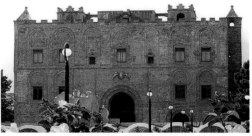

Castello della Zisa

At one time the beautiful planned gardens held rare and exotic beasts, although today they are somewhat drab. Inside are beautiful Islamic mosaic designs and an impressive collection of Islamic art and artifacts. Keep an eye out for the beautiful crafted screens and a 12th-century bronze basin. (Piazza Guglielmo il Buono, ☎ 091-652-0269, Mon-Fri 9 am-7:30 pm; €3).

★★Convento dei Cappuccini

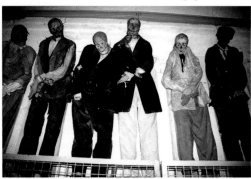

Convento dei Cappuccini

This macabre attraction contains the mortal remains of 8,000 corpses embalmed until 1881 in the crypt of the 17th-century Capuchin monastery. It's not a place you'll want to visit alone. There is an eerie chill to the underground vault, filled with grinning corpses. The corpses are divided according to social and professional status, which is clearly identifiable by clothing such as religious robes, suits or simply Hessian sacks. However, many also have tags identifying names, birth dates and places. Signs also lead to a baby girl of just two years, perhaps

Palermo

the most heart-wrenching. Catch bus 327 from Piazza Indipendenza to the Catacombs. (Via Cappuccini 1, ☎ 091-212-117, 9 am-12 pm, 3-5:30 pm; €1,50).

■ Adventures

On Foot

The **Qanat** (draining tunnels) are underground passages that distributed water in ancient times. You can visit the Qanat Gesuitico alto (Fondo Micciulla) and the Qanat Gesuitico basso (Vignicella) with guides. No minimal level of fitness is required but don't do it if you suffer from claustrophobia! Daily tours are run by **Sciclando** (Via P.pe di Pantelleria 37, ☎ 091-7541-626, www.siciclando.com, 9 am-1 pm, €25) and **Centro Servizi Turistici SottoSopra** (☎ 091-580-433, www.cooperativasolidarieta.org, one hour, €10).

The "**A as in Albergheria**" tour departs daily in Piazza San Saverio through the Albergheria district (Via Vesalio 1, ☎ 091-651-8576, 9 am-3:30 pm, €8), visiting churches, markets, local artisans and more. Other companies leading city tours include **AAPIT** (☎ 091-605-8339) and **Compagnia Siciliana Turismo** (Via Emerico Amari 124, ☎ 091-582-294, cstmail@tin.it).

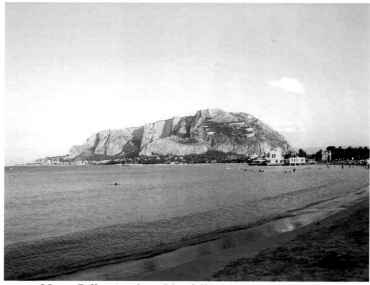

Monte Pellegrino from Mondello (www.spaghettitaliani.com)

A two-hour route of 7.7 km starts from Parco della Favorita near the Casa Natura to the Santuario di S. Rosalia in the **Riserva Naturale Monte Pellegrino** (☎ 091-671-6066, www.riservamontepellegrino. it). **AMAT** (☎ 091-690-2690, www. amat.pa.it) bus 806 stops here. The route starts out along the Valle del Porco following red paint markers. When you hit the road, cross the tarmac and take the left track. After the drinking trough, go straight at the fork and right at the next junction. Turn onto the tarmac up to the

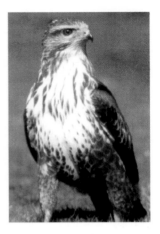

statue of Santa Rosalia and a splendid lookout. Go back down the road and turn left at the junction to the Santuario di Santa Rosalia. A chapel marks the cave where the saint spent time in meditation. From the sanctuary AMAT bus 812 return to Piazza Sturzo in Palermo. You can descend via the Scala Vecchia, a stepped path that twists from the road by the sanctuary to Le Falde, near the exhibition ground, Fiera del Mediterraneo.

The **Capo Gallo** reserve between Mondello and Sferracavallo has a number of beautiful walks from the Marinella entrance beyond Torre Mondello and Via Tolomea (Mondello) or Sferracavallo.

On & Under Water

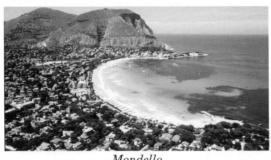

Mondello

Mondello is the place for windsurfing and boating. **Albaria** (Viale Regina Elena, Mondello, ☎ 091-453-595, www.albaria. it) rents equipment and gives boating lessons. They also coordinate with a diving school at Sferracavallo to visit caves, walls, beautiful rocky areas and

an interesting wreck. **Mare Nostrum Diving Centre** can also assist you (☎ 091-684-4483, www.marenostrumdiving. it). They run excursions and training courses from Mondello. However, Ustica is the dive capital of Sicily and just over an hour from Palermo.

On Bicycles

 The narrow alleyways of the city neighborhoods are a good place to meander, as are the tracks in Parco della Favorita, especially those near the Casa Natura. The **Nature Association** (☎ 091-308-847) arranges rides here on Sundays (11 am) and Wednesday and Saturday (both 3:30 pm). At the end of the park follow signs to Mondello (11 km from Palermo) and Capo Gallo – a beautiful coastal ride with a view of the hills surrounding Palermo.

The climb to **Monte Pellegrino** on the old road to Santuario di Santa Rosalia is steep but the views make it worth the effort. You can continue on to Mondello or loop back to Palermo via the Grotte d'Addaura. **Monreale** (8 km south-west) is a climb and the mosaics will take your breath away if the exertion to get here did not!

Palermo Bike Affair (Via E Toti 83, ☎ 0914-26908, www. bokos.it/bikeaffair) does regular rides of Palermo and surrounding areas. They promote three itineraries in the hills west of the city, including Pizzo Manolfo, Monte Palmeto and Montagna Longa. They also can provide maps and may even come along. You will need good fitness for these routes and the better part of a day, unless you have vehicle access to the start of the routes.

You can rent bikes from:

- **Toto Cannatella**, Via Papireto 14, ☎ 091-322-425
- **Kursaal Kalhesa**, Foro Umberto I 21, ☎ 091-616-2828
- **Bio Eco Ambiente**, Via Marchese Ugo (in front of Giardino Inglese)
- **Bici Rent**, with three locations in Giardino Inglese, Via Magliocco and Piazza Unita d'Italia (9 am-7 pm)
- **Western Union** office, cruise terminal, €6/day
- **Hotel Letizia**, Via dei Botai 30, ☎ 091-589-110

There are three Palermo hotels that are part of Albergabici and offer discounts to FIAB cyclists. These are **Hotel Letizia** (Via dei Botai 30, ☎ 091-589-110, www.hotelletizia.com, €€€€) who also rent bikes, **Cristal Palace Hotel** (Via Roma 477/a, ☎ 091-611-2580, www.shr.it, €€€€) and **Shr President Hotel** (Via F Crispi 230, ☎ 091-580-733, www.shr.it, €€€€).

Palermo is linked to the national cycling route produced by BicItalia (www.bicitalia.org) which leaves the city and heads to Trapani.

Siciclando (☎ 091-754-1626, www.siciclando.com), in conjunction with Palermo Tourism (editoria@palermotourism.com), produced a book of cycle itineraries in the Province of Palermo. None of the itineraries starts close enough to the capital to do on a day-trip unless you have your own transport. Siciclando conducts day-tours outside Palermo (8:30 am-7 pm, €60).

On Horseback

For a sedate journey around Palermo, consider a horse-drawn cart ride for €50. The carriages line up on Via Maqueda at Piazza Pretoria. The APT tourist office (☎ 091-7020-289, www.palermotourism.com) can put you in contact with regional farms that offer horseback riding. **Sciclando** (Via P.pe di Pantelleria 37, ☎ 091-7541-626, www.siciclando.com) has a three-hour itinerary to the Grotte della Gulfa (8:30 am-6:30 pm, €80).

In the Sky

If you want a bit of adrenalin, take a skydiving course, or go hang gliding, ultralight free climbing, bungy jumping, base jumping or para flying with the **Associazione Skybrothers Sicily** (Via S. Spinuzza 51, ☎ 091-662-2229, www.extremeplanet.biz) in and around Palermo.

Culinary Adventures

Sciclando (Via P.pe di Pantelleria 37, ☎ 091-7541-626, www.siciclando.com) has one-day cooking courses (8:30 am-5 pm, €80), four-day/three-night (€350) and five-day/four-night packages (€450) in and out of

the city. The city package begins each day with shopping in
the city markets like every good Sicilian mother.

Archaeological Adventures

Journey back to Palermo's early days by checking out the ruins of ancient **Panormos**. Panormos (meaning all-harbor)
was a Phoenician city established in the seventh century BC
and based around the harbor. It served as a base for the

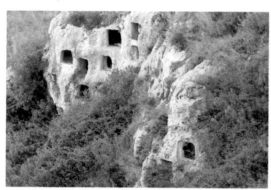

Carthaginian
navy in the
conflict with
the Greeks of
Sicily (480 BC)
but fell to a Ro-
man fleet in
254 BC. The
most signifi-
cant ruins are
at Piazza Vit-
toria (Villa
Bonano) where
three Roman

Grotta di Addaura

houses have been recently restored (Mon-Sat 9 am-1 pm) with
beautiful mosaic floors. Another part of the city is a sixth-century cemetery, **Necropoli Punica** (Caserma Tukory, Corso
Calatafimi 100, ☎ 091-590-299, Mon-Fri 9 am-7 pm, €2).
Southeast of Mondello, Stone Age tools and carved figures
were found in the **Grotta di Addaura** at Monte Pellegrino
(Via Gualtiero da Caltagirone, ☎ 091-696-1315). Other historic locations include **Antica Cortina Muraria** (Piazza Bellini and Piazza Celso) and the **Grotta Niscemi** (Parco della
Favorita, ☎ 091-696-1319).

■ Where to Stay

Visit the APT for accommodation recommendations
or see their website at www.palermotourism.com.
They produce a handbook called *Guida
dell'Ospitalita* listing hotels, B&Bs, campgrounds and hostels
in the province. Most of Palermo's budget accommodation is
between the train station and the Quattro Canti. Women
traveling alone should be careful in this area at night.

The best budget options are some distance out of the city and therefore it may be worth sticking with a central location for convenience. The HI hostel **Baia del Corallo** (Via Plauto 27, ☎ 091-679-7807, www.ostellionline.org, €) is

HOTEL PRICE CHART	
€	Up to €25 per day
€€	€26-€55
€€€	€56-€85
€€€€	Over €85

two km from Tomasso Natale train station. Catch 628 bus to near the hostel. From Palermo Centrale take bus 101 to the stadium and then bus 628.

The other budget option is **Camping International Trinacria** (Via Barcarello 25, ☎ 091-530-590, www. campingtrinacria.it, €) 10 km from Palermo and just east of Sferracavallo, toward Capo Gallo. Open all year.

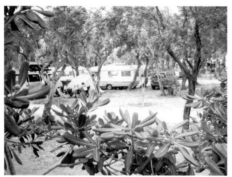

Camping La Playa

Camping La Playa is at Isola delle Femmine (Viale Marino 55, ☎ 091-867-7001, www.camping-laplaya.net, €), 800 yards from the train station.

The other **youth hostel** is in the Capo Gallo Nature Reserve (Via Spinasanta 210, €€).

In August the **Student's Hostel San Saverio** opens its doors while its students are away (Via G. Di Cristina 39, ☎ 091-626-2363, www. ballaro.org, €). Prices include breakfast. They also have a guesthouse with four apartments in Via dei Biscottari (July-September).

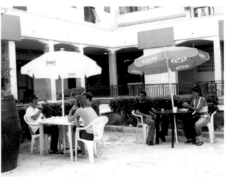

Courtyard at San Saverio

Palermo

Moderate choices include the popular university hostel **Casa Marconi** (Via Monfenera 140, Zona Ospedale Civico, ☎ 091-657-0611, www.casamarconi.it, €-€€). It is often full, so book ahead. It is 300 yards from the metro Orleans.

I Florio B&B (Via Villa Florio 87, ☎ 091-652-4809, www.i-florio.com, €€€) is run by the delightful Nunzia, near Castello Zisa, with three spotless bedrooms.

Giorgio's House (Via A. Mongitore, ☎ 091-525-057, www.giorgioshouse.com, €€€) is all about space, with large rooms, and service. The hosts provide free day/night tours and fitness classes during the day! They also have a free meeting service at the train station.

A Casa di Amici (Via Volturno 6, ☎ 091-584-884, www.acasadiamici.com, €€€) gets good ratings with clean bathrooms and two bedrooms. They accept pets, allow smoking and rent bikes.

Zed & Momo Guesthouse (Via La Farina 11, ☎ 338-876-0290, www.zedmomo.com, €€-€€€), close to Via Liberta, is accessible by bus 101 from the central station. Clean, colorful rooms are named after exotic cities and the hosts are relaxed.

Hotel Sicilia (Via Divisi 99, ☎ 091-616-8460, €€€) in an elegant old building has small but comfortable rooms.

Hotel Elena (Piazza Giulio Cesare 14, ☎ 091-617-0376) is convenient for travelers, next to the train station and with an airport bus stop outside.

Hotel Letizia (Via Botai, ☎ 091-589-110, www.hotel-letizia.com, €€€-€€€€) is close to the Quattro Canti offering tasteful rooms with antique furnishings and family atmosphere. It is part of Albergabici and gives discounts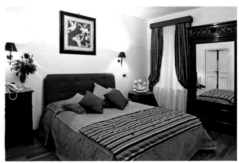

Hotel Letizia

to FIAB cyclists. It's half a mile from Giulio Cesare station.

Grande Albergo Sole (Corso Vittorio Emanuele 291, ☎ 091-604-1111, www.ghshotels.it, €€€€) is near the Quattro Canti with the usual swankiness to match the price tag.

■ **Where to Eat**

You can't go wrong eating out in Palermo with a fine array of local ingredients like swordfish, pine nuts, red chilies, sardines and capers. Local specialties include *pasta con le sarde* (pasta with sardines) or *pesce spada alla ghiotta*

DINING PRICE CHART	
Price per person for an entrée, including house wine.	
€	Up to €12
€€	€13-€25
€€€	€26-€35
€€€€	Over €35

(swordfish with onion and tomato sauce). It's also affordable dining where a few euros can net you some squid, pasta and local wine.

Bars, Cafes & Gelaterie

If you have just arrived by train in Piazza G. Cesare, cross toward Via Roma where a bar on the right corner serves traditional *cassata* and *cannoli*. It should get your taste buds going.

Palermo

Easter Celebrations with the Martorana

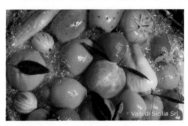

In Palermo you will see *frutta martorana* – sweets shaped and colored like oranges, mandarins, lemons, watermelon or banana. These are in fact marzipan sweets colored with vegetable dyes. They are said to have originated at the Monastero di Martorano when nuns decorated empty fruit trees with marzipan fruit to impress an archbishop. You can find them at **Confezionando** (Corso Vittorio Emanuele 299, Mon-Sat 9 am-1 pm, 4 pm-8 pm).

In Via Principe di Belmonte (#108) there are a number of good cafés. **Coffee and Chocolate** (Mon-Fri 7:30 am-8 pm, Sat 7. 30 am-1 am, Sun 10 am-8:30 pm) serves hot chocolates and coffee or you can choose from an array of fine chocolates. On

the other side of street is **Antico Caffé Spiannato**, established in 1860, serving lavish pastries, almond cakes, tea, chocolate, fresh salads, grills, seafood pastas and cocktails in the evening. *Lungomare* is where you find the oldest gelatarias. **Al Pinguino** (Via Ruggero Settimo 86, closed Mon) is near the APT and serves frappes, *arancine*, *gelato*, *caramelo*, *cassata* and drinks. The **Antica Focacceria San Francesco** (Via A. Paternostro 58, ☎ 091-320-264, www.afsf.it, closed Sun) is one of the city's oldest eating venues, dating from 1834. Their most famous snack is a *panino* (bread roll) with *milza* (veal innards) or fresh ricotta.

If you're looking for a quiet or even not-so-quiet drink, try the trendy **091 Wine Bar** (Piazza Magnone 12) opposite the park. **Piazza del Carmine** is another good spot for a beer on a summer evening, or try **Via Candelai** near the Quattro Canti or the bars in Piazza Olivella. **Enoteca Cana** (Via Alloro 105, ☎ 091-610-1147), just off Piazza Marina, is a good place for Sicilian wines.

Pizzerias

Panormus Pizzeria (Via Torino, Piazzetta Santa Spino) is a bar-cum-pizzeria of moderate price. Ristorante Pizzeria (Al Cortile Santa Caterina, ☎ 091-662-2094, €€) is down a small alley near the Quattro Canti. Ristorante Peppino (Piazza Castelnuovo 49, 12-4 pm, 7 pm-1 am, €) near the APT has good value pizzas starting at €5. **Antica Trattoria del Monsu** (Via Volturno 41, ☎ 091-327-774) is another pizzeria with good local ambience.

Trattorias

Trattoria Antaria (Via di Benedetto Fratelli 6, ☎ 091-612-931) just off Via Torino has typical Sicilian plates.

Ai Corsari (Via Francesco Crispi 104, ☎ 091-582-060, €-€€), is near the port on the corner with Via Mariano Stabile. It's good value with big plates of *spaghetti alla vongole* for €10.

Trattoria Primavera (Piazza Bologni 4, ☎ 091-329-408, €-€€), is a local favorite for genuine Sicilian dishes, with plates from €7 or pay €18 for a fixed menu.

Il Bagatto (Piazza Marina 24, ☎ 091-611-6383, closed Sun, €€€) has bow-tie service and a pleasant garden area for its

seafood dishes. **La Cambusa** at number 16 (☎ 091-584-574, closed Mon, €€€) has seafood lunches for two including wine for under €35. Cross the road afterwards to **Café Luca** for a *sorso* in the tea room.

★**Osteria di Vespri** (Piazza Croce dei Vespri 6, ☎ 091-617-1631, www.osteriadeivespri.it, closed Sun, €€€) has tables on the pretty square outside or cozy seating inside surrounded by hundreds of fine Italian wine selections. Set menus for €45.

Casa del Brodo (Corso Vittorio Emanuele 175, ☎ 091-321-655, closed Tues, €€) is an old favorite near the Quattro Canti. Specialties include swordfish and veal rolled in a tight ball with a garlic sauce. The *antipasto* is marvelous.

Trattoria Trapani (Piazza Giulio Cesare, €) near the train station next to Albergo Elena has cheap squid, pasta and wine.

Trattoria da Bill Boll (€) is a no-frills place in the Vucciria with an interesting atmosphere and typical Sicilian food. Lunch is the best time to come so you can appreciate the market. **Trattoria Shanghai** (Vico Mezzano 34, ☎ 091-589-702, €) is another reasonable option in this area. If you eat in the Vucciria, food tends to be of the fried variety.

■ Around Palermo

Monte Pellegrino

This mountain north of the city was first occupied in 7000 BC and remains from this period have been found in the Grotta d'Addaura on the northern slopes. Incised drawings remain in the cave while tools and other finds are in the

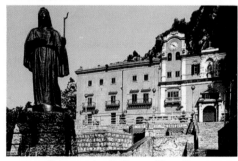

Santuario di Santa Rosalia

Museo Archeologico. Monte Pellegrino is primarily a Sunday picnic spot but is popular with pilgrims visiting the shrine of the city's patron saint, St Rosalia; and with walkers and bik-

ers (see *Adventures*). The **Santuario di Santa Rosalia** (7 am-7 pm, free) is rather tacky, with souvenir stalls selling religious paraphernalia, cafés and a museum of the saint's life. Rosalia's bones were discovered in 1624 in the cave where a chapel now stands. It's also where the saint had lived as a hermit. Get AMAT (☎ 091-690-2690, www.amat.pa.it) bus 812 from Piazza Sturzo.

Mondello

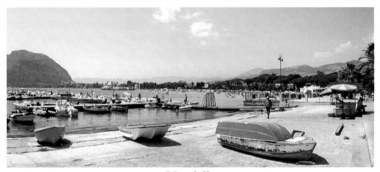

Mondello

Mondello is one of the closest beaches to Palermo and it's busy and crowded in summer. If you want to spend time by the sea you'd be better off heading to Scopello or San Vito Lo Capo farther afield. But it's a good day-trip, with fine dining and pleasant seaside activities. On the waterfront opposite the Mondello Palace Hotel is a floating island with the Charleston Restaurant and diving center where you can rent canoes, surf boards, surf skis and small sailing boats. Buses (614) for Mondello and Sferracavallo leave from Piazza A Gasperi.

Ricci (sea urchin) is a specialty in Mondello and you can see it being prepared in the open kitchens of some restaurants. They serve food on large ceramic plates doused with lemon. **Da Cologero** (Via Torre Mondello 22, ☎ 091-684-1333, €€) is a particularly interesting place to watch this. Look for the octopus sign and waiters in bright shirts. Plates with *vongole* (clams) or *cozze* (mussels) start from €6. **Bye Bye Blues** (Via del Garofalo 23, Valdesi Mondello, ☎ 091-684-1415, www. byebyeblues.it, closed Tues, €€€) is part of the esteemed Le Soste di Ulisse restaurant group. Chef Patrizia has developed a menu based on recipes handed down to her. The menu

changes according to the season. Main courses €7-10. Cheaper options include **Le Lunette** *panini* on the riverfront and **Peppi's Pizza** (Via Torre 16, ☎ 091-684-3020), which has pizza and spaghetti dishes.

For accomodation try **Pomelia B&B** (Via Saffo 23, ☎ 340-696-1742, www.pomelia.com, €€€) set back from the beach with three bedrooms, a kitchen and bathroom. Other options are **Conchiglia d'Oro** (Viale Cloe 9, ☎ 091-450-032) and **Mondello Palace Hotel** (Viale Principe di Scalea, ☎ 091-450-001, 139-265) with its own beach and park. They have standard rooms and suites.

★★★ Monreale

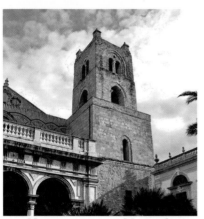

Norman tower at Monreale
(Galen R Frysinger, www.galenfrysinger.com)

The famed 12th-century cathedral (8 am-12:30 pm, 3:30-6:30 pm, free), eight kilometres southwest of Palermo, should not be missed on any account. It is awe-inspiring, with the finest examples of Norman architecture in Sicily and of Christian medieval mosaicwork in the world. The cathedral owes its existence to King William II, who built the cathedral to curb the growing power of the Sicilian papacy and the powerful archbishop of Palermo, Walter of the Mill. The cathedral is impressive even from the outside, but nothing quite prepares you for the interior. The aisles, sanctuary, apses, ceiling and every spot in between are entirely covered in gilded mosaics – a job that only took 10 years, which speaks volumes for the skill of the Greek and Byzantine craftsmen. It's hard to know where to start looking but if you cover the mosaics systematically you can get an overall biblical picture.

Your eyes are immediately drawn to the 66-foot-high figure of Christ in benediction in the central apse. The two side apses are dedicated to Saint Peter (right) and Paul (left), even displaying their martydom in graphic terms. The nave mosaics

Palermo

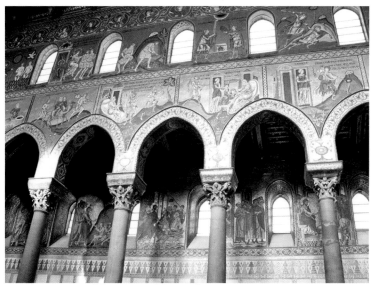

Mosaics at Monreale (Galen Frysinger)

relate the story of Creation and the aisle mosaics depict the teachings of Jesus. You'll easily recognize biblical scenes – Jesus washing his disciples feet, Adam and Eve in the garden of Eden, Noah making the ark and more. It's like a story book for children.

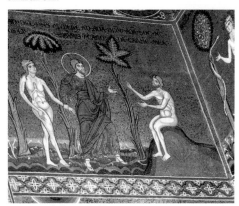

Adam & Eve (Galen Frysinger)

The **Terrazze del Duomo** (9 am-6 pm, €1,50) at the back of the church offers a panoramic view up 180 steps of the cloister outside (9 am-7 pm, €6), which is part of William's original Benedictine monastery. The 228 twin columns are all different, depicting plants, animals and other motifs. If you don't want to pay, enter the **Monastero dei Benedittini** (Mon-Sat, 8 am-12:30 pm, Sun, 8 am-12 pm, 3-7 pm). Go up-

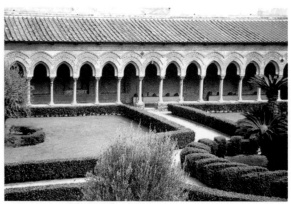

Monreale cloister (Joanne Lane)

stairs and turn right at the end for a view of the cloister below. Friendly staff may also show you the room where the monks once ate.

There are a number of mosaic laboratories in Via Arcivescovado or you can visit the Istituto Statale d'Arte per il Mosaico south of the parking lot during term times. **Siculi and Sicani** (Via Chiesa degli Agonizzanti 2/4/6, ☎ 3389-813-345, www.siculiesicani.it, €€-€€€) is a food museum worth a browse or even a bite to eat. They sell organic wine, liquors, jams and sauces and serve Nebrodi *cinghiale* (wild boar), *tonno* (tuna) and pesto made from pistacchios. Bus 309 or 389 run from Piazza dell'Indipendenza to Monreale.

Where to Eat & Stay

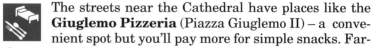

The streets near the Cathedral have places like the **Giuglemo Pizzeria** (Piazza Giuglemo II) – a convenient spot but you'll pay more for simple snacks. Farther away in Piazza G. Mateotti, there are two choice places in the pretty fountain courtyard. **Cafe Arancio** and **Taverna del Pavone** (Vicolo Pensato 18, ☎ 091-640-6209, www.tavernadelpavone.it, €€) have medium-priced meals or you can make a selection from the wine and beer menu. **Picolo Rifugio** (Piazza Vittorio Emanuele 38, ☎ 091-640-2391, closed Mon, €-€€), opposite the church, has basic dishes from €5-6. **Bricco and Bacco Brasserie** (Via B. D'Aquisto, ☎ 091-641-7773, closed Mon) is a trendy place with €13 lunch and €20-30 dinner menus. **Dietro L'Angolo** (Via

Chiasso Piave 5, ☎ 091-640-4067) is a quiet choice with a balcony offering fantastic views of the valley. Decorations inside include old stamps and prints, antique objects, mosaics and souvenirs. **Trattoria Mizzica** (Via Cappuccini, ☎ 091-640-8643) also has fine views.

La Ciambra B&B (Via Sanchez 23, ☎ 091-640-9565, www.laciambra.com, €€) sits just off Via Arcivescovado in a quiet, plant-filled lane.

Ustica

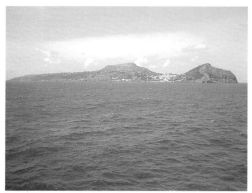

This beautiful island 60 km north of Palermo is a tranquil settlement and the perfect getaway from the bustle of the capital for a daytrip or a few days. It is best visited between June and September, but in August huge crowds drive up the prices. The far side of the island has been partially declared a marine reserve and the limpid clear waters are known for the best diving in Sicily.

Ustica island (Peppe)

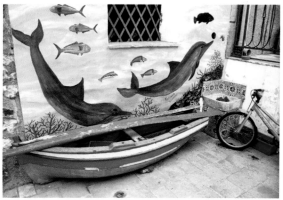

A house in Ustica (Joanne Lane)

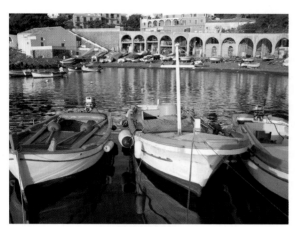
Ustica harbor

Ustica Town is the arrival point for ferries and where most people stay. It's more a village than a town, with a series of interlocking squares leading up to a church. You'll definitely get fit wandering the steep streets. A series of murals decorate the façades of the buildings and there's the usual array of flower pots hanging from window terraces. There's a tourist office (Piazza Umberto 1, ☎ 091-844-9456, Mon-Fri 8 am-1 pm, 4-6 pm; Sat-Sun 8 am-2 pm) that can advise on good snorkeling spots and dive centers. Shops in the main street sell snorkels and fins. Orange minibuses make an island circuit every 30 minutes from the town hall (2½ hours round-trip, €1). In summer agencies and hotels rent scooters and bicycles.

Ships (two hours, €11.75) and hydrofoils (one hour, €18.45) serve Ustica from Palermo. There is also a hydrofoil from Napoli in summer (four hours). The first **Siremar** (Via Roma 2, ☎ 091-582-403, www.gruppotirrenia.it/siremar) hydrofoil leaves Palermo at 8:15 am, the last returns at 5:15 pm. **Ustica Lines** (www.usticalines.it) has services from Favignana (6:55 am, two hours, €19), Levanzo (7:10 am, two hours, €19), Napoli (3 pm, four hours, €66) and Trapani (6:30 am, three hours, €19). Departures are Monday, Thursday, Friday and Saturday in July and August; and Monday, Thursday and Saturday in June and September.

The Torre Santa Maria houses the **Museo Archeologico** (9 am-12 pm, 5-7 pm; €3) with exhibits and fragments from the ancient city of Osteodes, now submerged beneath the sea a mile off the coast. Other artifacts like anchors and amphorae were recovered from wrecked ships.

Palermo

Adventures

On Foot

 Ustica's name comes from the Latin *ustum* or burned – an accurate description of its blackened, volcanic rock. In the center of the island are the remains of two volcanic cones, **Monte Guardi dei Turchi** (813 feet) and **Monte Costa del Fallo** (768 feet). A series of paths cross the island. There is a coastal route (three-four hours) that starts near the cemetery and hugs the cliffs on the island's north side past the Bronze-Age archaeological site of Farraglioni as far as the Marine Reserve at Punta di Megna. Farraglioni dates from the 14th century BC and contains the foundations of 300 stone-built houses. From Punta di Megna you get a view to the offshore rock Scoglio del Medico where snorkeling is fantastic. Contine along to the battered old tower at Punta Spalmatore and natural pools at the *torre* or Punta Cavazzi. Rejoin the main road back across the island to the port.

Another interesting walk is to the **Rocca della Falconiera** (515 feet, two hours), a site of Roman habitation dating from the third century BC. It starts near the Carabinieri and passes an ancient area used for burial with 150 tombs carved into the mountain and a late Roman necropolis. You also pass two Bourbon fortresses built in the 1760s to protect the island from pirate raids. The **Forte della Falconiera** is just before the summit, where there are stairs, water cisterns and shops excavated in the volcanic rock.

Culunneda is an archaeological site on Guardia dei Turchi (one or two hours) that has not yet been excavated or developed for tourism. However the walls of habitation are evident and there are a few tombs. To reach the summit take Via B. Randaccio to the right of the church. Turn left at the top and then right and you'll reach the Municipio. From here, turn left along Via Tre Mulini. Follow the cobbled path and cut off to the left when you reach the stepped path for the summit.

An easier walk is the 20-minute climb to the remains of the **Castello Saraceno** above the town. The old fort has numerous water cisterns. To get here, find Via Calvario and turn left at the cross.

On Wheels

 The following itinerary can be undertaken by bicycle or scooter around the perimeter of the island (12 km, half a day). Rent bikes/scooters in town (€24-33/day). From the main square, turn right at the church and follow signs to Faraglioni and then the main road for Piana di Tramontana past cultivated fields. Climb up towards Passo della Madonna and then down to Punta di Megna, where you can swim at Cala Sidoti. The route continues on to Punta Cavazzi and the lighthouse, one of the most beautiful points on the island. From here, it's two hours back to town.

On Water

Ustica's jagged coastline is packed with creeks, bays, caves and inlets and best explored by boat. You can rent a boat in town (€45/day), do a tour (€15/2½ hours) or accompany local fishermen. If you have your own boat leave the port and head toward **Capo della Falconiera**, where you can see the lighthouse of Punta Omo Morto. Follow the point around to the opening for **Grotta dell'Oro**. Continue around the coast past volcanic rock towards **Scoglio del Medico**, where legend says a Saracen King left his doctor to die of hunger because he could not cure his daughter. The section from here to Punta dello Spulmatore is part of the Marine Reserve and entry by

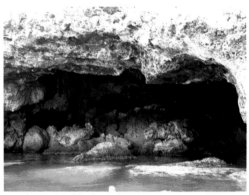

Ustica grotto (Fabrox)

boat is forbidden. Keep well clear of the shoreline until you pass Punta dello Spalmatore. There are two inlets here, one leading to a small beach and the other to a point directly beneath the lighthouse at Punta Cavazzi. Turning around the island, the southern side has various half-submerged caves like **Grotta Pirciata**, **Grotta del Tuono** and **Grotta Verde** immediately after Punta dell'Arpa. This last cave is particularly beautiful. After Punta Galera and Punta San Paolo is

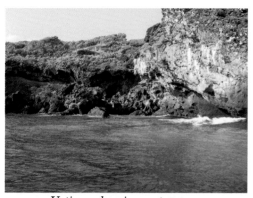

Ustica volcanic coast (Fabrox)

the **Grotta delle Barche**, a small inlet enclosed by black rock where fishermen anchor during storms. A pyramid-shaped rock signals the opening to the **Grotta della Pastizza** (stalactites) and the **Grotta dell'Accademia**. Below Hotel Grotta Azzurra is the opening to the well known **Grotta Azzurra**. The best time to visit is in the afternoon when the light penetrates the cave, causing an irridescent glow in the water. The Cala Santa Maria port is just beyond. You can rent boats from:

- **Da Gaetano** (Via C. Colombo, ☎ 091-844-9605)
- **Carmela Tranchina** (Via C. Colombo, ☎ 349-242-7960)
- **Da Umberto** (Piazza Vittoria 7, ☎ 091-844-9542)
- **Profondo Blu** (Via Cristoforo Colombo, ☎/fax 091-844-9609, www.ustica-diving.it)

Dive centers include:

- **Profondo Blu** (Via Cristoforo Colombo, ☎/fax 091-844-9609, www.ustica-diving.it)
- **Mare Nostrum Diving Center** (Via Cristoforo Colombo, ☎/fax 0922-972-042, www.marenostrumdiving.it)
- **Barracuda Diving Center** (Punta Spalmatore, ☎ 091-844-9132, www.barracudaustica.com)

Where to Eat

The obvious choice for dining in Ustica is fresh seafood. **Schiticchio** (Via dei Tre Mulini, ☎ 091-844-9662, 1-3 pm, 7:30 pm-2 am, €€) is a good choice for grilled frish, homemade pasta and fresh ingredients. Main courses €8-12. **Trattoria Clelia** (Via Sindaco I, 29, ☎ 091-844-9039) and **Trattoria Da Umberto** (Piazza della Vittoria

7, ☎ 091-844-9542) come recommended by travelers for rustic local meals. **Da Mario** (Piazza Umberto I, 21, ☎ 091-844-9905, 12:30-3 pm, 8:30-10:30 pm) serves squid, crabmeat, swordfish, grilled fish and homemade pastas with local wine. Courses €8-10.

Where to Stay

 Some hotels offer affordable weekly accommodation and dive packages. The shoulder seasons of April-June and September are cheaper as prices double in August. There are many apartments and country houses for lease or rent on Ustica. See www.usticaholidays.com, www.isoladiustica.com or go into a bar to ask for *camere*. The prices listed here are for double rooms in high season; out of season they are much lower.

Caminita Vittorio (Via Tufo 1, ☎ 091-844-9212, €€) is run by a friendly individual who'll most likely find you near the main square to scout business or have a chat. His two self-contained rooms are just minutes from the church and the prices are among the best in town.

One- and two-star hotels include:

Diana (Contrada San Paolo, ☎ 091-844-9109)

Hotel Patrice (Via Refugio 23, ☎ 091-844-9053)

Hotel Stella Marina (Via Cristofo Colombo 33, ☎ 091-844-9014)

Pensione Clelia (Via Sindaco I, 29, ☎ 091-844-9039, €€€€) was one of the first places on the island to receive visitors and is still going strong with a central location and reasonable prices. The rooms are small but additional services include a shuttle bus, scooter and boat rentals and specials for diving. Prices drop out of season.

The Hotel Grotta Azzurra (Contrada S. Ferlicchio, ☎ 091-844-9048, fax 091-844-9396, www.framonhotels.com/en/hotels.htm, €€€€) is the top hotel in Ustica, with a unique spot on terraces by the sea. The breakfast area is beautiful but they have an unfortunate excess of concrete.

Solunto

Another pleasant day-excursion from Palermo are the remains of the Hellenistic-Roman town of Solunto (March-October 9am-7.30pm, €2). Solunto is 20 km east of the city and ac-

Palermo

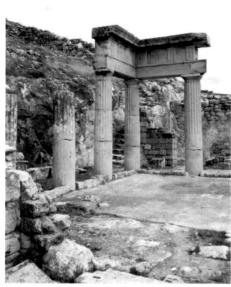
A temple at Solunto

cessible by train, although the Santa Flavia-Solunto-Porticello station is a 30-minute walk. Solunto was originally Solus, an eighth-century BC Phoenician settlement. It was resettled in the fourth century BC and later Hellenized before it surrendered to Rome and changed to Solentum. The site is dramatically located on Caltafano Feriale mountain overlooking the sea – bring a picnic and enjoy the view. Remains of main streets, houses with original mosaic floors, a theater, gymnasium, public toilet and the Casa di Leda have been uncovered – all largely from the Roman period. It's like a graveyard of stones and columns. Ceramics, hooks and nails, hair pins made from bone, marble statues taken from the houses and funerary items from the site can be seen in a small museum on site.

Piana degli Albanesi

Another easy day trip from the capital is this quiet 15th-century Albanian town perched above a peaceful lake. The Albanians first settled here after taking flight from the Turkish invasions. The town was called Hora (city), then Piana dei Greci and finally Piana degli Albanesi in 1941. Many of the inhabitants have retained their traditions following an Orthodox rite and speak a version of their language. You'll notice many streets have Albanian signs and church services are in Greek. There's not a lot to see. The **Museo Civico di Nicola Barbato** (Via P. G Gazzetta, ☎ 091-857-1787, Tues-Sun 9 am-

1 pm, 3-7 pm) is in the Comune, 70 feet from the main piazza. In the narrow streets are small shrines, long arches and you can hear prayers coming from the houses. There is a tourist office in the library (Piazza Vittorio Emanuele, ☎ 091-857-1787). The best time to visit is at Easter or Christmas when the locals wear splendid costumes typically embroidered with gold and silver. Most processions rally before the churches of Santa Maria Odigitria, San Giorgio and San Demetrio.

Prestia & Comande buses leave from Stazione Centrale in Palermo (Piazza D. Peranni 9, ☎ 091-586-351) and continue to Santa Cristina Gela. The last bus to Palermo leaves at 4 pm

 from Viale 8 Marzo. For accommodation you could try the **Istituto SS Salvatore** (☎ 091-857-1046) where beds are sometimes available on request.

 There are only a handful of restaurants in town, including:

La Montagnoa, Cda Brigna, ☎ 091-857-71831
Le Due Gare, Viale 8 Marzo, ☎ 091-875-589
Trattoria San Giovanni, Via Matteotti, ☎ 091-857-1070
Red Parrot, Viale 8 Marzo (slightly out of town)
Antico Bar Sport, just before Piazza Vittorio Emanuele, has good pastries and coffee and can make you a *panino*.

Adventures

On Foot

 The artificial lake three kilometres south of town is an easy walk. Follow signs to the WWF Oasis and their small *sentiero* track 'Mone' which skirts the lake.

Four kilometres from Piana is a mountain pass southwest of town, **Portella della Ginestra**. In 1947 11 people were killed and 55 wounded here as they took part in May Day celebrations. A stone memorial marks the spot. In spring the pass is covered in thickets of *ginestra* (broom).

There are two walks signposted from outside the DESPAR supermarket. One leads past the lake toward Ficuzza (25 km) passing Rifugio Val dei Conti (six hrs 30 mins) and ends at Rifugio Alpe Cucco (☎ 091-820-8225) near Rocca Busambra. The other heads in the other direction to Dammusi (five hrs, 15 km).

Another lesser-known route starts from the modest Chiesa dell'Odigitria at the top end of town where you'll find a signpost marking walking trails. Follow path 17 below the church to **La Pizzutta** mountain (3,886 feet, one hr 30 min) for a birds-eye view over Portella della Ginestra. From the saddle follow the markers north-northwest to another saddle, a ruined stone house and bomb craters and ascend **Portella Garrone** (3,280 feet, two hrs 20 min). Follow the trail signs back to town (three hours, 7½ km).

★ Monte Iato

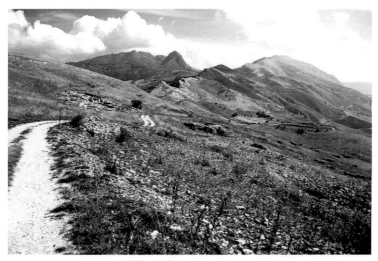

Monte Iato (Joanne Lane)

Monte Iato (2,794 feet) is 30 kilometres west of Palermo. Its rocky, steep slopes made it a perfect area for early settlements and the remains of the ancient cities that existed can still be found here. The ruins aren't as amazing as Selinunte or Segesta but the mountain location is beautiful. **AST** buses from Palermo run to San Cipirello and San Giuseppe Iato, both beneath Monte Iato. In San Cipirello is a tourist office (Corso Trieste 26, ☎ 091-858-1017, Mon-Fri 8:30 am-1:30 pm, Mon and Thurs 3:30-5:30 pm, sancipirello.turismo@libero.it).

The ancient city known as Jaitas to the Greeks, Ietas to the Romans, Giatas to those in the early Middle Ages and now Iato, has origins dating back to the ninth century BC. How-

ever most of the major monuments were erected in the fourth century BC, including the 4,400-seat theater, *agora*, sanctuary and several elegant Hellenic type dwellings. In the wake of Carthaginian ocupation the Romans took over for

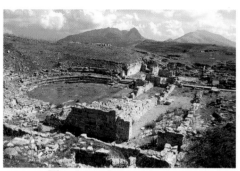
Theater at Iato (Joanne Lane)

several centuries but it then slid into insignificance. More recently it was frequented by shepherds and farmers, many of whom helped clear away the rubble. Excavations are still continuing.

There is no public transport to the site (open Tues, Thurs & Sat 9 am-7 pm; Mon, Wed, Fri & Sun 9 am-1 pm, ☎ 340-706-8876) which is some distance from town. The first access route is along Via Roma but it's not terribly well marked. Eventually you come to *Vauso a morte*, a slab of rock where coffins would be rested temporarily by bearers en route to the former sanctuary of San Cosmo to the east. Farther along are remains of houses, the theater and agora, with various fluted columns and much debris. The route across the top eventually leads to the other entrance, a 2½-kilometre trek back to town. A *navetta* used to run from this entrance to the *porta antica Iato* which saved a good half-hour hike each way. Try to encourage them to bring it back.

In town you can visit the **Museo Civico** (Via Roma 320, ☎ 091-857-3083) which contains finds from the site, including four capitals of women from the *casa peristilio*, jugs,

pots, ceramics and pieces of mosaic pavement. If you need something to eat ,there's **Wonder Pub** (☎ 091-857-3105) and **Al Tropical Bar** in Piazza Vittorio Veneto. Or **Ristorante Apud Jatum** (Corso Trento 49-51, ☎ 091-857-6188). There is no accomodation in town but if you call ahead these nearby places should be willing to pick you up: **Agriturismo Casale del Principe** (Contrada Dammusi, ☎ 091-857-9910), **Casale dello Jato** (Contrada Percianotta, ☎ 091-857-2175) and **Agriturismo Feudo Chiusa** (Contrada Chiusa, ☎ 338-767-6884).

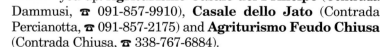

Palermo

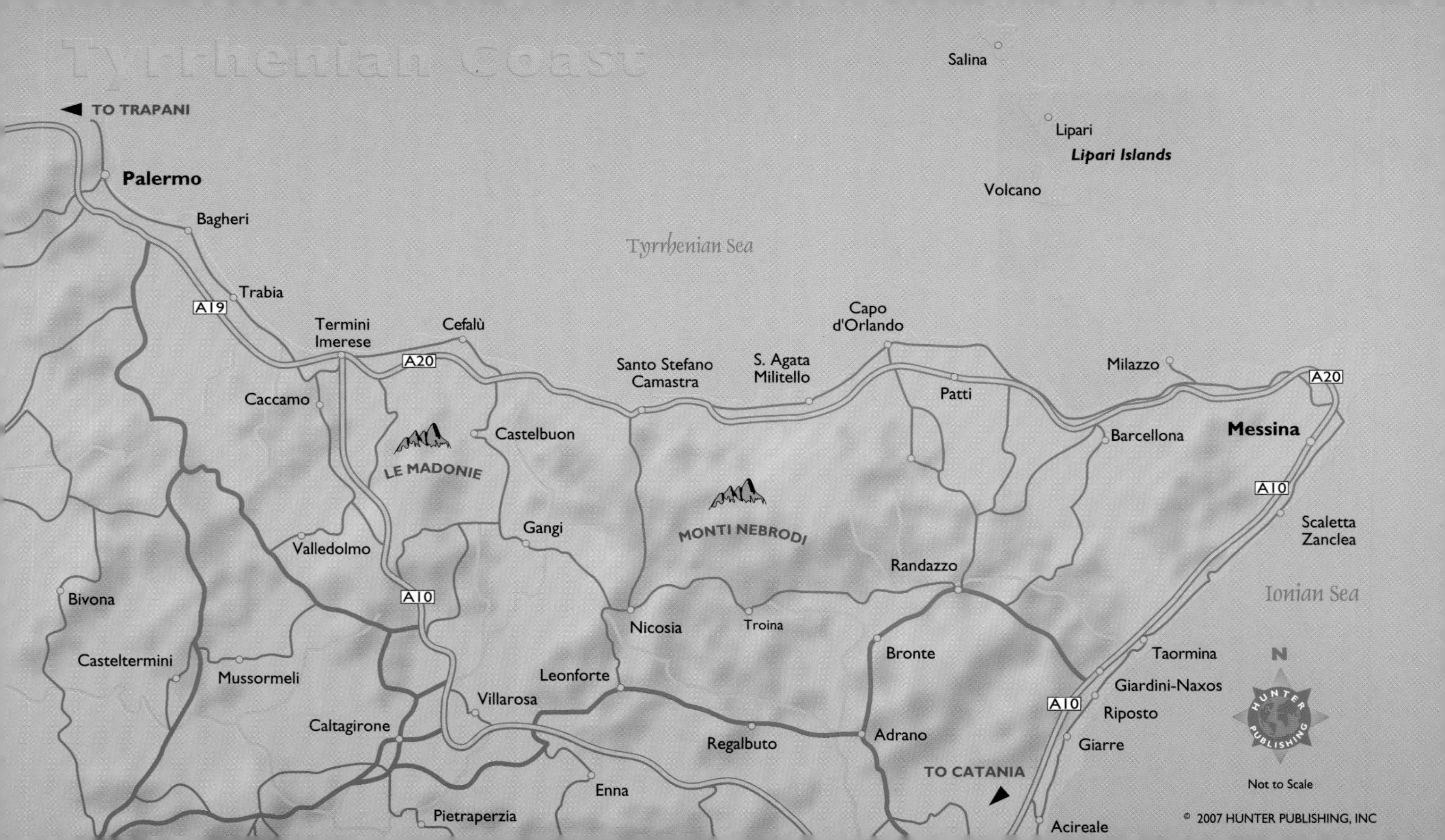

Tyrrhenian Coast

TO TRAPANI

Palermo

Bagheri

Trabia

A19

Termini
Imerese

Caccamo

Cefalù

A20

LE MADONIE

Castelbuon

Gangi

Valledolmo

A10

Santo Stefano
Camastra

S. Agata
Militello

Capo
d'Orlando

Patti

Tyrrhenian Sea

MONTI NEBRODI

Nicosia

Troina

Leonforte

Villarosa

Enna

Pietraperzia

Caltagirone

Mussormeli

Bivona

Casteltermini

Regalbuto

Adrano

Bronte

Randazzo

Milazzo

Barcellona

Messina

A20

A10

Taormina

Giardini-Naxos

Riposto

Giarre

Acireale

Scaletta
Zanclea

Ionian Sea

TO CATANIA

Salina

Lipari

Volcano

Lipari Islands

N

Not to Scale

© 2007 HUNTER PUBLISHING, INC

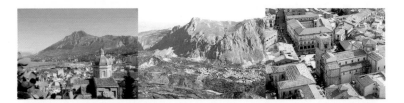

The Tyrrhenian Coast

An Islanland within an island. The Tyrrhenian coast runs almost the entire length of Sicily's northern shore and is an uninterrupted line of resorts, beaches and little towns. This is all about vacationing and it can be congested. But, once you head inland, the crowds thin and at any other time of year there's plenty of room to maneuver.

Cefalù is the major attraction along the coast, with a

pretty town and beach set below a rocky outcrop. After

Cefalù

Taormina, it's the busiest of Sicily's coastal resorts. The **Parco Madonie** rises behind Cefalù and is popular with skiers in winter and hikers during the summer months. East of Cefalù is a great stretch of coast towards **Milazzo**, with a pretty series of lakes at **Oliveri**. The Tyrrhenian coast is also dotted with archaeological sites, including **Himera**, **Tyndaris**, **San Marco d'Alunzio** and **San Biagio**. Behind Sant Stefano di Camastra and bordered by Mistretta, Cesaro and Randazzo, the **Parco dei Nebrodi** is a good spot for nature lovers.

The Tyrrhenian coast is very accessible via a good train service and regular buses to inland destinations. However, a car is particularly useful for the interior and the two park regions.

HIGHLIGHTS OF THE TYRRHENIAN COAST

- Cefalù's Christ Pantokrator mosaic
- Nebrodi driving tour or mountain biking
- Skiing the pistas of the Madonie
- The picturesque Oliveri *laghetti*
- Roman and Greek ruins at Himera, Tyndaris, San Marco d'Alunzio and San Biagio
- Following the castle trail to Caccamo
- Playing golf on the slopes of the Madonie mountains
- Loading your suitcase with ceramics in Santo Stefano d'Camastra

■ Termini Imerese

This is the first stop of interest between Palermo and Cefalù. Unfortunately it is bordered by some rather ugly industry but there are a few interesting places nearby.

The town derives its name from the two neighboring Greek settlements of Thermae and Himera. It was settled by Greeks from Zancle (Messina) in the seventh century BC and grew in importance as it absorbed the survivors from Himera, renamed Thermae Himerensis. The Romans took over in 252 BC and it became famous as a thermal spa, which it still is. Until the 19th century the town was enclosed within protec-

tive walls but is now spilling out into the countryside. The most interesting parts of town inlcude a few good Baroque churches and the museum containing finds from Himera. You could also base yourself here to visit Caccamo.

Getting Here & Around

The train station is 400 yards southeast of the town center. The town is on both the Palermo-Messina and Palermo-Agrigento lines. Local and long distance buses arrive from outside the station. **SAIS Trasporti** runs between Termini Imerese and Palermo and Cefalù.

To get from the train station to the town center, turn right outside the station, walk past Piazza Crispi and down Corso Umberto. This becomes Via Roma and climbs to the upper town. It's a bit of a walk! Alternatively, local buses will bring you up here. Buses leave from the train station to Himera.

Information Sources

The **Assessorato Turistico** (☎ 0918-128-279, Mon and Wed 8 am-2 pm, 3-6 pm; Tues and Thurs-Fri 8 am-2 pm) is in the upper town off Via Mazzini in Cortile Maltese. For information on the community, see www.comune-termini-Imerese.pa.it.

Sightseeing

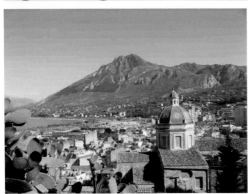
Termini Imerese

The heart of the upper town is **Piazza del Duomo**, a spacious piazza with the 17th-century Duomo. Inside are sculptures from the Gagini school and various frescoes. Near the altar are paintings of the disciples. Opposite the cathedral is the **Museo Civico** (Via del Museo, ☎ 0918-128-279, Tues-Sun 9 am-1 pm; Wed, Thurs, Sat and Sun 3-7 pm; free). Three sec-

tions inside are devoted to archaeology, art and natural history. In the nearby **Palazzo Municipio** (8 am-2 pm), ask nicely to see the frescoes (as it's not a tourist location) in one of the bottom rooms. They give detailed information on the destruction of

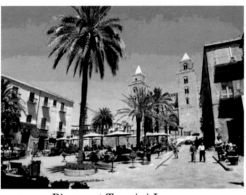

Piazza at Termini Imerese

Himera and construction of the new city. Start in the right hand corner as you enter to follow the sequence of events. Beyond the Duomo, Via Belvedere leads to a wonderful panorama of the lower town and port. There are also the remains of a *castello* (9 am-10 pm daily, free) up some steps. There's a bar up here, **Le Terrazze delle Muse** (☎ 338-632-3094), a good spot for a pint at night. Beyond this is the church of **Santa Caterina d'Alessandria**. It is often closed (ask at the Duomo to get in) and has splendid frescoes. The public gardens, **Villa Comunale** (8 am-9 pm, free), contain Roman ruins, including an *anfiteatro* where it is thought gladiators competed, although there are no documents to prove it. Go through the gardens to the exit back onto Via Garibaldi. Nearby is **Porta Palermo**, the former entrance to the city. More Roman remnants are visible on the road to Caccamo in Contrada Figurella, where part of an ancient aqueduct with double arches is still visible.

 The Carnevale celebrations before Lent here in February are particularly interesting.

Ancient Himera

Himera (9 am-6 pm daily, free) was founded in 648 BC by Greeks from Zankle (Messina) and named after the River Imera that flows nearby. It was the first Greek settlement here and was to be an advance post against the Carthaginians. Instead it worked as a bit of a flash card and in 480 BC a battle was held here between the two foes. The combined armies of Theron of Agrigento and Gelon of Syra-

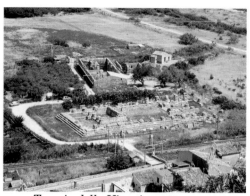
Tempio della Vittoria (Clemensfranz)

cuse defeated Hamilcar's Carthaginian army. But his nephew Hannibal came back in 409 BC and destroyed the town to revenge his uncle's death.

There's not a lot left of the once important site (9 am-6 pm daily, free), except for the massive **Tempio della Vittoria** near the railway tracks. It was built to commemorate the defeat of the Carthaginians. The **Acropolis** lay to the south of the temple, inland beyond the **Himera Aquarium** (Mon-Sat 9 am-6 pm, Sun 9 am-1 pm, €2). The museum contains the usual finds from the site, mainly cracked vessels. Much of the collection is in Termini Imerese and Palermo.

If you need something to eat, there is the **Baglio Himera** nearby, serving pizza. There's also accommodation at the **Himera Polis Hotel** (SS 113, Contrada Buonfornello, ☎ 0918-140-566), near the station, and **Villaggio Himera Camping** (☎ 0918-140-175), just before Buon Fornello. To get to Himera, take a train to

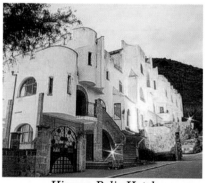
Himera Polis Hotel

Buon Fornello, then head to the *statale* road and turn left. Buses run from Termini Imerese from in front of the train station four times daily.

Where to Stay

Hotel Il Gabbiano (Via Liberta 221, ☎ 0918-113-262, www.hotelgabbiano.it, €€€) is about one km from the station. They have rooms and a restaurant. Meals are €15-20.

Grande Hotel delle Terme (Piazza delle Terme, ☎ 0918-113-557) is one of the limited options in the upper town. You can get water treatments from the town's ancient spas.

For camping see previous page.

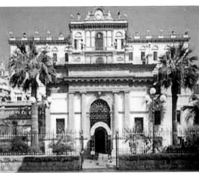
Grande Hotel delle Terme

Where to Eat

 The **Bar del Duomo** (Via Belvedere 16, ☎ 0918-112-978) has a friendly proprietor and a lovely seating, either outside with a view of the Duomo or in the atmospheric interior. There's a big screen TV, old bottle lampshades, wine barrels and Sicilian carts. Plates of spaghetti cost just €5 or get a *panino* (sandwich) to take out.

Trattoria Santi e Pescatori, near Hotel Gabbiano, is recommended by locals for good seafood but is some distance from the upper town.

■ Caccamo

Caccamo is a popular day-trip from Termini Imerese for its amazing **Norman castle** that dominates the townscape. It's only 10 km away and the only inland town in this area of note. It was a Carthaginian stronghold and a thorn in the side for Greek Himera during the fifth century BC. The town was only officially founded in 1093, when the Normans began to build the castle.

Getting Here

 Buses from Palermo arrive four times daily in Caccamo. **Autolinee Randazzo** (☎ 0918-148-235) runs to Termini Imerese and Cefalù nine times daily.

Information

 The **Ufficio di Turismo** (Piazza Matrice, Mon-Fri 9 am-1 pm, Tues and Thurs 3-6 pm) can give you a map of the town. **Sicila e Dintorni** (Via Amilcare 10,

☎ 0918-121-312, www.siciliaedintorni.it) can also provide tourist information and itineraries, particularly of local castles.

Sightseeing

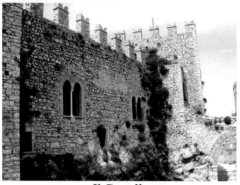

Il Castello

The ★*Castello* (Via del Castello, 9 am-1 pm, 4-8 pm, €2) is the main drawcard and feature in town and well worth a look. A steep path leads through three gateways to the main keep. The walls and original fortifications are particularly interesting.

Below the castle **La Bottega della Roccia** (Via del Castello 8, ☎ 091-812-1312, 9 am-1 pm, 3-6 pm) is the 100-year-old house of a farmer who had five kids. It's now a store selling Sicilian products. There's honey, jam, liquors, Marsala wine and Grappa.

Across from the Bottega next to La Locanda del Principe is the **Associazione Culturale Sicilia e Dintorni** (Via Amilcare, ☎ 091-812-1312, www.siciliaeditorni.it, siciliaeditorni@tiscali.

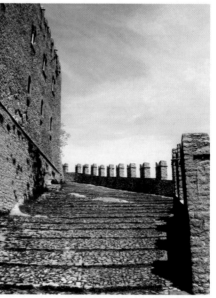

Il Castello

Tyrrhenian Coast

it) with a photographic display of Sicilian castles and models. It's free to enter but an offering is appreciated.

The rest of the town is a jumble of houses and squares. Have a wander – it's impossible to get lost because it's so small. Eventually head down to the fine Piazza del Duomo behind the castle crag. The tourist offices are here, as is Caccamo's **Duomo** (9 am-12 pm, free). The 11th-century building has been remodeled twice. It was originally Norman, but is now heavily Baroque. There are lovely carvings on the door and inside. To the left of the Duomo is the **Chiesa dell'Anime del Purgatorio** (Mon-Sat 9 am-12 pm, free). The custodian will happily show you the catacombs where skeletons of the townspeople lie in niches in the wall. The other church is the **Chiesa di San Benedetto alla Badia**, wth Baroque grating and a beautiful majolica floor.

Where to Eat

A Castellana (Piazza dei Caduti 4, ☎ 0918-148-667) is just beneath the castle walls.

La Locanda dei Principe (Via Amilcare 13, ☎ 0918-122-182, www.lolocandadelprincipe.com, Mon-Sat evening, Sun lunch and dinner, €€) is near the castle entrance.

■ Cefalù

★★Cefalù is a small fishing port tucked under a shelf of land and beneath a crag known as La Rocca. The medieval streets, historic sights and pleasant harbor have made it a popular tourist resort, though some hotels are very high-priced during the height of summer. It's an easy day-trip from Palermo or stay here and face the tourist pinch. It's also a good location for visiting the natural park of Madonie.

A small Greek settlement existed here from the fifth century BC, but it only really made its name when it was captured by the Romans, who used it as a key port. It was famous in antiquity for its abundant waters and fortifications and grew particularly splendid under the Normans, who set about destroying traces of the previous Arab occupants. Roger II commissioned the town's impressive cathedral in 1131, one of the most lovely in Sicily, that grew in power with important bishoprics.

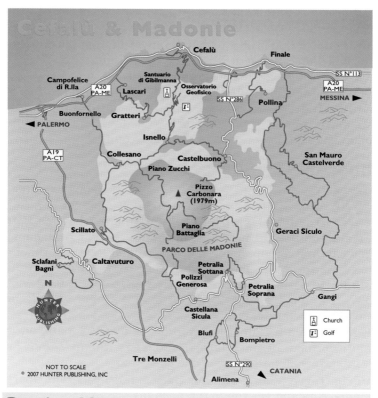

Getting Here

Cefalù is just over an hour from Palermo by train or bus. Trains run frequently along the coast and are the best way to get here. **SAIS** buses leave from Palermo twice daily and arrive at the square outside the station. Other connections go to Gangi, Geraci, Castelbuono, Collesano, Trabia, Termini Imerese and Caltanisetta in the interior.

Sommatinese Viaggi (Via Cavour 2, ☎ 0921-424-301, Segreteria.sommatineseviaggi@gvv.it) connects to Gibilmanna (three times daily) and Grateri (four times daily).

AST has connections to Turno, Castello, Isnello, Collesano, Campo Fellice Rocce, Campofelice Stazione, Erice, Termini Immerse and Palermo.

Autolinee Randazzo (☎ 0918-148-235) runs to Caccamo and Termini Imerese nine times daily.

From Cefalù you can also get a hydrofoil to the Aeolians islands with **SNAV** (☎ 091-631-7900, www.snav.it).

Getting Around

The train station is about a 10-minute walk from the city center and Corso Ruggero where the main sights are. You can leave your luggage at the station deposit.

Scooter for Rent (Via G. Matteotti, 13 bis – c/da S. Lucia-Club Med, ☎ 092-142-0496, 338-230-9008, www.scooterforrent.it) rents scooters (€20/day) and mountain bikes (€10/day). Weekly rentals are discounted.

Information Sources

 The tourist office (Corso Ruggero 77, ☎ 0921-421-050, www.cefalu-tour.pa.it, Mon-Sat 8 am-7:30 pm, Sun 9 am-1:30 pm) has helpful information for both Cefalù and its surroundings, including the Parco Madonie. You can find a map, hotel information and local bus timetables. However, for more information on the **Parco delle Madonie**, visit their offices (Corso Rugero 118, ☎ 0921-923-327, 8:30 am-1:30 pm, 2:30-7:30 pm). A useful website on Cefalù is www.cefalu.it.

Kultur Forum (Corso Ruggero 55, ☎ 092-192-3998, www.kulturforum.it, 9 am-1 pm, 4-7 pm) offers Italian lessons for €120/€75/€65 for groups of one/two/three.

Porta Terre Viaggi (Piazza Garibald 12) can rent apartments, cars and get you to the Aeolians.

Scicil Travel (Piazza Garibaldi 9, ☎ 0921-420-090) has similar services.

Tracce Sican (☎ 0921-427-113, www.traccesicanet.it) has guided 4WD and trekking excursions.

Sightseeing

★★**Duomo di Cefalù** (8 am-12 pm, 3:30-6:30 pm, free) is the main drawing card away from the sands and worth going to first thing in the morning to avoid the summer crowds. The duomo was commissioned by the Norman Count Roger II in 1131 and befits his position as one of Sicily's most influential rulers. The superb Norman edifice may also have been designed to curb the growing influence of the papacy in Palermo. It sits at the top of stairs in the pleasant Piazza del Duomo with a rocky crag towering above it. The main entrance is through a courtyard to the right of the façade, a massive for-

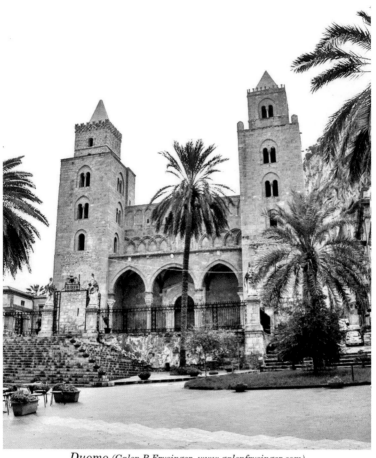
Duomo (Galen R Frysinger, www.galenfrysinger.com)

tress-like exterior with twin towers linked by a double row of arches. Inside is mostly plain except for the apse and vault, which have some of the most beautiful mosaics in Sicily and Italy. It is worth noting that they were completed some 20 to 30 years before those of Monreale. They are also from a different artistic tradition with a more Byzantine influence. They feature the gigantic figure of Christ Pantokrator (All Powerful). Christ has a really human expression and holds an open Bible bearing the inscription from John 8:12: "I am the light of the world; he who follows me shall not walk in darkness." The Duomo is closed to tourists during mass (well worth attending). There's also a lovely 14th-century wooden cross in the apse.

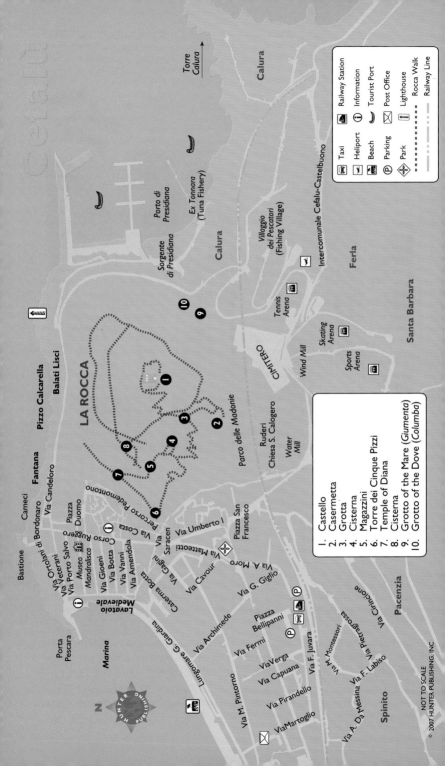

Cefalù

Torre Calura

Calura

Legend:

🚖 Taxi	🚂 Railway Station
🚁 Heliport	ⓘ Information
🏖 Beach	☾ Tourist Port
Ⓟ Parking	✉ Post Office
✧ Park	🔦 Lighthouse
····· Rocca Walk	
—·—·— Railway Line	

Porto di Presidiana

Ex Tonnara (Tuna Fishery)

Sorgente di Presidiana

Villaggio dei Pescatori (Fishing Village)

Intercomunale Cefalù-Castelbuono

Calura

Ferla

Santa Barbara

Balati Lisci

Pizzo Calcarella

LA ROCCA

Tennis Arena

Skating Arena

Wind Mill

Sports Arena

Bastione   Cameci

Fantana

Via Candeloro

Parco delle Madonie

CIMITERO

Ruderi Chiesa S. Calogero

Water Mill

Porta Pescara

Marina

Via Ortolani di Bordonaro

Via Veterani
Via Porto Salvo

Museo Mandralisca

Corso Ruggero

Piazza Duomo

Via Gioeni
Via Botta
Via Vanni
Via Amendola

Via Saracen

Via Costa

Percorso Pedemontano

Via Gaglio

Via Matteotti

Piazza San Francesco

Via Umberto I

Lavatoio Medievale

Caserma Botta

Via Cavour

Via A. Moro

Lungomare G. Giardina

Via Archimede

Piazza Bellipanni

Via Fermi

Via G. Giglio

Via M. Pintorno

Via Verga

Via Capuana

Via Pirandello

Via Martoglio

Via F. Juvara

Via M. Montessori

Via A. Da Messina

Via F. Labiso

Via Pietragrossa

Via Ciminna

Pacenzia

Spinito

NOT TO SCALE

© 2007 HUNTER PUBLISHING, INC.

Numbered locations:

1. Castello
2. Casermetta
3. Grotta
4. Cisterna
5. Magazzini
6. Torre dei Cinque Pizzi
7. Temple of Diana
8. Cisterna
9. Grotto of the Mare (Giumenta)
10. Grotto of the Dove (Columba)

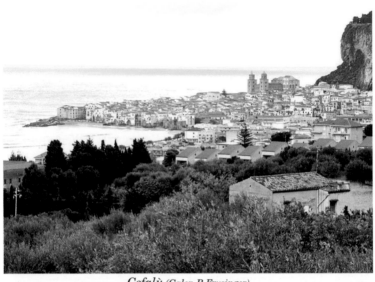

Cefalù (Galen R Frysinger)

Opposite Piazza del Duomo is **Via Mandralisca**. Walk down past the 15th-century Monte di Pieta – locked and barred – on

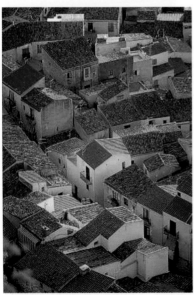

Cefalù rooftops

to the **Museo Biblioteca Mandralisa** (Via Mandralisa 13, 9 am-7 pm, €4,20), which has a collection of Greek ceramics and Arabic pottery and paintings. If you're passing by but don't want to stop, peek into the ticket office to see the mosaic.

Walk down to the end of the street and turn left on Via Vittorio Emanuele for the *lavatoio*, a 16th-century wash house built over a spring. The spring was known even in Arab Norman times and has good water, so feel free to fill up your water bottle. The wash

house has a series of basins cut into the rock with canals leading to the sea.

Go back down Via Vittorio Emanuele in the other direction via Porta Pescara where colorful fishing boats are pulled up on the beach. Make sure you wander and have a look at the designs. Piazza Marina has a number of good eating options. From here you could walk down Via C.O di Bordonaro for evening dining choices to Piazza Crispi where there's a view over the sea.

If you want to see a *pupi* (puppet) performance, go to the **Teatro dei Pupi a Cefalù** (Corso Ruggero 92, Wed and Fri-Sun 6 pm, €5) for nightly shows.

The **Osterio Magno** on the corner of Via Amendola and Corso Ruggero is a curious mix of a medieval palace and a tower house that was once the residence of Roger II.

Adventures

On Foot

The massive crag of 912 feet called **La Roccha** is a popular climb for views of the town and coast. Steps lead up from the Banca di Sicilia on Piazza Garibaldi. After 20 minutes you will reach the **Tempio di Diana** of the fifth century BC. Keep to the left of the temple and the path continues to the

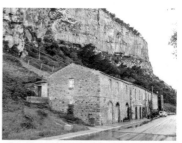

La Rocca (Galen R Frysinger, www. galenfrysinger.com)

top of the crag. There's not much left of the Norman castle that once existed on top but you are rewarded with good views. It should take an hour round-trip.

In Water

The seas around Cefalù are very pictur-esque and there are op-

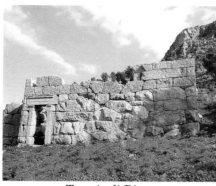

Tempio di Diana

portunities for swimming and snorkeling in the beautiful bays and coves along the coast. Boat tours of 4½ hours with **Turismez** (Corso Ruggero 83, ☎ 0921-421-264, €25) leave from the Cefalù port at 9 am and 2:30 pm.

For a chance to fish along the coast join **Coop Nettuno's** (Via Pietragrossa 32, ☎ 338-230-9141) professional fishermen. There are three departures at 9 am, 3 pm, and 9:30 pm for a five-hour fishing and

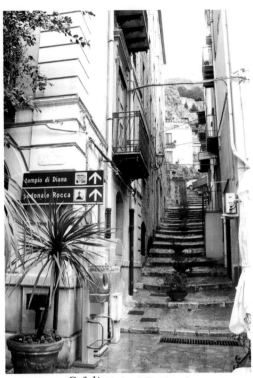

Cefalù (Galen R Frysinger)

eating excursion (€45). Another option includes dinner at Café Duomo for €60.

Where to Stay

Camping

Camping options are the only budget choices in the area.

Camping Costa Ponente (Contrada Ogliastrillo SS 113, ☎ 092-142-0085, fax 092-142-4492, www.camping-sizilien.de) is two km west of town. Take the La Spisa bus from the train station. It has a panoramic position above a rocky cliff right at the entrance to Cefalù and has been managed for 28 years by the same German owner. Open mid-March to mid-October. **Camping San Filippo** (Contrada

Ogliastrillo SS 113, ☎ 0921-422-504, campingsanfilippo@ libero.it) is next to Costa Ponente.

B&Bs

Dolce Vita B&B (Via C.O di Bordonaro 8, ☎ 0921-923-151, www.doclevitabb.it) is in the historical center and close to the beach, with elegant rooms.

B&B Case Ruggero (Corso Ruggero 54, ☎ 0921-922-259, €€-€€€), just before the information center, is a set of three apartments in an old Cefalù house.

Hotels

Astro Hotel (Via Nino Martoglio 8, ☎ 0921-421-639, www. astrohotel.it, €€€-€€€€) is a small place, with well equipped rooms.

La Giara (Via Veterani 40, ☎ 0921-421-562, www.hotel-lagiara.it, €€€€) is very central and close to the Duomo.

Rival del Sole (Via Lungomare 25, ☎ 0921-421-230, €€€€) is not too pretty from the outside but has good rooms and is right on the beach.

Where to Eat

Cafés & Bars

La Galleria (Via 25 Novembre 22/24, €€) is a bar, restaurant, bookshop and Internet café with photo-graphic exhibitions and art shows that change every 20 days. You eat in the garden courtyard.

Café del Molo (Piazza Marina) has pleasant tables in the shade and you can see the beach from the bar.

Bar Duomo (Corso Ruggero 120, ☎ 0921-922-348) serves on tables in the square.

Restaurants on *Lungomare*

Ristorante Vecchia Marina (Via Vittorio Emanuele 73, 12-3 pm, 7-11:30 pm, €€€) has tables overlooking the water and live fish in the tank! There are boats, ropes, nets, and paint-ings of fishermen to set the scene.

Le Covo del Pirata (Via Vittorio Emanuele 59, €€) has a balcony over the sea and cheap meals.

Restaurants on Via C.O di Bordonaro

Via C.O di Bordonaro has a number of good restaurants with terraces looking out over the sea.

Lo Scoglio Ubriaco (Via C.O di Bordonaro 2-4, ☎ 0921-423-370, €€€), meaning the drunken rock, has good fish specialties.

Trappitu (Via C.O di Bordonaro 96, closed Thurs, €€) stands out for its blue colors. Pizza is served in the evening; try the *trappitu* with tomato, mozzarella, porcini mushrooms, rocket and parmesan cheese. There are tourist menus for €18-20.

Al Porticciolo (Via C.O di Bordonaro 66, closed Wed, €€) has fixed menus from €15-30 and good pizza.

Restaurants by the Duomo

Ristorante Caffe Duomo (Piazza Duomo 24, ☎ 0921-921-271, €€€), on the right side of the square, offers snacks and drinks or you can eat inside. It's a posh establishment with a nice upstairs balcony for eating.

La Corte dei Bolosu or **Bolosi** is an *enotecha* nearby that's good for an evening drink.

Osteria del Duomo (Via Seminario 3, ☎ 0921-421-838, €€€€) is right in front of the cathedral at the bottom of the steps. The smoked fish is good and the *carpaccio* of fish or beef is renowned.

La Brace (Via 25 Novembre 10, ☎ 0921-423-570, €€€€) is a Michelin star restaurant not far from the Duomo. The cuisine has Sicilian and Asian touches.

■ Parco Naturale
Regionale delle Madonie ★★★

Cefalù is surrounded by the Parco Naturale delle Madonie – a land of high mountains, woods and hillsides dotted with small villages and beautiful monuments of the Arab and Norman era. These mountains are the second-oldest and -highest geologic group in Sicily after Etna. The reserve is 112,000 acres and, while it accounts for just 2% of the surface area of Sicily, half the plant species on the island can be found here. You can combine walking, biking, horseback riding and other pursuits with touring the interesting towns. Visitors should always be

Tyrrhenian Coast

equipped for the extremes of weather in the Madonie mountains with warm jackets and waterproofs.

Getting around is easiest with your own car, but there are bus connections from the coast and Palermo, mostly with SAIS and AST. Cefalù's tourist office has some maps of paths in the area, as does the Parco delle Madonie office (see *Information Sources, Cefalù*). There is also an office in Petralia Sottana at Corso Paolo Agliata 16 (☎ 0921-644-011). The Cefalù-Madonie (1:50,000) map is available at the offices, detailing 30 walking itineraries in the park.

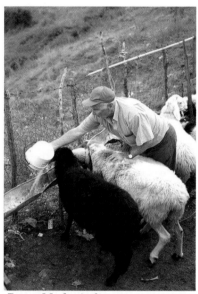

Parco Madonie farmer (Joanne Lane)

If you do plan on doing any hiking, make sure you get a good map and full information about the itinerary you are using. The tourist office in Cefalù should be able to help. You could also get a list of the local refuges. The routes described here are walking suggestions and should not be your only source of information.

See www.parcodellemadonie.it for more information. They have downloadable itineraries in pdf format online (in Italian only). Another good resource is *The Madonie Park* by Francesco Alaimo (Fabio Orlando Editore).

MADONIE CUISINE & CRAFTS

Each of the Madonie villages has a strong gastronomic and craft tradition. A lot of the holiday farms prepare organic products, including oil and wine. Here are some of the items to look out for while you're exploring the area:

■ The award-winning wines from around Castelbuono.

■ Fresh pasta in Caltavuturo and Petralia Sottana. Petralia Sottana produces excellent durum grain pasta sold all over Italy.

■ *U'sfuoghhiu*, a cheese-baked cake from Polizzi Generosa.

■ The typical Madonie black pigs that you see out grazing in herds and running across the road are farmed and served as part of tasty first and second courses in local restaurants and holiday farms.

■ Fresh and salted ricotta.

■ Seasoned goat's cheese called *caciocavallo*.

■ Mozzarella and *caciotta* (soft cheese).

■ Typical Madonie crafts – ceramics, fine hemming in macrame, wrought iron and wood and stone products.

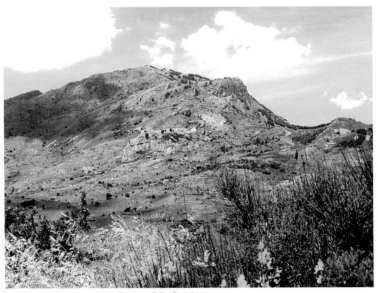

Parco Madonie (Martin Teetz)

Santuario di Gibilmanna

This 17th-century church (8 am-1 pm, 3-8 pm; free) is a good day-trip from Cefalù or can be one of your first forays into the

park. It's commonly a pilgrimage site for those praying to the shrine of the Virgin Mary. Visitors flock here on September 8 each year but there are usually quite a few people here muttering prayers, picknicking under

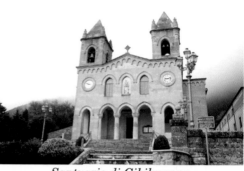

Santuario di Gibilmanna

the trees or admiring the view from the terrace. You can see the Madonie mountains and maybe even the peak of Pizzo Carbonara. A path leads into the woods from the car park, with plaques showing the stages of the cross. There's a museum beside the sanctuary (8 am-1 pm, 3-8 pm, €1.50) with artifacts from churches, convents and monasteries nearby. A local bus from Cefalù's Via Umberto 1 gets to the *santuario* in 20 minutes. If you need something to eat, there is a pizzeria and bar. The **Fattoria Pianetti** (☎ 0921-421-890) has a restaurant and rooms with baths. They also have a number of activities, including guided horseback riding and walking tours into the woods, with information on the flora. In particular they run excursions to Gratteri, Castelbuono and Gangi.

Gratteri & Isnello

Gratteri and Isnello have classic Madonie scenery with green hills, rocky mountains and clouds! Both villages have their nucleus in their piazza and central church. Here you'll still see farmers out with their sheep or goats and authentic Madonie life. There are a few interesting ruins, including the old castles of Isnello. AST (☎ 0916-800-030) buses run from Cefalù to Isnello and La Spisa (☎ 0921-424-300) and connect Gratteri to Cefalù.

Adventures

On Foot

■ *Isnello to Gratteri (3½ hours, 8½ km)*

This is a fairly strenuous walk on a medium-altitude mountain ridge. It starts from a path curving past the

cemetery across the field and over the watercourse to the forestry area. Go through the gate and up the lane. The path
climbs to near Monte Grotta Grande, then turns southwest to
Pizzo Dipilo and the lovely elongated pastoral valley known
as the Vallone San Giorgio. The track enters Gratteri near the
evocative eighth-century castle underpass, which leads
around to the adjoining church of the Matrice Vecchia.

■ *Gratteri to San Giorgio Abbey (1.7 km)*
From the highest part of Gratteri near the ruins of the castle,
take a narrow track heading south in the direction of a big
valley. This leads to the beautiful remains of the San Giorgio
Abbey. The solitary ruins are the only settlement of the
Premonstratensian Order of the Reformed Augustinians. The
abbey was founded in 1140 by Duke Roger. The track beyond
the abbey eventually leads to Collesano.

In Caves

■ *The Wind Cave*
This is one of the most interesting and complex of the
Madonie caves. It is over four km long and rich in concretions
and underwater pools. There are splendid views from the entrance to the cave. Due to its length and depth you would be
well advised to contact a proper guide before attempting to explore the cave. Check with the Cefalù tourist office for recommendations or contact Club Alpino Italiano (Via Agrigento 30,
Palermo, ☎ 091-625-4352) or Associazione Nisida (Via
Agrigento 67, Palermo ☎ 091-301-663).

■ *Grotta Grattara (30 minutes)*
The Grattera cave is an easy walk through thick pine woods
to two enormous rock arches, moulded by erosion. Inside, a
depression has been formed by the trickle of water. To find the
path, turn left on the first road into Gratteri, which runs behind the town to the *forestale* entrance maintained by the
commune. You'll find a small wooden hut and a stone wall.
The pathway beyond it is manned 9 am-6:30 pm daily and on
weekends in winter. The entrance fee (€1.50) goes toward
maintaining the paths. Contact Soc. Cooperitiva Hollywood
(Corso Umberto 1, 83, Gratteri, ☎ 333-179-2973) for information. They can also organize mountain bike or donkey and
pony rides. The route beyond the cave continues to Isnello.

Tyrrhenian Coast

Where to Stay & Eat

 Nta'Chiannara (Via Garrotta 3, closed Mon, ☎ 092-142-9633, 348-871-9780, €€) is a popular spot for a meal on the road into Gratteri. They also have three rooms. **D'Agostaro Francesca** (Via delle Scuole 26, ☎ 0921-429-242) rents rooms in town, or stay at the **Agriturismo Fattoria Pianetti** (Contrada Pianetti, ☎ 0921-421-890) outside of town.

La Villa (Via Carrozza 68, ☎ 092-142-9497) is a bar and restaurant and the **Bar del Corso** at the end of the main street serves snacks.

In Isnello the options are **Bonafede Manzella Vincenza** for rooms in town (Via Roma 36, ☎ 0921-662-179) or **Piano Torre Park Hotel** (C. da Piano Torre, www.pianotorreparkhotel.it, ☎/fax 092-166-2671, 092-166-2672) out of town. For meals go to Pizzeria Santa Lucia (Via Dante 32, ☎ 0921-662-374).

Piano Zucchi

Climbing to 3,625 feet. this pretty karst tableland can often be covered in clouds during the summer and snow in the winter. There's also a beautiful little church, **San Paolo Apostolo**, with a pleasant combination of stone and wood that fits into the landscape. In the summers the pleasant lawn area is perfect for camping (see *Where to Stay & Eat*) and the start of good walking itineraries to Collesano and Piano Battaglia. During summer, locals can often be spotted looking for mushrooms.

Accomodations include the **Park Hotel** (☎ 092-162-671, 092-162-672), just before Piano Zucchi on the main road. It also has a restaurant.

Club Alpino Siciliano Rifugio "Orestano" (Piano Zucchi, ☎/fax 092-166-2159, www.rifugiorestano.com) is a large chalet-like structure with a huge St Bernard dog roaming around – completely harmless. Inside is warm and cozy, with a fireplace and plenty of useful information on walks. They can sleep up to 120 people and provide breakfast lunch and dinner (€18). They can also provide guides for walkers.

Following page: Piano Zucchi (Joanne Lane)

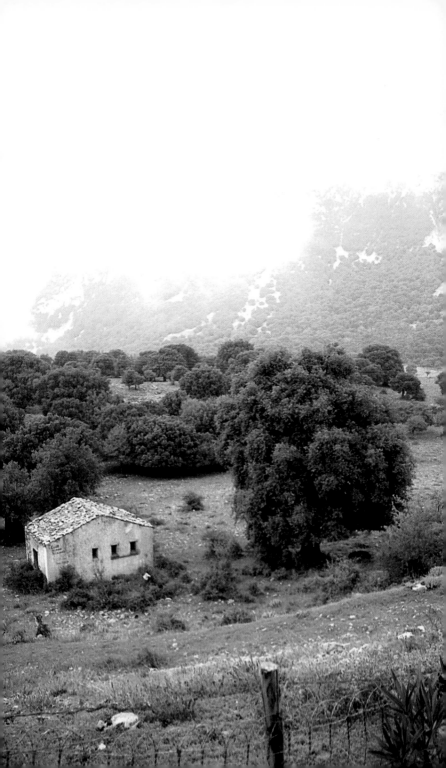

Piano Battaglia

This tableland at 5,200 feet is also of karst origin. It is surrounded by rich beech woods and is a relaxing place in spring and summer as well as being a renowned skiing resort. In the winter three km

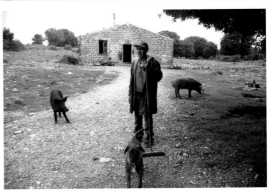

Madonie farmer (Joanne Lane)

of tracks on the north slopes of the Monte Mufara give ski enthusaists the opportunity to enjoy the snow. There are also plenty of accommodations.

Adventures

In Snow

Skiing is possible at Piano Battaglia in January and February for a longer period than elsewhere in Sicily thanks to very cold winds from the north. There are two ski lifts to the ski runs. The Mufara skiing complex goes up to 6,800 feet above sea level and serves 3½ km of runs. There are five *pistas*, with easy, medium and three black runs. The Mufaretta is southwest and reaches 5,435 feet, with a run about half a kilometre. It is possible to do cross-country skiing here too. **Ski World** (☎ 335-727-9110) rents equipment if you don't have your own.

On Foot

- *Piano Battaglia – Pizzo Carbonara*
  (2 hours 45 minutes, 5.8 km)

★★This itinerary entails the ascent of Pizzo Carbonara, the highest peak in the Madonie – although Pizzo Antenna is only six feet lower! In clear conditions the views are amazing, but don't hold your breath – thick mists are frequent and can be disorienting. The walk is not difficult, but a sense of direction and a compass do help.

If the weather is not great when you start you may want to hold off for another day.

The route starts from Piano Battaglia, climbing past the Ostello. At the next junction, turn left and park on the ensuing curve. A clear path strikes out towards a saddle. Pass a ruined house and keep left at the fork and the following one. There are occasional splashes of red paint to show you the way. You should be able to spot Pizzo Antenna due north and admire the fossils of corals, sponges and shells in the rock base. The path skirts Pizzo Antenna and the path all but peters out. But you're close to the saddle here. Head northwest up the mountainside to a modest pass and then keep right for a peak marked by two poles (6,343 feet) and then due north to the sizeable cairn of Pizzo Carbonara (6,494 feet, 1½ hours). If it's clear, you'll have an amazing view. Return the way you came to the modest pass but then continue southish to another saddle, where you keep left alongside some beeches. There is no path, but you follow the depression left towards a hut. From here, there's a faint path southwest that joins a clearer route left and eventually drops back down to where you started.

■ *Piano Battaglia to Piano Sempria (three hours)*

From Rifugio Ostello della Gioventu take path number two heading north to Pizzo Scalonazzo (6,242 feet) and an unattended refuge. The path snakes northwest by Pizzo Carbonara (6,490 feet) and then west to a fork. Take the left path to the refuge and wind around to **Rifugio Francesco Crispi** (☎ 0921-672-279) at Piano Sempria.

There are *sentieri geologico* (geological walking tracks) that explain some of the natural phenomena of the area with boards by the roadside or on the ski runs during summer.

MADONIE RIFUGI

At the time of writing this was the list of mountain cabins in the Madonie.

■ Rifugio Luigi Orestano (Piano Zucchi, ☎ 0921-662-159).

■ Rifugio Ostello della Gioventu Piero Merlino (Piano Battaglia, ☎ 0921-649-995).

■ Rifugio Francesco Crispi (Piano Sempria, ☎ 0921-672-279).

- Rifugio Marini (Piano Battaglia, ☎ 0921-49994) closed at the time of writing.

The following are unmanned:

- Rifugio A Saverino gia Scalonazzo (Isnello).
- Rifugio Melchiorre Morici (Castelbuono).
- Rigugio del Vicaretto (Geraci Siculo).
- Rifugio Monte Cervi (Isnello, ☎ 091-581-323).
- Rifugio F Tropea (Petralia Sottana, ☎ 0921-680-496).

With Mushrooms

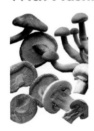

The Madonie *funghi* are a prized culinary item and you'll find them on menus throughout the park. The summer months are ideal for hunting mushrooms and you'll see people pulling in by the roadside to do their own troweling. It's best not to attempt this alone unless you know the types of mushrooms that are edible! If you would like to look for mushrooms, contact **Gruppo Micologico Siciliano** (Via Isidoro La Lumia 79, Palermo, ☎ 091-331-978) or ask one of the locals doing a spot of *cercando* (searching) if you can join them.

With Golf

★★At Contrada Bartuccelli (Collesano), **Le Madonie Golf** (☎ 0921-934-387, www.lemadoniegolf.com) offers an 18-hole course on 123 acres of turf. The golf course is open year-round, with a beautiful sea view. There's a bar and restaurant on-site and 31 cabins. The agricultural farm produces a number of biological products available for sale.

On Horseback

The Madonie mountains are an ideal place for horseback rides at altitudes that are not common on the island.

Tenuta Luogo Marchese (SS 286, Contrada Luogo Marchese, Pollina, ☎ 0921-910-029, www.tenutaluogomarchese.it has horses and does trips in the Madonie Park. The school uses indigenous horses that are characteristically docile, patient and proud.

★**L'Agriturismo Arione** (Contrada Pozzetti, Collesano, ☎ 347-476-3738, www.agriturismoarione.it) is one of the best places to find a riding itinerary. They have a six-day excursion taking in Piano Zucchi, Piano Cervi, Piano Grande, Petralie and Piano Sempria. If you are into horseback riding, this is the itinerary for you.

Fattoria Pinetti (☎ 0921-421-890) at Santuario di Gibilmanna, also provides lodging and riding.

Rifugio Francesco Crispi (Piano Sempria, ☎ 0921-427-703) has six horses and does excursions in the park.

Hotel Baita del Faggio (Isnello, ☎ 0921-622-194) has up to 10 horses.

Ranch San Guglielmo (Contrada San Guglielmo, ☎ 0921-671-150).

Cavallo Natura (Contrada Selia, ☎ 0921-672-740).

On Wheels

 If you want a good cycling path through the Madonie Park you can make your own itinerary with a good map. using the accomodation options along the way. Bike riders from Castelbuono frequently ride to Piano Battaglia in about three hours.

Donalegge (Polizzi Generosa, www.donalegge.com, ☎ 0921-562-289, €€€€) has bikes available for guests.

Hotel Kalura (Via Vincenzo Cavallaro 13, Cefalù, ☎ 0921-421-354, www.hotel-kalura.com) rents mountain bikes for €25/€130 per day/week and runs guided tours to Castelbuono (56 km), Gratteri (43 km), Isnello (66 km) and Pollina (56 km).

Other places to contact about bike riding in the Madonie are:

- **Federazione Ciclista** (Palermo, ☎ 091-671-8711).
- **UISP** (Via Napoli 84, Palermo, ☎ 091-611-3645).
- **Associazione Toto Cannatella** (Via Papireto, Palermo ☎ 091-322-425) for bike rental and guided tours or personal itineraries.
- **Gatto** (Vicolo Pantelleria 37, Palermo, ☎ 091-688-1484) promotes mountain biking.
- **Azienda Agrituristica Arione** (Contrada Pozzetti, Collesano, ☎ 0921-664-003) rents mountain bikes and provides itinerary ideas or can accompany riders.

Where to Stay

Hotel Baita del Faggio (C. da Fontanone, Piano Zucchi, Isnello, ☎ 092-166-2194, www.baitadelfaggio. it, €€€) is on the road three km before Piano Battaglia. Full- and half-pension deals are available. There is more accommodation here than at Piano Battaglia with 92 beds. Open all year. They also have horses (see *Adventures on Horseback*).

Rifugio Marini (☎ 0921-649-994) was closed at the time of writing.

Ostello della Gioventu P Merlino (Piano Battaglia-Isnello, ☎ 0921-649-995, €€€) is a warm, cozy chalet-style lodge offering fantastic Madonie meals around a fireplace and comfortable accommodation. They only have 12 rooms so book ahead. In winter it's €55 for rooms and two meals (full pension). In other seasons they do *mezzo pensione* for €40. Meals use local Madonie products – wild boar, mushrooms and cheese. It's busy in winter with skiiers; cyclists and motorbike riders come here at other times.

Castelbuono

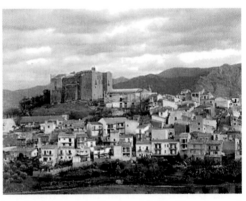

Castelbuono is an easy day-trip from Cefalù, just 40 minutes ride up the green valley. It's also on the SAIS bus route from Cefalù's train station. This is a lovely little place in the lower reaches of the mountains with some delightful central squares, friendly locals, a pleasant hill climate and good food. The tourist office is in Piazza Margherita (Mon-Sat, 9 am-1 pm, 4-8 pm, Sun 4-8 pm).

The **Associazione Naturalistica** (☎ 320-666-1849, 329-107-5054) can give you information on trekking and excursions in the region. The website www.castelbuono.com has useful details about the town.

Sightseeing

Above the tourist office you can visit the **Torre dell'
Orologio** (clock tower) on weekends. Outside in the piazza is
the **Matrice Vecchia** (9 am-1 pm, 4:30-7 pm), rather dark
and gloomy, but with some beautiful frescoes, particularly in
the crypt (€.50).

Il Castello de Ventimiglia (☎ 092-167-712, Tues-Sun 9 am-
1 pm, 4-7 pm; €1,50) is a squat 14th-century castle which
houses the **Museo Civico** (same hours). It sits at the top of

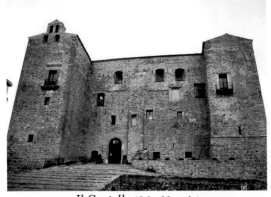

town directly up
the hill from the
tourist office.
The entrance
takes you into a
courtyard with
small barred
cells. Up the
stairs you enter
the first rooms,
with finds from
the castle, in-
cluding terra-
cotta pots,
coins, carved

Il Castello (John Mazzola)

stone and ceramic jugs. On the second floor is a collection of
religious paintings, processional wooden relics, jewelery, altar
boxes, candlesticks and other religious clothing. There is also
a small chapel with beautiful stuccos on the walls, the work of
Giacomo Serpotta. Outside the castle is a square where concerts are held in summer and there is a good restaurant.

Handicrafts and traditional foods are still very much alive in
Castelbuono. You may well see woodwork and wrought iron
objects, embroidery of lace, woven objects and confectionaries.
(See *Where to Eat*).

Adventures on Foot

You can walk from Castelbuono up to Piano Sempria
and to the **Rifugio Francesco Crispi** in two hours.
To find the start of the path, leave Castelbuono on the
SP 9 (the road leading above the town) and follows signs for
San Giuglielmo and Rifugio Sempria. The route is about 3½

km. From Piano Sempria you can continue to Piano Battaglia (three hours).

Where to Stay

Hotel Ariston (Via Vittimaro 2, ☎ 0921-671-321) is right in town.

4 Cannola B&B (Via Dafni 7, ☎ 0921-671-587).

Albergo Milocca (Contrada Piano Castagna, ☎ 0921-671-944, €€€) has a pool and ponies for rent.

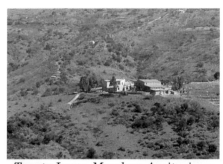

Tenuta Luogo Marchese Agriturismo

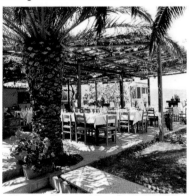

Tenuta Luogo Marchese terrace

Tenuta Luogo Marchese Agriturismo (SS 286, Km 4,700, Contrada Luogo Marchese, ☎ 0921-910-029, www.tenutaluogomarchese. it), towards Cefalù, has accommodatiosn and horseback riding.

★**Relais Santa Anastasia** (www.santa-anastasia-relais.it, ☎ 092-167-2233, 092-167-2092, fax 092-167-2288, €€€€) is on the road to Cefalù in a restored abbey. There are 25 rooms and three suites furnished with extreme care. A beautiful pool has a view over the property's extensive vineyards. There's a billiard room, conference

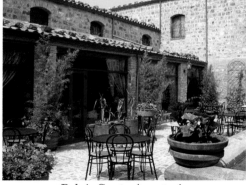

Relais Santa Anastasia

room, restaurant, bar, reading room, lounges and even a church.

Where to Eat

 Palazzaccio (Piazza Castello 2, ☎ 092-167-3664, open for lunch and dinner, closed Mon, €€) has a prime location right under the castle.

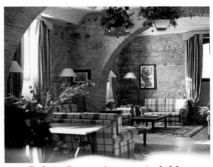
Relais Santa Anastasia lobby

Along Via S. Anna are a series of cafés and restaurants that make the most of the atmospheric street. **Ristorante U'Trappitu** (Via Sant'Anna 27, ☎ 0921-671-764, closed Mon, €€) is recommended by locals for fast service and good pizzas.

Nangalarruni (Via Alberghi 5, ☎ 0921-671-428, www.ristorantenangalarruni.it) is renowned for its use of Madonie ingredients like wild fennel.

In Piazza Margherita a number of the cafés have tables out in the square. Try ★**Fiasconaro** (Piazza Margherita 10, ☎ 0921-677-132) for traditional sweets, jams, cakes and liquors. They've also developed a product called Mannetto, which they promote as a new taste of the area. Basically it's it's made from local trees and mixed with white chocolate as a topping for cakes or for chocolates and is delicious. You are bound to walk out with a lot more than you bargained for here. The friendly staff will let you taste some of the specialties; ask to try *torroncini alla manna*.

Romittaggio (Località San Giulelmo Sud, ☎ 0921-671-323, €€€) is five km south of Castelbuono and specializes in simple mountain food. The restaurant is inside a monastery from the Middle Ages. Prices are €25-30.

■ Castel di Tusa

The village of Castel di Tusa lies 25 km east of Cefalù and is on the train line and Interbus route. It has the remnants of a defensive castle and some good rocky beaches – a good alternative to other coastal spots. Just above the town are the ruins of a castle that give the resort its name.

Tyrrhenian Coast

Lo Scoglio campsite (☎ 0921-334-345, €) offers budget accommodations. Otherwise, take the road down to the seafront to find ★**Atelier sul Mare Albergo Museo** (Via Cesare Battisti 4, ☎ 0921-334-295, www.ateliersulmare.com, €€€€). It's more an artistic creation

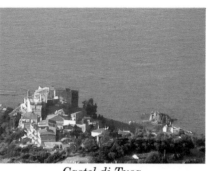
Castel di Tusa

by a restless owner than a hotel and is open to the public 12-1 pm for €4 when the rooms are vacated. With a fantastic location right by the seafront, the first room sets the scene –

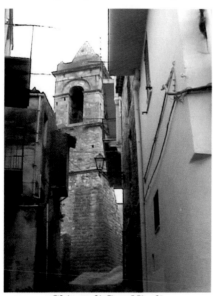
Chiesa di San Nicolò

completely covered in newspaper clippings, with the statement "Devozione alla bellezza" (devotion to beauty). The rooms are an incredible blend of color and style, but not really comfort. *Il Cosmo* has a bathroom like a carwash where water sprays from holes in the pipes.

Le Lampare (Via Cesare Battisti, ☎ 091-334-258) lies beyond the hotel at the end of the road beneath the old castle walls. It's a great spot for an afternoon drink or to watch the sunset. You can eat dinner on the terrace by the sea.

Three km away are the sparse ruins of **Halaea**, a fifth-century BC Sikel settlement. You can make out the streets, the *agora* and foundations of two third-century BC temples.

■ Santo Stefano di Camastra★

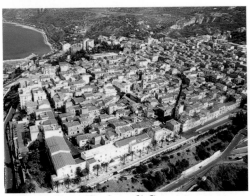

Santo Stefano di Camastra

You will have seen the colorful ceramics of Santo Stefano di Camastra all over Sicily long before you arrive here. If you haven't, you'll soon understand what the town is famed for. Every corner of Santo Stefano contains ceramic shops and there are some real bargains. If you're going to take home some gifts this is the place to buy them.

Ceramiche Desuir (Via Nazionale, ☎ 092-133-1156, www.desuir.it), just before town, has a huge series of warehouses where you can watch the artists at work. They also give fantastic discounts for bulk purchases.

The **Museo della Ceramica in Palazzo Trabia** (Via Palazzo, Tues-Sun 9 am-1 pm, 4-8 pm; free) has more displays. Or you can walk around the town to see the houses numbered with plates, street signs and just about everything else made of ceramic.

Café Belvedere is a small place with a great view at the end of Via Vittorio Emanuele. Sberna buses operate to Santo Stefano and it's on the train line.

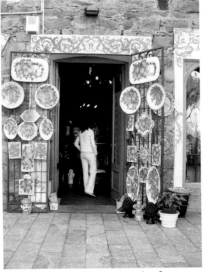

Santo Stefano ceramic shop

■ Parco Nebrodi★★★

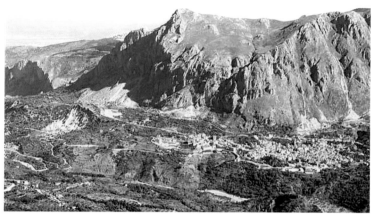

Parco Nebrodi

The Nebrodi mountains span 240,000 acres, of which 140,000 acres are woods. It was only set up in 1993 and protects a variety of trees and animals. The mountains extend from the Peloritani range in the east to the Madonie range east of Palermo. Mt Soro is the highest point at 6,000 feet.

Nebrodi comes from the Greek word Nebros, meaning fawns or young deer, which were once abundant in this area. The region contains 21 towns (17 in Messina province, three in Catania and one in Enna). SS 289

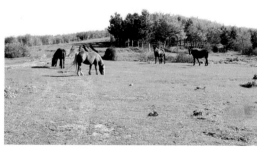

Horses graze in the park

cuts through the heart of the park, linking Cesaro behnd Mt Etna to Sant'Agata di Militello on the Tyrrhenian coast. Nebrodi is a protected area, but hunters do roam the woodlands looking for game. If you're driving along SS 289 you'll

spot various types of animals – try not to hit them! Wild pigs are common and in the lower stretches there are San Fratello horses, unique to this area.

Unlike the Madonie park, the Nebrodi is largely unpopulated. You're more likely to hear cow bells than sounds of human habitation. You can explore for days on end without meeting another soul. It's also incredibly misty in the high reaches, which can be disorienting. Mist and rain can also alter the conditions of trails, making them impassable or at least unpleasant. Don't expect to find information centers and well marked trails; apart from a few centers (listed below) and accomodations, there's not a lot of tourist infrastructure. However, there are good biking, walking and horseback riding opportunities.

The Touring Club Italiano produces a useful map of the area, *Il Parco dei Nebrodi* (1:50,000), if you can find one in stock. Tourist offices are notorious for running out of copies. With any luck the official seat in Messina (Via Ruggero Orlando 126, Messina, ☎ 0921-333-211) or in Alcara Li Fusi (Via Ugo Foscolo 1, ☎ 0941-793-904) will have some.

Recommended guides for the Nebrodi:

- **Hotel Kalura** (Via Vincenzo Cavallaro 13, Cefalù, ☎ 0921-421-354, www.hotel-kalura.com) rents mountain bikes for €25/€130 per day/week and runs guided tours.

- **Emilio** (Via dei Colonna 16, Cesaro, ☎ 095-773-2011, 328-047-6573) has a 4WD and does off-road excursions. He can meet you if you have no transport.

- **Nebro Tours** (Via Liberta 83-85, Castell'Umberto, ☎ 0941-438-730).

You will need your own car to do any exploration in the park or you'll have to arrange to be dropped off somewhere. One bus a day travels from Sant'Agata across to Cesaro.

Tyrrhenian Coast

NEBRODI CRAFTS & CUISINE

Nebrodi people are industrious and creative. On your travels through the region you're likely to see hand-embroidered clothes and sheets, cane or rush baskets, agricultural items made of wood or reed, stoneware and wrought iron objects, ceramics and multicolored mats and rugs (*pizzare*) made with ancient looms.

Of the foods, cheeses are a favorite. There's the mild or spicy *canestrato*, the tasty *pecorino* or *provola* and shepherds still make *ricotta* by hand.

The Nebrodi pigs also make good eating and the meat is seen on many menus. Olive oil, honey, hazelnuts, pistachios, fruits, mushrooms, tomatos and eggplant are all abundant. Almonds form the base for a number of biscuits and sweets.

Adventures

On Wheels

SS 289 cuts through the heart of the Nebrodi mountains and is a good way to explore its reaches if you don't have a lot of time. You can start from the Tyrrhenian coast at **Sant'Agata di Militello** and cut through to Cesaro, skirt Mount Etna and be in Catania in a day (a lot of driving!)

From Sant'Agata the first town of note is **San Fratello** (15 km). The town was once populated by a Lombard colony and – if you're a language whiz – you'll notice traces of the accent in the local dialect. There's a colorful festival

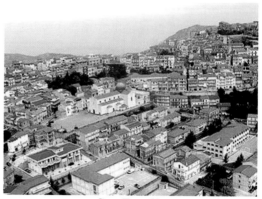

San Fratello

here one week before Easter called the **Festa dei Giudei** (Feast of the Jews), worth getting to if you're in the region. It's fairly quiet at other times. Bars, gelaterias, banks and men playing cards wearing berets line the main road through town. There are a few churches in town but **Mount San Fratello** is what will catch your eye. This isolated rocky outcrop lies below the town. Perched on top is a **Norman sanctuary** overlooking Sant'Agata di Militello. It's a superb loca-

tion for a picnic or a trudge from town if you want to stretch your legs. The sanctuary is dedicated to three brothers horribly martyred by the Romans. There are also the ruins of the ancient city of **Apollonia**, a Sicilian city occupied by the Greeks. You should be able to spot some San Fratello horses in the surrounding fields.

There's not a lot else going on in town but if you need somewhere to eat there's a *rosticceria* and supermarket on the main street and the **Albergo Monte Saro** (Via Saverio Latteri 23, ☎ 094-179-4120, €€) has rooms and a restaurant on the first floor.

THE SAN FRATELLO HORSE

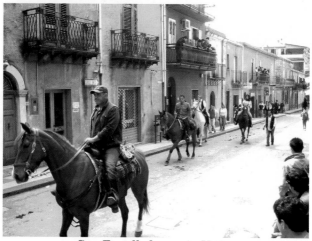

San Fratello horses in Ustica

Seven km beyond San Fratello on your right is the **Centro Ristoro Cooperative Spazi Verdi** – a mouthful for the small shed offering wonderful Nebrodian game food. On the road beyond is the **Istituto Incremento Ippico per la Sicilia**, where you can see the San Fratello horses, famous in these parts. They don't do excursions but are happy for you to view their fine stallions and may even take them out into the yard from the dark stalls so you can get a better look. They're frisky but beautiful. Usually someone is there from 7 am to 12 pm and 3:30-7 pm, but call first (☎ 333-980-2978 or 095-551-925). Ask to speak with Zafuto or Bendivegna.

Tyrrhenian Coast

On Wheels & On Foot

★★★Mistretta to Floresta (three days, 57 km)

It is possible to hike, bike or Jeep the entire breadth of the Nebrodi from a point just south of Mistretta on the S117 that cuts right through the park to Floresta on the S116. If you're in a car it needs to have high ground clearance. And you are advised to get the Touring Club Italiano map that marks this itinerary clearly. The route takes you past lakes of interest and the highest point of the park, Monte Soro. But there won't always be views because of the frequent mist. You're also guaranteed sightings of various animals includ-

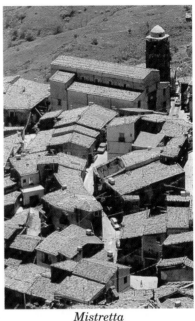

Mistretta

ing horses and pigs. Be wary of dogs guarding sheep as they can be aggressive. If you don't have a vehicle, you could complete the route to Monte Soro from the Villa Miraglia at Portella lla della Miraglia on foot. The access to the *sentiero* is

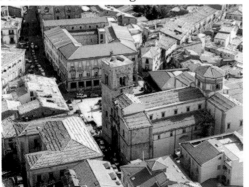

Mistretta's Centro Storico

near San Fratello. The road to Monte Soro is about 10 km. Alternatively, you could trek the seven km to Lago Maulazzo and three km beyond to Lake Bivere di Cesaro. This lake turns red in the summer months from microalgae.

The walk is suitable for those of medium walking ability. The time frames correspond to a walking speed of four km every hour. Each day the walk ends near one of the Nebrodi towns, so you can stop the excursion there if you prefer.

Mistretta, where the eastern section starts, lies just to the west of Santo Stefano. It's the first and biggest of the Nebrodi hill villages and can be reached by Interbus from Santo Stefano. There's not a lot to detain you in Mistretta, but it is a good base if you plan to tackle the route to Floresta.

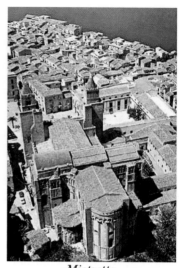
Mistretta

Piazza Vittorio Veneto is the main square, with wrought iron balconies and a central church. The **Albergo Sicilia** (Via Liberta, ☎ 0921-381-463) has rooms, a bar and pizzeria.

Day 1: Mistretta - Portella dell'Obolo (21 km, six hours). The access to the *sentiero* is south of Mistretta on the SS117 at Serra Merio. The route is of medium difficulty and if you wanted to end the trail here the road from Portella dell'Obolo runs south to Capizzi or north to Caronia. The route takes you past **Urio Quattrocchi**, a circular lake popular for spotting waterbirds, turtles, small mammals and rodents. Beyond are beautiful beech woods.

Day 2: Portella dell'Obolo - Portella Femmina Morta (23 km, six hours). The second day passes close to the Sorgente Nocita, where fresh drinking water is available. **Monte Pelato** (5,140 feet) is one of the most beautiful peaks, with a breathtaking panorama towards Monte Soro and Etna. You could stay the night at **Villa Miraglia** or end the route here and take the SS289 to Cesaro or Sant'Agata Militello.

Day 3: Portella Miraglia - Case Cartolari (23 km, seven hours). The third day passes Lago Maulazzo and Lago Biviere and continues all the way into Floresta, where the journey ends. You could also take an excursion to the top of Monte Soro, the highest Nebrodi peak, near the start of the trip.

Tyrrhenian Coast

Alcara Li Fusi

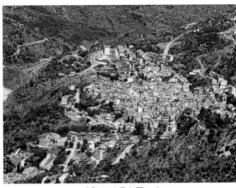

Just 16 km from Sant'Agata Militello on the coast, Alcara Li Fusi could be a world away, nestled into part of the mountain above the river in the Valle del Rosmarino. It's a sleepy place, best visited for access to the Rocche del Castro.

Alcari Li Fusi

There are a few things to see in town, including the *lavatoio* in Piazza Abate, where seven water channels gush out into a long line of stone washing tubs. The Chiesa Matrice is in the main square.

Sberna (☎ 0941-701-023) departs from Sant'Agata Militello for Alcara at 8 am, 11 am, 1:30, 3:15 and 5 pm. If you need somewhere to stay, **Castel Turio** (Via della Rinascita, ☎ 0941-793-788) has rooms. For tourist information, call ☎ 0941-793-010 and the **Ente Parco dei Nebrodi** (Via U Foscolo, ☎ 0941-793-904).

Rocche del Castro

This enormous rock is located between Longi, San Marco d'Alunzio and Alcara Li Fusi. It's a majestic formation with deep cracks where birds of prey nest. The summit has beautiful views. Walking routes from all three locations will get you there. From Portella Gazzana (Longi) on the SS157 it's a seven-km walk of about 2½ hours. From Alcara Li Fusi (Contrada Lemina) it's 9.2 km and from San Marco d'Alunzio start from near the *sorgento* Maliro for a seven-km hike.

Where to Stay & Eat

★The **Centro Spazi** (Contrada Cicaldo, ☎ 094-179-4683, 094-179-4838, 339-639-2355, €€), seven km up from San Fratello on the right hand side, is open March to November for lunch and dinner. It's popular with local hunters and farmers. This is little more than a shed, but

you'll get amazing *salsiccia, maccheroni freschi al sugo* and *grigliata di pecora castrato* for just €15-20. Plus you're guaranteed some first-rate local company. Call first to make sure it's open.

Beyond San Fratello the only place to stay is the ★★**Villa Miraglia** (SS 289 Cesaro, www.villamiraglia.it, ☎ 095-773-2133, €€€€). They are open all year, but reserve ahead for lunch and dinner, especially in August. There are five doubles and one twin. Half/full pension is €50/€62 per person. It's a fantastic rustic place, usually misted over by Nebrodi clouds, with salt-of-the-earth ownership and popular with locals and hunters. They can help you out with details of itineraries to Monte Soro nearby (see *Adventures on Foot*), arrange for or recommend a guide or let you leave your car while you take excursions through the woods. From here the road drops down into Cesaro.

■ San Marco d'Alunzio

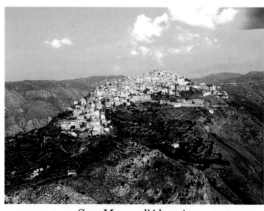
San Marco d'Alunzio

San Marco d'Alunzio is another day-trip well worth making away from the coast. It is impressively sited high above the coastal plain and is a delightful town with narrow streets. You could easily wander around here for half a day or even stay overnight. Camadra and Drago buses come here. There's an information office in Via Aluntina (☎ 094-179-7339, 9 am-1 pm, 3:30-8 pm, www.ufficioturistico.aluntino.virgilio.it), which is very helpful and will encourage you to visit all of its 22 churches and two museums.

The town was founded by the Greeks in the fifth century BC and later occupied by the Romans. The **Tempio di Ercole** is

the first build-
ing you'll notice
as you come into
town, with a
wonderful loca-
tion making it
appear to hang
suspended over
the sea. A roof-
less church was
built on the tem-
ple's red marble

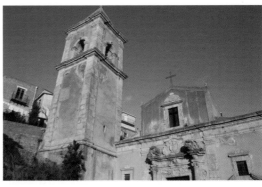

base, called **Chiesa Normannia di S. Marco Alunzio**.
Many of the San Marco buildings are built with this same red

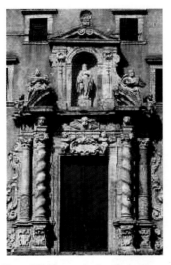

marble, giving them a picturesque look, particularly at sunset. In town there are scant remnants of a Norman castle and
some beautiful churches, including **Chiesa S. Antonio**, **Chiesa
SS Salvatore** (once a Roman
chapel) and the **Chiesa di
Santa Maria delle Grazie**. The
Museo Arte Sacre (☎ 0941-
797-045, 10 am-1 pm, 4-8 pm,
€2.60) has keys to all the other
churches. If you pay €3.10 they
will take you on a tour of the
churches. The museum contains
religious paintings and artifacts.

If you need something to eat,
Bar Tiffany is in the piazza where the buses arrive. Near the
Chiesa Madre is **Number One Pizzeria** (☎ 0941-797-627)
and **Le Fornace** (Via Cappucini 115, ☎ 094-179-7297). If you
need somewhere to stay, ask at Le Fornace for *affitacamere*.
They start at just €20 per person.

L'Angolo delle Delizie is a fantastic shop with typical products from all over Nebrodi, including salami made from
Nebrodi pigs.

■ The Coastal Route to Milazzo

Adventures

In Archaeology

■ *Patti*

Patti is a fairly unin-
teresting town but
most people come
here for the remains
of the **Villa Romana**
(9 am-7 pm, €2) that
lie directly under the
autostrada. They're
nothing exciting but
something to do on a
wet day. The site
seems to be a mix of

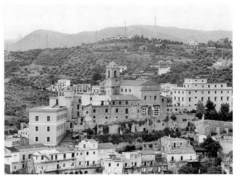

scaffolding, a few mosaics and the remains of a bathhouse.
You can buy a ticket for the ruins at Tyndaris for €3. Patti has
train and AST bus connections to the rest of the coast.

■ *Tyndaris*

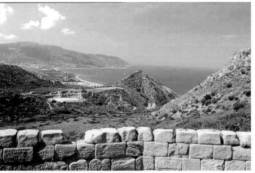

Looking from Tyndaris toward the bay

The ruins of the
ancient city of
Tyndaris are on a
rocky promon-
tory overlooking
a beautiful bay
about six km east
of Patti. This was
one of the last
Greek settle-
ments in Sicily,
built and forti-
fied by settlers
from Siracusa as a defense against the old enemy, the
Carthaginians. There are about three SARI buses from
Patti's main square that come here daily, which is useful as
the train station is a few km away. AST and SAIS services
from Messina go to Patti. The bus drops you at the bottom of
the hill. It's a steep climb to the top or you can make use of the

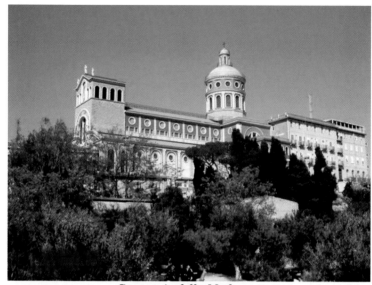
Santuario della Madonna

minibuses plying the route for €.50 (9 am-7:30 pm). Parking is €2/day down the bottom.

At the top of the hill is the **Santuario della Madonna** (6:45 am-12:30 pm, 2:30-9 pm). This 1960s church houses the much revered *Madonna Nera* (Black Madonna), thought to have been made in Asia Minor and come to Sicily by sea. A plaque boasts *Nigra sum, sed Hermosa* (I am black but beautiful). She is supposed to have performed several miracles and pilgrims are always on the site muttering prayers and taking part in mass. It can be quite an interesting experience, especially once you've meandered past the religious trinkets for sale outside. Inside the church are a series of splendid tiled mosaics on the walls under the arches.

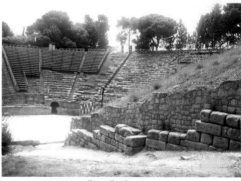
Greek theater

The archaeological site (9 am-7 pm, €2) lies beyond all this. Most of the remains are Roman, including the basilica at the entrance. There's also a Roman house in quite good condition with mosaic floors. At the other end of the street is the **theater**, that was Greek but later modified by the Romans for their inevitable gladiator combats. Parts of it were later dismantled to build the city wall. A museum contains finds from the excavations, including a bust of the emperor Augustus.

Opposite the entrance is the **Ufficio Azienda Soggiorno Turismo** (8 am-2 pm, ☎ 094-136-9023, 094-136-9184).

If you need something to eat, there's the **Ristorante Tyndaris** outside the church bar. There's a great view from outside the church over the Marinello reserve.

- *San Biagio*

If you still haven't satisfied your archaeology appetite, there are the modest remains of a first-century AD **Roman villa** on the SS113 at San Biagio. The villa (open 9 am to one hour before sunset, €2) also provides information on the construction of baths. There are vivid mosaics with ocean scenes.

Oliveri

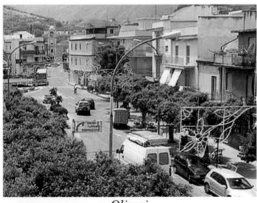
Oliveri

Oliveri is a good base for visiting Tyndaris and the *Santuario* but most especially for the beautiful series of lakes lying below the cliff face that are part of a marine reserve. The town is a pleasant beach resort with small-time tourism. The train station Oliveri-Tindari is not far from the reserve. Turn right from the station and follow the signs. Messina-Patti SAIS buses stop at Oliveri.

The seven ★★*laghetti* (small lakes) under the headland make for a superb itinerary on foot or for fishing or swim-

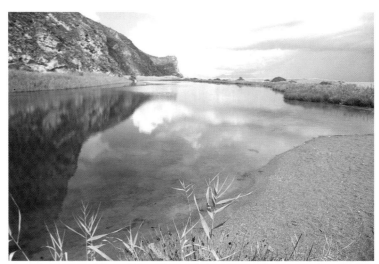

One of the Oliveri lakes (Joanne Lane)

ming. They are part of the Riserva Naturale Orientata
Laghetti di Marinello. Each has its own biological characteristics. The largest is **Marinello Lake** with both land and
marsh vegetation. **Mergolo Lake** and **Green Lake** have salt
water, while the interior ones are fresher. Once you've explored the lakes, find the path that ascends up to the Rocca
Femminina. You can sunbathe, fish, rent a boat, windsurf or
dive near the campgrounds.

There are numerous options for eating along Via Cristoforo
Columbus.

Marinello Camping Villaggio (Via del Sole 17, ☎ 0941-313-
000, fax 0941-313-702, www.villaggiomarinello.it €-€€) has a
superb position right near the lakes. There are cabins and
tent grounds, a bar, restaurant, grocery shop and sports, such
as tennis, basketball, volleyball, wind-surfing and diving.
They also offer excursions to the Aeolian Islands.

■ Milazzo

Most people that come to Milazzo make a beeline for the ferry
terminal and are on a boat within an hour to the Aeolian Islands. However, there are a lot of surprising features in this
seaside town and you could do worse than spend a few hours
here or even make an overnight stop. It does have some layers

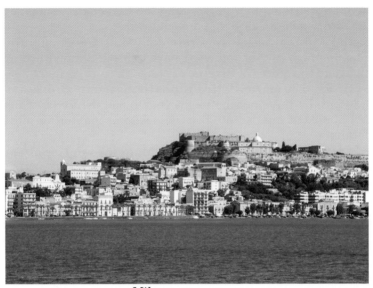

Milazzo (Clemensfranz)

of industrial development but there's a good *lungomare*, lively fishing marina, a rambling old castle, and good biking and walking itineraries out to Capo Milazzo. It deserves more credit than it's usually given.

Milazzo has historically been one of the most fought-over towns in Sicily due to its location. The Greeks arrived in 716 BC and later Milazzo was hotly contested by the Carthaginians and the Aragonese. Even the British made a base here during the Napoleonic Wars and Garibaldi himself won a victory here that led to his later conquest of Italy. In recent history it was used as a prison in WWI and during the Fascist period.

Getting Here & Around

Trains connect Milazzo to the Palermo-Messina line, although the station is three km south of the town center. Regular AST buses leave from outside the station to the quayside. Buses, including **AST** (☎ 0906-74386, 840-000-323, 0906-62244) and **Giuntabus** (☎ 0906-73782), run from Piazza della Repubblica along the quayside.

Tyrrhenian Coast

If you are driving to Milazzo, take the *lungomare* and enjoy the nice sea views as you approach town.

Sailings to the Aeolians operate daily and are usually frequent enough so that you won't have to book. Simply turn up and go to the offices of **Siremar** (Lungomare 18, ☎ 0909-283-242, 6 am-6:30 pm) or **Ustica Lines** (Lungomare 33, 5:30 am-7:30 pm) by the quayside to get your ticket. **Snav** (☎ 0909-284-509) is at number 40. See the *Aeolians* chapter for more details.

You can even rent a car at the port. **Maggiore national car rental** has offices just past Ustica lines on *lungomare*.

Information Sources

The **Azienda Autonoma di Soggiorno e Turismo** is in Piazza Caio Duilio (☎ 0909-222-865; Mon-Fri 9 am-2 pm, 3-6 pm and Sat 9 am-2 pm).

Sightseeing

From the port it's a pleasant 15-minute walk north along Lungomare Garibaldi up to the old town. The higher you climb the older the buildings become. The *Castello* at the top (10 am-12 pm, 4-7 pm, closed Mon; €3. 20) was constructed by Frederick II in the 13th century and enlarged

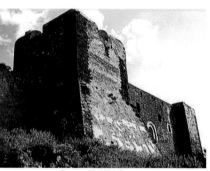

Castello Milazzo

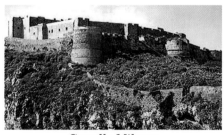

Castello Milazzo

by Charles V in the 15th century. The Norman keep remains intact and there's also the *Antico Duomo* (old church, closed) inside. The massive walls are magnificent and were erected by the Spanish.

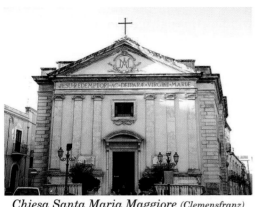

Chiesa Santa Maria Maggiore (Clemensfranz)

Directly opposite the castle is the Dominican **Chiesa del Rosario**, built in 1538 and once seat of the Inquisition. This is a lovely part of town with colorfully painted houses, narrow streets with stone arches and a number of churches. It's a good place to enjoy an evening meal. Walk around the back of Chiesa SS Salvatore to stairs that lead down to the *lungomare* or stroll back down to the old town where the main site is the **Duomo Nuovo**, with its excellent Renaissance paintings.

The ancient maritime quarter of **Vaccarella** was previously inhabited by fishermen and sailors. There's an old *tonnara* (fish processing facility) here, the Baia di Tono and a small harbor, rocky cove and beach. And a cute little *chiesetta*, **Santi Filippo e Giacomo**, from 1686.

Adventures on Wheels & on Foot

From Milazzo the headland extends out to Capo Milazzo. You could probably walk out to the first bays near Hotel Riviera Lido but you're better off taking a bus that leaves from the quayside around to the Punta Capo Milazzo. By car or bike it's an easy itinerary. Stop off at beaches along the way and then leave your wheels to undertake this small walking itinerary.

From the car park outside Il Faro restaurant, a small path leads down below to the **Santuario Rupestre di S Antonio**. At the bottom of the path is a little chapel with a rock ceiling. It is usually open in the daytime; if not ask in the restaurant. There's a statue of the saint and a shrine. From here you can follow the path along the sea to a tower, **Torre del Palombaro** (1900) and then follow a set of stairs up to a viewpoint on your right or down to rockpools on your left where

Tyrrhenian Coast

you can swim. From the viewpoint the track cuts across the top of the headland winding through olive groves and *ficche di india* (prickly pears) to the restaurant. The whole circuit should take less than an hour. Allow more time for swimming. If you follow the route the other way around, look for signs to Punta Capo Milazzo from behind Il Faro restaurant. The views from the cape on a clear day are spectacular – you can see the boats heading out to the Aeolians in the distance.

Where to Stay

 There are a number of pleasant hotels near the port and in town, such as:

Piazza Roma B&B (Via B Pistorio 1, ☎ 320-726-0946, www.bbpiazzaroma.it).

Eolian Inn Park Hotel (Salita Cappuccini, ☎ 0909-286-133).

If you have a car or don't mind being a little farther away there are campsites and an agriturismo on Capo Milazzo. Buses depart for the cape from the quayside stop. The driver can drop you off at the right spot. The three campsites are **Villaggio Turistico Cirucco** (☎ 0909-284-746), **Villaggio Turistico Smeralda** (☎ 0909-282-980) and **Agritourist** (Localita S Antonio, ☎ 0909-282-838) and they are dotted around the cape.

HOTEL PRICE CHART	
€	Up to €25 per day
€€	€26-€55
€€€	€56-€85
€€€€	Over €85

There's also the **Agriturismo La Baronia** (☎ 0909-286-688) at Punta Capo Milazzo, where the bus stops.

Where to Eat

 Check out the **morning fish market** on Via Peschera (7 am-1 pm). Another weekly market is held on Thursdays on Lungomare di Ponente.

There are numerous bars and restaurants on *lungomare*, such as **Lo Spizzico Pizze-**

DINING PRICE CHART	
Price per person for an entrée, including house wine.	
€	Up to €12
€€	€13-€25
€€€	€26-€35
€€€€	Over €35

ria Rosticceria, which does a roaring business next to the
Ustica Lines office. Walking back into town near the post office, the superb **Ritrovo Diana Café** (Lungomare Garibaldi,
☎ 090-928-6945, €) has good meals for just €5. They also have
a bar and *pasticceria*.

However, if you have any time you should wander up to the old
town and try any of the *pizzerias* or *birrerias*. About half way up
are two good *locale* sharing the square by the faded ruins of S.
Gaetano's church (also across from Chiesa SS Salvatore). They
are **L'Angolo Degli Aragonesi** (Via G. B Impallamomeni 69,
☎ 090-922-4927, www.langolodegliaragonesi.com, Sat and Sun)
and the **Caffe Antico**. The Caffe has live music in summer on
Wednesday, Thursday and Sunday.

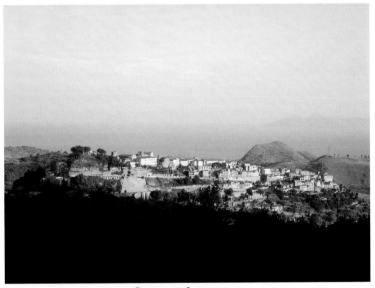

Castroreale (Ressaven)

■ Castroreale

Castroreale is a good detour inland from the coast on your
way east to Milazzo or west towards Capo d'Orlando. The medieval town is a quiet little center with creaky old streets,
pocked walls, stone houses, the ruins of buildings and a view
to the sea. **AST** buses make the climb from Barcellona which
is on the coastal train line. There's a Pro Loco (local tourist office) in Via Trento 2 (☎ 0909-746-673, 9 am-12 pm).

Frederick II of Aragon used to come here for hunting and
there's a fragment of his fort remaining which houses the

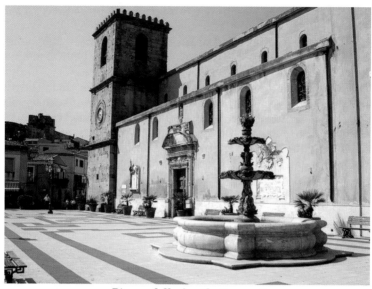

Piazza delle Aquile (Ressaven)

youth hostel. The castle was built in 1324 but ruined in an earthquake. The 17th-century **Duomo** is the main site with access from Piazza delle Aquile next to the 16th-century bell-tower. Inside is a strong scent of incense and even birds in the rafters! If you catch someone doing organ practice it adds to the atmosphere. A line of arches leads to the central altar.

There are two museums. The **Museo Civico** (Via G Siracusa, 9 am-1 pm, 3-7 pm, closed Wed afternoon, €1.03) contains historic items from town, including a 1450 crucifix, a marble piece where monks once washed their hands, along with photos and information about the town. The **Museo degli Argenti** (€2), in a church at the end of the same street, contains religious silver items. If you want to see any of the other churches, ask at the Museo Civico. Piazzetta S. Agostino has a great view of Milazzo and Capo Milazzo.

One of Sicily's few hostels, the **HI Ostello delle Aquile** (Via Annunziata, ☎ 0904-745-050, €) was closed for restoration at the time of writing. If it ever opens again it's a superb location at the end of town in the remains of the old castle. It's still worth a stroll up here for a peak at the tower.

Apply to Antonino Bellivia (☎ 0909-746-219) for other rooms or ask at Bar Aquila (Corso Umberto 1, 2, ☎ 0909-746-039) about **Bucca Pensione**.

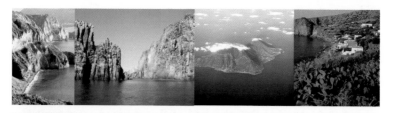

The Aeolian Islands

These seven delightful islands lie off the north coast of Milazzo between Italy and Sicily. Each is different, featuring steaming volcanoes, luxurious mud baths to wallow in, crystal-clear waters full of fish and caves to explore, beaches to relax on, pleasant island walks and some serious

trekking to reach the volcanic craters. However, they also share the same great weather in summer, fertile soils, beautiful blue waters, wonderful vistas and waves of day-trippers and vacationers. Don't be under any illusion – these islands have been discovered, but if you come on either side of July and August the weather is still fine and the crowds have either just left or are yet to arrive. The farther out you go on the islands too, the more you'll escape the summer hordes.

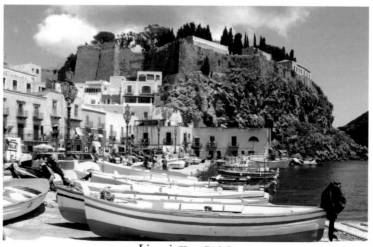

Lipari (Hans Bickel)

In winter, the weather can turn ferocious, pummeling the small islands with wind and water. It's not a good time to visit. And, historically, the volcanoes have not always been so dormant. It is no coincidence that the ancient Greeks named one of the islands after the god of fire, Vulcan, and that the god of wind, Aeolus, gives the archipelago its name.

The first settlers on the Aeolians exploited the volcanic resources, trading them far and wide. Refugees from the wars between Segesta and Selinus arrived in 580 BC and were welcomed by the residents. The Greeks cultivated the land and settled the smaller islands. They allied with Carthage during the First Punic War but were later wiped out by the Romans in 251 BC as a result and the islands became part of the Roman province of Sicily. Later they were abandoned to the frequent attacks of North African pirates. After Italian unification, they were used for political exiles until WWII. Mussolini's own daughter Edda Ciano was detained here in 1946. Emigration reduced the Aeolian population in the late 1950s, until the arrival of the first hydrofoil signaled the beginning of salvation –in a sense – by tourism.

HIGHLIGHTS OF THE AEOLIANS

■ Take a sulphorous mud bath on Vulcano.

■ Climb Stromboli's volcano at night amid the steaming vents.

■ Hang out with the bearded locals at the remote hamlet of Ginostra.

■ Join the élite, well-heeled crowd on elegant Panarea.

■ Taste Malvasia wine at Salina.

■ Explore prehistoric sites on Filicudi.

■ Getting Here

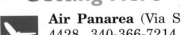

Air Panarea (Via S Pietro, Panarea, ☎ 090-983-4428, 340-366-7214, www.airpanarea.com, elic@inwind.it) is based on the island of Panarea, offering helicopter flights over Stromboli and Etna volcanoes. They also have a scheduled flight from Reggio Calabrea airport ev-

ery Friday and Monday to coincide with the scheduled flights of Alitalia and Airone.

Sicilwing (Via Provinciale 233, S. Venerina, Catania, ☎ 095-532-003, www.sicilwing.com) operates flights over the the Aeolian Islands at €902.50 for up to three persons in a Cessna 172. The flight is 2½ hours and departs from the Catania international airport. They also have flights to the Agrigento temples and over Mt Etna.

You can also reach the Aeolian Islands from Milazzo by ship or *aliscafi* (hydrofoil). Most of the services run to Lipari and on to other islands, but services to some are less frequent, unless you change in Lipari. Major operators on this route include **Siremar** (☎ 091-749-3111, www.siremar.it) and **Ustica Lines** (☎ 090-364-044, www.usticalines.it). Their websites both have full timetable listings. In summer there are numerous services per day; in other seasons they can drop to a few weekly services. It is possible to get to the Aeolians from Messina, Palermo, Cefalù, Capo d'Orlando and Sant'Agata Miltello, although such routes are longer and less frequent.

Ferries are cheaper but also slower. However, the hydrofoils can be prone to cancellation due to bad weather. You cam simply turn up at the ferry terminal and buy a ticket for an immediate departure. Ticket offices are usually right near the port.

Snav (☎ 081-428-5555) runs a fast boat from Napoli to the Islands once daily.

Navigazione Generale Italiana Traghette (Via dei Mille 26, Milazzo, www.ngi-spa.it) runs from Milazzo to the Aeolians in July and August only.

On all the islands you can rent boats by the hour, day (€25-50) or week. There are often bikes, scooters and cars for rent.

■ Lipari

Lipari is the largest of the islands, as well as the most popular and diverse. Lipari town is a thriving port with typically Mediterranean houses huddled around its two harbors beneath an impressive castle. There are four other towns accessible on a road circling the island. There are plenty of accommodations and, if you return here after visiting more remote places in the Aeolians such as Ginostra on Stromboli, it will feel as if

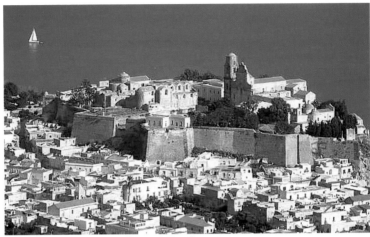

Lipari Castle (Herander)

you are coming back to civilization. For major services such as banks and the Internet, this is where to get them. If you're coming during the summer months, book ahead.

The original inhabitants of Lipari were expert miners and traded obsidian. They called the island Meligunis, meaning "gentle slopes." Today Lipari's minerals are still a money spinner; there is a thriving pumice industry in the north of the island. The original Greek settlement lies between the two harbors, where the remains of the Norman cathedral now stand.

Getting Here

Hydrofoils arrive at Marina Lunga and ferries at Marina Corta on either side of the castle. **Siremar** (☎ 0909-811-312), **Snav** (☎ 090-985-2230) and **Ustica Lines** (☎ 0909-812-448) have offices to help you.

Getting Around

Local Urso buses circumnavigate the island, leaving from the port front. Tickets cost €1.30 anywhere or you can buy an *abbonamento* for 10 tickets at €9.80. In summer they can be horribly crowded and, unless you get on at the initial departure poimt, you'll be lucky to squeeze on at all – especially with bags.

No part of the island is more than 30 minutes away. Timetables are available from **Urso** (Via Torr Cappuccini 29, ☎ 090-981-1026, www.ursobus. com) offices at the port, but are not always terribly accurate from other points on the island in summer, depending on delays. The same company also operates tours of the island in summer – handy if you're pressed for time to get around.

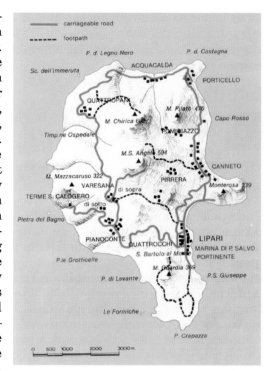

They stop at Quattrocchi lookout, Pianoconte, Quattropani lookout and Canneto Bay.

Noleggio a Lipari (☎ 090-981-1489) rents scooters, cars, bicycles and boats from near the port. Scooters are €18/day, cars from €45/day and mountain bikes €10/day.

Da Marcello (Via Tenente Amendola, ☎ 0909-811-234, www. noleggiodamarcello.com) also rents bikes and scooters. In Canneto try **Nautic Center** (Marina Garibaldi, ☎ 0909-811-656).

Touring the island by boat is a great way to get around and see out-of-the-way places where there are fewer people.

Eolian Crociere (☎ 090-922-2209, www.eoliancrociere.com) does a seven-day cruise on seven islands, departing from Milazzo or Lipari on Saturday. There are eight cabins, with basic commodities. The ship visits Stromboli, Vulcano, Alicudi, Panarea, Filicudi, Salina and Lipari.

Vulcano Navigazione (Via Piano Greco, ☎/fax 090-985-3105, ☎ 347-821-8588, 340-463-3076, www.vulcano-

navigazione.it) does full-day excursions to the islands (€20-30) and a tour of Vulcano island (€13) every day.

Pignataro (Via Prof. Carnevale 29, ☎ 0909-811-417) has excursions to all the islands.

Information Sources

 There is a tourist office at Via Vittorio Emanuele 202 (☎ 0909-880-095), which can give you sailing schedules, accommodation options and more. There is a bag deposit in the port ticket office, €3 per bag, €5 for overnight.

Sightseeing

The citadel or upper town containing the castle and Duomo is where Lipari town existed until the 18th century. Walk to the upper town from Via Garibaldi for the most impressive approach on long steps cut through the thick walls. You will find the **Cattedrale di San Bartolomeo** (9:30 am-7 pm) at the top. The 17th-century church was built to replace the original Norman cathedral. There are a number of other rather dilapidated Baroque churches up here and excavations in the southern part of the citadel in a park (9 am-7 pm). There are Greek and Roman tombs, a modern Greek theater where plays are performed and a good view of the port and town.

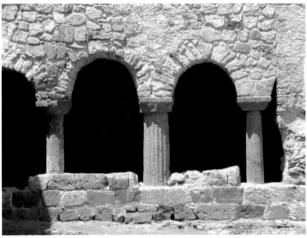

Lipari Cathedral Cloister

SAN BARTOLO

A prominent figure in the history of Lipari is the early Christian martyr San Bartolo, who met a gruesome end in Armenia (flayed, then decapitated). Somehow his coffin miraculously washed up on the shores of Lipari in 264. During the Arab invasion in 838 AD his remains were flung into the sea. However, the persistent saint appeared in a dream to monks who were instructed to gather his bones shining luminously in the dark water. The body was transported to Benevento for safekeeping, but the cathedral still boasts a fragment of arm and a thumb. He is venerated as the protector of the islands and has been credited with many acts sparing the islands population – no one was killed during the 1693 earthquake that struck the rest of Sicily, during a famine he guided a phantom ship loaded with foodstuffs to their aid and he also helped in times of plague.

The **Museo Archaeologico Eoliano** (9 am-1 pm, 3-6 pm, €4.20), housed in buildings near the Duomo, will better explain the excavations in the park. The finds here are very important, allowing archaeologists to uncover almost 2,000 years of history through the layers of occupation, from the Neolithic to the Roman age. It has also en-

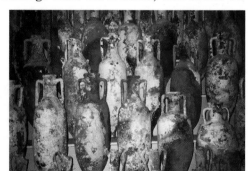
Amphorae in the Museo Archaeologico

abled them to date other Mediterranean cultures. If you're an archaeology or history nut, this is unmissable.

Other points of interest in town include the **Parco Archaeologico** in Contrada Diana, west of Vittorio Emanuele. It contains part of the original Greek walls and some Roman

houses. Tombstones are still visible in the southwestern part of the park.

Canneto is three km north of Lipari Town, with a good beach and accommodation options, including the island's only campsite and hostel (see *Where to Stay*). This is a good alternative to staying in Lipari, with regular bus services linking the town and ready access to the beach. Just beyond Canneto is the popular beach, **Spiaggia Bianca**. There are pumice quarries north of Spiaggia Bianca where you can have a lot of fun sliding down the hillside into the water below. This featured in the classic film *Kaos* that was made here in 1984.

Other bus stops on this route include **Porticello**, with a small beach and tiny village below in the bay. Beyond is the terminus of this bus route – **Acquacalda**.

You can also reach the areas west of Lipari Town by buses from Marina Lunga. **Quattrocchi** (Four Eyes) is a panoramic spot about three km away (see *Adventures on Foot*). Another km is the village of **Pianoconte**, where you can get to the Roman baths of **San Calogero** (turn off before the village – see *Adventures on Foot*). These baths were famous for their thermal spring. The last stop on the route is **Quattropani**, the start of a walking route to Aquacalda (see *Adventures on Foot*).

Adventures

On Foot

■ *Mt Pilato (one km)*

The crater of Mt Pilato (1,560 feet) looms above Campobianco. This is the source of the pumice found in the area and you can climb to the crater via a path from the northern end of Campobianco. It's a short 1.2 km. Don't worry about eruptions – the last one was in AD 700.

■ *Quattropani – Aquacalda (five km)*

Catch the bus from Marina Lunga to Quattropani, then walk five km north to Aquacalda, where you can get a bus back to Lipari. You could continue on to Porticello (30 minutes) for views of the azure waters and pumice quarries.

■ *Lipari – Quattrochi*

If you don't mind a hike, you could walk to Quattrocchi instead of taking the bus (see *Sightseeing*) for one of the best

vistas of the Aeolians. From this viewpoint you can see Vulcano and other rocks off the coast.

■ *San Calogero Spa*

From Quattrocchi continue walking to Pianoconte on the road, but turn off to the old thermal baths at San Calogero – the oldest spa structure in the Mediterranean. This is a pleasant walk across a valley and skirting cliffs to the baths at the end of the road. The original spa looks a bit like an igloo. The sauna-like interior is fitted with stone benches and a trickle of 140°F water still flows along the ancient channels. Continue on to **Quattropani** (one hour 45 minutes, 5½ km) for more fine views, passing the ruins of a Saracen watchtower and the windswept Punta Palmato. Catch a bus back or continue five more km to **Aquacalda**.

■ *Lipari – Monterosa (one hour 30 minutes)*

The pinkish promontory to the northwest of Lipari is easily accessible from a track on the Marina Lunga waterfront, heading due north from the port. The path initially climbs beside the road for Canneto but turns east for the panoramic summit.

■ *Lipari – Southern headlands (two hours 40 minutes)*

From Marina Corta, follow the waterfront south away from the *castello* and take the *salita* San Giuseppe to the lovely church of **San Giuseppe**. Walk up through the alleyways past Hotel Villa Meligunis, where you turn left to Via Maddalena. Take Via Dante on the right and then turn left onto Via Sant'Anna. Turn right on a dirt track where the road heads to Hotel Carasco. The lane passes through a deep valley and emerges on tarmac at **Capistrello** (25 minutes). Descend south on the concrete ramp to **Punta della Crapazza** (45 minutes), with a good view of rock pinnacles rising from the sea. Take the path on the right to the crest of **Capparo**, around a modern villa and veer left to the **Osservatorio Geofisicio**. From here you can see Alicudi and Filicudi to the northwest and Salina to the north-northwest. Extend the walk to a viewpoint beyond Falcone on the headland or turn back along the track. Don't take the path you came from but continue to another junction where you go left for the tiny old church of **San Salvatore**. A lovely narrow path follows a side-valley in the shadow of Monte Guardia. You'll soon see Lipari

and the *castello* again. Continue straight on, descending slowly towards the township.

For running trails, contact the **Mandala Trek** agency (Viale A. Doria 69, ☎ 0955-08959, www.mandalatrek.com) about the Volcano trail over Vulcano, Lipari, Salina, Stromboli and Etna.

Under Water

 Diving opportunities in Lipari abound. Two high-lighted spots include **Punta Castagna** and **Pietra del Bagno**. Punta Castagna is from 30-120 feet and a difficult dive. The initial platform is covered with white pumice from the mines above and drops to deep channels. Pietra del Bagno is 30-120 feet depth and of medium difficulty. The dive circumnavigates the rock to see all the sea life.

Get scuba diving information at **Centro Nautico Eoliano** (Salita San Giuseppe 8, ☎ 0909-812-691).

Diving Center La Gargonia (Salita S Giuseppe, ☎ 0909-812-616, www.lagorgoniadiving.it) has single dives from €30.

On Water

If you decide to rent a boat, make the excursion to the Faraglioni rocks, portruding from the sea, and to Pietra del Bagno on the far side of the island from Lipari town.

With Photography

 Villa Meligunis (Via Marte 7, ☎ 090-981-2426, fax 090-988-0149, 335-625-3914, www.villameligunis.it) has photography workshops run by the brother of the manager, who has produced a wonderful book on Aeolian life. You may have seen it in the bookshops. Ask about the workshops ahead of time as he is not always in Lipari.

Where to Stay

 The youth hostel and only campsite are on the beachfront at Canneto. The **Baia a Unici** (Via Marina Garibaldi, Canneto, ☎ 0909-811-540, www.liparicasevacanze.it, €) will pick up new arrivals

HOTEL PRICE CHART	
€	Up to €25 per day
€€	€26-€55
€€€	€56-€85
€€€€	Over €85

from the port and a friendly driver called Cosmo provides a

Aeolian Islands

cheap bus service at other times. The dormitories are divided for males and females and include kitchens. Even in the busy season there are usually beds available. The campsite is next door. Walk out the front door and you're on the beach. There's also a bus stop outside.

If you haven't booked ahead note the offers at the port on arrival or wander down the main street looking for signs that say *affita camera* (rented rooms).

La Nardo (Vico Ulisse 32, ☎ 090-988-0431, €€€), down an alleyway off the Corso, has rooms starting from €60 in peak season. The owner may insist you stay more than one night.

Villa Meligunis (Via Marte 7, ☎ 090-981-2426, fax 090-988-0149, 335-625-3914, www.villa-meligunis.it, €€€€) is a beautiful hotel in a quiet street behind the port, with fabulous sea views from the rooftop pool and restaurant.

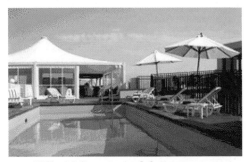

Villa Meligunis pool & restaurant

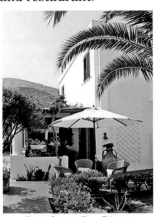

Residence La Giara

Residence La Giara (Via Barone, ☎ 090-988-0352, www.residencelagiara.it, €€-€€€€) has apartments just 650 feet from the Marina Lunga. Rentals are week long.

Vulcano Consult (Via Vittorio Emanuele 20, ☎ 090-981-3408, www.vulcanoconsult.it) has vacation houses on all the islands.

Rocce Azzurre (Via Maddalena 69, ☎ 0909-811-035, €€€-€€€€) is 10 minutes south of the center on a secluded beach.

Where to Eat

 Trattoria da Bartolo (Via Garibaldi 53, www.trattoriadabartolo.com, €€) is rather touristy but moderately priced.

Trattoria del Vicolo (Vico Ulisse, ☎ 090-981-1066) is *casalinga*-style restaurant, with a basic menu, and a few moments from the *acropoli*.

DINING PRICE CHART	
Price per person for an entrée, including house wine.	
€	Up to €12
€€	€13-€25
€€€	€26-€35
€€€€	Over €35

Ristorante Al Pescatore (Piazza Ugo San Onofrio, ☎ 090-981-1537, 333-714-3504, www.alpescatorelipari.com, €€€) serves typical Sicilian and Eolian foods right on the piazza.

La Cambusa (Marina Corta, Via Garibaldi, www.lacambusalipari.it, €€) is a real classic family-run spot and they'll send you the recipes afterwards if you liked the food.

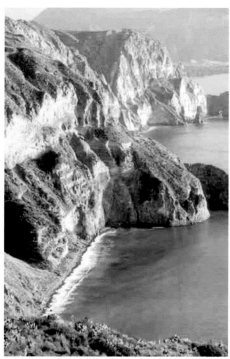
Lipari coast

Filippino (Piazza Mazzini, ☎ 0909-811-002) is the best known restaurant on Lipari. It opened in 1910 and has local dishes such as antipasto with vegetables preserved in oil, local capers and pecorino cheese. For main dishes, try Aeolan lobster in caper sauce.

La Nassa (Via G. Franza 41, ☎ 0909-811-319, €€€), run by a mother-son team, serve local fa-

vorites, notably seafood. For dessert try cookies with Malvasia wine.

Marina Corta is a good spot for night entertainment. **Chitarra Bar** (☎ 0909-811-554), the **Kasbah Café** (☎ 0909-811-075) or **La Precchia** (☎ 0909-811-303) all have live music.

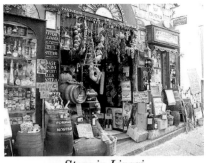
Store in Lipari

Ristorante Pizzeria (Pianoconte, ☎ 0909-822-387) is a good option in Pianoconte. It's a bit like a farming museum with equipment and housewares dotted around the rooms.

■ Vulcano

Vulcano is the first port of call for ferries and hydrofoils from Milazzo. It's also an easy day-trip from Lipari with ferries departing regularly for the short crossing. There are three volcanoes on the island – Vulcano Piano, Vulcanello and Fossa di Vulcano (also known as Gran Cratere). This last volcano is still active, expelling egg-smelling gases that you'll detect on arrival and that will linger in your clothes and hair for days!

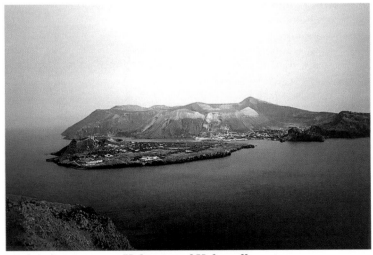
Vulcano and Vulcanello

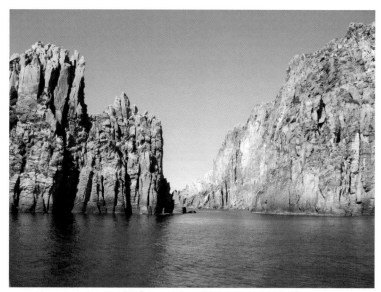

Vulcano island (Luis C. Ho)

Historically, the island inspired respect and fear; no one lived here, in fact, before the 18th century. However, the volcano's last bout of activity was between 1886 and 1890. Today, there are villas, hotels and restaurants on the island and many people visit for the famed sulphur baths. It's a good choice as a day-trip or you can stay and enjoy some of the archipelago's best beaches and walks.

Ferries and hydrofoils dock at Porto di Levante. There's a tourist office in the port and ticket agencies for **Ustica Lines** (☎ 090-985-2230) and **Siremar** (Piazza Vulcano Levante 3, ☎ 0909-852-149). Buses also run from dockside to Piano. You can rent boats, scooters and yachts for getting around. Mountain bikes and scooters are available from **da Paolo**, 75 feet from the port. For scooters there's **Noleggio Sprint** (Porto Levante, ☎ 0909-852-208) and **Romeo Paolo** (Porto Levante, ☎ 0909-852-112).

Sightseeing

Porto di Levante is the little harbor, backed by a few streets containing restaurants, villas and shops. Go straight ahead from the landing dock and you'll find the famed ★★**mud**

baths (6:30 am-8:30 pm, €2). Well actually you'll probably smell them first. The sulphorous egg smell can be off-putting but it's actually quite a lot of fun to wallow around in the mud.

From Porto di Levante you can bus 15 km south to **Gelso**, meaning "mulberry" in Italian and they are cultivated here. You can also bike it or hire a boat. There are trattorias (casual restaurants, where you sit at a common table) in Gelso, so stop for lunch and take a dip at the beach. The best spot is **Spiaggia dell'Asino**, a larger cove you pass on the way into Gelso.

The best beach on Vulcano is considered **Spiaggia Sabbia Nera** at Porto di Ponente. It's smooth and sandy with rocks jutting upward. You can rent paddle boats here.

Adventures

On Foot

★★★The walk to Vulcano's **Gran Cratere** (11 km, two hours, 15 minutes) is one of the easiest and safest walks on the Aeolians to a live volcano. If you only do one walk on all the islands this is a good choice, since you don't need a guide. From the Porto di Levante, follow the main road southwest for about 500 yards until you come to signs for the crater. From here it's a 50-minute walk to the top (40 min-

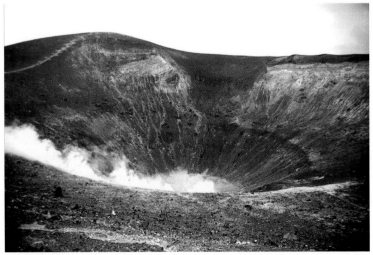

Gran Cratere (Joanne Lane)

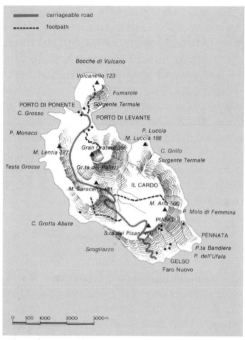

utes from the small office where you pay a €3 entrance fee). The track climbs up through lava soil that is grainy, sandy and rather difficult to grip (bring good shoes). There is a small canteen a few minutes farther up, offering cold drinks and seating, but bring your own water in case it's closed. At the top billowing smoke makes for spectacular photos down into the depths of the crater. but don't descend into it! You can circumnavigate the crater if there is not a lot of wind or smoke blowing. Use extreme caution and mind children carefully. It takes another hour to travel all around the top of the crater. The volcano is open for walking from 6:30 am to 7 pm in summer.

Under Water

Vulcano's best dive sites include:

- Capo Grosso
- Scoglio Quaglietto
- La Parete della Sirenneta
- Capo Testa Grossa
- La Franata dell'Arcipelago

Alternatively, if you boat trip around the island, stop off at **Grotta del Cavalo** (Horse Grotto) and **Vulcano Gelso**. Other interesting caves are the **Allume** group.

Where to Stay & Eat

 Porto di Levante has plenty of options for staying, including the campsite **Togo** (☎ 0909-852-128). It's run by the same management as **Camping Vulcano Togo Togo** (☎ 0909-852-128, www.campingvulcano.it, €) at Ponte di Ponente. The other campsite is **Eden Park** (Ponto Ponente 37, ☎ 0909-852-120).

Farraglione (☎ 0909-852-054, €€€€€) and **Rajas Bahia Hotel** (☎ 0909-852-080, €€€) are options for hotels in Porto di Levante. In Porto Ponente there are more choices. The **Eolian** (☎ 0909-852-151) has good out-of-season discounts.

Da Maurizio (Porto di Levante, ☎ 0909-852-426, €€) has a shady oasis and typical Aeolian meals.

Ristorante Belvedere (Via Reale 42, ☎ 0909-853-047, €€) is a little cheaper.

Il Palmento (Via Porto Levante, ☎ 0909-852-552 €-€€) serves cheap pizza and there's good seafood as well.

■ Salina

The quiet island of Salina is easily recognizable for its two towering trademark volcanoes. Both are long-extinct, but they appear to split the island in two. Salina has actually been shaped by six different volcanoes which have helped create a fertile landscape encouraged by fresh spring water. The name Salina comes from the salt pans that once existed at Lingua on the southernmost point.

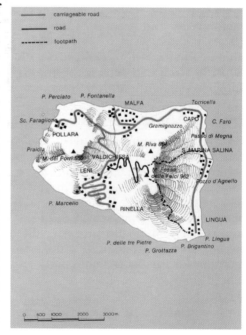

Aeolian Islands

These are now a lake where migratory birds stop over.

The famous Aeolian capers and the grapes used to make Malvasia wine can be found here. This is one of the least-visited islands of the archipelago but there are enough tourism services to make it feasible to stay here.

Salina has been inhabited since the Bronze Age. The first real settlement dates to the fourth century BC at Santa Marina Salina. It was a farming center and grew until the eighth century AD with new arrivals escaping the volcano on Vulcano.

Getting Here

 You can get a hydrofoil or ferry to either Santa Marina Salina or Rinella from the other islands. Services also run between the two towns. There is a **Siremar** office (Piazza SM Salina 2, ☎/fax 0909-843-004) or you can call **Ustica Lines** (☎ 090-984-3003) for information.

Getting Around

 Buses for all ports on the island stop just outside the Siremar offices. **CITIS buses** run to Lingua, Malfa, Rinella, Pollara, Valdichiesa and Leni. You can rent motorcycles and scooters from **Antonio Bongiorno** (Via Risorgimento 240, ☎ 0909-843-409). Scooters are also available in Rinella. Go to **Eolian Service** at the port (☎ 0909-809-203). You can rent boats from **Nautica Levante** (Via Lungomare, Santa Marina Salina, ☎ 0909-843-083).

Sightseeing

Santa Marina Salina, where you dock with the hydrofoil or ferry, is the main port. There's not a lot to do here but you can swim off the stone beach. **Lingua** is three km south of Santa Marina (it's a pleasant walk or you can bus it). There's even less to it than Santa Marina Salina. At the end of the road is the salt lagoon from which Salina takes its name. The remains of a Roman villa have been discovered near the narrow beach. A small ethnographic museum faces the lagoon with examples of rustic art and island culture. It is may well be closed when you are there.

Malfa is the island's biggest town, located on the northern side of Salina. It has a good beach and the **Museo**

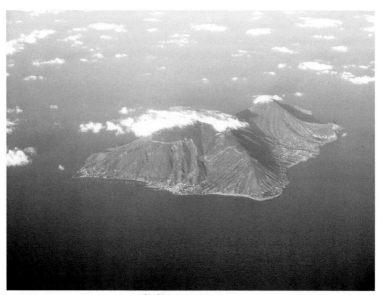

Salina (Salvatore 88)

dell'Emigrazione Eoliana (☎ 0909-844-373, 9 am-1 pm, free), which gives visitors an idea of how imigration has effected the Aeolian islands.

★★**Pollara** is more secluded and where much of the movie *Il Postino* was shot, both in the town and on the narrow beach at the base of cliffs below the village. The beach is unbeatable and worth coming for. Buses run to Pollara from Santa Marina Salina.

Rinella is popular for spearfishing and good swimming from the rocks near the **Tre Pini** campsite (see *Where to Stay*). Boats arrive here too so it's a good place to base yourself. Unfortunately, it's a long way from other places and can make you reliant on buses. You could walk as far as Leni, three km higher up on the slope.

Adventures

On Foot

Walks on Salina are particularly nice because of the rich vegetation.

★**Monte Fossa delle Felci** (7.2 km, 3½ hours)

Ths walk up the mountain to the extinct volcano of Monte Fossa delle Felci is on a clear forestry track and a series of paths. At the peak are unbeatable views over the islands. Bring a wind jacket for the peak and good shoes. Food and water, of course, will also be needed. Get a **CITIS bus** (☎ 0909-844-150) from Santa Marina Salina to the **Madonna del Terzito sanctuary** where the walk starts. This sanctuary lies in the valley separating the two volcanoes and is a place of pilgrimage, particularly around **Ferragosto** on August 15. Take the track around the church to climb through the vineyards above. Climbing gradually, you reach the peak (3,149 feet) after one hour and 45 minutes. The crater is 1,640 feet in diameter, at least 330 feet deep and choked with trees and heather. Follow the path down to Santa Marina Salina.

Other walks criss-cross the island, linking Santa Marina with Leni and the south coast at Rinella. You can also head up to Monte Fosse from Lingua (follow signs for Brigantino).

Where to Eat

 Santa Marina di Salina has several *alimentari* along Via Risorgimento if you are cooking for yourself. By the dock, you could try **Portobello**, serving fish fresh out of the sea. **Da Franco** (€€€) is also popular, about 20 minutes walk away at the top of the village (up Via Risorgimento, left up Via F Crispi and turn right at the top).

Where to Stay

 Most accommodation is at Santa Marina Salina, where the boats dock, or in Rinella, a fishing hamlet on the southwest coast. **Campeggio Tre Pini** (Rinella, ☎ 0909-809-155, www.trepini.com) is the only campsite in Rinella.

Hotels include **Santa Isabela** (Via Scalo, Malfa, ☎ 0909-844-018) and **Punta Scario** (Via Scalo 8, Malfa, ☎ 0909-944-139) in Malfa. In Santa Marina Salina, **Punta Barone** (Via Lungomare Notar Giuffre 8, ☎ 0909-843-161, €€€) and **Mamma Santina** (Via Sanita 40, ☎ 0909-843-054) are good options.

■ Panarea

Tiny Panarea is beautifully picturesque, with an elegant little township at **San Pietro**, clusters of outlying islets for good swimming, pleasant walks and archaeological remains. Only electric cars and three-wheelers are allowed on the quiet streets, making it peaceful and tranquil.

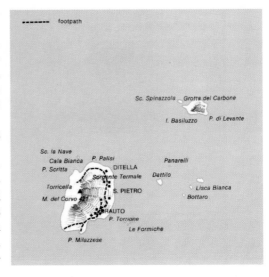

The three major hamlets of **Ditella**, **San Pietro** and **Drauto** are still where most of the population lives. Boats dock at San Pietro, where most of the accommodation and services are found.

Getting Here

Ferries dock in San Pietro's harbor. There's a **Siremar** ferry office (Viale S Pietro 3, ☎/fax 0909-830-007) or you can call **Ustica Lines** (☎ 090-983-3344) for information.

Getting Around

The island is served by taxis (☎ 338-493-1207 or 333-313-8610). There are no buses. You can rent boats in the port for about €50 a day. Look for signs saying *noleggio barche*. Rides to the islets are about €8.

Eolie Mare Panarea (Via Umberto 1, ☎ 090-983-328, 333-721-5118, 338-330-7562, 338-995-5182, www.cafarella.it) rents boats and also has excursions of the islands.

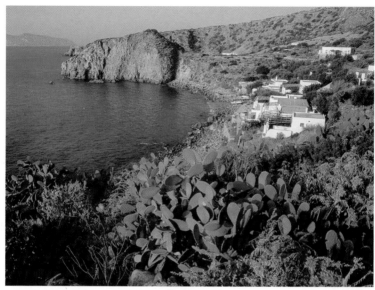

Panarea

Information Sources

There's a **Pro Loco** (local tourist office) in Piazza
Cavour (☎ 0923-911-838).

Sightseeing

The quiet lanes of Panarea are worth a stroll but it won't take
you long to sniff them all out. The whitewashed streets and
Greek-like styles are pretty but there aren't many of them.
Head to **Chiesa M. San Pietro** and continue to **Drautto** (15
minutes), where you can swim or rent a boat in a rocky cove.
Try **Nautillus** (☎ 090-983-074, 330-849-295, alessi.rosario@
tiscali.net). The water is refreshing, but the beach access is
better at **Spiagetta Zimmari**, five minutes farther on. The
sand is more brown than white but it's a popular spot. A terrace restaurant overlooks the beach and you can rent canoes
and pedalos. If you can't walk back, call Paolo and Angela for
a taxi (☎ 333-313-8610).

Facing page: Drautto, Panarea (Joanne Lane)

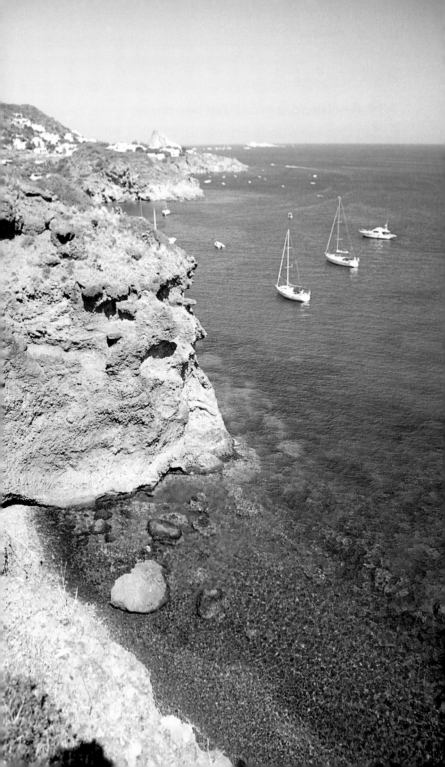

Adventures

★★Archaeological Adventures

- *San Pietro – Villagio Preistorico (2½ km, 70 minutes)*

A simple walk follows the road out of town towards the beach of Draulo and down to the **Punta Milazzese**, where a Bronze Age village was discovered om 1948. The oval foundations of 23 huts are visible on the pretty headland. It is thought that this site was occupied since the 14th century BC. Pottery found here (now in Lipari's museum) has a Minoan influence, lending credance to the theory that there were ties between Crete and the Aeolians. It also suggests evidence of commerce. There are superb views from here to Vulcano and Lipari, west to Salina and beyond to Filicudi.

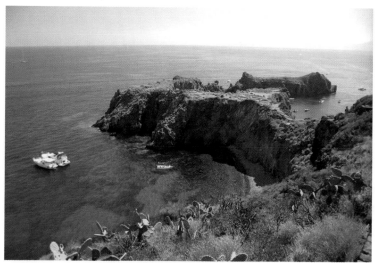

Punta Milazzese (Joanne Lane)

Steps below descend to **Cala Junco**, a pleasant stony cove perfect for swimming and snorkeling. Meander around to the headland to explore all the caves.

- *San Pietro – Punta del Corvo (four km, three hours)*

This loop runs past **Punta Milazzese** first (70 minutes), from where it's another two hours up to Punto Corvo and back to San Pietro. The track after Punta Milazzese is overgrown and

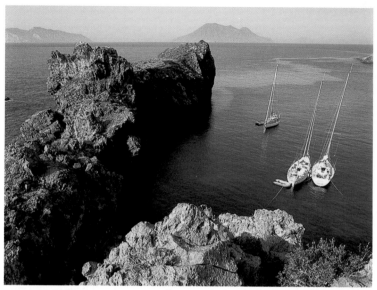

Panarea

it's a reasonably steep climb up to the top. But the climb is worth it for the stunning views. You won't want to attempt it in the heat of the day, however. The route back down into San Pietro is better-marked.

Other walking itineraries are signed on noticeboards in San Pietro.

On Water

 Panarea's own archipelago of six islets makes a good trip. The largest islet, **Basiluzzo**, used for caper cultivation, is the most distant. At the back of the island is the wreck of a Roman ship. Nearest to Panarea is **Dattilo**, with a jagged finger-like rock and miniscule beach. **Lisca Bianca** has better swimming (there's also good diving – see *Adventures Under Water*). Boat tours can take you out here or you can rent your own boat. **Da Diego** (Via Iditella, ☎ 338-293-1533) rents 25 hp wooden and rubber boats for €50/day for two people, €70/day for more than two people.

Under Water

 Diving around Panarea starts at €50 for one dive. It's also possible to do dives farther afield, for example at Stromboli. Usually operators give you discounts if you do more than one dive. **Hotel Cincotta** (Via San Pietro, ☎ 347-555-3198) is a good place to try as they have no minimum numbers for a dive. Another is **Amphibia** (Via Iditella, ☎ 0909-83311).

Lisca Bianca has good scuba diving around the wreck of an English ship that sank in the 19th century. To find it, proceed past the tiny beach and continue around the sharp point of the island. The wreck lies at about 130-165 feet depth.

In Air

 Icarus Helicopter Tours (☎ 090-983-33, 348-133-4972, www.elicotteri-icarus.it) operates from Panarea, offering helicopter flights over the Aeolians. Stromboli (€120) seen from the air is fantastic. The flights usually need a minimum number of people. They post last-minute specials on their notice boards. For example, you could get a flight to Reggio di Calabria for as little as €150 per person.

Where to Stay

 ★**Hotel Quartara** (Via S Pietro 15, ☎ 090-983-027, www.quartarahotel.com, €€€€) is a family-run hotel set amid other whitewashed houses at the end of a lane with a superb terrace view to the sea. The hotel is named after the jug famed in the area for storing oil and wine. Note the handmade furniture from Melanesia and China, as well as the old Sicilian bed covers. The restaurant is superb and part of the Le Soste di Ulisse fine food group (www.lesoste-diulisse.it). Food is served by two of the sis-

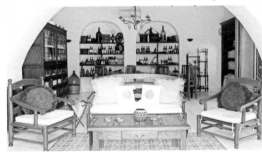
Hotel Quartara

ters who own the property. **Hotel Cincotta** (Via San Pietro, ☎ 0909-93014, €€€€) has a good view of the port and on the higher end of the scale, as is the even higher-priced **Raya** (Via San Pietro, ☎ 0909-93013, €€€€)

La Terrazza (Via San Pietro 20, ☎ 090-983-033, €€€) and **La Sirena** (Via Drautto, ☎ 090-983-012, €€€) rent rooms and are a little farther into town. They offer good off-season discounts. La Terrazza has a good restaurant.

Where to Eat

Ristorante da Modesta (Via S Pietro, www. paginegialle.it/ristorantemodesta, ☎ 090-983-306) is behind the Hotel Concetta.

Da Pina Ristorante (Via San Pietro, Panarea, ☎ 090-980-3032, 090-983-324, fax 090-983-147, www.dapina.com).

Hotel Quartara (Via San Pietro 15, ☎ 090-983-027) is a dining experience you will remember for a long time. Immaculate, friendly service and great food.

Da Francesco has a panoramic spot down at the port.

Ristorante o Palmo has a €20 tourist menu and is one of the cheaper options on Panarea.

If you're really hurting, there is a mini-market on the front wharf.

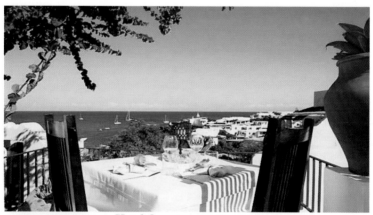

Hotel Quartara restaurant

■ Stromboli

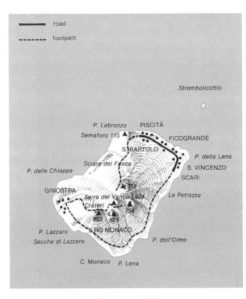

Stromboli's active volcano of the same name completely dominates the island – in fact the entire island is little more than a volcanic cone. It is the farthest north of the Aeolian group and the name is derived from the Greek *Stronglyle*, meaning "rounded," for the shape of the summit. The unceasing smoke and intermittent fiery output of lava has earned it the name "lighthouse of the Mediterranean." Unfortunately, a lack of naturally occurring fresh water means supplies of tank-collected rainwater or water from the mainland are required. Residents have dwindled in recent years with

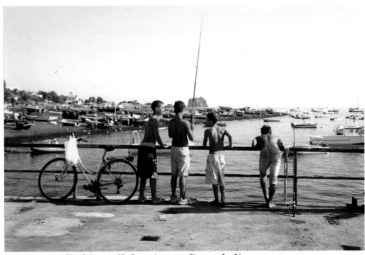

Fishing off the pier on Stromboli (Joanne Lane)

immigration, particularly in the 1930s when an eruption led to the departure of many of the 5,000 inhabitants to Australia.

Apart from the village and port of Stromboli on the easternmost corner, there is only the backwater hamlet of **Ginostra**, with a skeleton population. However, it's immediately enticing, with a real back-of-beyond feel.

Getting Here

 Stromboli might be remote and far away but getting here by ferry is not a problem during summer. In winter or in bad weather, however, services can be disrupted or cancelled.

Getting Around

 There are no bus services on the islands and cars are not allowed. But electric taxis do operate, which are so quiet they can sneak up on you – keep right and stay alert. You will see signs for these everywhere. Call ☎ 338-460-3340 or 333-292-5434 or 335-520-7158. Most hotels will meet you on arrival, or there are taxis waiting. If not, it can be a steep climb up to town with your bags.

To get to the hamlet of Ginostra you can follow a very rough track linking it to San Pietro or take advantage of the ferry services. There are only a few each day so you'll need to check the schedule carefully or you could be stranded in Ginostra for the night.

Information Sources

 The helpful website, www.stromboli.net, should be able to answer most of your questions. **Ustica Lines** (☎ 090-986-003) and **Siremar** (Via Roma 74, ☎ 0909-860-016) can help with schedules. There's a ticket office at the port.

See *Adventures* below for information on guides to the volcano.

Sabbia Nera (Via Marina, ☎ 0909-86390, www. sabbianerastromboli.com) is a good place to stop in on your way from arrival at the port. They can book accommodations

and rent you just about anything you want. They also have a left-luggage deposit. It costs €3 per bag per day or overnight.

Sightseeing

Ferries and hydrofoils arrive at the port, where you can swim on the lava black beach. The town itself spreads up over the lower slopes of the volcano and the island's beaches for about two km. The town has narrow lanes, whitewashed houses, buckets of flowers, restaurants and a few churches. **San Vincenzo** is the largest of the churches and has a square with a good view of the sea and **Strombolicchio**. For a closer look at this tower rock rising out of the water, wander down to **Ficogrande Beach**. Volcano guide offices lie at the bottom of the stairs below the piazza and just around the corner on Via Vittorio Emanuele III. Follow this road to a second church of **San Bartolo and Piscita**, where another path to the crater starts. There's an ashy beach here and another one at **Ficogrande**. The only "sight" in town is the house where Ingrid Bergman lived with director Roberto Rossellini in 1949 while filming *Stromboli: Terra di Dio*. The scandal of the liaison created much talk. The house is pink and just after San Vincenzo church on the right, before Barbablu restaurant.

★★★Ginostra

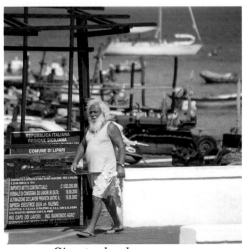

Ginostra local (Joanne Lane)

Ginostra, on the far end of the island, is a solitary community where donkeys are still used to cart rubbish down to the port and off the island, plumbing is still rather basic and electricity does not yet connect to all the houses (although there is solar power). It's a bit of a timewarp but

rather fascinating. The people here have a much rougher appearance and you'll see the older men sporting craggy beards – most unusual for Sicily. It's the perfect spot for an artist's hideaway and mostly visited, if at all, by daytrippers.

There's an old post office, a church and a local shop, **Bazar Ginostra** (10 am-1 pm, 5-8 pm), that sells a bit of food and can rent boats, canoes and organize excursions. Snorkeling is particularly good in the rocks below. Cactus and *ficche di India* (prickly pear) grow profusely in the gardens.

There are a couple of eating/staying options. **L'Incontro** (☎ 090-981-2305) is a restaurant and bar, open 7 am-12 pm, but with meal times specified for lunch (1-3:30 pm) and dinner (8-10:30 pm). They have three rooms at the **B&B Luna Rossa** (☎ 0909-812-305, www.ginostraincontro.it, €€-€€€) and their prices drop after August. They have a good café serving cakes and coffee.

Puntazzo Ristorante Bar (☎ 090-981-2464, puntazzoginostra@virgilio.it), farther into the village, has a bar and restaurant open all year. Make a reservation if you want dinner. They can reserve basic rooms throughout the town for €15-30.

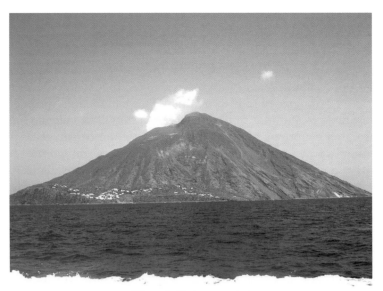

Stromboli (Denis Barthel)

Adventures

In Water

 You can enjoy a limited view of the volcano's fireworks display from boats moored below the Sciara del Fuoco in the evening. You will see tours for this posted all over the Aeolians, but it's best to book them from Stromboli. Generally, tours leave the port at 10 pm and return at 11 pm. Contact **Botteghino Port** (☎/fax 0909-86135, 338-985-7883). **Ippo Boat Rental** does a tour of the island leaving the port at 10:30 am and 3 pm, returning at 1 and 5 pm (€15). Departures on request can also go to Spiaggia Lungo, Scalo Balordi, Villagio Stromboli and Ficogrande. **Ristorante Le Terrazze di Eolo** (☎ 338-505-1543) rents kayaks.

For diving, contact **La Sirenetta Diving Center** (Via Marina 33, ☎ 0909-86025) or **Sotto l'Acqua del Vulcano** (Via Marina Scari, ☎ 0909-96390).

Boat excursions are offered from the port. Strombolicchio is a popular spot on any of the tours.

On Foot

★★★Ascending the Volcano

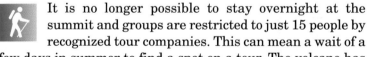 It is no longer possible to stay overnight at the summit and groups are restricted to just 15 people by recognized tour companies. This can mean a wait of a few days in summer to find a spot on a tour. The volcano has isolated eruptions of great intensity about once per year; in other words, statistically speaking, it's more dangerous to drive a car than visit the volcano. The only rescue missions have been of lone trekkers who have not correctly judged the dangers.

Magmatrek (Via Vittorio Emanuele, ☎/fax 090-986-5768, www.magmatrek.it, 10 am-1 pm, 4-6:30 pm) is probably the best choice to arrange your trek. They give out brochures explaining the dangers of the climb for those with health

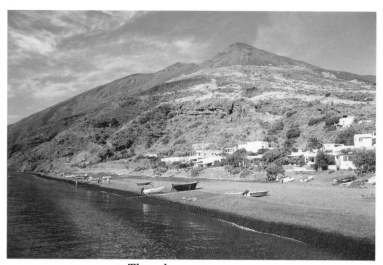

The volcano (Joanne Lane)

problems, heart, asthma, dizziness and kids under 10 years old. They also get you to check that you have the right equipment: socks, trekking boots, an electric torch with alkaline batteries, wind jacket, water, sandwhiches, chocolate or dried fruit, a comfortable backpack, short pants for the climb and long ones for the top, a change of t-shirt and a handkerchief or bandanna for the dust. Their groups leave at 5 pm from outside the church (€25). They are a popular agency and are often booked up to a week ahead.

Stromboli Guide (☎/fax 090-986-211, 090-986-263, 330-965-367, 368-664-918, www.stromboliguide.it, Mon, Wed, Sat, Sun) is the agency below the church and has been operating for some years. But they don't seem to take as much care with equipment or give as much information. It's more like follow the leader. The group leaves from the church at 6 pm and returns about midnight.

Totem Trekking (http://totemtrekking.tripod.com, totemtrekking@hotmail.com, ☎ 090-986-5752, 10 am-1 pm, 4:30-9 pm), outside the San Vincenzo church, can rent you all the equipment you need for the ascent. Boots are €5 and you can also get a pack, torch or other equipment. The office stays

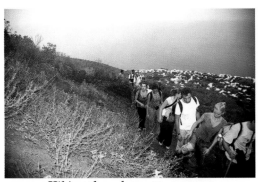
Hiking the volcano (Joanne Lane)

open until you return. They also have fax and Internet (€2.50/one hour).

The walk to the crater is an experience. While the walk is open to everyone, a certain level of fitness is recommended. If you've just spent a few weeks inertly wallowing in the waters of the islands, your body might find it a rude shock to do some work. Be prepared; it's a hike – though it's certainly not as bad as the Jules Verne's characters had in *Journey to the Center of the Earth*, trekking through the crater of Stromboli itself.

Alternative to the Summit

Climb up to the **Chiesa di San Vincenzo** and either turn right behind it towards Piscita or do a short circuit up to the *cimetero vecchio* and *cimetero nuovo*, which will bring you back down to the road to Piscita. The road passes the **Chiesa di San Bartolo**, the island's patron saint, and heads downhill to the sea. The beach at **Piscita** is fine black sand and pebbles edged by sculpted lava that halted at the sea edge. A road up beyond Piscita leads you to a height of 1,312 feet, the maximum distance allowed without a registered guide.

Ginostra – Stromboli (3½-4½ hours, six km)

If you get stuck in Ginostra for the night or would prefer to walk back, this tough route is an option. It is best to ask for conditions of the trail in L'Incontro and find out if you'll need someone to guide you before setting out. The route skirts around the coast to Stromboli past the Secche di Lazzaro, Punta Lena and Punta dell'Omo. There are some difficult passages, including two 13-foot rock faces to climb. It is not recommended for the inexperienced.

Where to Eat

 Bar Il Malandrino (Porto Scari, ☎ 0909-86376, €) serves hot and cold snacks down at the port.

Il Ristorante Zurro Osserva (Via Marina, ☎ 0909-86283, 338-719-465, 1-2:30 pm, 7-11 pm, €€€), beyond the harbor, has fresh seafood and the special *spaghetti alla strombolana*.

Punta Lena (Marina Ficogrande, ☎ 0909-86204, €€-€€€) has a terrace opening to the sea. It's a good walk from the center of town but worth it.

Il Canneto (Via Roma 64, ☎ 0909-86014, €€) always serves fresh fish.

La Taratana Club (☎ 0909-86025) is near the Sirremar office, serving all meals, with a happy hour before dinner. Buffet meals available at lunch.

La Sirenetta (Via Marina 33, ☎ 0909-86025, €€€€) has a restaurant with a renowned chef. It's elegant and you pay for it.

Where to Stay

★**Giovanni Stanco** (Via F. Natoli 1, ☎ 090-986-087, €€€) and his wife are an Italian couple who moved to Australia long ago. But they return to Stromboli six months every year and open rooms in her grandparent's home. The private rooms just above the pharmacy are very simple and share two communal bathrooms downstairs. But it hosts a lot of travelers and the couple will help you out with anything you need in town. Open April-September. They are located just below the pharmacy.

The Secret Garden B&B (Via Francesco Natoli, ☎/fax 090-986-211, 036-866-4918) is

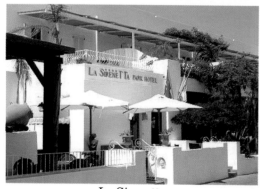

La Sirenetta

run by Antonio, a volcano guide attached to the Stromboli Guide office. It's three minutes walk from the center with a large garden and good views.

Hotel Ossidiana (Via Picone 18, ☎ 0909-86006, www. hotelossidiana.it, €€€€) is right on the beachfront.

La Sirenetta (Via Marina 33, ☎ 0909-86025, www. lasirenetta.it, €€€€) is well maintained and the island's best place to stay. It sits on Ficogrande beach in front of Strombolicchio.

■ Filicudi

Filicudi is the bigger of the two minor westerly islands and the favorite of many visitors to the Aeolians. Arrival at the harbor is fairly disenchanting, however, so don't be put off. Once you're out of the port, the rest of the island is beautiful and easily accessible on foot.

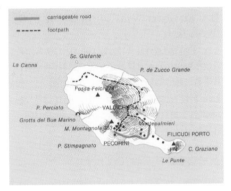

There aren't a lot of services to Filicudi even in summer and they can be cancelled if there are rough seas. You could find yourself stranded here. Given the distance (1½ hours by fast ferry from Lipari) you'll need to assess whether you have the time and money to get here. **Ustica Lines** (☎ 0909-889-949) and **Siremar** (Via Porto 7, ☎ 0909-889-969) can help you with schedules.

Adventures

In Archaeology

From Filicudi Porto take the road south to the archeological site, the **Villagio Preistorico** at Calo Graziano. The remains of circular Bronze Age huts have been found here that predate Panarea's Punta Milazze. You can walk down to a stone beach for a swim.

On Foot

To see the rest of the island, take the steep steps in the port to the left of the hotel. Turn right at the fork about 10 minutes up to the **Valdichiesa**, a little vil-

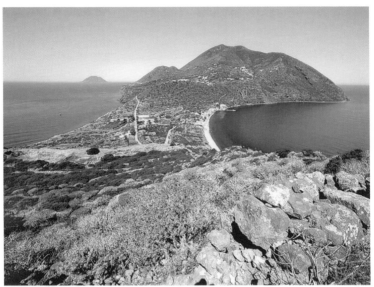

Filicudi

lage on a hillside terrace. Catch your breath by stopping to look at the views. The church is rather pretty if a little dilapidated. Above the church and village is **Fossa dei Felci** (2,540 feet). You can climb it by a path that runs through the terraces, or more easily by just walking straight up!

Zucco Grande is 50 minutes walk from Valdichiesa. Take the signposted path at the turn below Valdichiesa. It's a rewarding hike. Beyond it and south is **Pecorini**, a tiny village grouped around a church. You could continue down to the little harbor of **Pecorini Mare**.

On Water

If you don't enjoy the exertion of getting around Filicudi, consider renting a boat from the port. They are usually about €20 for a two-hour trip. With a boat you can consider visiting the uninhabited northern and western coasts. **Punta Perciato** to the west has a fine natural arch. Nearby is the **Grotta del Bue Marino** (Cave of the Monk Seal). The cave is 121 feet long and 98 feet wide and named for the seals that once lived here. They were all harpooned years ago by local fishermen. To the northwest,

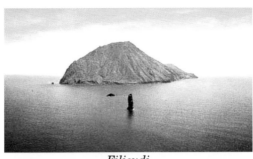
Filicudi

Scoglio della Canna is a long thin stack of rocks 233 feet tall that looks rather like an obelisk.

The small islands of **Elefante** and **Montenassari** are worth exploring by boat. You can also access the beach below Capo Graziano and walk up to the prehistoric village on top.

Where to Stay & Eat

La Canna (Via Rosa 43, ☎ 0909-889-956, €€€€) and **La Sirena** (Pecorini Mare, ☎ 0909-889-997, €€€) are among the few options. Both drop their prices before and after August.

■ Alicudi

The flood of tourists in the Aeolians never makes it to this out-of-the-way place, one of the most isolated spots in the entire Mediterra-

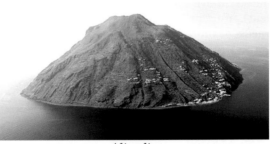
Alicudi

nean. But maybe that will tickle your fancy. Mafia prisoners were sent here for some time. Now it's used by a handful of farmers and fishermen who only received electricity in the 1990s.

The island forms a perfect cone, like a pimple, with its shores punctured by caves. **Alicudi Porto** is the only settlement – a clump of white houses on terraces overrun with the heather known as ericusa, which was the ancient name of Alicudi.

Getting Here & Around

 There aren't many services to and from Alicudi. As with Filicudi, services can be intermittent even in summer when high seas can lead to cancelations. There aren't any buses on Alicudi so getting around is on foot or by boat.

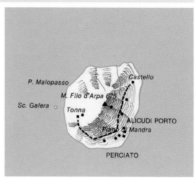

Information Sources

 Siremar (Viale Reg. Elena 5, ☎ 0909-889-912) and **Ustica Lines** (☎ 0909-889-795) can give you timetable information.

Adventures

On Foot

 The central peak of Alicudi is **Filo dell'Arpa** (String of the Harp) at 2,204 feet. It's a hard two-hour hike to the top up a rocky path with panoramic views. Bring water and start early.

The rocky shore to the south of the port is the best place to swim or laze about. If you have a boat, you could stop off at the **Scoglio della Galera** rocks and **Timpone delle Femmine** to do just that.

Where to Stay & Eat

 Ericusa (Localita Perciato, ☎ 0909-88902, €€€).

Casa Mulino (Via Regina Elena, ☎ 0909-889-681, €€) has five rooms.

B&B Da Rosina (Via Principe Umberto 13, ☎ 0909-889-937, €€) has just two bedrooms, with a shared bathroom.

map

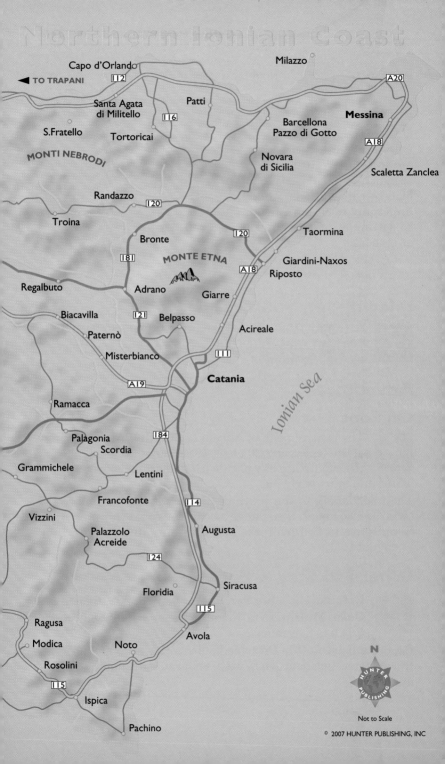

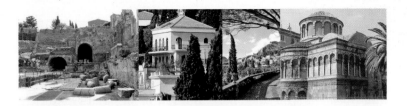

The Northern Ionian Coast

The Ionian coast offers stunning sea views, luscious vegetation, hill-top villages, natural woodlands, spectacular gorges and numerous old towns. Above it all looms the smoking, rumbling specter of **Mount Etna**. To the north is

Messina, the first port of call for travelers to Sicily. Down the coast are pleasant beachside resorts peppered with Norman churches and castles. Off the coast, **Savoca** and **Forza d'Agora** are worth making the foray inland to the woods and craggy uplands. The **Alcantara Valley** and its spectacular gorge, as well as the heights of **Castiglione di Sicilia**, are worth another inland expedition southwest of the area's most illustrious resort, **Taormina**.

HIGHLIGHTS OF THE IONIAN COAST

■ Sipping a granita in the Godfather town of Savoca.
■ The view of Mt Etna from Taormina's Greek theater.
■ Plunging into the Alcantara Valley gorge.
■ Snorkeling at Isola Bella.

■ Messina

For those crossing into Sicily from the mainland, Messina may be your first view of Sicily. And it's not a bad one, with a fine hooked harbor (from which the city got its Greek name, Zancle or Sickle) stretching along the seafront and views back across the straits to the forested hills of Calabria. Messina

has much natural beauty and, in fact, Shakespeare actually used it for the setting of his play, *Much Ado About Nothing*. There are some vestiges of the Greeks, Romans, Byzantines and Normans who ruled here. But few of Messina's historical buildings are left now, due largely to the devastation wreaked by invaders, plagues, bombings (the most bombed Italian city of WWII) and earthquakes. The 1738 and 1908 earthquakes destroyed much of the town, with the latter killing 80,000 people. Messina is best used as an orientation point on arrival and for itineraries nearby.

Getting Here

By Boat

 Car ferries make the crossing to Messina frequently from Villa San Giovanni on the mainland in about half an hour. In summer months there can be longer delays. The **Ferrovie dello Stato** or FS Italian Railways (☎ 892-021, www.trenitalia.com) operates 30 car and passenger train ferries daily (one to two per hour, 40 minutes). The private firm **Caronte Ferries** (☎ 090-641-6352, www.carontetourist.it) is free for passengers on foot, €19 for small cars. Departures are every 10 minutes. For a quicker passage, there are hydrofoils taking passengers only (no cars) from Reggio di Calabria. **SNAV**, **Meridiano Lines** and **FS** operate on this route. In summer SNAV connects Messina to the Aeolian Islands. **Aliscafi Ustica Lines** (Via Cortina del Porto, ☎ 090-364-044) also operates to the Aeolians.

By Train

 If you are traveling overnight from the mainland, stay on the train, as it dismantles and is loaded onto the FS ferry. But in the day you may wish to leave the train at Villa San Giovanni station and follow the signs for the ferries to save time. If you continue to Messina's Stazione Marittima by train, it's a good idea to disembark and walk the 100 yards to Stazione Centrale, as it takes a good hour to reassemble the trains. From here long distance buses are available. Regular train services connect Messina to Catania, Taormina, Syracuse, Palermo and Milazzo. However, buses are generally faster.

By Bus

Interbus (Piazza 6, ☎ 090-661-754) has services to Catania. There are numerous buses to towns along the Ionian coast and around Taormina. Buses to Milazzo for connections to the Aeolian islands are with **Giunta** (Via Terranova 8, ☎ 090-673-782).

Getting Around

By Car

Driving into and through Messina is a nightmare and parking is difficult. If you have a car you'd be better off parking it and setting out on foot. Parking in blue zones is €1/hr from 8:30 am-1 pm, 3:30-8:30 pm. Alternatively, see if your hotel can make recommendations. If you want to rent a car, contact any of the following offices:

- **Avis** (Via Garibaldi 109, ☎ 090-679-150)
- **Europcar** (Via Vittorio Emanuele II, 77, ☎ 090-661-365)
- **Hertz** (Via Vittorio Emanuele II, 113, ☎ 090-344-424)
- **Maggiore** (Via Vittorio Emanuele II, 75, ☎ 090-675-476)
- **Sicil Car** (Via Garibaldi 187, ☎ 090-46942)

If you need a taxi, phone:

- **Radio Taxi Jolli**, ☎ 090-6505
- **Piazza Carioli**, ☎ 090-293-4880
- **Piazza Republicca**, ☎ 090-293-6880
- **Viale Liberta**, ☎ 090-44492

By Bus

ATM buses (☎ 800-880-013, www.atmmessina.it) depart from Piazza della Republicca for destinations around the city. Tickets can be purchased at *tabbachi* or ATM agents and cost €.80 for a 60-minute ticket or €1.60 for two hours. There are daily tickets for €2.60 or you can buy weekly or monthly combinations. The city buses are a good way to get around. Most leave from Piazza della Repubblica, Piazza Carioli and Via Garibaldi. Useful bus numbers to know for getting around include 78, 79 and 80 for the museum, Duomo and Ganzirri. Number 81 goes to Mortelle and the campgrounds.

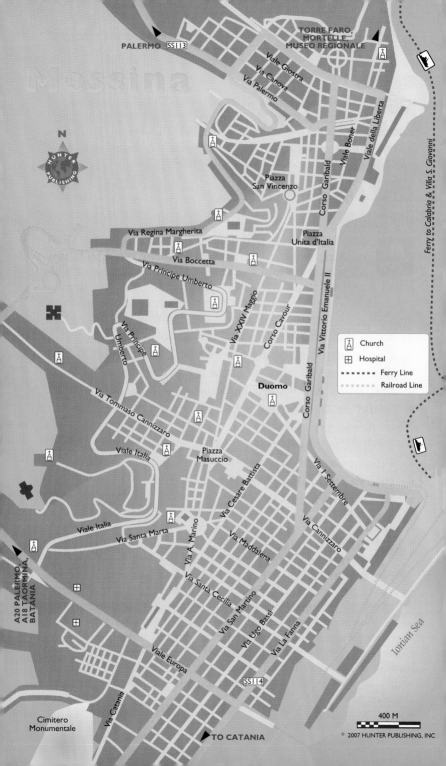

Messina

PALERMO SS113

TORRE FARO;
MORTELLE,
MUSEO REGIONALE

N

Viale Giostra
Via Canova
Via Palermo

Viale Boner
Viale della Libertà

Corso Garibald

Piazza
San Vincenzo

Ferry to Calabria & Villa S. Giovanni

Via Regina Margherita

Piazza
Unità d'Italia

Via Boccetta

Via Principe Umberto

Via XXIV Maggio

Corso Cavour

Via Vittorio Emanuele II

Via Principe
Umberto

Duomo

Corso Garibald

Via Tommaso Cannizzaro

Via I Settembre

Viale Italia

Piazza
Masuccio

Via Cesare Battista

Via Cannizzaro

Viale Italia

Via Santa Marta

Via A. Marino

Via Maddalena

Via Santa Cecilia

Via San Martino

Via Ugo Bassi

Via La Farina

A20 PALERMO,
A18 TAORMINA,
CATANIA

Viale Europa

SS114

Via Catania

Cimitero
Monumentale

TO CATANIA

Church

Hospital

---- Ferry Line

····· Railroad Line

Ionian Sea

400 M

© 2007 HUNTER PUBLISHING, INC

By Tram

The **ATM** (☎ 800-880-013, www.atmmessina.it) tram runs from the terminal at Piazza Carioli to the downtown center and harbor area. It connects to the main train station.

Information Sources

There are two useful information offices. The **AAPIT** office (Via Calabria 301, ☎ 0906-74236, 8:30 am-6:30 pm, closed Sun) and **AAST** (Piazza Carioli 45, ☎ 0902-923-292, Mon-Thurs 9 am-1:30 pm, 1-5 pm; Fri 9 am-1:30 pm) near the station. Both offices should be able to provide town maps, hotel lists and information on the Aeolian Islands. See www.messinacitymap.com for city listings on transport, sights and maps. Other options are www.messinacity.com and www.provincia.messina.it.

Events

Ferragosto celebrations in Messina are worth seeing. The festivities start on August 12. Two plaster giants are wheeled around town and then stationed near the port opposite the Municipio. On August 15 a carriage with papier mâché angels, the Christ and Mary are hauled through the city to the Piazza della Republica. At night a huge fireworks display is held on the seafront.

Sightseeing

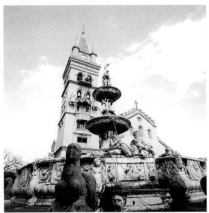

The Duomo & Fontana di Orione

The **Duomo** is Messina's major monument (Piazza del Duomo, open daily 7:30 am-12 pm and 4-6:30 pm; free) although it's actually a copy of the original 12th-century Norman cathedral that was destroyed by the 1908 earthquake and a firebomb in 1943. Today it's a case of the phoenix rising from the ashes. The interior is massive

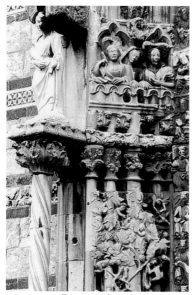

Duomo detail

and suitably impressive with a marble floor and elaborately painted wooden ceiling. There are three sets of mosaics in the apses. In the **Tesoro** (Mon-Fri 9 am-1 pm, 4:30-7 pm, Sat 9 am-1 pm, ☎ 090-675-175, €3) there are valuable candlesticks, chalices and gold reliquaries. Outside in the square, take a moment to notice the clock tower, which houses a rather extraordinary astronomical clock deemed to be the world's largest. Come on the hour to see the machinery moving, best at noon when the lion roars out the hour. In front of the cathedral is the 16th-century

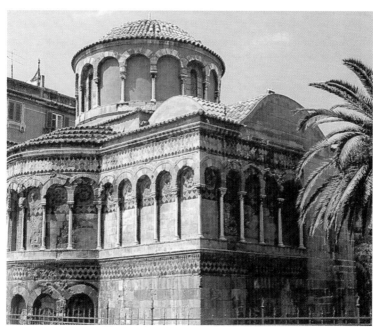

Chiesa Annunziata dei Catalani

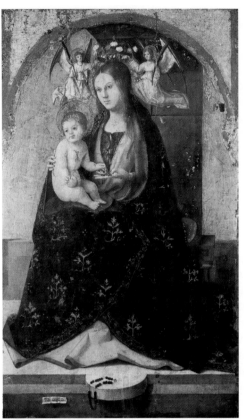

Madonna (Antonella da Messina, 1473)

Fontana di Orione, depicting the city's mythical founder Orion with cherubs, nymphs and giants.

Nearby in Piazza Catalini the **Chiesa Annunziata dei Catalani** (8 am-12 pm, 4-6:30 pm; free) has had better fortune over the years than the Duomo. It is Messina's only surviving example of an Arab-Norman church building.

The **Museo Regionale** (Via della Liberta 465, Tues-Sat 9 am-1:30 pm, 4-6:30 pm, Sun 9 am-12:30 pm; €4.50) houses many of Messina's and Sicily's greatest art works, including the Madonna above and those rescued from the earthquake rubble. To get here, take an ATM bus or walk down from the church along the port side.

Adventures on Wheels

If you have a car, consider the drive north from Messina to **Capo Peloro** and farther east. It's a pretty coastal route with beaches to stop at and views of the Italian mainland. It could easily be done by bicycle as well.

Where to Stay

 The budget choices are a little too far out of the city to make them an option if you need access to Messina.

HOTEL PRICE CHART	
€	Up to €25 per day
€€	€26-€55
€€€	€56-€85
€€€€	Over €85

The campsite, **Il Peloritano** (Localita Rodia, ☎ 0903-48496, €), is quite a long way out; take bus 81 to Rodia from Via Calabria. There's also **Nuovo Camping dello Stretto** (Circuito Torre-Faro, ☎ 0903-223-051). Camping is possible as well in Milazzo or south in Sant'Alessio; both are 40 minutes away.

If you insist on staying in the city, the **Mirage** (Via N.Scotto 3, ☎ 0902-938-844, €€) is a cheap option, but you get what you pay for. It is three blocks south of Piazza della Repubblica.

Touring (Via N. Scotto 17, ☎ 0902-938-851, €€-€€€) is near the Mirage. The rooms are bare but spacious, with TV and telephone. Rooms without bath are cheaper.

Grand Hotel Liberty (Via I Settembre 15, ☎ 0906-409436, fax 0906-409340, www.framon-hotels.com, €€€€) is popular with business travelers and rather luxurious.

Grand Hotel Lido di Mortelle (SS 113, Mortelle, ☎ 0903-21017, www.giardinodellepalme.com, €€€€) is north of the city at Mortelle, offering small units with bathrooms.

There aren't a lot of B&B options in Messina but you could try: **Oasi Azzurra** (Via Lungomare S. Saba, ☎ 0908-46034, €€€) or **San Giorgio** (Via Urna 53, ☎ 0908-43067, €€€).

Where to Eat

 You won't have trouble finding good eating in Messina or nightlife at affordable prices. The best places for a selection of restaurants are in and around Piazza Cairoli and Piazza del Popolo, Cristo Re and Montalto. In summer there are often concerts behind Cristo Re or Piazza del Duomo. Or go up to the lake area of Ganzirri or Mortelle for some fine dining – this is where everyone goes in summer.

Cafés & Bars

Le Brasserie (Via Ugo Bassi 83) is a popular *birreria* open til late. They also serve pasta, *panini* and chips. It is closed in summer.

The Duck (Via Pellegrino) is a popular English-style pub. It has a range of German bottled beers and Stones bitter. Closed Mondays and in summer.

DINING PRICE CHART	
Price per person for an entrée, including house wine.	
€	Up to €12
€€	€13-€25
€€€	€26-€35
€€€€	Over €35

Cheap Eats

Café d'Italia (Piazza Carioli 33, €) has some cheap fixed menus.

One of the cheapest eats is the self-service bar beyond the tourist office outside the train station.

Astral (Via XXVII Luglio 71, ☎ 0907-71087, €) offers a full meal menu for under €10. Astral is just off Piazza Ciaroli.

Restaurants

Alberto (Via Ghibellina 95, ☎ 0907-1711, €€€€) is one of Messina's best seafood restaurants, but you pay for the privilege. Try the swordfish *involtini* (rolled and stuffed) and *cassata siciliana*. You should reserve ahead in summer and weekends and definitely dress up.

Further down on the expense scale is **Il Gatto e La Volpe** (Via Ghibellina 154, €€). This *trattoria* features local specialties daily in a rustic brick interior.

Pizzeria del Capitano (Via dei Mille 88) has basic pizzas and fast services.

Ristorante Casa Savoia (Via XXVII Luglio 36/38, ☎ 090-293-4865, www.ristorantecasasavoia.it, €€) is rather old fashioned and decorated with Oriental rugs and antiques. They specialize in swordfish here and pasta with fried zucchini.

Piero (Via Ghibellina 119, ☎ 0906-409-354, €€) is well known and serves traditional Sicilan foods. The *antipasti* buffet is good.

Outside of Messina

Ganzirri is a pleasant town about 10 km north of Messina where the city's youth go during the hot summer months. The town is based around a lake that is used for mussel-farming. You'll find very good seafood here. In

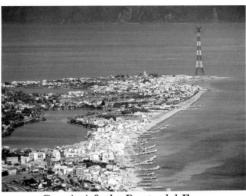

Ganzirri & the Punta del Faro

fact there are *trattorie* wedged all along the lakeside. Many offer similar options and prices. We've recommended a few but you could eat anywhere.

La Sirena (☎ 093-912-68) and **La Taverna sul Lago** (☎ 090-393-222, closed Sun evening) have plates for about €7. **La Conchiglia** (Via Pantano 72, ☎ 090-391-160) is similarly priced farther along – look for the yellow shell on the right side.

Continuing along the road to the Punta del Faro or Capo Peloro, is a small community with a pleasant church and harbor. **Il Pescatore** (Via Ist Palazzo, 16 Torre Faro, ☎ 090-326-029) is a superb place to sit right near the church with a view of the Straits of Messina and the fishermen working the waters. Their specialty is *paella*. There are a handful of other restaurants, along with a *gelateria* and *birreria*.

At the end of the road is the **Punta del Faro** – the eastern tip of Sicily. In the Torre Faro is a tourist and cultural center, **Parco Horcynus Orca** (Località Torre Faro, Capo Peloro, Castello Ruffo, www.horcynusorca.it, ☎ 090-325-236, fax 090-322-3038, 10 am-1 pm, 4-8 pm, closed Mon, €7). The center is housed inside an ancient fortress with original medieval foundations that have recently been unearthed. Exhibits include an archaeological museum, contemporary art, cinema library, photographic works and marine science section. Guides accompany you through the tower so you don't get lost! Prices change depending on the exhibits.

Adventures

In Water

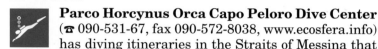 **Parco Horcynus Orca Capo Peloro Dive Center** (☎ 090-531-67, fax 090-572-8038, www.ecosfera.info) has diving itineraries in the Straits of Messina that are historically interesting. There are wrecks to explore in these depths and abundant sea life. You can rent equipment, do PADI-certified courses or take advantage of the *immersioni* (dives) offered.

They can also arrange for you to go out with fishermen hunting swordfish in traditional local boats known as *feluche*.

■ The Coastal Route to Taormina

Savoca★★

This beautiful town four km inland from Santa Teresa di Riva has a cluster of houses, a handful of medieval churches and what remains of a tattered castle. The streets are mostly deserted and you can enjoy a stroll in a preserved medieval atmosphere and not have to share it with anyone. If you're coming from Taormina, this will be a welcome change. **Jonica** buses (☎ 0942-751-566) departs from outside Bar Il Vitello to Antillo, Messina (four daily), S. Teresa and Taormina (once

Northern Ionian Coast

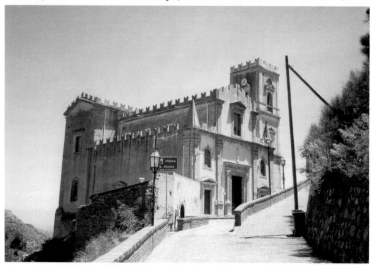

Chiesa San Nicolo (Clemensfranz)

daily). Once you get to S. Teresa there are connections to other places along the coast. **CST** (Corso Umberto I, 101, ☎ 094-262-6088) in Taormina has half-day excursions on Monday to Savoca and Forza d'Agora (€26).

Most people tend to congregate around ★ ★ ★**Bar Il Vitello** at the entrance to the town where scenes for Francis Ford Coppola's *The Godfather* were filmed. The bar was used for Michael Corleone's bertrothal to Apollonia. The owner, Maria D'Arrigo, is almost as famous as the film, an elderley *signora* close to 80 years old who still serves behind the bar. The bar interior is pure vintage with an array of old objects, including sewing machines and beaded curtains, along with pictures from the movie on the wall and and local products that are for sale. The *granita* is famed and also the *liquori di limone* (€3. 50). In summer, lines can curl out the door.

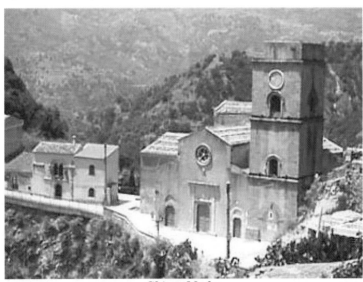

Chiesa Madre

Once you leave the bar behind, the crowds disperse and you can wander the town in peace. There are two roads through town leading to the Chiesa Madre and Chiesa San Michele. The **Chiesa Madre** is stunningly located and worth the walk to admire it between the hills. On the way you will pass the **Museo Comunale** (9 am-1:30 pm, 3-8 pm, €1) in the Chiesa San Nicolo. The museum has two floors; the first dedicated to the farming world, poetry and popular culture and the second

to history and nobility. Other signs back near the bar will point you towards the ★**Cappuccin monastery** and the *cripta* (9 am-1 pm, 4-7 pm, closed Mon, donations requested). The catacombs are currently being restored but the 32 mummiess from the 17th century are still on display in a room. They still look rather gruesome but lose a bit of their goulish quality away from the eerie catacombs.

If you've built an appetite walking around, there are a couple of food options. **Ristorante La Pineta** makes *tagliatelle* on the premises and is around the corner from Bar Il Vitello towards the monastery. Meals are about €15-20. **Pizzeria Ristorante del Parco** is a little out of the center beyond the *cripta*. They make their own *maccheroni*. You can get pizza for €4-8 or a meal for around €15.

Forza d'Agora ★

A corkscrew road leads the few km off the coastal stretch north of Taormina to the pretty little hilltop center of Forza d'Agora. It's a good day-trip fromTaormina and usually quiet. Interbus connections link Agora to Taormina and Letojanni and pull into the main piazza. From here a road leads to the 14th-century cattedrale **Maria SS Annunziata** and up increasingly narrow, more tumble-down streets to a crumbling **Norman Saraceno** *castello* of the 12th century. The main entrance to the castle is closed, although a local will be able to show you a way past the prickly spines of cacti to see what remains of the old fortifications. Once you've pattered up, here meander the streets to see a handful of churches and piazzas with views of the surrounding valley. Find a good spot and you'll likely have only the company of local cats and the dong of bells.

Hotel Souvenir on Via Belvedere (☎ 0942-721-078, €€), **B&B Carnabuci** (Via De Joannon 10, ☎ 347-008-6806, €€€) and **B&B Casa Mia** (☎ 349-504-1501) are accommodation options.

L'Abbazia (☎ 0942-721-226, closed Mon) is located on a terrace with great views, serving some local specialties. There's also **Pizzeria Il Priore** (☎ 094-272-1607) and **Osteria Agostiniana**.

CST (Corso Umberto I, 101, ☎ 094-262-6088) in Taormina have half-day excursions on Monday to Savoca and Forza d'Agora (€26).

■ Taormina★★★

Sicily's best known resort is set high on Monte Tauro with sweeping views to the sea and Mt Etna. The long high season from April to October means budget travelers feel the pinch, but you'd make a mistake to avoid it all together.

There's a lot that's seductive about Taormina and it's still possible to see the old-world charm that first attracted the high-end tourist set. Goethe and DH Lawrence were also besotted with Taormina, and for good reason. The picturesque streets adorned with bougainvillea trees contain some real delights. There's Sicily's best view of Mt Etna from the stunning Greek theater, good walks in the heights of Castelmola and some of the coastline's best beaches.

Getting Here & Around

 The best way to get to Taormina is by buses that arrive directly in town. Interbus leaves from Messina and Catania (?4,20, one hour). Taormina is well connected with all the towns in the immediate area. Trains arrive on the coast at Taormina-Giardini station. Regular Interbus buses make the journey (€1.30) about every 30 minutes up the steep hill to the center of town.

Local buses in Taormina will be handy for getting to and from your hotel if you don't want to walk up the steep streets. Several go up to Castelmola every day. You could also make use of the *funivia* (cable car) to get to the beaches at Isola Bella and Mazzaro. See the Catania chapter about tours leaving from Taormina to Mt Etna.

Information Sources

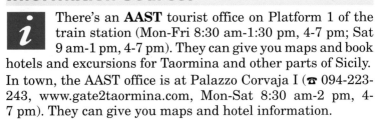 There's an **AAST** tourist office on Platform 1 of the train station (Mon-Fri 8:30 am-1:30 pm, 4-7 pm; Sat 9 am-1 pm, 4-7 pm). They can give you maps and book hotels and excursions for Taormina and other parts of Sicily. In town, the AAST office is at Palazzo Corvaja I (☎ 094-223-243, www.gate2taormina.com, Mon-Sat 8:30 am-2 pm, 4-7 pm). They can give you maps and hotel information.

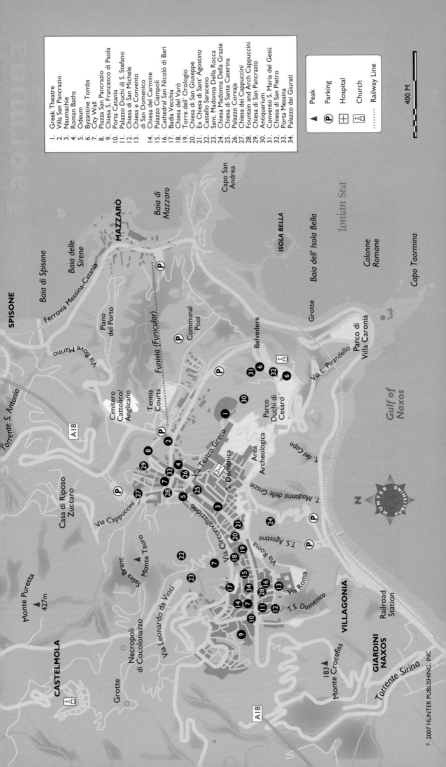

Taormina

1. Greek Theatre
2. Villa San Pancrazio
3. Naumachie
4. Roman Baths
5. Odeum
6. Byzantine Tombs
7. City Wall
8. Piazza San Pancrazio
9. Chiesa S. Francesco di Paola
10. Porta Catania
11. Palazzo Duchi di S. Stefano
12. Chiesa di San Michele
13. Chiesa e Convento di San Domenico
14. Chiesa del Carmine
15. Palazzo Ciampoli
16. Cathedral San Nicolò di Bari
17. Badia Vecchia
18. Chiesa del Varò
19. Torre dell'Orologio
20. Chiesa di San Giuseppe
21. Ex Chiesa di Sant' Agostino
22. Castello Saraceno
23. Sant. Madonna Della Rocca
24. Chiesa Madonna Della Grazie
25. Chiesa di Santa Caterina
26. Palazzo Corvaja
27. Chiesa dei Cappuccini
28. Fountain and Arch Cappuccini
29. Chiesa di San Pancrazio
30. Antiquarium
31. Convento S. Maria del Gesù
32. Chiesa di San Pietro
33. Porta Messina
34. Palazzo dei Giurati

▲ Peak
Ⓟ Parking
⊞ Hospital
Ⓐ Church
········· Railway Line

400 M

© 2007 HUNTER PUBLISHING, INC.

Sightseeing

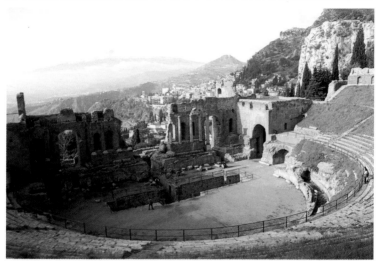

Taormina's Greek Theater (Joanne Lane)

The most famous sight is undoubtedly the ★★★**Greek The-ater** (Teatro Greco, ☎ 0942-23220, 9 am-1hr before sunset, €4.20). It was built in the third century BC but heavily re-modeled in the first century AD by the Romans. Today it's an essentially Roman structure. The Greeks had chosen the site for the amazing views of Mt Etna and the Bay of Schiso, but the Romans must have largely obscured this with their col-umns and gladia-tor-style arrange-ments. You can wander up and down the seating and poke around in the high vaulted rooms where animals were once kept for show. In July and August the theater hosts an international arts festival.

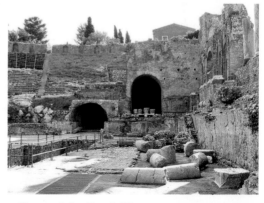

Stage of the Greek Theater (Galen R Frysinger, www.galenfrysinger.com)

There are events at other times of the year. These will give you some idea of the original role the theater played, hosting the great tragedies of antiquity.

Behind the tourist office is the **Roman Odeon**,

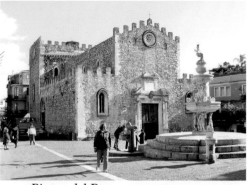

Piazza del Duomo (Galen R Frysinger)

a small theater partly covered by Chiesa

Santa Caterina was constructed in AD 21 and is much smaller than the Greek theater. It was discovered in 1892 by a blacksmith digging in the area. The **Santa Caterina church** was built in the mid-17th century and sits on a piazza at the highest point of Corso Umberto I. It is open daily 9 am-12 pm, 4-8 pm. Farther along Corso Umberto is the **Piazza del Duomo** and **cathedral**, currently closed for renovations.

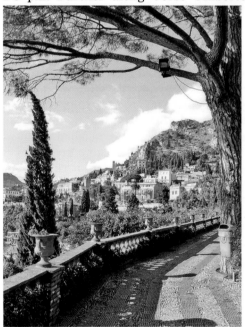

There are two museums in town. The **Museo Archeologico di Taormina** (Palazzo Badia Vecchia, ☎ 0942-620-122, Tues-Sun 9 am-1 pm, 4-8 pm, €2.60) is set on the site of Roman baths and where all the archaeological remnants discovered around the city are stored. The other museum is the **Museo Siciliano**

Taormina (Galen R Frysinger)

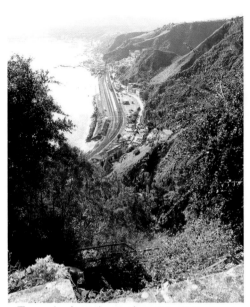

Taormina's train station (Galen R Frysinger)

di Arte e Tradizioni Poplari (Palazzo Corvaja, Piazza Santa Caterina, Corso Umberto I, ☎ 0942-23243, Tues-Sun 9 am-1 pm, 4-8 pm; €2.60). It has 18th-century oil portraits, donkey carts and embroidery. You can enter the ground floor of the palace at no charge to go to the tourist office.

The **Villa Commune**, or **Parco Duchi di Cesaro**, is a beautiful park with rich flora. It's perfect for a picnic or for great views over the bay below.

There are other stately buildings along Corso Umberto but Taormina is really more about strolling, window-shopping and admiring the views. One place you can do that is from **Piazza IX Aprile** by the **Torre dell'Orologio**.

The most popular beach, **Lido Mazzaro**, is reached via a cable car that leaves from Via Pirandello. Tickets are €1.80/3 one-way/return (www.asm.taormina.me.it) and it runs every 15 minutes from 8 am-1:30 pm, 9-1:30 am. At the Lido, past the Capo Sant'Andrea headland, is the prettiest cove on the coastline and the tiny ★★**Isola Bella islet**. If you come down with the *funivia* you will see stairs that take you down to the beach. The small cove and beach is packed during the summer, but is fun for exploring with a snorkel or swimming. You can rent pedal boats here during the summer. There are plenty of eating options along the coastal route. Hotels also line the *lungomare*.

Adventures

On Foot

■ *Castello Saraceno (two hours)*

Start from the railway station and walk up via the Madonna delle Grazie to Piazza IX Aprile to extend the walk, or start in town at this latter point. Take Vicolo Stretto, a tiny arched alleyway, towards Porta Messina. Continue along to find the next flight of stairs. Cross Via Circon-

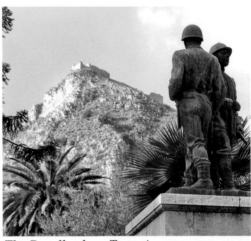

The Castello above Taormina (Galen R Frysinger)

valazione and then start up the old mule track for the Castello Saraceno and Via Crucis. You get views of the Greek Theater, town center, Ionian Sea, the Castle Rock and the Middle City Wall. At the end of the stairway is the **Madonna della Rocca**, a 16th-century church built into the limestone bastion. Around the corner is the last leg to the castle. The 12th-century castle occupies the site of the acropolis built in classical times. There is still defensive walling, a tower and the remains of a cistern. Unfortunately it is usually closed.

■ *Castelmola (two hours)* ★ ★

The dizzy perch of Caselmola is reached from Porta Messina, a short distance uphill from the bus terminal and cable car. Take Via Costantino Patricio in gradual ascent, turn right onto Via Cappuccini and onto Via Dietro Cappuccini, then onto the signed Salita Branco. The track cuts below the Castello Saraceno and then crosses the tarmac road for Castelmola. Continue on the track to enter the main piazza of Castelmola.

To return to Taormina, follow signs for the Pizzeria Le Mimose down the steps. Cross two minor roads and continue

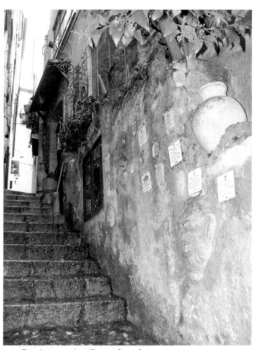

Stairway in Castelmola (Galen R Frysinger)

along a panoramic path windng through gardens. You pass ancient tombs of the Sicel necropolis dating back to the 10th-seventh centuries BC.

Castelmola is thought to have been the site of an ancient acropolis called Tauromenion. There are ruins of a medieval castle and some lovely views. It's a good break from busy Taormina and you can also stay up here. **Panorama di Sicilia** (☎ 0942-28027, €€), **Villa Sonia** (☎ 0942-28082, €€€€), **Villa Regina** (☎ 0942-28228, €€€) and **Villa Pace B&B** (☎ 0942-28202) are the options. There's also a fine bar in the Lilliputian piazza. Most of the bars serve *vino alla mandorla* (almond wine). **Le Mimose** (Via Tutti i Santi, Terrazza Panoramica, ☎ 0942-28216) is 160 yards from Piazza Duomo and has menus for €11-12.

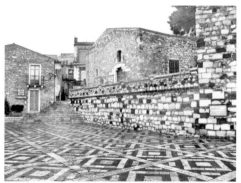

Castelmola (Galen R Frysinger)

Buses from Interbus come up here several times daily.

Where to Stay
Hostels & Camping

There are two youth hostels in Taormina. The popular **Odyssey** (Trav A. Di Via G. Martino 2, ☎ 0942-24533, www.taorminaoddyssey.it, €) has beds from €14-16.

Ulisse Youth Hostel (Via San Francesco di Paola 9, ☎ 094-223-193, ostelloulisse.taormina@email.it, €) gets mixed reviews. You may be accosted by them down at the train station.

The nearest campsite, **Campeggio San Leo** (☎ 0942-24658), is near the beach next to the Grande Albergo Capo Taormina.

B&Bs

Il Leone (Via Bagnoli Croce 127, ☎ 0942-23878, €€) has plain rooms with some good views.

Casa Grazia (Via Lallia Bassia 20, ☎ 0942-24776, €€) is another no-frills budget option.

Hotels

Elios (Via Bagnoli Croce 98, ☎ 0942-23431, €€€) has nice rooms with bathrooms.

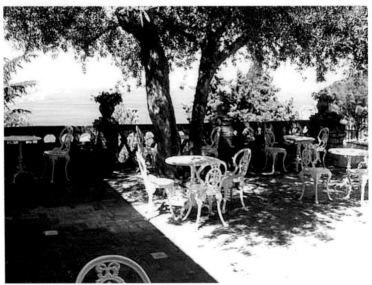

Villa Fiorita

Villa Fiorita (Via Luigi Pirandello 39, ☎ 0942-24122, www.villafioritahotel.com, €€€€) is close to the cable car station.

★★**Romantik Hotel Villa Ducale** (Via Leonardo da Vinci 60, ☎0942-28153, fax/☎0942-28710, villaducale@tao.it, €€€€€) is an elegant old Sicilian villa that was transformed into a hotel and is as romantic as its name suggests. The breakfast is hard to beat – an amazing spread with an unsurpassed view over flowers and fields to Mt Etna.

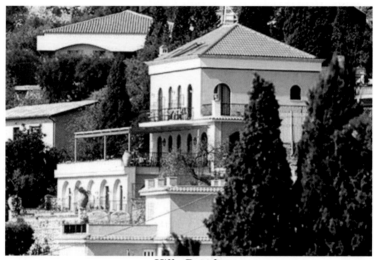
Villa Ducale

Villa Belvedere (Via Bagnoli Croce 79, ☎ 0942-23791, €€€€) is near the public gardens and has good views to the sea.

Where to Eat
Bars & Cafés

 Rosticceria Pigghia e Potta (Via di Giovanni 23, €) has great pizza by the slice. **Mediterraneo Café** (Via di Giovanni) is a trendy spot for a drink, with jazzy music until late. **Mocambo** (Piazza IX Aprile) has seats on the corso.

Time Out (Via San Prancazio 19) has a pleasant garden and lively crowd, with draft Guinness and other beers and snacks.

Restaurants

Gambero Rosso (Via Naumachie 11, ☎ 0942-24863, €-€€) is a busy spot with fast pizza and cheap meals.

Al Giardino (Via Bagnoli Croce 84, closed Tues, €€) serves fresh pasta across from the Giardino Pubblico.

Granduca (Corso Umberto I, 172, ☎ 0942-24983, €€€) is an atmospheric choice, entered through an antiques store. Eat in beautiful gardens with a view over the bay.

Casa Grugno (Via Santa Maria de Greci, ☎ 0942-21208, www.casagrungno.it, €€€€) has an Austrian-born chef and mixes Sicilian food with some more European sensibilities. Set-price menus will help cut the cost.

Al Duomo (Vico Ebrei 11, Piazza Duomo, ☎ 0942-625-656, www.ristorantealduomo.it, €€€€) enjoys poll position in the square outside the cathedral.

■ Giardini Naxos

This town five km south of Taormina is a good alternative to the resort town – everything is cheaper here, from accommodations to eating – and there's good swimming on the wide, curving bay. This was the site of the first Greek colony in Sicily. A settlement started in 734 BC, named Naxos after the Greek island from which the colonists came.

Getting Here & Around

 Buses run regularly between Giardini and Taormina's bus terminal until about midnight in summer and 10:30 pm in winter. You can also reach Giardini Naxos by train. The Tourist Office is on Via Tysandros 54 (☎ 0942-51010, www.aast-giardini.naxos.it, Mon-Fri 8:30 am-2 pm, 4-7 pm; Sat 8:30 am-2 pm).

If you want to rent a bike or scooter contact:

- **Rent Scooter** (Via Vittorio Emanuele 1266, www.mcracing.it, ☎ 094-253-905).
- **Sicily by Car** (Via Recanati 21, ☎ 0942-54045).
- **Etna Rent** (Via Casarsa 27, ☎ 0942-51972) for bikes and cars or mopeds.

Northern Ionian Coast

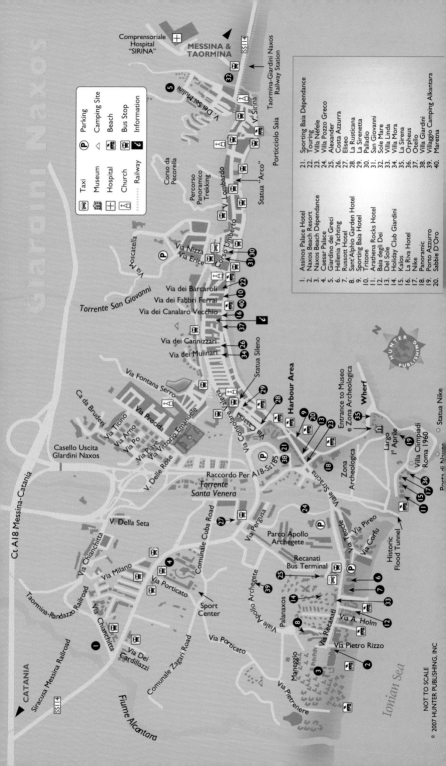

Giardini Naxos

Comprensoriale Hospital "SIRINA"

MESSINA & TAORMINA

←SS114

←Taormina-Giardini Naxos Railway Station

V. Dei Sei Mulini

V. Sirina

Porticciolo Saia

Corso da Pecorella

Percorso Panoramico Trekking

V. Lombardo

Statua "Arco"

Via Moscatella

Via Nizza

Via Erice

Corso Umberto

Via A18 Messina-Catania

Torrente San Giovanni

Via dei Barcaroli
Via dei Fabbri Ferrai
Via dei Canalaro Vecchio

Via dei Cannizzari
Via dei Mulinari

Statua Sileno

Via Fontana Serro

Ca da Bruderi

Via Ticino
Via Procida
Via Arno
Via Po
Via Praie
Via Vittorio Emanuele

Casello Uscita Giardini Naxos

Raccordo Per A18-Ss 185

Torrente Santa Venera

Via Corso Vittorio Emanuele

Harbour Area

Entrance to Museo e Zona Archeologica

Wherf

Largo 1° Aprile

Villa Climpiadi Roma 1960

Zona Archeologica

Viale Scacina

Porto di Naxos

Statua Nike

V. Della Seta

Via Pergusa

Parco Apollo Archegete

Recanati Bus Terminal

Via Teocle
Via Pireo
Via Corfu

Historic Flood Tunnel

Viale Apollo Archegete

Palanaxos

Via Recanati

Via A. Holm

Via Pietro Rizzo

Sport Center

Via Milano

Via Porticato

Via Chianchitta

Taormina-Randazzo Railroad

CATANIA

Siracusa Messina Railroad

SS114

Via Dei Cardillazzi

Via Porticato

Maneggio

Via Pietrenere

Comunale Zagari Road

Comunale Cuba Road

Fiume Alcantara

Ionian Sea

NOT TO SCALE

© 2007 HUNTER PUBLISHING, INC

HUNTER PUBLISHING

Legend

☒ Taxi	℗ Parking
🏛 Museum	△ Camping Site
✚ Hospital	🏖 Beach
⛪ Church	☒ Bus Stop
Railway	⚓ Information

1. Assinos Palace Hotel
2. Naxos Beach Resort
3. Naxos Beach Dependance
4. Caesar Palace
5. Giardino dei Greci
6. Hellenia Yachting
7. Russott Hotel
8. Sant'Alphio Garden Hotel
9. Sporting Baia Hotel
10. Tritone
11. Arathena Rocks Hotel
12. Baia degl Dei
13. Del Sole
14. Holiday Club Giardini
15. Kalos
16. La Riva Hotel
17. Nike
18. Panoramic
19. Porto Azzurro
20. Sabbie D'Oro
21. Sporting Baia Dépendance
22. Touring
23. Villa Néfele
24. Villa Pozzo Greco
25. Alexander
26. Costa Azzurra
27. Eliseo
28. La Rusticana
29. La Sirenetta
30. Palladio
31. San Giovanni
32. Sole Mare
33. Villa Linda
34. Villa Mora
35. La Sirena
36. Orpheus
37. Otello
38. Villa Giardini
39. Villaggio Camping Alkantara
40. Maretna

Sightseeing

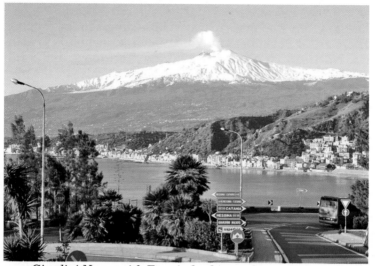

Giardini Naxos with Etna in background (Galen R Frysinger)

The excavations of the **Greek settlement** (9 am-1 hour before sunset, €2.10) are not as stunning as at other places in Sicily, athough they do lie right on the end of Capo Schiso. They contain a stretch of ancient lava-built city wall, two covered kilns and a temple. There's also the **Museo Archaeologico** on-site, housing fragments of amphorae and anchors. To get here, take the bus from Taormina or walk along *lungomare*.

Where to Stay & Eat

Campeggio Maretna (Via Pietralunga, ☎ 0942-52794) and **Camping Alkantara** (Via Porticato, ☎ 0942-576-031) are both rather inconvenient for travelers without a car. One is directly behind the tourist office beyond Via Pietralunga. The other is the on the far side of the archaeology area back off the coast.

Il Pescatore B&B (Via Naxos 96, ☎ 347-104-7878, www.b-bilpescatore.com, €€€) has pleasant rooms and a garden terrace. **Pensione Otello** (Via Tysandros 62, ☎ 0942-51009, €€€) has plain rooms overlooking the sea. **Hotel La Riva** (Via Tysandros 52, ☎ 0942-51329, €€€) is next to the tourist

information office. **Villa Mora** (Via Naxos 47, ☎ 0942-51839) has its own restaurant, colorful ceramics and balconies, but no sea view.

The *lungomare* becomes a busy strip of diners in the evening. There are lots of options on Via Tysandros, including **Trattoria Nettuno** (☎ 0942-571-278) **La Lampara** and **Lido d'Angelo**. **La Cambusa**, at the end of Via Schiso by the pier, has good pizzas and seafood right on the beach.

■ Alcantara Valley

The pretty Alcantara Valley lies inland from Taormina on the SS 185. The highlight is the series of modest lava gorges known as the ★★**Gola dell'Alcantara**. Alcantara derives from the Arabic *al cantara*, meaning "bridge." The gorges are a few km short of **Francavilla** (itself a pleasant destination). **Interbus** has eight daily buses from Taormina to Gola dell'Alcantara and Francavilla. Four buses come from Randazzo.

It's a bit commercalized at the top of the gorge, with a car park, bar and restaurant. You can walk or take the lift down to the gorge below from the entrance (☎ 094-298-5010, www. golealcantara.it, €2.50). There is a free access path for those in the know a few hundred yards up from the entrance.

Adventures

In Water

You can trek through the gorge to an interesting series of waterfalls, the **Vasca di Venere** (Venus Falls). The water is freezing (50°) and you special clothing is needed. Groups of 10-15 are led through in *salopetti* boots, neoprene suits and shoes, crash helmets and fluvial life jackets by a guide daily from March-September. There are four routes, from 20-60 minutes (€2.50) to two hours (€40). Route D requires a little daring. The first tours start at 9:30 am.

You can raft the Alcantara river with **Acquaterre** (Via Antonino Long 74, Catania, ☎ 095-503-020, www.acquaterra.it) between January and March (three hours, €40). Or on a type of body board known as a hydrospeed (three hours, €40, November-April). They also do canyoning (three to four hours, €40) **SAT** (Corso Umberto I 73, ☎ 094-224-653, www.sat-group.it), in Taormina, has bus tours of Etna via the Alcantara region. (See *Taormina*.)

Facing page: Gola dell'Alcantara (Joanne Lane)

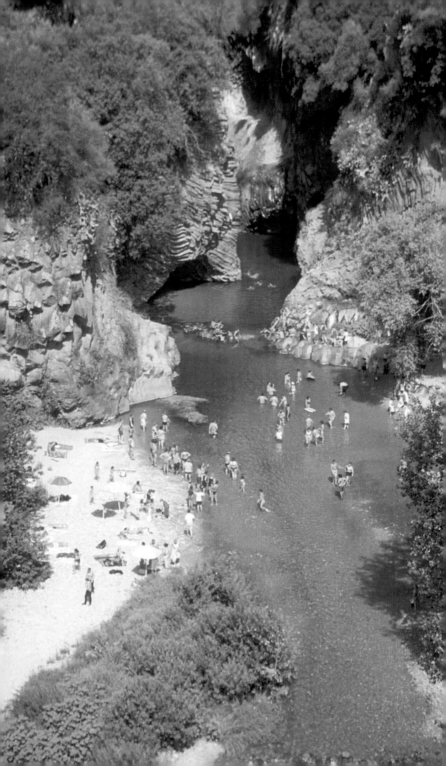

If you want to stay in the region, ask at the entrance (☎ 094-298-5010, www.golealcantara.com) for an overnight farm stay at **La Casa delle Monache**, **Il Poggio** or **Il Borgo**.

Francavilla di Sicilia

Four km along the river is the pleasant town of Francavilla di Sicilia. Wait for an Interbus connection from the Gola dell'Alcantara or walk to the town. This was the site of one of the bloodiest battles fought in Sicily when the Austrian Army engaged the Spanish in 1719. Eight thousand died. Today it's a quiet community nestled in the Alcantara Valley and particularly pretty in the autumn.

The 16th-century **Convento dei Cappuccini** across the river has a little museum (11 am-1 pm, 3:30-7:30 pm; ☎ 329-056-7480, donations appreciated) shows how the monks passed their time – baking, brewing and crafting. Helpful staff will allow you to taste their products. You can buy honey, grappa and other liquors.

If you want to stay in Francavilla, **D'Orange d'Alcantara** (☎ 0942-981-374, www.hoteldorange.itgo.com) is a popular option.

Castiglione di Sicilia★★

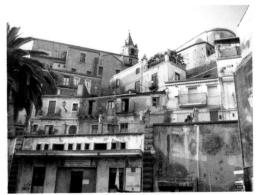

Castiglione di Sicilia

Five km above Francavilla is the medieval hill town of Castiglione di Sicilia, one of the hidden gems in this part of the Valley. It is immediately inviting as you enter town for its many church spires and the ruined castle of rock, **Fortezza Greca**. You can wander up to this castle for sweeping views of the countryside.

Castiglione had its beginnings in the 12th century, when the Normans drew the Arabs out of the valley and founded countless cities and monasteries. Castiglione was surrounded by

defense walls and divided into districts. The original nine gates are now scarcely visible.

For tourists the town offers a quiet option away from the busy coastal area around Taormina and the chance to explore the surrounding Alcantara valley or Etna region on foot, bike, horse or jeep. Wine is particularly good in this region too.

Getting Here & Information Sources

Tourism infrastructure is growing in Castiglione and you'll find some of the most organized information offices in the province with lots of new initiatives starting.

Ufficio Informazioni Turistiche (Piazza XI Febbraio, ☎ 0942-980-348) is the place to go. **Etna Travel** (Piazza XI Febbraio 17, ☎ 094-298-0386, 328-617-9118, 328-414-6447, www.jaro.it/etnatravel, 7:30 am-8 pm) can help arrange itineraries for you. **Etna Alcantara** (Piazza Il Febbraio 13, ☎ 333-298-1651, ☎ 094-298-0526, www.etnalcantara.net) arranges walking, biking, horseback and other itineraries in the area.

Unfortunately there are no bus services to Castiglione. You can get to Francavilla, but then it's a five-km walk to Castiglione.

Sightseeing

The quiet, narrow streets of Castiglione immediately invite a wander past crumbling churches and turrets with views of the surrounding hillside. The **Fortezza Greca** (9 am-8 pm, ☎0942-980348 free) is the main attraction, with great views from the top over the town's piazzas and squares and to Etna and the Alcantara Valley

Adventures

With Wine

A very good *spumante* wine is produced in the area and is also the first *spumante* in the Etna zone. Ask in the tourist office for a list of wine *cantine* to visit in the area. You can get an independent itinerary or go with a guide.

On Foot & on Wheels

There were a number of *sentieri* being developed at the time of writing. Ask in the tourist office for full details about the trek down to **Fiume Alcantara** (three

hours), starting from Piazza Febbraio. There are also routes along the old railway line.

One route from Castiglione along Via Rosario Cimino does lead to the old railway line, which you can follow. After a few km, a road through hazelnut groves and vineyards leads to **Monte Miramare**. From the top there are beautiful views.

A pleasant walk to Francavilla to pick up the bus takes around an hour and passes the sturdy medieval bridge and the ruins of a Byzantine church.

The **SAT bus** company (Corso Umberto I 73, ☎ 0942-24653, www.sat-group.it) in Taormina visits the Alcantara Gorges and then continues to Randazzo and via Circumetnea train to Adrano. From here a bus takes you to **Rifugio Sapienza** (Etna). It is €37 or €75 if a jeep ride to the main crater on the mountain is included. Departure is 7 am. They have a second option at 8 am for €33 that goes to Alcantara, Randazzo and Etna North.

With Golf

 For a golf course with a difference try the 18-hole ★★**Il Picciolo Golf Club** at Castiglione di Sicilia (Via Picciolo, 1 Castiglione di Sicilia, ☎ 0942-986-252, www.ilpicciologolf.com, 18 holes €55, nine holes €38). The course only opened in 1989, but you could not picture a more dramatic setting. It is actually located on the slopes of Mt Etna between old lava fields and a former hazelnut farm. The old farmhouse was renovated into a clubhouse with restaurant, bar, bridge room and television lounge. Il Picciolo also offers single and double rooms for bed and breakfast (€110) or for half- or full board.

Where to Stay & Eat

 Ostello Regina Margherita (Via Abate Coniglio 7, ☎ 0942-984-956).

B&B St Caterina (Via S. Ten Mazza 10, ☎ 347-441-7473).

Casa Conti B&B (Via Rosario Cimino 20, ☎ 0932-983-248).

The best choice for eating in town is **Belvedere d'Alcantara** (Via Abbate Coniglio 44) for the rooftop terrace, taking in the full views from the town.

Le Chevalier in Piazza Popolo has coffee and snacks.

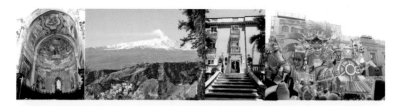

Catania

Catania is Sicily's second-largest city and is often the first place where foreign tourists arrive on the island. Lucky for them, as it's one of the island's most intriguing centers. If you get past its commercial aspects, you'll immediately sense a vibrancy and liveliness that's not so apparent in the capital. It's the best of both worlds. The pandemonium of Palermo is not here and yet the piazzas and markets are still busy, there's fantastic student nightlife with cheap food and music, some of Sicily's most pungent markets and glorious historical buildings.

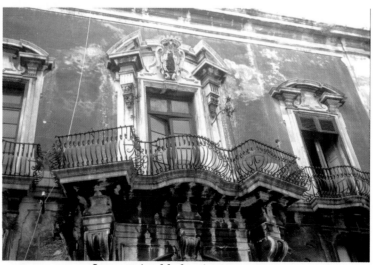

Lava-stained balconies (Joanne Lane)

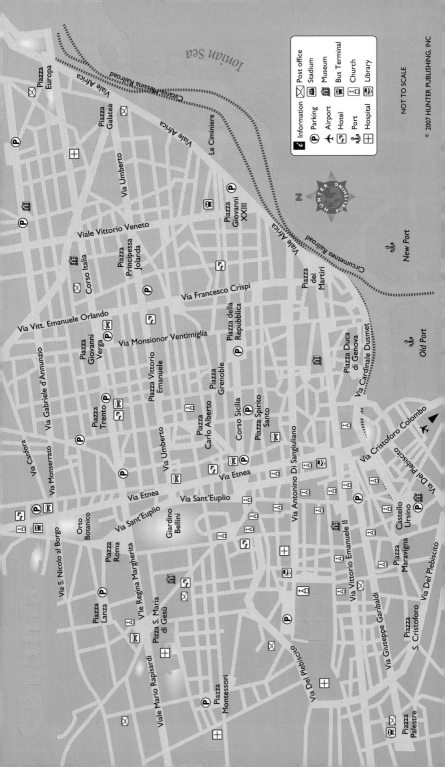

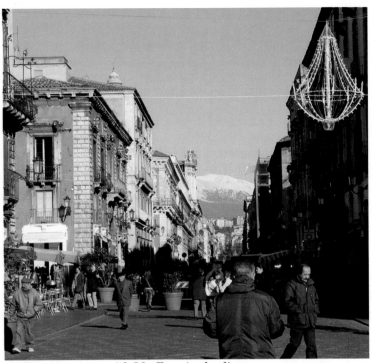

Catania street, with Mt. Etna in the distance (Galen R Frysinger)

It's one of those cities with a bit of everything. The main streets have air-conditioned shopping centers, Internet cafés, banks and Gucci shoes. But turn down any side-street and it's a different story – age-old markets compete in the squares and alleyways; water is still collected from street fountains; and old shoe cobblers hammer your worn soles into place. There's also variety everywhere, with Asian and Africans competing for phone and Internet business, next to century old Sicilian bread shops.

Catania is also a fantastic base from which to visit Mount Etna. The city lives very much in the shadow of the volcano, which not only dominates the skyline but has also pervaded the city. Lava is the local building material and you can find lava-encrusted Roman relics and Baroque structures streaked with volcanic ash. These grand architectural structures give the city a noble, lofty air, although they do look slightly run-down. It would be easy to blame their decayed

condition on the polluting effects of Mt Etna's vulcanizing smoke or on age, but the streaks on the outside must also be dirt. You will find rubbish in the streets, an enormous population of scabby dogs and feral cats and an equal number of shabby balconies overwhelmed with flapping laundry. However, it seems to give the city a mysterious air rather than a shady one.

Catania was one of the first Greek colonies on the island in 729 BC and became very influential in the colonies of Magna Graecia. The city was one of the first to fall to the Romans, but it also prospered greatly in their time and has many ancient Roman relics to this day. Catania's patron saint is Agata, who is supposed to have saved the city from complete volcanic destruction in the 17th century. She was put to death by the praetor Quintianus when she rejected his advances and was later canonized. However, despite her protection, the city was engulfed in lava in 1669 and an earthquake devastated the city in 1693. For more information on Etna, see the section later in this chapter.

CATANIA HIGHLIGHTS

- An ice cream at Scardaci on Via Etnea.
- The hectic morning *pescheria* market by the Duomo.
- Baroque buildings stained with Etna's polluting dust.
- A saucy, delicious plate of *spaghetti alla Norma*.
- The Ciclopi islands at Aci Trezza.
- *Café concerti* entertainment during the summer months.
- Sipping a beer in Piazza Scammacca and watching the soccer on big screens, crying *forza* when your team scores!

■ Getting There

By Air

 The **Fontanarossa airport** (☎ 095-723-9111 or 095-340-505, toll free 800-605656, www.aeroporto.

catania.it) is seven km south of the city and has domestic and European flights (usually via Rome or Milan, but also Palermo and Naples). Major carriers include **Alitalia** (☎ 848-865-641, 06-2222, www.alitalia.com), **Meridiana** (☎ 06-478-041, 199-111-333, www.meridiana.it) that operates from both Milan and London, and **Volare Web** (☎ 800-454-000, 199-414-500) from Milan and Venice. Other airlines using Catania include **Air Berlin** (☎ 848-390-054, www.airberlin.com), **Air Malta** (☎ 095-345-311), **Air One** (www.flyairone.com), **Austrian Airlines** (www.aua.com), **British Airways** (www.britsihairways.com), **Helvetic** (www.helvetic.com), **Lufthansa** (☎ 199-400-044, www.lufthansa.it), **Luxair** (☎ 06-650-1880, www.luxair.lu), **My Air** (☎ 899-500-060, www.myair.com), **Transavia** (☎ 02-6968-2615, www.transavia.com), **Virgin Express** (☎ 848-390-109, www.virgin-express.com) and **Windjet** (☎ 095-340-227, 899-809-060, www.volawindjet.com).

A taxi from the airport to the city center should cost about €19 (**Radio Taxi**, ☎ 095-330-966). Alternatively, catch the **Alibus** leaving from outside the terminal every 20 minutes (5 am-midnight) for Piazza Stesicoro (Via Etnea) and Stazione Centrale. The journey takes 20 minutes and tickets (€2.30) can be purchased from the *tabacchi* on the first floor of the departures hall or from a kiosk near the bus stop if it's open.

By Train

Catania is connected by frequent trains to Messina and Syracuse (both 1½ hours) and less frequently to Palermo (three hrs 25 minutes), Enna (one hour 45 minutes) and Agrigento (four hours). See www.trenitalia.com for details on schedules. Here are some common route prices:

Catania-Caltanisetta €6.45
Catania-Giarre €2.25
Catania-Taormina €3.15
Catania-Milazzo €6.70
Catania-Palermo. €11.25
Catania-Siracusa €4.80
Catania-Agrigento €11.25

Catania

By Bus

See the *Getting There* section at the beginning of this guide for information about arrival in Sicily from the Italian mainland. The numerous bus companies serving Catania can depart from different places in the city, although most terminate in Piazza Giovanni XXIII across from the train station. Many also stop at Piazza Borsellino, which may save you a walk if you're going to a destination on Via Etnea. **SAIS** (Via d'Amico 181, ☎ 095-536-168 or 095-536-201) runs services to Messina (€6.20), Taormina, Noto, Syracuse, Palermo (€12.50, two hours 40 minutes), Agrigento (€11, 8 daily, three hours), Enna (€6.40) and Rome (€38.75, departs at 8 pm). **SAIS Autolinee** (☎ 095-536-168) runs 24 buses daily to Messina (1½ hours, €6.70) and 17 buses to Palermo (two hours 45 minutes, €13). **AST** (Via Luigi Sturzo 220, ☎ 095-531-756, 095-746-1096) runs the same services but also goes to smaller provincial towns around Catania including Nicolosi (via Belpasso, €1.95), Acireale (three daily, €1.95), Zafferana Etnea/Sant'Alfio (€3), Siracusa (€4.50), Caltagirone (€4.70), Palazzolo Acreide (€5.55), Pozzallo (€7.45), Modica (€6.95), Piazza Armerina (two to three daily, €6.95) and the cable car on Mt Etna. For more details on getting to the volcano see the Mt Etna section.

Buda (Via Lisi 23, Giarre, ☎ 095-931-905) has links from Catania to Giarre, Calatabiano and lots of Etnean towns. **Giuntabus** (Via Terranova 8, Messina ☎ 090-673-782) links Catania to Milazzo. Giamporcardo (Via Matteotti 150, Vittoria, ☎ 095-536-201) has services to Vittoria and Comiso.

Interbus Etna Trasporti (Via d'Amico 181, ☎ 095-532-716, 095-746-0111) has services to Piazza Armerina (one hour 45 minutes, €7), Aidone, Ragusa (two hours, €6.60) and Gela (€6.40). Other bus routes also stop at the airport, including those that go to Siracusa (70 minutes, €4.50), Taormina (one hour, €4.20), Ragusa, Agrigento, Enna (€6.50) and Palermo. Other services run direct to Messina (2½ hours) and Milazzo. See the timetables at the right side of the arrivals hall.

By Car

The A18 connects Catania to Messina; the A19 goes to Palermo. Signs for the center of Catania from either *autostrada* bring you into Via Etnea.

By Boat

 Catamarans from Malta dock on Molo Centrale off Via Dusmet. You can take bus 427 to the center and Stazione Centrale or walk the short distance to Piazza del Duomo. **Virtu Ferries** (☎ 095-535-711, www.virtuferries.com) run between Malta and Catania from March to October. Cars can be transported on some services. They run at least three days weekly with numerous trips on some days (three hours, €28 single passenger). **TTT Lines** (☎ 095-734-0211, www.tttlines.it) departs for Napoli Friday and Sunday at 7:30 pm (€25-38 on the deck, €35-55 for a chair). **Societa Adriatica** (☎ 095-281-816) departs for Ravenna three times a week at 8 pm.

■ Getting Around

By Car

 Catania is not a good place to drive unless you know it well. Traffic is congested, there are set times when you can drive down some streets and parking can be difficult unless you're good at worming into spaces two inches longer – or shorter – than the length of your car (this has to be seen to be believed!)

You can't drive down Via Etnea at any time of the day unless you want to attract the attention of ever-present traffic *vigili* (wardens). At night a lot of streets in the center are closed to traffic from 8-2 am. Roadblocks are set up to ensure this. If you do have a car, your task should be to ask your hotel where to leave it. Alternatively, there are numerous parking options around town. White lines mean free parking and blue lines require a payment (€.52/hr; 8:30 am-1 pm and 3:30-8 pm). At other times you may see parking wardens with whom you can negotiate a price for the time you are away. Some are custodians from a local restaurant, others are people in the street who give advice and you pay them. If you have to leave your car somewhere for a few minutes only, leave your lights flashing or a note inside with a telephone number to call. Usually your best alternative is to find the first good spot you come across and walk the rest of the way on foot. If you want to rent a car you should do it the day you leave the city. It is better to do it in the city than at the airport so as to avoid surcharges.

Hollywood Rent has two offices on Piazza Cavour 12 (☎ 095-442-720) and Via Luigi Sturzo 238 (☎ 095-530-594). They offer some good deals for car and bike rental, starting from €25 per day for a Fiat Panda. Other rental offices include:

Argus Rentals (Piazza Giovanni Verga, www.argusrentals. com, Mon-Fri 9:30 am-7:30 pm, Sat 8 am-1 pm).

Meridiana Auto e Moto Noleggi (Via Milano 94/a, ☎ 095-711-0176, www.meridiananoleggi.it). Scooters, cars and vans for hire.

Etnasicily Rent (☎ 095-434-688, www.etnasicilyrentacar. com). Fiat Puntos from €175/week.

Bellomo Rino Katane Rent (☎ 338-714-8680, katanerent@ hotmail.it).

Il Moto Noleggio (Viale Raffaello Sanzio 4, ☎ 095-552-610). Motor scooters from €15/day, two-seater cars from €50/day

By Bike

You can rent bikes from the following places. See *Adventures by Bike* later in this chapter for itinerary ideas.

Vassallo Agatino, Via Monserrato 52, ☎ 095-447-101.

Rent Bike (Acireale, ☎ 346-231-7451, www.rentbike.it). €13/ day for city and mountain bikes.

Acquaterra Adventure Shop (Via Antonino Longo 74, ☎ 095-503-020) has 20 bikes.

By Taxi

CST (☎ 095-330-966) operates a 24-hour taxi service. You can find taxi ranks at the following places:

■ Stazione Centrale, ☎ 095-532-269
■ Piazza Cavour, ☎ 095-439-580
■ Piazza Duomo, ☎ 095-715-0515
■ Via Fattorini 40, ☎ 095-386-794
■ Piazza Manganelli, ☎ 095-316-650
■ Piazza Santa Maria di Gesu, ☎ 095-316-630
■ Piazza Stesicoro, ☎ 095-316-670
■ Piazza Trento, ☎ 095-322-673
■ Piazza Verga, ☎ 095-447-970
■ Villa Bellini, Via Etnea, ☎ 095-316-770

By Train

 Stazione Centrale in Piazza Giovanni XXII (☎ 848-888-088 or ☎ 095-730-6255) is where all main-line trains pass. There are left-luggage facilities open daily from 7 am-10 pm.

Catania has a metro system that operates every 15-30 minutes between 7 am and 8:45 pm. The tickets cost €.80 for unlimited travel within a 90-minute period. You can purchase tickets at *tabacchi* shops. Remember to punch your tickets before boarding the train. The route runs from the train station south to Catania Porto and northwest to Catania Borgo (Via Piazza Galatea, Corso Italia and Via Vincenzo Giuffrida), where you can get the Circumetnea (Via Caronda, ☎ 095-541-250, www.circumetnea.it). This narrow-gauge train does a long circuit around Mt Etna (see *Adventures by Rail*).

By Bus

 Catania has a small center and you will probably make little use of the city buses unless you're heading out to the airport or to a campsite. The **AMT** city buses (☎ 800-018-696, 095-736-0111, www.amt.ct.it) stop outside Stazione Centrale. Useful routes include 1-4 and 4-7 from the station to Via Etnea via Piazza Duomo. The **Alibus** from the airport stops at Piazza Stesicoro and terminates at the train station. Line 410 is a dedicated tourist route starting from Piazza Giovanni XXIII and taking in major stops like the Duomo, University, Piazza Stesicoro, Teatro Greco, Castello Ursino, Porta Garibaldi and more. The round-trip ticket is the cost of a one-way fare (€.90) but is made by appointment only; call ☎ 095-736-0247. In summer service D runs from points in the city, including Piazza G Verga and Piazza Duomo to the sandy beaches or Sanzio Lidi Playa to the east and west. Circolare Ognina-Mercati takes you to Ognina Beach and campsites (see *Where to Stay*).

Bus tickets can be purchased from *tabacchi*, newsagents inside the Stazione Centrale or from the booth outside and are valid for any number of journeys within 90 minutes for €.90. Daily tickets, *Biglietto Turistico* or *Giornaliero Biglietto*, are €2 for one day's unlimited travel. Monthly tickets are also available. You must punch the ticket on the first ride.

Catania

■ Information Sources

Inside Stazione Centrale on platform 1 is a small **APT** tourist office (☎ 095-730-6255, www.apt. catania.it, Mon-Sat 8 am-8 pm, Sun 8 am-2 pm). Ask here for accommodation and free maps of the city. Their main office is at Via D. Cimarosa 10 (☎ 095-730-6211, 095-730-6233; 9 am-7 pm, Sun 8 am-2 pm). They offer free guided tours of the city every day with to literary, musical or architectural themes (9 am-11:30 am). See the *Adventures on Foot* section later in this chapter.

The *comune* also runs another information office on Via Vittorio Emanuele 172 (☎ 800-841-042 or 095-742-5573, www.comune.catania.it; Mon, Wed, Fri and Sat 8:15 am-1:30 pm, Tues and Thurs 8:15 am-7:30 pm). Alternatively, if you arrive at the airport, a handy information desk with maps, accommodation lists and bus timetables can help you (☎ 095-730-6266 or 095-730-6277, 8 am-9 pm).

Lapis and *Ciao Catania* are monthly bulletins issued by the tourist office listing special concerts, festivals, movies or nightclubs. These are available at hotels and bars throughout the city.

Useful Websites
- Catania official website – www.comune.catania.it
- Province of Catania official website – www.provincia.ct.it
- Tourism portal for Catania – www.turismo.catania.it
- All about Catania – www.catanialive.it
- Guida culturale della città – www.cormorano.net/catania/
- Catania civic network – www.catania.virtuale.net

Events

Etna Fest (www.etnafest.it) is a festival of music, dance and theater running through the summer and featuring national and international acts.

Catania Tango Festival (www.caminitotango.com) is held in mid August.

The **Festival of Sant'Agata**, February 3-5, has been taking place for the last 500 years, with parades, traditional music and candle-lit processions.

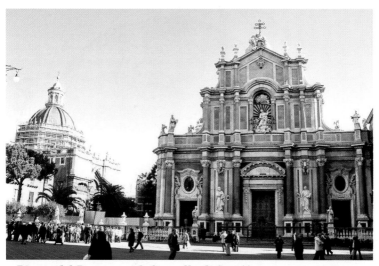

Piazza del Duomo, with Cappella di Sant'Agata (Galen R Frysinger)

■ Sightseeing

Catania is a walkable city with only a few major sights. The city's main thoroughfares, Via Etnea and Via Vittorio Emanuele II, both converge at ★★**Piazza del Duomo**. The piazza was rebuilt in the first half of the 18th century and is surrounded by elegant buildings, created largely by the architect Vaccarini. These structures include the 1735 **Fontana dell'Elefante** (Elephant Fountain) made from lava, the **town hall** in Palazzo degli Elefanti, the **Duomo** and the abbey church **Badia di Sant'Agata**. The Duomo (☎ 095-320-044, 7 am-12 pm and 4:30-7 pm) is Vaccarini's grandest Baroque project. It was originally founded by Count

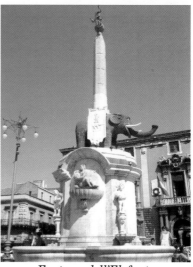

Fontana dell'Elefante

Catania

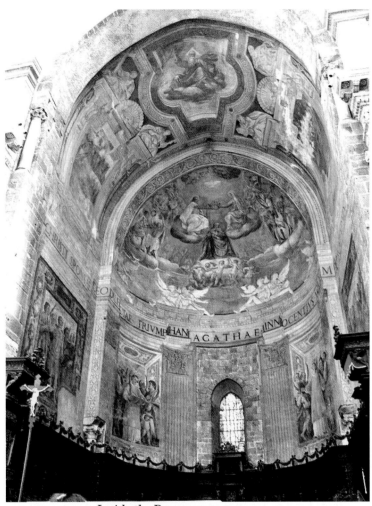

Inside the Duomo (Galen R Frysinger)

Roger in the 11th century, but only the medieval apses crafted from volcanic rock survived the 1693 earthquake. For a glimpse, peer through the gate at Via Vittorio Emanuele 159. The Duomo was built on the ruins of Roman baths and also survived a lava flow in 1169. So if it's a case of nine lives, the Duomo is fast using them up.

Much of the Duomo was under renovation until recently, but the work is now finished. The **Cappella di Sant'Agata** is to

the right and houses the relics of the saint, which are brought out on the saint's festival days. The Duomo is actually dedicated to Sant'Agata. There's also a fresco in the sacristy that depicts the 1669 eruption of Etna. You may also see the tomb of the composer Vincenzo Bellini on the right as you enter; it's the first of many glimpses you'll get of him around Catania. The APT has a walking tour of Bellini-important sights in Catania (see the *Adventures on Foot*).

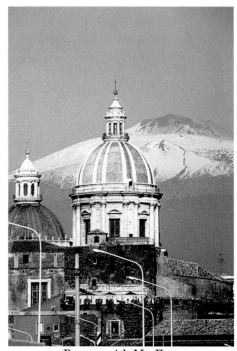

Duomo with Mt. Etna

Catania

FESTA DI SANT'AGATA

The Festa di Sant'Agata, from Febrary 3-5, brings the city to life during the throes of winter. A golden statue of Sant'Agata is paraded through the streets while fireworks explode in Piazza del Duomo and street stalls in Via Etnea sell traditional sweets. The procession of the *Cannaroli* (long candles up to 20 feet high) is the highlight. They are carried by groups representing different trades and a prize goes to those who hold out the longest.

The **Museo Diocesano** is next to the Duomo, by the Porta Uzeda (☎ 095-281-635, www.museodiocesano.it, Tues-Sat 9 am-12 pm, 4-7:30 pm, closed Mon). It contains a collection of religious art and silverware, 15th-century sculpture and a gallery of paintings, some dating from the 14th century. They are closed the first two weeks of August.

Sant'Agata Convent (Mon-Sat 8 am-5 pm), opposite the Duomo, is another Vaccarini creation, although the interior dates from after his death. The entrance is just off the main road on Via Raddusa. If you like his style you can find a Vaccarini façade on **Chiesa San Giuliano** in Via Crociferi. The APT office has a walking tour taking in the key Vaccarini sights (see *Adventures on Foot* later in this chapter).

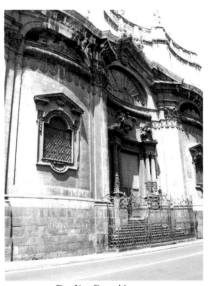

Badia Sant'Agata

Via Vittorio Emanuele II is the main road at the end of the Corso that runs beside the Piazza del Duomo. You could sidetrack down this road towards the train station for a moment to **Piazza San Placido** on your right and the 18th-century church of the same name. This is Catania's red light district. Look across the road to no. 140, the house of the 19th-century erotic poet Domenico Tempio; you'll see figures of men and women on the balcony playing with themselves.

Catania's open-air food market ★★★**La Pescheria**, is one of the island's best. Take the stairs down by the marble fountain in the southern part of Piazza del Duomo and you'll be

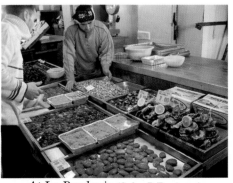

At La Pescheria (Galen R Frysinger)

suddenly thrown into a heaving tangle of slabs and buckets full of twisting crustaceans and other sea animals for sale. You may well discover something unusual and be offered a taste! It's at its best early in the day when locals come down to here the fast sales

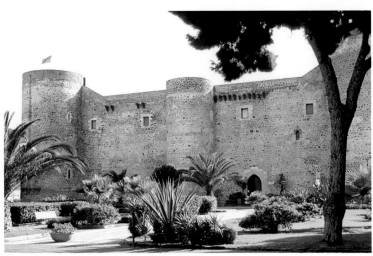

Castello Ursino

pitches of the fishermen. There are also lanes of vegetables and fruits and a few *trattorie* (see *Where to Eat*).

Via S. Calogero by the market leads to the 13th-century **Castello Ursino** in Piazza Federico di Svevia. It was once the proud fortress of Frederick II, but has been landlocked since the 1693 earthquake that shifted the land. Inside is the **Museo Civico** (☎ 095-345-830, Tues-Sun 9 am-1 pm and 3-7 pm, €4 if there is an exhibition). The museum is currently closed for renovations but the guards may let you see the first room if you ask nicely. Previously, the museum held mosaic fragments, stone inscriptions and tombstones. The region around the Castle is one of the poorer neighborhoods of Catania and you'd be well advised not to wander alone or at night.

Returning to the Piazza del Duomo and then turning down Via Vittorio Emanuele, away from the train station, you come across Catania's favorite son Vincenzo Bellini again. This time it's the **Museo Belliniano** (☎ 095-715-0535, 9 am-1:30 pm, Tues and Thurs also 3-6 pm; free), where the composer was born in 1801. The famed Sicilian composed his first work at age six. The pasta dish, *Spaghetti alla Norma*, is named after one of his operas. Opera fans will love this museum, which has been visited by Pavarotti and contains the original folios of his operas, his death mask, harpsichords, the piano he used as a child and even the coffin in which his body was transferred.

Catania

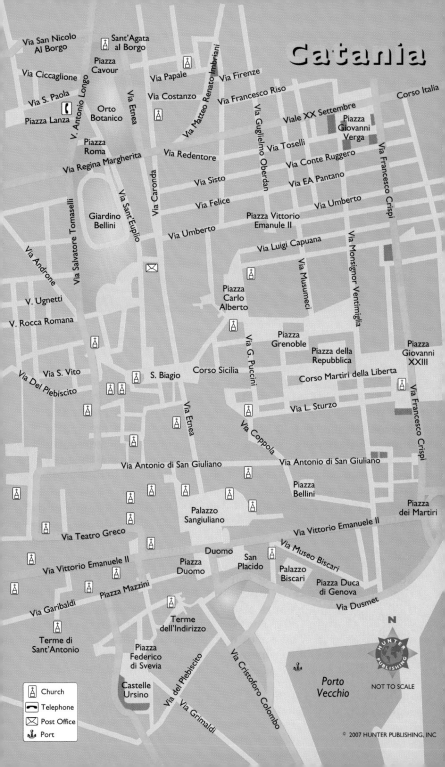

Farther along from the Museo is **Teatro Romano** (Via Vittorio Emanuele II, 226, Mon-Sat, 9 am-1 pm and 3-7 pm, Sun, 9 am-1 pm, €2.10), one of the few Roman relics in Catania that survived the 18th-century Etna eruption. It was built of lava in the second century AD on the site of an earlier Greek theater, Teatro Greco. The seating and underground passages largely remain, although the marble

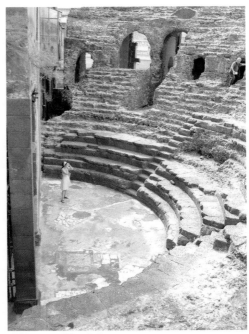

The Odeon (dumbfoundling)

casing is long gone. The **Odeon** adjacent to it was used for music and recitations. It was built between the second and third centuries AD.

At the back of the square containing the Teatro Romano is **Via Teatro Greco**. Heading farther west on it you will across **Piazza Dante**, a crescent of houses where workshops of cabinetmakers and metalworkers open to the pavement on the ground floor. Opposite the crescent is the biggest church in Sicily, **San Nicolò All'Arena** (Piazza Cavour, ☎ 095-438-077, Thurs 5-7:30 pm, Sun 11 am-1 pm; free) at 344 feet wide and 203 feet high. The façade is still unfinished and studded by six enormous columns. Inside, is rather bare and often described as spooky. It has an 18th-century organ, a meridian line to catch the sunlight at noon (although it now occurs at 12:13 pm due to land shifts).

Via Etnea is the main artery of Catania, running from the Piazza del Duomo straight up through town towards the foothills of Mt Etna. Along the road there are many churches, squares, palaces, gardens and other buildings. The **Univer-**

Catania

sity, founded by the Aragonese Kings in the 15th century, has a courtyard designed by Vaccarini. Farther up is the enormous **Piazza Stesicoro**, which contains the Anfiteatro Romano (9 am-1 pm and 3-7 pm, free). If it is open do go in and wander down through the cold lava walls. It dates from the second or third century AD. Much of it is now concealed by other buildings but its lava blocks could once seat 16,000 spectators.

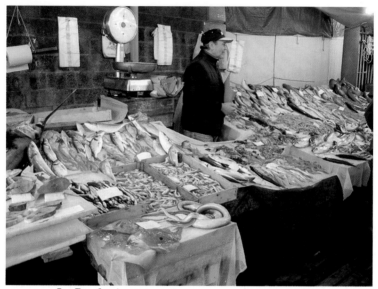

La Pescheria (Galen R Frysinger, www.galenfrysinger.com)

Markets

The two main food markets in Catania are **La Fiera** (also called 'A fera 'o Luni by locals) in Piazza Carlo Alberto and **La Pescheria** fish market in the streets near Porta Uzeda. Both markets are held every day until lunch time and are worth a browse even if you have no need of fish or food. The daily La Fiera market has a variety of fresh fruit stalls, cafés and snack bars. But on Sunday the square fills with antiques, electronics, puppets, old radios, lamps, batteries, books, plants, record players, statues, taps, plastics, coins and other useful and junky paraphernalia.

Parks

Catania has a few small parks. **Via Bellini** is the largest public garden, in the center of the city on Via Etnea. In the summer concerts take place in the bandstand. The looping ring road through the park is about a quarter-mile around and the only place to run if you want a jog in the city. At the northern end of the park is **Orto Botanico** (Mon-Sat, 9 am-1 pm).

Villa Pacini, at the southern end of Via Etnea, through the Piazza del Duomo near the bus station, is open until 8 pm at night. During the day it's full of children on swings and old men by the fountains but is a little seedy.

Beaches

The closest beach to the city is **Jonio**. However, don't picture white sands and clear water – there are rocks (*scogli*), jellyfish and huge crowds. Plus the water this close to the city is not so clean. But it is popular for nightlife. The other good seaside spot is **San Giovanni Li Cuti** where there are some *locale* popular with the Catanese (see *Where to Eat*). This little rocky port is a pleasant place to watch fishermen, enjoy the views and dine in the evening. AMT bus 443 from Stazione Centrale goes to Piazza Europa, from where it's a short walk.

Shopping

Via Etnea is the place to do your shopping in Catania. It's good for browsing or having a coffee in one of the bars. The liveliest section is between Piazza del Duomo and the Villa Bellini.

■ **Where to Eat**

There are plenty of gustatory experiences in Catania worth savoring and, because of the large student population, meals are very affordable. Catania's proximity to the sea means seafood plays an important role. Some Catanian specialties include *Spaghetti alla Norma* (see the recipe earlier in this chapter);

DINING PRICE CHART	
Price per person for an entrée, including house wine.	
€	Up to €12
€€	€13-€25
€€€	€26-€35
€€€€	Over €35

Catania

spaghetti cooked with tomato and aubergine/eggplant (*melanzane*); *crispelle* (fritters of flour, water, yeast and ricotta or anchovies); and soda water and crushed lemon with or without salt (*seltz e limone con/senza sale*). You will also find a lot of traditional sweets and snacks in market stalls during the Festa di Sant'Agata in February.

Cafés & Gelaterias

Via Etnea is lined with numerous eating places. Down the northern end near the gardens of Villa Bellini are two of Catania's oldest and most famous cafés. The ★**Spinella** (Via Etnea 300) has a covered outdoor seating area (costs extra) and delicious traditional sweets like cannelloni and cassata. If you are game, try an almond-flavored granita. Next door, the **Savia** (Via Etnea 302/304), open since 1897, is a stand-up café bar that's usually packed. And if you can get past the crowds, order a *granita*, *arancine* or any of the mouth-watering pastries and you'll soon see why. Farther up the street is Dolceria Mantegna, a family-run favorite favored by locals. There is excellent *pasta di mandorla* and *cassata*. Halfway down Via Etnea back towards the Duomo, **Scardaci** (Via Etnea 158) has one of the best gelati selections in Catania with almost 50 flavors to choose from. Still farther along is the popular **Al Caprice** (Via Etnea 30/32/34, ☎ 095-320-55) near Piazza Università with tables spilling into the streets for its snacks, sandwiches, *tavola calda* meals and gelati. **Caffé del Duomo** (Piazza del Duomo) has nuts, ice cream, pizza and traditional sweets; and arty lights and mirrors in the ceiling. You can eat in the bar or outside in the piazza. The **Cathedral Bar** (Via Garibaldi 1) has outdoor chairs near the Duomo square and is popular with some interesting older characters. **Pane e Dolcezze** (Via Galvagna 5, closed Sun), next to Trattoria Aldo, offers every kind of bread you might want. And, if you want a night-time dessert **Nirja Creperia** (Via Montesano 27, 9 am-11:30 am and 3-8 pm) has fantastic crêpes and other sweets. This area is popular for outdoor eating.

Pizzerias & Ethnic Food

Just off Via Etnea, with a terrace overlooking the church, is **La Collegiata** (Via della Collegiata 3, ☎ 095-321-230, €), open for lunch and dinner and a popular student hangout.

The settings are rustic, either upstairs on a balcony overlooking the street or downstairs near the open kitchen. There are a handful of good eateries tucked around the streets off Via Pancini, one of Catania's multi-ethnic areas. ★**Il Sale Art Café** (Via S. Filomena 10/12, ☎ 095-316-888, ilsale@globalcom.it, closed Tues, €i) has little tables in the street where you dine by candlelight. Pizza, good wine, funky music and an art gallery make this a top affordable choice. The nearby **Vico Santa Filomena restaurant** (Via S. Filomenia 35, ☎ 095-316-761, closed Mon, €€) also serves pizza or you can get it by the slice at the small take-out **Pizza Cotto** in the same street on the corner with Via Pacini. **Ristorante Net** (Via S. Filomenia 55) down the other end of the street is a restaurant with fixed and wireless Internet connections. The menu has spicy food such as Mexican paella, Texas ribs or buffalo chicken wings. Or you can sip a cocktail from the bar if you just want a drink while you surf. There is a big Chinese population in this area and a number of Asian diners. One that is easy to find is **La Grande Muraglia** (Via Pacini 83, ☎ 095-312-535, dinner only) on the left side just before the square. **Pizzeria del Centro** (Via Montesano 11, ☎ 095-311-429, closed Mon, €) serves dinner at 6-12 pm nightly and lunch in summer. Pizzas range from only €2.50-4.50, with all the usual varieties like *calzone*, *capriciosa*, *quattro stagione* and *quattro formagio*, but also some local specialties such as *Vesuvio*, *Ragusana* and *Etna*.

Restaurants by the Pescheria

The restaurants around La Pescheria offer a lot of good deals on incredibly fresh seafood produce that has probably been flipping around in a bucket moments before arriving on your plate. If you come here at lunch time you can enjoy the chaos of the market but at night the streets come alive with activity as restaurants spill tables out into the streets. **Ristorante Ambasicata del Mare** (Piazza Duomo 6, ☎ 095-341-003, 12:45-3 pm, 8-12 pm, closed Mon, www.ambasciatadelmare.com, €€) is right on the edge of the square near the fountain – you can hear it splashing – above the market. On nearby Via Pardo there are a couple of good options. Trattoria La Paglia (Via Pardo 23, ☎ 095-3460838, Mon-Sat 12:30-2:30 pm and 8-11 pm, €€) is a rustic, cheap trattoria. Try the specialty, *tonno con cipollata* (broiled tuna with onions and vinegar). **Osteria**

Antica Marina (Via Pardo 29, ☎ 095-348-197, Thurs-Tues 1-3 pm and 8-12:30 am, €€-€€€) offers a view of the market from behind plate-glass, but it still conveys a sense of the teeming activity outside! At **Antiquus Locus** (Via Bottino 13, ☎ 340-978-6869) Christian and Carla serve seafood on wood chairs in the street. The other good option in this area is the restaurant at the **Agora hostel** (Piazza Curro 6, ☎ 095-723-3010, €-€€), where main meals start at just €6. There is often excellent live music and young local Catanese provide a good atmosphere.

Trattorias

Sicilia in Bocca (Piazza Pietro Lupo 16-18, ☎ 095-746-1361, closed Wed, €€) is close to the Teatro Massimo Bellini off Via Ventimiglia. It's a good place for seafood and quite lively. They serve dinner only through the week but also do lunch on Sunday. **Trattoria de Fiore** (Via Coppola 24, closed Mon, ☎ 095-316-283, €€) offers good basic cooking. **La Siciliana** (Viale Marco Polo 52a, ☎ 095-376-400, www.lasiciliana.it, Tues-Sun 12:30-3 pm, Tues-Sat 8-11 pm, €€€-€€€€) is renowned for its pasta dishes and desserts. It is located in north Catania in a 19th-century villa. **I Crociferi Ristorante** (Piazza S. Francesco d'Assisi 14, ☎ 095-715-2480, 340-109-9226, fax 095-310-623, closed Tues, lunch and dinner, €€€) is on the corner opposite the magnificent Santuario San Francesco d'Assisi. The tourist menu is €27 with all plates. **Trattoria Da Aldo** (Piazza G. Sciuti, ☎ 095-311-158, closed Sun, €) is well-known for its lunch-time grills and *casalinga* meals. **Osteria I Tre Bicchieri** (Via San Giuseppe al Duomo 31, ☎ 095-715-3540, www.osteriaitrebicchieri.it, closed Mon and Sun lunch, €€€-€€€€) is another of the high-quality restaurant group, Le Soste di Ulisse. It's also considered one of the finest dining spots in Catania, with a quiet location near the Duomo. You can eat in the rustic room near the front entrance called the *cantina* (wine tavern) or in the vaulted high ceiling rooms at the back of the *cantina*. Try the *tagliatelle* with suckling pig, *triglia* (saltwater fish) with onion-stuffed artichokes or *gnocchi* with Ragusan cheese. The wine list has 1,000 Italian vintages, mostly from Sicily.

Dining at San Giovanni Li Cuti

San Giovanni Li Cuti (see *Beaches* previously in this chapter) at Lido Jonio is a good spot for pizza or seafood by the beach. Most dining here is mid-range from €20-30. The name *Li Cuti* translates to something like rocks smoothed by water. There are three well known dining places here. **Andrew's Faro** (Via S. Giovanni Li Cuti 55, ☎ 095-382-642, lunch and dinner) serves pizza and seafood with a view of the sea. **Porto San Giovanni Ristorante Pizzeria** (Via S. Giovanni Li Cuti 36, ☎ 095-376-377, 095-722-5623, www.siciliaholiday.it, closed Tues) has fantastic wood-fire pizza. **Pizzeria Cutilisci** (Jonio 69, ☎ 095-372-558, www.cutilisci.it, closed Mon, €€-€€€) has an international and local menu. For snacks, there is the **Gelateria Alicuti** on the same street or ★**Ernesto** (Viale Ruggero di Lauria 91, Lungomare Ognina, ☎ 095-491-680, fax 095-712-7484, gelateriaernesto@infinito.it), a block back on the main road. Ernesto was the first owner of the shop back in 1974 and established a tradition of *gelati* (ice cream) and *dolce* (sweets), with traditional decorations like Sicilian *carrozze* (carts) and *pupi* (puppets). Not surprisingly, this place is listed in *Gambero Rosso*, the guide to good Italian eating. You won't find *gelati* like this elsewhere in Catania with real bits of nuts and biscuit added to the tantalising selection of flavors.

Bars

Catania has a large student population, which means the bars are fairly lively and open until late, especially in the summer months. The *comune* arranges ★★*cafe concerto* periods in summer in the streets and squares of the old town between Piazza dell'Universita and Piazza Bellini from 9 pm to 2 am, when the streets are closed to traffic. The bars in the area put out tables and chairs in the street and some have large screens to watch the latest soccer matches or live bands. Most of the music does not start until 10 pm. Popular spots include **La Cartiera Pub** (Via Casa del Mutilato 8), a student bar on the northeastern side of Piazza Bellini, and **Il Picasso** (Piazza Ogninella 4) and **L'Altro Picasso** (Piazza Scammacca 1b), which face each other in the old town. Anywhere along Piazza Scammacca you will find large TV screens, live bands and almost anything to eat from steak to

Catania

pizza. Two popular spots include **The City Jazz Bar** (Piazza Scammacca 1/b, ☎ 347-734-7157, closed Mon and Tues) and the **Taarna Irish Pub** (Piazza Scammacca 4, ☎349-195-0228, www.vivicatania.net). **Waxy O'Connors Irish Pub** (Piazza Spirito Santo 39) and the **Joyce Irish Pub** opposite are two other good locations in another part of the city. Alternatively, down near *La Pescheria*, you could try the **Hardrock Café** (Via C. Colombo 10, ☎ 095-723-4856158, store open 10 am-1 pm, restaurant 12-12:30 am, www. hardrock.com/Catania).

■ Where to Stay

 It is advisable to book as much in advance as possible if you want to stay in Catania during the summer. Try to stay close to the main sights but be aware that petty crime is prevalent in some parts of

HOTEL PRICE CHART	
€	Up to €25 per day
€€	€26-€55
€€€	€56-€85
€€€€	Over €85

the center so take care at night. Be wary also of leaving valuables in your room.

Camping

All the campsites are located just out of the city and many offer bungalows in the summer. There are three campsites on Viale Kennedy, on the long beach south of Catania. From the airport take the Alibus and then bus D (red or black). Or take either bus 427 from Stazione Centrale or Porta Uzeda, or 538 from Piazza Borsellino. If you have a car, follow the signs to Lidi Playa.

Internazionale La Plaja (Viale Kennedy 47, ☎ 095-340-880, €) is popular near the beach with a disco and horseback riding. **Villagio Souvenir** (Viale Kennedy 71, ☎ 095-341-162 or 095-355-440, open May-Sept, €) is the cheapest and smallest of the campsites. **Villagio Turistico Europeo** (Viale Kennedy 91, ☎ 095-591-026, www.villaggioeuropeo.it, May-Sept, €) has more facilities and is slightly pricier.

Camping Jonio (Via Villini a Mare 2, Ognina, ☎ 095-491-139, €) is five km north of the city and open all year. There are tent sites and bungalows. To get here, take bus 24 from the

airport, then change in Piazza Duomo for bus 34. By car it's on the SS114.

Hostels

The only hostel in town is the easy-going **Agora** (Piazza Curro 6, ☎ 095-723-3010, http://agorahostel.hypermart.net, i), an alternative, modern-retro establishment by the morning *Pescheria* market. Dorm beds are €18-20, doubles are €45 per room. All prices include breakfast. The bar downstairs goes until all hours but offers fantastic meal deals. Other facilities include kitchen, Internet and washing. Meals start at just €6.

Hotels

Roma (Via della Liberta 63, ☎ 095-534-911, €€) is a good option if you are arriving late from Stazione Centrale. The rooms are small but adequate and the price is budget. **Hotel Centrale Europa** (Via Vittorio Emanuele 167, Piazza Duomo, ☎ 095-311-309, fax 095-317-531, www.hotelcentraleuropa.it, €€€) is right on Piazza del Duomo. The rooms contain old photographs and paintings of Catania and the area as well as en-suite bathrooms. Singles/doubles are €50/€85 including breakfast.

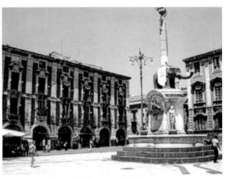
Hotel Centrale Europa

Catania

The **Politi Residence** (Via Politi 12, ☎ 095-715-0957, www.politiresidence.com, €€) offers fully furnished private apartments, singles, private and even dorm rooms close to Piazza Duomo. Children stay for free with their parents.

Royal (Via Antonio di San Giuliano 337, ☎ 095-313-448, fax 095-325-611, €€) has a good location west of Via Etnea with quiet and comfortable rooms.

Hotel Gresi (Via Pacini 28, ☎ 095-322-709, www.gresihotel.com, €€-€€€) is centrally located just off Via Etnea near the Villa Bellini. There are 24 rooms in this 18th-century building

with simple furniture and a small bathroom, but the frescoed ceilings make it stand out.

Hotel del Duomo (Via Etnea 28, ☎ 095-250-3177, €€€) has comfortable rooms with a view over the square and Duomo. There are often business, family and other specials on offer.

Hotel Mediterraneo (Via Dottor Consoli 27, ☎ 095-325-330, €€€€), near the tourist office, has uncomplicated rooms typical of all Best Western hotels, of which this is one.

Hotel Nettuno (Viale Ruggero di Lauria 121, ☎ 095-712-2006, www.hotel-nettuno.it, €€€€) is a large-scale hotel by the sea-front but within easy access of the city center.

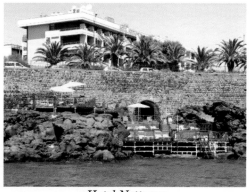

Central Palace (Via Etnea 218, ☎ 095-325-344, fax 095-531-007, €€€€) is Catania's top hotel. It is right on the main street

Hotel Nettuno

with eating, drinking and shopping close by. July and August are more heavily priced.

Katane Palace (Via Finocchiaro Aprile 110, ☎ 095-747-0702,

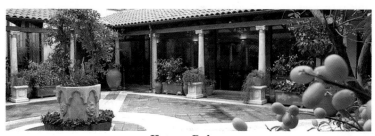

Katane Palace

www.katanepalace.it, €€€€) is centrally located with a pickup service from the airport, a restaurant and meeting center.

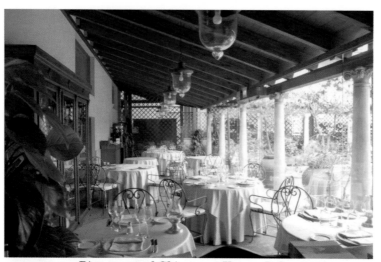

Ristorante sul Chiostro at Katane Palace

B&Bs

Yancu e u'sali (Via S. Filomena 25, ☎ 340-625-9589, www. yancueusali.it) is a bed and breakfast just off Via Etnea near Villa Bellini. This is one of the quaintest areas of Catania right near *La Fiera* market.

B&B Stesicoro (Via Neve 7, ☎ 095-311-178, www. bbstesicoro.it, €€€) is on the second floor, with views of the Roman amphitheater.

B&B Bellini (Via Auteri 26, ☎ 095-340-545, www. bandbbellini.com, €€) is at the end of Via Crociferi, Catania's famous Baroque street. It's comfortable and homey. Breakfast features local organic produce.

■ Adventures

On Foot

Catania is an easy city to explore on foot. A good city itinerary could start at the **Piazza del Duomo** and cross to the noisy open-air food market down the marble steps. Narrow streets from here lead through to **Piazza Federico di Svevia**, where Castello Ursino once stood. Visit the **Museo Civico**. Follow **Via Uteri** north through **Piazza Mazzini** and an interesting tangle of churches, streets and

archaeological remains from **Via Garibaldi** up to **Via Vittorio Emanuele II**. Turn into **Via Crociferi** with its interesting religious and secular buildings. Back on Via Vittorio Emanuele II there is the **Teatro Romano** to the west and the **Odeon** theater. **Via Teatro Greco** to the west leads to **Piazza Dante**, a crescent of houses with workshops on the ground floor. Opposite is **San Nicoló**, the biggest church in Sicily (see *Sightseeing* previously in this chapter for more details).

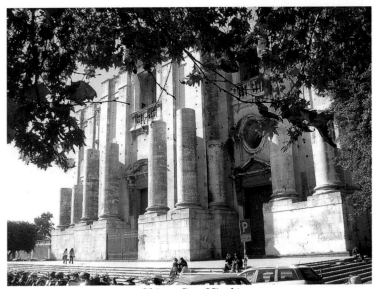

Chiesa San Nicoló

Another walking itinerary could be along the busy **Via Etnea**, which runs north from Piazza del Duomo and out of the city. You could follow it all the way to the foothills of Mount Etna. There are plenty of notable buildings, churches and gardens, particularly on the west side of the street.

Another option is to start at **La Fiera market** at the end of Via Pacini. From the **Santuario di Carmino** walk past the **Cripta S. Gaetano** on Via G. Puccini, the first Catanese church, built in 261 AD, the Roman period of Catania. If you come in the morning you'll be hard-pressed to spot the crypt in the thronging streets closed to traffic. There is a large Chinese community here. Exit on **Piazza Stesicoro** where a

statue is dedicated to the composer Vincenzo Bellini. The steps up to Bellini have carved musical notes, if you can see them under the pigeon poop. Cross Via Etnea to the **Anfiteatro**,

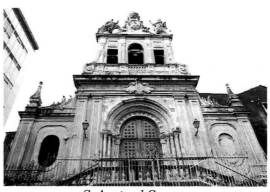

S. Agata al Carcere

past the wedding shops to 18th-century **Chiesa di San Biagio**, also known as the **Chiesa di Sant'Agata alla Fornace**, where Catania's patron Saint Agata was martyred – killed in the furnace. The **Church of S. Agata al Carcere**, rising behind the square, is supposed to have been built on the site of the jail where she was imprisoned in 251.

Turn left into Via Manzoni where there are carnevale costume shops, take the first right into **Via Penneinetto** and up the slope into **Via Crociferi**. On Saturdays in summer there are numerous weddings in this street and it can feel like continual replay of confetti and rice throwing as you stroll down towards **Santuario San Francesco d'Assisi**. Most of the time

Catania

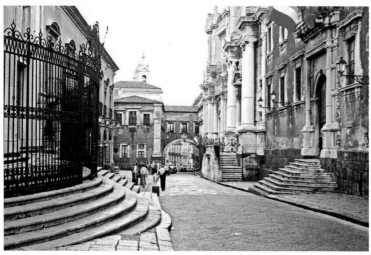

Via Crociferi

the churches seem closed, except during mass. However, Santuario San Francesco d'Assisi opens 8 am-12 pm and 5:30-8 pm. Via Crociferi is regarded as Catania's Baroque street *par excellence*. As the name *crociferi* (crucifixes) suggests, many of the magnificent buildings are churches or religious complexes. There are great wrought iron gates, crosses and other religious markings.

■ *APT Walking Itineraries*

The APT tourist office runs daily walking tours through Catania from 9-11:30 am celebrating the 'city of arts.' Simply turn up at Via D. Cimarosa to join the free group. If you have more than 25 people you should reserve at least one week in advance. You will have to pay entrance fees for some monuments and venues. The weekly schedule at the time of writing was:

Monday: *In praise of Bellini* (9 am-11:30 am) visits the places synonymous with the famous composer's life, including Piazza Vincenzo Bellini and Casa Museo V. Bellini.

Tuesday: *Giovan Battista Vaccarini and the architects of rebirth*, taking in the buildings Vaccarini worked on and other architects of the Baroque period in Catania.

Wednesday: *From Antiquity to Byzantium*, which includes a visit to the Anfiteatro Romano, various churches, piazzas and Gothic arches.

Thursday: *Literature and Cinema* features Catanian locations in film and literature.

Friday: *Monte Vergine Acropolis* visits the church of Sant'Agata, the city's patron saint, and the Monastero dei Benedittini.

Saturday: *From the Origins to the Baroque* shows you the city's Roman origins through to Baroque times. Highlights include Teatro Greco, Via Crocifieri and Castello Ursino.

Sunday: *In Search of the Divine: Through the City, Lava and Faith Tours* many of Catania's great churches.

It is possible to book a guided tour on Tuesday and Thursday for the morning tour *Between Nature and Culture* and Fridays *Illuminating the Baroque*, which is a night-time itinerary from 9-11 pm.

By Bike

 Acquaterra Mountainbike (Piazza Cavour 14, Catania, ☎ 095-438-954, http://web.tiscali.it/ acquaterrabike) meets every Thursday evening from

October to June at their office. They do mountain-bike trips
every three weeks for eight months of the year. There are
more regular summer programs and tours of national parks
in Sicily. They also have night tours of Catania's monuments.
There is a membership fee to join any trips.

Montainbike Sicilia (☎ 095-434-859, Via Napoli 45,
Catania, www.montainbikesicilia.it/) promotes both city, off
road and children's riding through a number of excursions
and activities. There seems to be a link between the two organizations but we weren't able to ascertain exactly what!

Acquaterra (Via Antonino Longo 74, ☎ 095-503-020, www.
acquaterra.it) is based in Catania but does cycling just about
everywhere in Sicily; the nearest place to Catania is the
Simeto Nature Reserve (see *Around Catania: South*). You can
rent mountain bikes from them for €8/half-day, €13/day or
€21/two days.

By Horse Cart

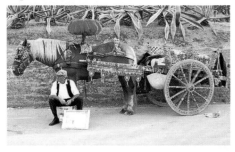

A traditional horse-
drawn Sicilian cart
makes its rounds of
the city in the summer
months driven by an
old man and his
grandson. It costs
about €50 to take a
turn along Via Etnea.
There is no number to
call; you just wave the man down in the street.

With Language

Catania's University gives Italian languages courses
for foreigners (Facoltà di Lingue e Letterature
Straniere, Monastero dei Benedettini, Piazza Dante
32, ☎ 095-710-2708, www.old.unict.it/slci/) in the atmospheric
Benedettini Monastery. Summer and winter courses are
offered over week-long or two-week periods. 40 hours of lessons cost €350 or personalized one-hour lessons for three students are €25.

■ Around Catania: North

The coast north of Catania towards Acireale is rocky and dominated by solidified lava, with little fishing villages and tour-

ist resorts. These towns can be easily reached by local buses, making it a pleasant day-trip for swimming, snorkeling and sunning.

Aci Castello

Aci Castello is the first of these towns, a popular vacation resort dominated by a turreted castle. The Norman fortress was erected in 1076 on an impregnable outcrop of rock by the sea and now houses the local civic museum. **Museo Civico Castello Normanno** (Piazza Castello Normanno, ☎ 095-737-3414, open 9 am-1 pm and 4-8 pm summer, 9 am-1:30 pm and 3-6:30 pm in winter, €1.50). Inside is a botanical garden, Byzantine chapel and the archaeological museum, with a large section devoted to minerals.

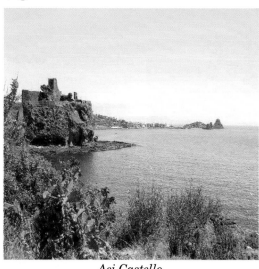
Aci Castello

There is a pleasant church in the square, beneath which weddings are held on summer weekends. Bars and gelati shops compete for space around the square, while boats, fishermen and snorkelers ply the waves around the castle. In summer, wooden platforms are erected on the sharp lava rocks for sunbathing. You could walk along the boardwalk from Ognina all the way to Aci Trezza. To get to Aci Castello take AMT bus No 334 from Piazza Borsellino.

A good place to eat is **Ai Muretti** (Via Fornace 47, Lungomare, ☎ 095-711-1064, €€€) just off the boardwalk. In summer they have tables closer to the water's edge, but they move inside after September.

Aci Trezza

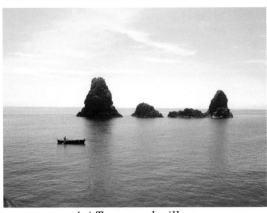

Aci Trezza rock pillars

You can see Aci Trezza from Aci Castello, the scene of the novel *I Malavoglia* by Giovanni Verga and the film *La Terra Trema* by Luchino Visconti. But its biggest attractions are the ★**Ciclopi Islands** (Lachea, Faraglione large and Faraglione small), which give the town its name – Aci Tezza means three needles. These tall

pillars of rock jutting out of the sea are part of a nature reserve of great geological interest. Snorkeling and scuba diving are popular here, with the sea home to many species of fish, seaweed, sponges and corals. There are a number of good trattorias on *lungomare*. They offer well-priced menus featuring *frutta di mare* (seafood). The **Pellegrino** (Via Marina 2/6, ☎ 095-276-680) is always open and is a good spot for an evening drink.

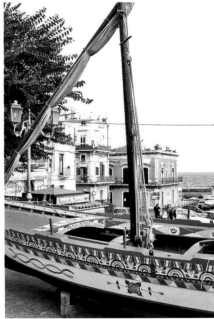

Aci Trezza harbor (Galen R. Frysinger, *www.galenfrysinger.com*)

THE ODYSSEY COMES TO ACI TREZZA

Aci Trezza is the place where the Cyclops Polphemus in the Odyssey threw huge boulders after he was blinded by Ulysses. Just up the coast is Ulysses Harbor, where legend has it that he landed his boat.

The major sightseeing attraction on dry land is the **Museo Casa del Nespolo** (Via A.S. de Maria 15, ☎ 095-711-6638, www.museocasadelnespolo.it, open 9 am-1 pm, 5-9 pm summer, 9:30 am-12:30 pm and 4-6 pm in winter, € 1.55), celebrating the life of the poet Gianni Verga who wrote the book *I Malavoglia* set in Aci Trezza.

Adventures on Water

 You can tour the Ciclopi islands by boats that leave from the Marina. Go down to the small booth in the port, which should be manned. If it's not – a good possibility – contact **Ministero dell'Ambiente e della Tutela del Territorio** (Via Provinciale 226, ☎ 095-711-7322, www.isoleciclopi.it) or ask a local fisherman to take you out. Another tour (☎ 095-711-6970) costs just €7 to Isola Lachea, I Faraglioni, Castello di Aci, Le Grotte di Ulisse, with departures at 10 am, 5, 8:15, 9:45 or midnight. The other tour is for Isola Lachea, La Baia di Capomulni, La Timpa di Acireale and Le Foci del Fiume di Aci, departing at 11:30 am and 6:30 pm.

If you'd like to do a bit of a paddle on your own you can rent kayaks and surf skis from **Chiosco ai Murretti** down by the water in front of Baia Blue in Aci Trezza. Kayaks (€6/hr), canoes (€8/hr) and pedal boats (€10/hr) are available from June-September. If you would rather go with a group, **Aquaterra Aquaterra** (Via Antonino Longo 74, ☎ 095-503-020, www.acquaterra.it) has excursions tp Acicastello and the marine reserve of Acitrezza (€40/day).

Centro Immersioni Acitrezza (Via Gondar 28, Acitrezza, www.isoledeiciclopidiver.com, ☎ 095-276-156, 9 am-8 pm) has PADI-accredited dives between 9 am and 12:30 pm daily. It costs €30 to rent a boat and equipment or €15 for equipment only. They access nine dive sites off the coast, including the Ciclopi Islands. Other dives visit the area under the lighthouse of Capo Molino and eight underwater archaeological sites.

Fishing

You can rent fishing equipment from **Euro Fishing** (Via Marina 213, ☎ 095-276-577, open 9 am-1 pm, 4-8 pm), who can also help you find the best local spots. Many people fish by the rocks at Aci Castello. **Tutto per la Pesca** (Corner Via Fontana Vecchia and Lungomare, ☎ 095-277-368) doesn't rent but you can buy any equipment you need and they'll also steer you in the right direction.

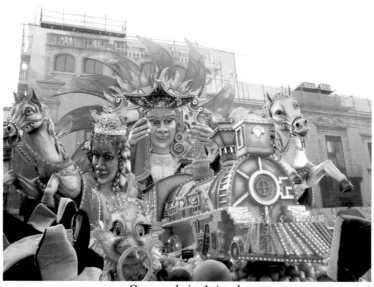

Carnevale in Acireale

Acireale

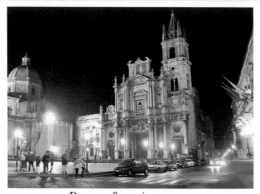

Duomo & main square

This elegant town is sited above the rocky shore, which you can view from a splendid piazza in the public gardens at the northern end of town. The town is well worth a day-trip from Catania for its magnificent Ba-

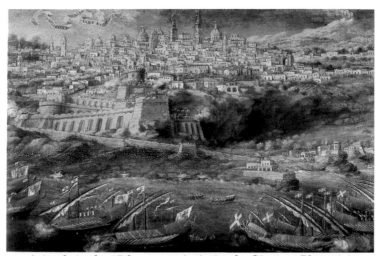

Acireale in the 17th century (painting by Giacinto Platania)

roque architecture and is especially colorful during the **Carnevale** celebrations (see *Holidays* in Introduction). Four towns have been built on this site, the latest established after the 1693 earthquake. The finest of the buildings is without doubt the extravagant **Duomo** (8 am-12 pm, 4-8 pm) in the handsome main square. There are in fact two churches in the square. You should also try to take in the long **Municipio** nearby on Via Romeo, the church of **San Sebastiano in Piazza Vico** and the grand **Palazzo Musmeci** in Piazza San Domenico. The other major attraction is the Roman spa, **Terme di Santa Venera** (Via delle Terme 47, ☎ 095-768-6111, www.terme.acireale.gte.it). Prices start at €13 for a sulphur bath or €20 for a mud and bath treatment.

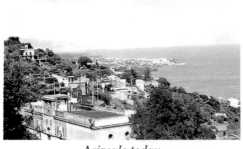

Acireale today

Traditional Sicilian **puppet theater** is a fixture in Acireale and there are a few places you can catch a show: **Cooperativa E. Magri** (Corso Umberto 11, ☎ 095-606-272); **Opera dei Pupi Turi Grasso** (Via Nazionale per

Catania 195, Capomulini, ☎ 095-764-8035). Thursday and Sunday nights at 9 pm (July 10-September 11). **Auditorium S. Giovanni** (Via Romeo, ☎ 339-410-3951).

You could also ask the **Azienda Soggiorno e Turismo** (Via Oreste Scionti 15, ☎ 095-892-129) for details. They offer daily excursions and guided tours of the city departing at 6 pm.

The only other point of interest in Acireale might be the art and historical collections in the **Biblioteca e Pinacoteca Zelantea** (library and picture gallery, Via M. di Sangiuliano 15-17, ☎ 095-763-4516, 9 am-1 pm and Mon-Wed 3:30-6:30 pm, closed Sun, free). You could also walk down to the communal gardens for a view over the sea.

To get to Acireale take one of the regular Interbus services from Catania to Messina. They depart every 30 minutes and arrive in Acireale's Piazza Duomo. Tickets are available from Piazza Al Duomo. The trains arrive well south of the town near the sulphur baths, making it a long walk to the center.

For something to eat, try **Gran Café el Dorado** (Corso Umberto 3-5, ☎ 0956-01464, www.el-dorado.it) near the Duomo for traditional sweets. **Pizzeria Bella** (Corso Umberto 16) has snacks and pizza.

Santa Maria La Scala, **Santa Tecla**, **Stazzo** and **Pozzillo** are all small hamlets by the sea near Acireale. The 16th-century **Sant'Anna lighthouse** tower built from lava blocks marks the promonotory of Capomulini, a good bathing spot on the road back to Aci Trezza. A cliff face by the water of over 460 feet runs for seven km past Santa Maria la Scala to Santa Tecia.

There are two campgrounds in this area. **La Timpa International Camping** (Via S. Maria la Scala 25, Acireale, ☎ 095-764-8155, www.campinglatimpa.it, €) and **Camping Al Yag** (Strada Provinciale Acireale-Riposto, ☎ 095-764-1763, www.campingalyag.it, €). The restaurant **Al Molino** (Via Molino 106 at Santa Maria La Scala, ☎ 095-764-8116, €€) has simply delicious seafood dishes at affordable prices.

Catania

■ Around Catania: South

The **Oasis of Simeto** lies just to the south of Catania. The best way to access the area is probably to tour it with **Aquaterra** (Via Antonino Longo 74, ☎ 095-503-020, www.acquaterra.it) by:

■ raft (January-March, three hours, €40). They provide the technical equipment, you bring your nerves!

■ 4x4 (year round, €70-80).

■ kayaking/canoeing (November-April, three hours, €40).

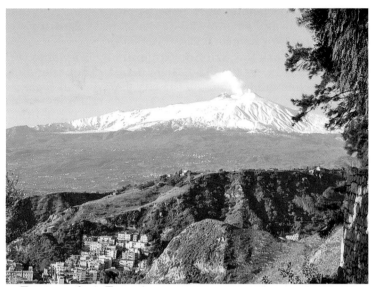

Etna seen from Taormina (Galen R Frysinger, www.galenfrysinger.com)

★★★ Mount Etna

The smoking giant of Mount Etna dominates most of the view of the eastern coast of Sicily, visible from as far south as Augusta, as far north as Taormina and from hilltop towns inland. Like a discontented old man, it huffs and puffs smoke into the air and glowers angrily at night from active lava flows. In 1987 Mount Etna and its surrounding slopes were protected by the establishment of the Parco dell' Etna, an area of 14,600 acres that contains Etna's central craters and lava deserts.

Mount Etna is one of the world's largest volcanoes at 10,900 feet high. The fact it is an active volcano is fascinating. But the danger of skiing, climbing, driving or touring on Mt Etna is considerable, so don't take a visit here lightly. Appropriately, the name "Etna" comes from the Greek word *aitne*, which means "I burn." Its local name is Mongibello, a combination of the Arab *gebel* and the Latin *mons* which both mean mountain. In ancient Roman and Greek mythology Mount Etna was the home of Vulcan, the god of fire, and the one-eyed monster Cyclops. It was thought that eruptions on Mount Etna were caused by his fiery breath.

RECORDED ERUPTIONS ON MT ETNA

There have been 135 eruptions recorded on Etna since 475 BC and some have been quite spectacular. In 1169, 1329 and 1381 the lava reached the sea, and in 1699 Catania was completely wiped out. More recently, in the 20th century, the Circumetnea railway was continually ruptured by lava flows, the towns of the foothills threatened and roads and farms destroyed. There have been 78 confirmed human fatalities from lava flow. Nine of these were from 1979 when tourists on the edge of the main crater were killed by an explosion. In 2001 the explosions caused no fatalities but the upper cable-car station was destroyed and the buildings around the Rifugio Sapienza were almost engulfed by lava. The eruptions in July and August of 2001 spewed forth from six vents on the mountain and far eclipsed those of the preceding decade in 1992, 1997 and 1998.

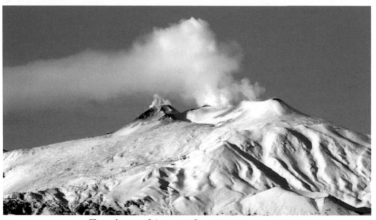

Etna's smoking peak (Galen R Frysinger)

Catania

Fiery breath or not, you can explore the fantastic **Parco dell'Etna** (Via del Convento 45, ☎ 095-821-111, www. parcoetna.ct.it) by cable train, mountain bike, bus or on foot. There is good skiing in winter and excellent hiking trails during the spring, summer and autumn months. If you are hiking, you will need a reasonable level of physical fitness but there are also walks for the less able. Unpredictable and ongoing eruptions on the volcano have undermined any perma-

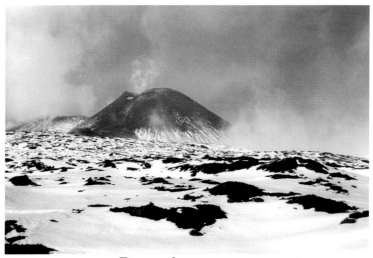

Etna up close (Joanne Lane)

nent infrastructure for tourists in the form of roads, ski-runs, ropeways and refuges. So all itineraries should be considered temporary and subject to closure or change at short notice. Remember that temperatures can plummet on the mountain top. Bring a thick sweater, wind- and rain-proof jackets and appropriate footwear. Jackets and boots can be rented locally. It can also be very hot, with sunlight reflecting off the snow, so bring sun glasses and sun screen.

WANT TO RUN OVER SICILY'S VOLCANOES?

This run covers over 110 km of rough ground on the Sicilian volcanoes of Mt Etna and those of the Aeolian islands. It's hard-core stuff so you'll want to be fit and brush up on Italian words like fire (*fuoco*), volcano (*vulcano*), lava (*lava*), tired (*stanco/a*) and difficult (*difficile*)! The week-long trail program starts by running 12 km up the central crater of Vulcano and Vulcanello, 24 km up the two volcanoes of Salina island, a 14-km leg on Stromboli to see the active volcano, and three on Etna of 18 km, 22 km and 18 km. There is also an equally challenging hiking program. If you think you're up to it, contact the Catania-based travel agency **Mandala Tour** (Viale Andrea Doria 69, ☎ 095-508-959, ☎/fax 095-504-029, www.mandala-tour.com).

Information Sources

 It is generally agreed that the best map of Mt Etna is *Parco dell'Etna* by the Touring Club Italiano (1:50,000, www.touringclub.it), available in souvenir shops, newsagents and bookshops both in Catania and on the mountain for €8.

Tourist Offices

All of the following offices will have information on skiing, trekking, driving and other activities on Etna:

- Etna Sud APT office, Rifugio Sapienza (☎ 095-916-356, daily).
- Azienda di Soggiorno e Turismo di Nicolosi (Via Garibaldi 63, ☎ 095-911-505. www.aast-nicolosi.it).
- APT, Piano Provenzana (☎ 095-647-352, April-Oct 9 am-6 pm, Nov-March 9 am-4 pm).
- Associazione Turistica Pro Loco, Linguaglossa (Piazza Annunziata 7, ☎ 095-643-094, www.prolocolinguaglossa.it, Mon-Sat 9 am-1 pm and 3-7 pm, Sun 9:30 am-12 pm).
- Ufficio Informazioni 'Etna Sud', Zafferana Etnea (Piazza Luigi Struzo 1, ☎ 095-780-8546).
- Pro Loco, Randazzo (Piazza Municipio, Corso Umberto I, ☎ 095-799-1611, open 9 am-1 pm and 2-8 pm).
- Tourism Office, Bronte (Via G. D'Annunzio 8, ☎ 095-774-7111).
- Pro Loco, Adrano (Via Roma 56, ☎ 095-769-2660).
- Pro Loco, Milo (Via Etnea 14, ☎ 095-955-423).
- Azienda Provinciale di Catania (☎ 095-317-722).

 Pro Locos are local tourist offices.

Useful Contacts

- **Guardia Forestale** (Via Etnea 107, Catania, ☎/fax 095-911-360, 1515 emergency) has bases in all of the main Etna towns: Zafferana Etnea (☎ 095-708-2065), Linguaglossa (☎ 095-921-224), Nicolosi (☎ 095-911-360), Bronte (☎ 095-921-124), Adrano (☎095-684-708).
- **Funivia dell'Etna Spa** or Cableway of Etna (☎ 095-914-141, www.funiviaetna.com).
- **Italian Association for Environmental and Excursionistic Guides AIGAE** (Via Riccardo Quartariaro 11, Catania, ☎ 095-333-543, www.gae.it).
- **Club Alpino Italiano** (Piazza Scammacca 1, Catania, ☎ 095-715-3515, www.caicatania.it).
- **Gruppo Guide Alpine Etna Sud at Nicolosi** (☎ 095-791-4755).

Events

For a celebration of Etna you may wamt to check out the **Festival Etna** in Scena (☎ 095-722-5340, www. etbox.it) that runs from late July to September. There is outdoor cinema, dance, music, concerts and more in towns all over the volcano.

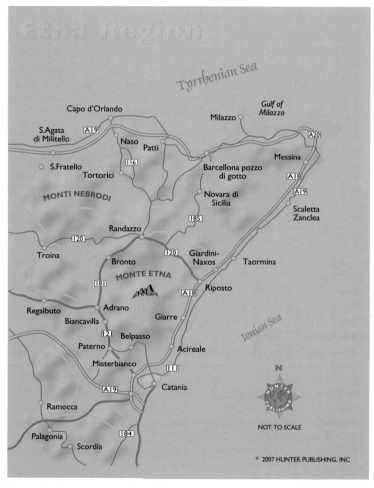

Excursions on Mt Etna

All excursions on Mt Etna should be treated with care as tourists and guides die on the volcano every year. Lava flows do change the tracks so make sure you have the most up-to-date

maps and guides. To fully appreciate Etna, you should consider a tour with a geologist, who can more accurately describe the phenomena you see as you explore. Alpine guides are recommended for climbing the main craters. AIGAE, listed above, is the governing body for environmental guides on Mt Etna and you should look for their credentials (*g.a.e.*) when seeking a guide. If you plan to stay out overnight on the mountain, bring a bivouac, plenty of food and water and/or a water filter. You should always check weather conditions before starting out and the condition of any *rifugio* you plan to use. The *forestale* should have that information.

- The **Parco dell'Etna office** (Via S. Nicola, Nicolosi, ☎ 095-822-111, Wed 9 am-1 pm, 4-6 pm and Fri 9 am-12 pm, www.parcoetna.ct.it) produces maps and brochures on Etna itineraries, but they often run out of copies later in the season. At the time of writing, the office planned to start a program of Sunday walks from September to November and March to July. To take part, call on Fridays from 9 am-12 pm to see if posts are available (20 people maximum, €5-7; add another €10 if you have to get the bus). The walks are during school time only and are half-day excursions, mostly from Piano Provenzana. Bring good walking shoes and a rain jacket

- **Gruppo Guide Alpine Etna Sud** (Via Etnea 49, Nicolosi, ☎ 095-791-4755) offers personalized excursions on foot to the craters.

- **Gruppo Guide Alpine Etna Nord** (Piazza Santa Caterina 24, Linguaglossa, ☎ 095-647-833, 095-643-430, 033-795-6124).

- **Gruppo Guide Alpine** (☎ 095-914-141)

- **Etna Trekking** (Piazza Cali Poeta 15, Linguaglossa, ☎ 095-647-592).

- **Mandala Tours** (Viale A. Doria 69, ☎ 095-508-959, ☎/fax 095-504-029, www.mandalatrek.com, www.mandala-tour.com) has a variety of excursions on Etna, including trekking, biking, bird watching and skiing.

- **NeT Natura e Turismo** (Via R. Quartarano 11, Catania, ☎ 095-333-543, natetur@tin.it) are university-prepared tourist and environmental guides who can offer advice and information in a variety of languages on the metereological conditions and behavior of the volcano. They arrange farm vacations and nature guides.

Independent Operators

- **Giovanni di Prima** (Via Cancelliere 121, Zafferana Etnea, ☎ 095-708-2302, 340-586-2739) is a guide recommended by the local tourist office.

- **Carmelo Ferlito** (☎ 338-219-7869, 095-716-7583, carmelozap@yahoo.com) is registered at the Sicilian Regional College of Alpine and Volcanologic Guides. He also speaks several languages,

Catania

including English, French, Spanish and Italian, and is a passionate supporter of Etna's environment and ecological tourism.

Grotto Excursions

- **Etneo Spelaeologic Center** (☎ 095-437-018) for trekking and grotto exploration.
- **Centro Speleologico Etneo** (Via Cagliari 15, ☎/fax 095-437-018, www.cse-speleo.it) is a non-profit association studying the volcanic grottos on Etna.
- **Gruppo Grotte Catania** (Piazza Scammacca 1, Catania, ☎ 095-715-3515, www.gruppogrottecatania.it).

THE NORTH OR SOUTH APPROACH?

You can ascend Mount Etna from the northern or southern side. Many prefer the north because it's cooler, has more forest and is richer in wildflowers. The southern side has had more eruptions in the last decade, is scarred by lava flows and has heavily used access routes. Most people come up this side because it's more accessible from Catania by public transport.

Museums

The informative **Volcanologic Museum** (Via Battiste 28, Nicolosi, ☎/fax 095-791-4589, www.etnaholiday.it/museo. htm, Tues-Sun 9:30 am-12:30 pm, Tues and Thurs 3:30-7:30 pm; free) contains pictures of the 2001 emergency works, a model of Etna with lights of the towns, volcanic rock exhibits and lava. An interesting section titled *Man and Etna* shows how locals have ingeniously used lava for house construction, pavement, buildings and even ashtrays. Unfortunately, much of it is in Italian and the staff at the time of writing didn't speak English.

Getting Here & Around

By Car

Car is the best way to get to and around Mt Etna. See the *Adventures on Wheels* section for details of itineraries. To reach Etna from Catania, take Via Etnea through the city into the outer suburbs and then follow signs for the mountain. Here are some of the major routes to Etna from other centers:

- Messina/Taormina – motorway Messina-Catania A18.
- Palermo – Palermo-Catania motorway A19.
- Siracusa – SS114 to Catania, take the ring road and follow indications to Nicolosi.
- Nicolosi – SP 92.
- Zafferana – SP 92 bis.
- Taormina – to get to Linguaglossa take the A18 south. After 12 km take the exit to Fiumefreddo, then, after .3 km, turn left and follow the SS120 to Linguaglossa.

By Bus

From Taormina

 SAT (Corso Umberto I 73, ☎ 0942-24653, www.sat-group.it) in Taormina runs daily excursions in summer to the north and south faces of the mountain. The Etna tour runs on Mondays from Taormina to Rifugio Sapienza allowing time to visit the Silvestri Craters (departs 8:30 am, €27 or €66 including the jeep to the main craters). On Tuesday and Thursday there are sunset tours leaving at 3 pm and returning at 10 pm (€67). During the winter months the only SAT tour goes to the Alcantara Gorge, Randazzo and Rifugio Sapienza (Thursday 8:30 am, €36).

CST (Corso Umberto I, 101, ☎ 094-262-6088, Mon-Sat 8:45 am-12:45 pm and 4-7:30 pm, closed Sat Oct-April.) in Taormina runs similar daytime tours on Monday to Fridays in summer. The tours cost €67 per person.

SAIS Tours (Corso Umberto I, 222, ☎ 094-262-5179) in Taormina runs excursions on Thursdays only that leave at 8 am and return at 4 pm. SAIS and FCE buses connect Linguaglossa with Fiumefreddo on the coast. From there you can get other SAIS services to Taormina, Messina and Catania. From Linguaglossa you probably will have to hitch hike unless there is a winter ski season or summer bus to Piano Provenzana.

From Catania

AST (Via Luigi Sturzo 230/232, ☎ 095-746-1096) operates a daily bus all year at 8:15 am from Catania's Piazza Giovanni XXII to the Rifugio Sapienza hotel. They have an office in Nicolosi at Via Etnea 32 (☎ 095-911-505, Mon-Sat 8 am-2 pm). The bus leaves the mountain top at 4:30 pm, returning at 6:30 pm (€5:15 round-trip). The trip takes you through green foothills, wooded slopes, volcanic debris and lava streams,

past spent craters and volcanic flowers. Other AST buses run 14 services daily to Nicolosi and to Acireale.

Zappala and Torrisi (Via Sconti 10, Acireale, ☎ 095-531-625) departs from Catania to Riposto; from Acireale to Giarre, Santa Venerina, Zafferana Etnea.

From Piano Provenzana

4WD bus excursions to the top of Etna also run from the main square of Piano Provenzana on the north side of Etna, operated by **STAR** (☎ 091-643-180). The round-trip lasts two hours and costs €37 for adults and €26 for children under 16 years. Departures are whenever business merits; in summer this is every hour.

From Other Centers

Other routes from major centers or towns on Etna's slopes provide access to the mountain. For example a service leaves Giardini Naxos for Linguaglossa daily at 2:55 pm. Zafferana Etnea is connected to Acireale, Giarre and Catania.

By Rail

From Giarre

 If you can get a train to Giarre (www.trenitalia.com) you can transfer to the Circumetnea train station and get a train to Linguaglossa. Accommodation options in Piano Provenzana or even farther up at Rifugio Brunek will come to get you if you give them a day's notice. The private Circumetnea train line circles Mount Etna. See the *Adventures on Rail* section later in this chapter.

Where to Stay

 Most people day-trip up to Etna using Catania or Taormina as a base. Accommodation is limited on top of the mountain but the towns around its slopes now have many options, offering both a taste of Etna and some authentic rural hospitality. The places noted below are listed by town.

Nicolosi

Etna Camping (Via Goethe, Pineta Monti Rossi, ☎ 095-914-309, fax 095-791-5186, Camping.etna@tiscali.net, €) is based just north of Nicolosi on the road towards the Monti Rossi craters (see *Adventures on Foot* later in this chapter). It is shaded and cool under pine trees and also has a pool.

Etna House B&B (Via Mompilieri trav. V, 7, ☎ 095-910-188, €€) has a pleasant garden and child-friendly facilities.

★**Etna Garden Park** (Via della Quercia 7, Nicolosi, ☎ 095-791-4686, fax 095-791-4701, www.etnagardenhostel.com, €-€€) is an HI affiliate with a hostel and hotel open year-round. The dorm rooms are segregated (€19) or you can choose from singles (€40), doubles (€60), triples (€85) or quads (€110). The AST bus stop is just 200 yards away and they offer discounts to local restaurants.

Bed and Breakfast Tomaselli (Via Giovanni Verga 39, Nicolosi, ☎ 095-914-445, www.bebtomaselli.it, €€€) has quad and double rooms; good for families.

Rifugio Sapienza

Corsaro Hotel (Piazza Cantoniera Etna Sud, ☎ 095-914-122, fax 095-780-1024, www.hotelcorsaro.it, €€) was built on the warm lava of the 1983 eruption. The management is brave, as the eruption destroyed a previous construction from 1946. The 20 rooms are fur-

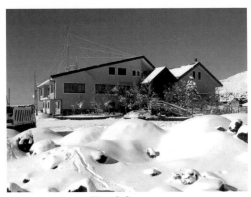

Hotel Corsaro

nished in wood with phones and TVs. There's a *casalinga*-style restaurant and it's a good base for excursions. The cableway and ski lifts are just 200 yards away.

Rifugio Sapienza (Piazzale Funivia, ☎ 095-915-321, fax 095-911-062, €€€) is right next to the cable car station and fills up very quickly all year round.

Rifugio Ariel (☎ 368-733-7966, open all year, €-€€) is run by a Dutch woman and her son. There are only 34 places in the dorm (€22-25) and private rooms (doubles €60-65), so book ahead. Mountain bikes are available to rent for €12/day with bike itineraries (see *Adventures on Wheels* later in this chapter) but check that they're available before you come. Breakfast, lunch and dinner are available for €18.

Catania

Piano Provenzana

Rifugio Nord Est (Via Mareneve, ☎ 095-647-922, €) is a hostel-like *rifugio* and offers simple accommodation. There are only 16 rooms so book well ahead.

La Provenzana (☎ 095-643-300) is just before the ski lift.

Rifugio Brunek (☎ 095-643-015) is five km from Pianzo Provenzana on the route to the craters (see *Adventures on Foot* later in this chapter).

Santa Venerina

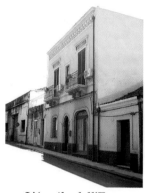

L'Aquila dell'Etna B&B (Via Stabilimenti 107, Santa Venerina, www.laquiladelletnabandb.it, €€€) can arrange riding trips on horses and ponies, mountain biking, walks, Land Rover trips and will even baby sit your kids if you want to take off for the day. The rooms are hotel-like in services, with air conditioning, fridge, TV, laundry and parking. They are part of the Albergabici (www.albergabici.it) organization, offering discounts for cyclists.

L'Aquila dell'Etna

★**La Casa di Pippinitto** (Via Pennisi 44, Santa Venerina, ☎ 095-953-314, www.lacasadipippinitto.it, €€€) offers some of Etna's warmest rural hospitality, with three units in little cottages on the farming property run by an affable couple, Cesare and Eugenia.

San Giovanni La Punta

Hotel Villa Paradiso dell'Etna (Via Per Grande 37, ☎ 095-751-2409, fax 095-741-3681, www.paradisoetna.it, €€€€) opened in 1929 and was the meeting place of artists and well known dignitaries, who enjoyed the magnificent setting beneath the volcano. It's still wonderful, with peaceful grounds, excellent terrace dining and elegant rooms. But it can get

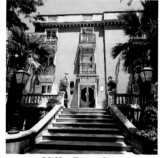

Villa Paradiso

noisy on weekends with wedding parties.

Randazzo

B&B Holiday in Sicily (Via dei Caggegi 27, ☎ 328-283-9279, www.hins.135.it, hins@email.it, €€€) is part of the Albergabici group, offering discounts to cyclists.

Ai Tre Parchi Bed and Bike (Via Tagliamento 49, ☎ 095-799-1631, www.aitreparchibb.it, €€€) is another member of Albergabici and actually offers bike tours to guests. Beautiful rooms with tasteful furnishings.

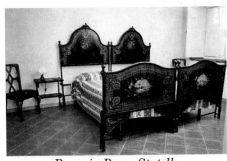

Room in Parco Statella

Parco Statella (Via Montelaguardia 2/s, SS 120, C. da Statella, ☎/fax 095-924-036, 347-409-7281, www. parcostatella.com, €€), run by the Fisauli family, is an agricultural farm with terracotta-tiled floors, antique beds with hand painted frames and spacious dining areas.

Zafferana Etnea

Sotto i Pini B&B (Via A. Diaz 208, Pisano, ☎ 095-956-696, 329-896-2962, www.sotto-ipini.it, €€) is an 18th-century villa in the center of Pisano. The three rooms are furnished with old wooden pieces and the 5.6 acres are cultivated with grapes. They have parking and

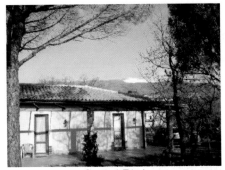

Sotto i Pini

accept animals. Breakfast is served on little terraces with typically local products. Many buses stop in Pisano (Catania-Acireale or Giarre-Zafferana Etnea). Call to book and someone will come and meet you.

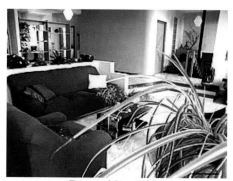

Poggiofelice lobby

Poggiofelice B&B (Via Chiesa Antica 11/ e Poggiofelice, ☎/fax 095-956-097, 347-945-3996, www.poggio-felicebeb.it, €€€) is a candy-pink new construction run by the Lupica family, with four elegant little rooms and a beautiful vine trellis along the outside walkway.

La Ginestra dell'Etna B&B (Via delle Ginestre 27d, www. ginestradelletna.it, ☎ 095-708-1302, 340-183-7748, €€€) has three spacious rooms with modern furnishings.

La Magnolia dell'Etna B&B (Via G. Mangano 36, Fleri, ☎ 348-799-3256, 349-714-0332, www.lamagnoliadelletna.it, €€€) is actually in Fleri just outside Zafferana Etnea.

Monte Ilice B&B (Via San Giovannello 46, Fleri, ☎ 095-313-798, 095-956-049, 333-377-5073, www.bbmonteilice.com, €-€€) is also in Fleri and a good budget choice.

Linguaglossa

Clan dei Ragazzi (Strada Marraneve 47, ☎/fax 095-643-611, €) is a campsite open year-round, 10 km outside Linguaglossa towards Piano Provenzana. They will do pickups from Linguaglossa if you call at least a day in advance.

Happy Day (Via Maraneve 9, ☎/fax 095-643-484, €€€) is 300 yards down from the train station on the right-hand side.

Villa Refe (Via Maraneve 42, ☎ 095-643-926, €), nearby, is a cheaper option.

Where to Eat

You will find restaurants and eating facilities in the major towns around the mountain. There are several cafés and restaurants around Rifugio Sapienza.

Rifugio Sapienza

There are a variety of restaurants and cafés on top of the mountain, all of which are similarly priced, offering *panini*,

café and souvenirs. To save money, consider getting some *panini* made in Taormina or Catania before you come.

Randazzo

Trattoria Veneziano (Via del Romano 8, ☎/fax 095-799-3314, ☎ 095-791-353, www.ristoranteveneziano.it, Tues-Sat 12-3 pm and 7-11:30 pm, Sun 12-3:30 pm, €€) serves *casalinga*-style hearty meals of fresh mushrooms, steaks, cured hams, and sausages.

Trattoria Da Antonio (Via P Nenni 8, ☎/fax 095-700-2534, 338-968-9152, trattoriadantonio@tiscali.it, closed Tues) serves a lot of their own produce – mushrooms, house wine, vegetables and cereals. Their menu includes specialties like *zuppa di funghi* (mushroom soup) and *pasta fresca con ragu di cinghiale* (fresh pasta with wild boar sauce).

Nicolosi

Dolce Vita Café (Piazza Vittorio Emanuele 31, ☎ 095-910-484) is a kitsch new joint in the center of town with pastries, gelati, wine and the regular bar food with bright tiles at the bar.

Hosteria al Palmento (Via Cesare Battisti 202/204, ☎ 095-911-689, www.hosteriapalmento.it) is where you come to dine well on local specialties in a restored building.

Trattoria Tipica da Alfio (Via Martiri d'Ungheria 93, ☎ 095-910-917), opposite the Forestale, is a pizzeria with a pleasant interior. Try anything with fresh Etna *funghi* (mushrooms).

If you're staying any length of time here, there's also a **Supermercato** in Via della Quercia and a fruit shop, **Eurofrutta**, in Via Longo 16-18.

Zafferana Etnea

Caracajada Pub (Via Roma 190, ☎ 329-619-4411, 347-350-9196, Tues-Sat from 4 pm, Sun from 9 am) is a pizzeria/trattoria with nice gardens and lawn.

Orchidea (Via Liberta 1, ☎ 095-708-2575, 338-761-5848, www.paginegialle.it/orchidearistorante) has been considered a specialist in Etna's *porcini* mushrooms for the last 35 years. Some of the dishes include *la zuppa di funghi dell'etna*, *caserecci e pappardelle ai funghi porcini*, *le grigliate di carne*, *grigliate di funghi porcini* and *il semifreddo alla mandorla*.

The pasta is home-made. They also have a home delivery pizza service.

Linguaglossa

Ristorante La Betulle (Etna Nord, ☎ 095-643-430, 12-3 pm and 7-9 pm, €€€) serves hearty meals in a cozy setting.

EATING ON ETNA

The lava-rich soil of Etna is extremely fertile and provides an interesting gastronomic tour. There are abundant peaches, kiwis, mangoes, oranges, lemons, almonds and pistachios. The mushrooms are also particularly rich and the ricotta from Linguaglossa and Randazzo is renowned in desserts. The world's first ice cream is also said to have been made by the Romans from the snow on the slopes of Mount Etna. It is believed that runners brought ice down from the mountain passes to rich nobles and flavored the ice for them to eat. Today the Sicilians still eat flavored ice or *granita*.

Adventures

On Foot

The best way to fully appreciate and experience Etna is on foot. This way you can study the volcano's surface under your feet, walk over the old lava flows, see the craters and foothills and watch how snow is melted by the heat of the rocks. You will require a reasonable level of physical fitness but a visit to the top of the craters is worth it for the views of Sicily, the Aeolian Islands and the Gulf of Augusta. The best time for hiking on Etna is normally high summer. Depending on the snowfall, you may only be able to do short walks into May. The major routes are often busy but anywhere off the beaten track can be quite isolated, so come well prepared.

The northern and southeastern foothills take you much closer to the summit than the towns on the Circumetnea railway route. So, for the best walks, take buses from Catania to places like Zafferana Etnea, Nicolosi or up to Rifugio Sapienza. The highest reaches are more fascinating but require more foot slog. The tracks are often rough and covered

in lava but safe if you stay within the limits defined. The opportunities for walking are both short and long, with five-day treks, day-walks and even short nature trails.

WARNING NOTE

Conditions on the mountain vary dramatically. At the time of writing all tracks were open, but some routes can become extremely dangerous or even impossible to climb, depending on volcanic activity. If you are planning an extended stay on the mountain, you are advised to check the status of your *rifugio* for water, wood and shelter, as their condition can vary. At the time of writing, Citelli was unsuitable. For detailed information about routes, see the list of offices in *Information Sources* previously in this chapter.

Here are just some of the options for walking on Etna:

★**Monti Rossi Craters**, Nicolosi (one-two hours, three km) – These craters just north of Nicolosi are considered the most important secondary craters on the volcano. The route around the three craters and the old lava flows of 1669 starts from an entrance past the campground. They are well signed with informative text along the way and maintained by the local school (www.scuoladusmetnicolosi.it). One sign indicates the fastest run around in 14 minutes. Regular buses leave from outside Catania's Stazione Centrale to Nicolosi.

★★**Monti Silvestri**, Rifugio Sapienza (one hour) – An erup-

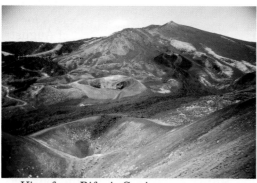

tion in 1892 formed these five eruptive cones near the Rifugio Sapienza Visitor's Center car park on the upper southern slope of Mt Etna. If you have limited time on the mountain these

View from Rifugio Sapienza (Joanne Lane)

are a good short walk option or picnic spot.

Catania

★★**La Grande Traversata Etnea** (five days, 80 km) – This trek follows paths that snake around four different fronts of the volcano. You cover roughly 12-15 km each day, a fantastic way to see the diversity of the volcano. There are several *rifugios* to stay in at night. The first day starts at Fornazzo towards Rifugio Citelli and Piano Provenzana (15 km).

Monte Gallo and Rifugio della Galvarina (three hours, 11 km) – This circuit starts on the Nicolosi-Adrano road at the entrance to Monte Gallo. The hike climbs to the Galvarina forest refuge (6,232 feet), the highest point, zig-zags through old craters before returning down to Monte Gallo.

Casa Pirao to Monte Spagnolo to Cisternazza (three-five hours, 10 km) – This hike through the Mount Spagnolo beech wood starts from Case Pirao on the northern slope, which you reach by turning off the Linguaglossa-Randazzo road just outside Randazzo. The beeches and the eruption of 1981 are the key features of this easy half-day hike.

Monte Nero degli Zappini Nature Trail (1½ hours, five km) – This was the first nature trail created in the park. It starts from Piano Vetore, not far from the Grande Albergo dell'Etna (just before the Osservatorio) and gives a view of some of the typical natural habitats of the area. It also passes old and recent lava fields dotted with natural woods and re-forested areas. The route is well signposted and has only slight changes in altitude, making it a popular walk for older people and children. It also passes the **Botanical Garden Nuova Gussonea** (☎ 095-553-273).

Monte Zoccolaro Nature Trail (1½ hours, two km) – This route starts six km from Rifugio Sapienza on the road to Zafferana Etnea and is one of the shortest but most interesting walks because it provides you with a history lesson of Etna over the last 2,000 years and the keys to the geological evolution of the volcano. It is quite a steep climb through apple orchards and beech woods up to the summit of Monte Zoccolaro. Viewpoints allow you to see the effects of the 1992 eruption, the diversity of vegetation on Etna, with patches of aspen and beech woods and the amazing seven-km depression of the Valle del Bove. There are some other walks in this area taking in the Valle del Bove.

Piano Provenzana - Monte Nero (one hr 20 min, four km) - **Grotta dei Lamponi** (three hrs 10 min, 10 km) – This walk

starts from Piano Provenzana at the rear of the souvenir stands near Rifugio Nord, leading into a pine forest. The first Rifugio, C.A.I M. Nero, is just 1.2 km into the route. The track continues to climb past ovile (sheep pens), passing small caves and open spaces where various cones circling Monte Nero have exploded in the past. This route reaches fairly high-altitude parts of the northeastern flank of Etna, so avoid the winter months to minimize chances of snow. The extension to the Grotta dei Lamponi is worth the extra effort. This "cave of raspberries" (they grow nearby) is a spacious, tubular cavity formed when lava streamed down from the summit in the 17th century. This is one of the finest and easiest to visit. Bring a flashlight for better viewing.

A three-day walk at **Rifugio Brunek** uses part of this route to Grotta dei Lamponi and continues to **Rifugio Forestale Saletti** (first day, 4½ hours, 14 km), then to **Rifugio Monte Scavo** (second day, four hours 12 km) and the final day to **Rifugio Sapienza** (third day, five hours, 14½ km).

Other Routes from Piano Provenzana – There is a 4½-hour walk to Voragine, one of Etna's central craters, from Piano Provenzana. It involves a lot of climbing and leads past Etna's highest craters, so it can be dangerous at times. Another route from Piano Provenzana hikes along the edge of the lava flow at 5,800 feet, circumnavigating some of the volcano. There are lava tunnels and lava flows to explore on the way down to Randazzo, and opportunities to stop and sample wines in local vineyards. The complete journey takes about six hours. The terrain is steep in parts. Go to the local tourist office in Piano Provenzana for more walking information.

■ *Up the Mountain*

If you want to climb up the volcano, you can approach from either the south or the north. Both routes offer different views. From Nicolosi to Rifugio Sapienza is through a barren, black and desert-like environment when compared to the lushly green section up via Piano Provenzana. One way to reach Piano Provenzana is from Fornazzo (four hrs 30 min, 15 km). Follow trail signs for Rifugio Citelli (two hrs 50 min) through birch wood and on to a shepherd's hut, then into the town. From Rigugio Citelli you could do a very interesting circuit around Monti Sartorio (pne hr 30 min, 3½ km), seven volcanic cones that came into being in 1865. The terrain is littered

with volcanic phenomena including over-sized cannon balls formed from lava flung out of the volcano.

★★★**From Rifugio di Sapienza** – Rifugio di Sapienza is the best base from which to access the upper reaches on the mountain. The weather conditions higher up can change so take warm clothes, a hat, good walking shoes and glasses. From the Rifugio you can visit the summit craters, active vents and the fumarole area and continue all the way across the mountain to Piano Provenzana (two hrs 30 min, 22½ km). This summit crater's path is easy to follow as the 4WD mini-buses cover this area constantly, making an obvious track. But it does require a lot of climbing. You can also attempt the track from the other direction. However, the itinerary is de-scribed here from Rifugio Sapienza as it is easier to reach with public transport. The first 15 km to Torre del Filosofo can be covered with a 4WD minivan or the cable car (see *Adventures on Wheels* later in this section) if you prefer. Or you could take the vehicle up and enjoy the walk down along the Piano del Lago, with a view of Valle del Bove from the Cisternazza. If you decide to walk all the way, you'll first pass La Montagnola towering above the track, the largest adventive cone on Etna that came into being after the 1763 eruption. Just after the cable-car station you'll find a detour to the Valle del Bove lookout and Belvedere (50 minutes round-trip). It's worthwhile taking this detour for the breathtaking views over the gaping former craters and valley flooded with layers of lava. The next significant landmark is the Torre del Filsofo (philosopher's tower), a dilapidated building used by guides but named after Empedocles, the fifth-century BC Greek phi-losopher who spent time here while studying the volcano. The section after this is a lunar desert and various craters from where flows have headed to both Bronte and Randazzo in the last 25 years. There is a path to the summit craters (one hour round-trip) after the Bocca Nuova that should only be at-tempted if conditions are favorable. Another detour at the broad saddle Piano delle Concazze leads to the Volcano Obser-vatory (30 minutes round-trip). From here the route goes di-rect to Piano Provenzana, although there are the gaping crat-ers of Umberto and Margherita (named for the King and Queen of Italy at the time in 1879). You could actually use Rifugio Brunek as a base, just five km from Piano

Provenzana. Another option is to continue descending after the Volcano Observatory to Rifugio Citelli. There is no path to follow, but it's easy to navigate your way down the open slopes. Head towards the telecommunications antennae (five minutes), and climb to the peak of Rocca della Valle (30 minutes) for a view of the Valle del Bove to the south. Change direction here and descend left (northeast) along another steep ridge. As you descend you will see Rifugio Citelli on the right and the buildings of Piano Provenzana on the left. It should take you 2½-3½ hours.

FOR THE DISABLED

Parco dell'Etna has created a *sentiero naturale* for children, the disabled and the elderly to enjoy around the Gurrida Lake on the Randazzo-Maletto road. The lake is accessed through a gate (Wed, Sat and Sun 9:30 am-5:30 pm, free). Allow one hour to cover the 1½-km route. Gurrida is a stop on the Circumetnea railway.

■ *Free Climbing*

Etna is also a fantastic base for free climbing. Try **Aquaterra's** (Via Antonino Longo 74, ☎ 095-503-020, www. acquaterra.it) half-day excursions (€ 40).

On Water

For a change of pace from volcanos and something for the kids, the **Parco Acquatico Etnaland** is an option with lots of pools, waterslides, toboggans and waterfalls. The park also has a zoo and dinosaur park. To get there take the A19 from Palermo to Catania and exit at Gerbini. Take the second exit for Misterbianco and the SS121 in the direction of Paterno and exit at Valcorrente. (Adults €19, summer 9 am-7 pm.)

On Wheels

Cable Car

The **Funivia dell'Etna** (☎/fax 095-914-141, www.funiviaetna.com) operates every 15 min-

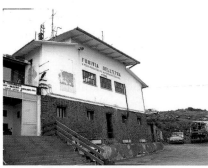

Funivia dell'Etna base

Catania

utes from Rifugio Sapienza (9 am-5 pm). The cable car starts at 6,307 feet and travels to 8,200 feet (€23) within 15 minutes. However, for €42.40 you can continue on in a car (€12. 50) and with a guide (€7) for a two-hour walk closer to the craters.

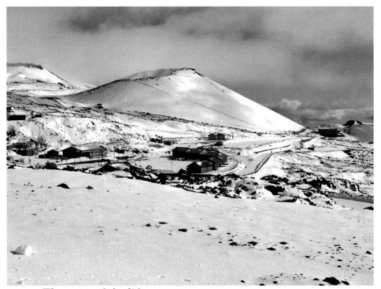

The start of the lift (Galen R Frysinger, www.galenfrysinger.com)

Mountain Biking

 Mt Etna and its territories are rich in flora and fauna, making it interesting for bike riding. If you're not joining a tour group you can rent bikes and choose your own itinerary. Here are some rental or repair options:

■ **Etna Touring** (Via Roma 1, Nicolosi, ☎/fax 095-791-8000, 347-783-8799, etnatouring@virgilio.it) has city and mountain bikes.

■ **Auto Moto Bike** (Via Martiri D'Ungheria 85, Nicolosi) has accessories for motorbikes.

■ **Rifugio Ariel** (☎ 368-733-7966), past Rifugio Sapienza, rents mountain bikes to tourists even if you're not staying there. They only have 20 bikes and they can be booked out by tour groups so you should call and check first. The bikes

are €12 per day and the owner's son can help you with itineraries.

There are also groups that arrange rides you can join, such as:

■ **Due Ruote**, Viale della Regione 106/b, S. Giovanni La Punta, ☎ 095-741-2072.

■ **Societa Ciclistica Fusion Sport**, ☎ 368-352-1477.

■ **Rent Bike** (www.rentbike.it) in Acireale rents city and mountain bikes for €13/day.

■ **Sole & Bike** (Via Marchese di San Giuliano 69, Acireale, ☎ 333-365-6518, www.solebike.it), operating from Acireale, offers various itineraries in the area and also organizes tours and accommodation for cyclists. They have two itineraries encompassing Etna, including *Le salite dell'Etna* (the Etna climb) of 134 km with two steep climbs and *Giro dell'Etna* (tour of Etna) of 127 km. Both routes are day-trips and cost €80.

Cyclists should consult **Albergabici** (www.albergabici.it) to note the accommodation choices offering discounts in the Etna region. There are Albergabici locations at Zafferana Etnea, Castiglione di Sicilia, Viagrande, Randazzo and Bronte.

Circuit Around the Volcano. The wonderful 165-km ride that loops in a ring around Etna takes four day and is easy to moderate in difficulty. The climbing day on the summit area of Mount Etna is by far the hardest. The biking route is the same as detailed in the *Adventures on Wheels* section for cars (later in this chapter). It can be attempted with a road bike ora mountain bike.

★★**De Manio Regionale Filiciusa** – Milia (one day, 40 km) or *pisto alto montana*. This high-mountain bike route can be covered in either one or two days (it could also be a good walking itinerary). If you intend to stay overnight you will need to check the conditions of the *rifugio* with the Forestale. You can bivouac for free in these *rifugios* but you should check to see if they have a roof or clean water. You will most probably need a water filter, plenty of warm and wet weather clothes and food. The track crosses different geological and botanic areas starting at the Corpo Forestale entrance 200 yards past Rifugio Ariel on your right. The first Rifugio Galvarina is eight km from the gate. The route is unpaved but in good condition and is used by the *Forestale*. It finishes in Piano Provenzana.

**Brunek – Grotta delle Palombe – Grotta dei Lamponi –
Siletta Step – Brunke** (six hours, 17 km). This mountain
bike route is of medium difficulty starts in Linguaglossa in
front of the Rifugio Brunek where accommodation is available
(Via Mareneve, ☎ 095-643-015, €26 including breakfast). The
route allows you to appreciate the changes in vegetation and
the unusual cave formations on the northern side of Etna.

Car/4WD

 For a different mode of adventure think about exploring Etna's craters and caves by quad. **Etna Travel**
(Piazza Lauria 17, Castiglione di Sicilia, ☎ 094-298-
0386, 328-6117-9118, 3284-146447, ebpantano@tiscalinet.it)
rents out quads for day excursions and can suggest itineraries. You'll want to enjoy a bit of rough riding and not mind the
mud for this one.

GeoEtna Explorer (Via Genova 49, Catania, ☎ 349-610-
9957, www.geoetnaexplorer.it) has a day-trip to the most recent lava fields, caves and even a house touched by lava. They
will pick you up from Catania-based hotels (€55 adults, €33
children, 9 am-3:30 pm). Taormina or Giardini Naxos pickups
are €75.

Northern Side. The best scenery on Etna is on the north side
and helpfully signposted Etna Nord. From near Taormina,
the road leads up from Linguaglossa, a 15-km winding road
that passes the Piano Provenzana ski slopes. Although from
here you have to leave your own car and take a 4WD minibus
(Jeep). See the *Getting There* section for more details.

If you headed south from Linguaglossa to Milo, you drive past
the old lava flows of 1852, 1950 and 1979 (Fornazzo). Milo is
15 km away and offers views of the Valle del Bove, an enormous chasm 20 km in circumference. This rent in the surface
of the volcano is about a sixth of the entire surface area of
Etna. Its walls are 2,952 feet high and streaked with lava
flows. If the road is open, continue northwest to the Rifugio
Citelli before going back to Linguaglossa. There are more fantastic views of the summit and the coastline below.

Rifugio Sapienza. Another 4WD minibus operates out of
the Rifugio Sapienza from April to October 9 am -5:30 pm. Departures are subject to weather conditions and demand. A
guide comes with you for the tour that costs €37.20. The minibus route leads up to recent lava at Torre del Filosofo. There is

a stop at 8,364 feet to view the cone of Montagnola 2 (Cono el Lago). Padded jackets and boots are available for rent from the guides for another €2.10. You may appreciate them as the weather can be different the higher up you get. On the way down, the minibus stops at Valle del Bove, an enormous chasm in the side of the volcano. This route can also be covered on foot (see *Adventures on Foot*).

The Complete Circuit (one day, 165 km). This circuit around Etna follows a similar route to the Circumetnea railway. It could also be attempted on bicycle and can be completed in either direction. By car, allow a full day, but start early to allow for more stops along the way. The route starts from Nicolosi and travels two km to the Monti Rossi craters formed in 1669. Continue along the SP 92 for four km following the indications for the Grande Albergo del Parco (18 km). Stop for a look around if you want and then continue to Rifugio Sapienza (6,265 feet, 22 km). In front of the *rifugio* is the *funivia* that departs every 15 minutes for the 8,200-foot-high point of Montagnola. The car itinerary continues towards Zafferana Etnea, with great views of the Bove Valley. From there the road goes to Milo, Fornazzo and Rifugio Citelli (63 km) for a beautiful view of the Alcantara Valley and Taormina. A deviation from the *Rifugio* goes to Piano Provenzana (5,937 feet, 68 km) one of the most popular tourist spots on the volcano. The road drops down to Linguaglossa (86 km) through luxuriant woodlands and continues on the SS 120 through small towns like Rovitello, Solicchiata and Passopisciaro to Randazzo. From Randazzo the itinerary continues to the high piano of Maletto heading towards Bronte and then Adrano and back to Nicolosi. You could combine the route with some wine tasting (see *Wine Adventures*) and some walking at Guridda near Maletto (see *Adventures on Foot*).

In the Air

One of the best ways to get a sense of Etna is from a bird's-eye view. **Sicilwing's** (Via Provinciale 233, S. Venerina, Catania, ☎ 095-532-003, www.sicilwing. com) one-hour flight takes in the main craters, lava flows and also descends to the coast of Aci Trezza, the Norman castle of **Aci Castello** and **Jonica** (one hour, €360, three passengers). Departures are from the Catania international airport. They

Catania

have flights over Agrigento (see page 487) and the Aeolian Islands (see page 228).

With Wine

The rich soil of Etna has been used for many years for wine cultivation and is now part of a tourist venture called the *Strada del Vino dell'Etna*, the Etna Wine Road (Via Nicola Coviello 15, Catania, ☎ 095-401-2961, www.stradadelvinodelletna.it). They detail four itineraries you can follow on your own. Enjoy these routes by bike, foot or car.

- **L'Agricola di Nunzio Cartillone** (Via Vico Tantalo 10, C. da Piana Cuntarati, Bronte, ☎ 339-422-3680, www.pistacchicartillone.it).

The **Milo Commune** (Www.comunedimilo.it, www.vinmilo.it) has a two week program of tastings, excursions to visit cantinas and taste local produce in late August to mid-September.

On Snow

Linguaglossa on Etna's northern slopes is a popular ski center. The equipment, ski schools and ski lifts are actually out of town, 15 km farther up the mountain at Piano Provenzana. There are five downhill ski lifts and a network of cross-country ski trails like the **Poiana ski run**. A day's ski pass costs €12.50 and ski rental is €10/day. Go to the Bernardo souvenir shop. For other skiing information go to the Linguaglossa Pro Loco office (see *Information Sources*).

Nicolosi Nord is another winter ski resort on the Etna slopes at 2,296 feet in altitude with 20 km of ski slopes and ski lifts that can take you as high as 8,200 feet. There are frequent AST buses to Nicolosi from Catania. Piano Vetore, 5,900 feet, near the Grande Albergo dell'Etna has 10 km of slopes.

You can rent equipment for skiing and other alpine sports at:

- **Etna Wall** (Via Garibaldi 61, Nicolosi, ☎ 348-280-9990, fax 095-791-5800, etnawall@aliceposta.it, mesh@interfree.it).

- **Scuola Italiana Sci Etna Nord** – Italian Skiing School Mount Etna North Side (☎ 095-643-094).

- **Scuola Italiana Sci Etna Sud** – Italian Skiing School Mount Etna South Side (☎ 095-780-9739).

THE FIRST SKIING EXCURSION ON ETNA

In the early years of the 1900s a group of people from Catania dressed themselves in scarves and put on wooden skis and decided to ski down the volcano. It wasn't until 1956 that the *funivia* was built for the public to make the most of this newly discovered Etna pastime.

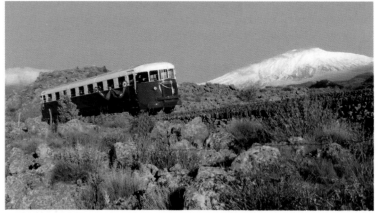
Circumetnea railway

Catania

By Rail

The ★★**Circumetnea railway** (Via Caronda 352a, ☎ 095-541-250, www.circumetnea.it) from Catania to Riposto is a fantastic and unique way of glimpsing Etna and its hinterland, especially if you're pushed for time to climb, bike or ski. The railway is a private line of 114 km following the base of the volcano and taking only three hours to complete (without stops). The landscape is surprisingly fertile in parts, with citrus plantations, vines and nut trees, but it also passes the strewn lava of recent eruptions. If you want to stop somewhere along the route for the night you should call ahead to book your accommodations as there are limited choices. See the accommodations options listed previously in this chapter.

The single-gauge train operates Mon-Sat from 6:30 am-9 pm. There are 11 daily departures, but you'll want to get going early to make the most of the stops. A round-trip ticket costs

just €5.65 to Giarre, although you must pay for the route back to Catania on the FS train line (www.trenitalia.com). A wine route utilizing the Circumetnea is described in *Wine Adventures*.

■ **Catania to Bronte**

The miniature railway terminus is on Corso delle Province 13 (☎ 095-374-842) opposite Corso Italia. To get there take bus 628, 448 or 401 from Stazione Centrale. Alternatively, take the *metropolitana* to Borgo or simply walk up Via Etnea. Helpful guards or the tourist office at the station will give you complimentary postcards and maps. To get to Riposto, at the other end, take a train or bus (from Taormina).

The first part of the route leaves Catania, stops at Misterbianco, then passes through citrus and olive groves to Paterno, where you can see Etna's southern slopes. You get a glimpse of Etna within the first few minutes. Paterno is a busy town in the valley of the River Simeto. There is a 13th-century medieval castle at the end of the main street. It was founded by Count Roger in 1073 and was used by the Germans in WWII. There's a great view from the terrace at the top. There is just one hotel in Paterno, the rather run-down **Hotel Sicilia** (Via Vittorio Emanuele 391, ☎ 095-853-604, €i), in a concrete building next to Giardino Moncada, with singles/doubles/triples.

Ten km farther down the line is **Biancavilla**, a town founded by Albanians in 1480. It is now an orange-growing area. Small side-roads run up through the orchards to the southwestern slopes of Etna. However, if you're limited for time, **Adrano** is a more interesting stop. It was built over the site of ancient *Adranon*, a town founded by Dionysius the Elder. You can still see the Greek lava-built walls in town although there are many other later fortifications. Adrano's squat, solid *castello* was built by Count Roger. It houses a small museum (open Mon-Fri 9 am-1 pm and 4-7 pm, admission free). Inside are finds from local sites, including early Bronze Age pottery. Next to the castle is **Chiesa Madre**. Make sure you note the 16th-century panels in the transepts. The old center of town features shady gardens, faded churches, bars and rustic restaurants.

The route from Adrano to Bronte is among the most scenic on the journey as the line climbs closer to the lava flows. Ask the conductor if you can join the driver in the front compartment for the best views of this terrain. **Bronte** was founded by Charles V in 1535 and its remaining battlemented and pointed belfries are all original. Today it's the center of Italy's pistachio-nut production, producing 85% of the country's output. The plantations lie around the town and are harvested in the early autumn of odd-numbered years. Buses leave Bronte for the Sicilian interior, including Cesaro.

■ *Bronte to Riposto*

After Bronte, the rail line leaves the pistachio area and enters walnut and chestnut country, also passing the huge lava flow of 1823 that almost destroyed the town. Farther on is Maletto, the highest point on the line. A minor road from Maletto leads west to the **Castello Maniace**. The Castello was founded originally as a convent in 1174 on the site of a victory over the Arabs. An earthquake in 1693 destroyed much of the building but the estate was given to Lord Nelson as part of his dukedom. Nelson never visited his Sicilian estate but his family only relinquished control of the property in 1978 and it now belongs to the *comune*. Inside the Castello is a 13th-century chapel with historical accounts of the castle. The floors are tiled and restored to their original pattern. There is a certain Englishness apparent in the gardens and the house (9 am-1 pm and 2:30-7 pm, €2.60).

Randazzo is the closest town to the volcano's summit but the locals have made the most of it and used the lava for building construction. Despite the proximity to the volcano, it has never been engulfed, although the lava flow from 1981 came perilously close. The Germans used Randazzo as one of the main forward positions during their defense of Sicily in 1943. Much of the town was heavily bombed but has been restored over the years since. In medieval times, Randazzo's three churches took turns acting as the cathedral. Today the largest of the three, **Santa Maria**, in Via Umberto I, is the sole titleholder. It's a severe Catalan-Gothic structure incorporating chunks of volcanic rock and a fine carved portal with vine decoration. In the interior are black lava columns – one serves as the altar. All that remains of Randazzo's castle is a blackened tower across the square that forms part of the old city walls. It was the prison until just 25 years ago. Now it houses the

Museo Vagliasindi (9 am-1 pm and 3-8 pm, €1.60). It has a collection of objects from a nearby fifth- to second-century BC Greek necropolis. Objects on display include Sicilian puppets, sporting armor, velvet cloaks and wine jugs. If you want to end the journey here, SAIS buses connect Randazzo with Taormina/Giardini-Naxos twice daily.

Farther east from Randazzo, the lava flows are clearly visible and the views of Etna are spectacular as the line passes within 15 km of the summit. The line passes near Castiglione di Sicilia and into Linguaglossa. This is the main tourist center on Etna's northern slopes. It is quiet during the summer, whereas in the winter it's a busy ski center (see the *Adventures on Snow* section).

Currently, the line ends at Linguaglossa while repairs are being made to a bridge. A bus at the station connects passengers to Giarre and the FS line back to Catania (www. trenitalia.it).

In Golf

For a golf course with a difference try ★**Il Pìcciolo Golf Club's** 18-hole course at Castiglione di Sicilia (Via Picciolo, 1 Castiglione di Sicilia, ☎ 0942-986-252, www. ilpicciologolf.com, 18-holes €55, nine holes €38). The course only opened in 1989 but you could not picture a more

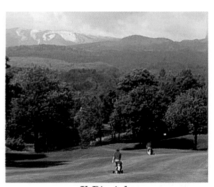

Il Picciolo

dramatic setting. It is actually on the slopes of Mt Etna between old lava fields and a former hazelnut farm.

Sicily Golf (Via Pantalemmi 11, c. da Mitogio, Castiglione di Sicilia, www.sicilygolf.com) organizes golf-related vacations in Sicily on this course and another one in the Madonie.

On Horseback

The following associations provide or arrange horseback or donkey treks:

■ **Internazionale La Plaja** (Viale Kennedy 47, ☎ 095-340-880).

- **Agriturismo Biologico dell'Etna** (Via G. Mameli n. 22, Trecastagni, ☎ 095-780-7670).
- **Coop. Coacri** (☎ 347-662-9378) – donkey treks.
- **APT Catania** (Via Cimarosa 10, ☎ 095-730-6211, www. apt.catania.it).
- **Associazione Asilandia Mondo degli Assini** (Contrada Miscarello Aranci, Milo, ☎ 333-527-5920) – donkey treks.
- **Hidden Trails** (http://hiddentrails.com/italy.htm) is a travel agent that arranges horseback itineraries on Mount Etna and other locations in Sicily including the *Traversata dell'Etna* (eight days and seven nights, €1,675).

These are some itineraries provided by the following providers:

- **Ippo Club Etna** (Via Enrico Fermi 7, Pedara - SP 92 about 4km from Nicolosi, ☎ 095-911-637) offers horseback rides lasting two and four hours with a packed lunch. The two main itineraries go up the side of the volcano in the Tarderia, Tre Monti and Monte Difeso districts.
- **Antica Cavalleria Rusticana** (c/o Azienda Casentino, c. da Olivo S. Cataldo 95, Mineo, ☎ 338-338-4945) has 10 horses available: indigenous Sicilian, San Fratello and Quarter. The *Ippovida del Grano* or Corn Ride (eight hours, 30 km, not for beginners) leaves from Raddusa through pine woods, cornfields, open fields and the ruins of old farms. There are sulphur mines, kilns and towers to explore and a stop for lunch at a dairy farm. The second itinerary, *Il Trekking della Storia* or Trekking through History (two days, seven hours per day, 40 km, for experts), heads out to an artificial lake – a refuge for migratory birds, a Sican archaeological site, a Byzantine necropolis and a night at an agricultural settlement that provides a breakfast of warm ricotta.
- **Centro Equestre Equites Maenarum** (Via Sottocastello 7, Mineo, ☎ 0933-981-415, www.sikania-horse.it) has a series of treks that incorporate rich vegetation, historical sites and Paleo-Neolithic caves.
- **Centro G.E.A. Sanconoese** (Via San Giuseppe 61, San Cono, ☎ 0933-970-883, www.geasanconese.it) has eight

Catania

horses. Their two itineraries are *Sulle trace dei Sicani* or In the Footsteps of the Sicans and *Le trazzere delle masserie* or The Farm Tracks. These are for riders of every ability. The first is a seven-hour circuit of 30 km starting from the center, climbing the sharp Monte Formaggio and passing Sican archaeological sites, small villages and farms.

Centro Ippico Amico del Cavallo (Via Gramsci 27, Misterbianco, ☎ 095-461-882, www.amicodelcavallo.com) has 30 stables for horses, 11 stalls, a saddlery and clubhouse. Three of the six riding horses are of Sicilian origin. They offer a seven-hour circuit of 25 km, *Ippovia dei Casali Etnei,* meaning Horse Trail Among Old Etna Farms, taking in views of Etna, lava flows, castles and stopping for a typical Sicilian lunch. It's suitable for every level of rider. Another itinerary, *Ippovia della risalita del Simeto* (two days, seven hours per day, 60 km), is slightly more advanced, starting from the riding center and following the Simeto river past WWII remains, castles and farms, before stopping the night at another farmhouse. They also offer *La Traversata dell'Etna*, The Crossing Etna Ride (five days, seven hours per day, 150 km, experts only). You spend each night in a Rifugio or Agricultural farm experiencing all sides of Etna, giving you a chance to see the woods, vegetation, old craters and lava flows.

Circolo Ippico Sikania (Via Pietro Carrera 4, Militello Val di Catania, ☎ 095-811-176, www.sikaniahorse.it) has itineraries focusing on the archaeological wealth of the area.

Equiclub Randazzo (Via Monteguardia 15, Randazzo, ☎ 349-325-1011) also offers *La Traversata dell'Etna* starting from their own property at Randazzo (experts only). They also offer a full-day itinerary (seven hours, 40 km, all riders) towards the terraced vineyards of Randazzo and across the Alcantara river to the panoramic summit of Monte Randazzo Vecchio. Another seven-hour itinerary of 40 km follows the same route but also visiting caves on the way, featuring a ride through the Ragabo pine forest (all riders).

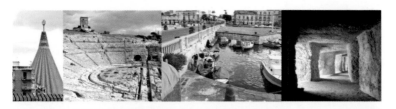

Siracusa & the Southeast

The southeastern corner of Sicily is a popular choice with travelers. Its historic towns, beautiful scenery and uncrowded beaches merit a substan-

tial part of any Sicilian itinerary. Two glorious epochs in history have helped make the southeast towns what they are today. The Greeks settled the region and it flourished for 500 years under them as a center of culture, learning and political power. The second epoch was made possible by a devastating earthquake that flattened towns and villages in 1693. As a result, it was rebuilt in the ornate architectural style known as Sicilian Baroque.

Siracusa is the major city in the region and the most visited, but there are plenty of other gems to discover in the wider province. Noto, Modica and Ragusa all feature the Baroque style; you could undertake some serious trekking at Pantalica's necropolis or Cava Grande in regions of immense beauty, bird watching at Vendicarri or explore Sicily's most southern point around Portopalo.

SIRACUSA HIGHLIGHTS

- Ortigia: This beautiful warren of streets combines ancient Greece and Baroque with a view of the sea from almost every lane.
- Piazza del Duomo: This is one of Sicily's great squares and the Duomo its best church and a prime example of Siracusa's polyglot character.
- Sicily's best granite, the famous icy drink.
- Take a dip in Cava Grande's waterfalls and refreshing pools.
- Pantalica's 5,000 tombs riddling the hillsides.
- The beautiful wetlands of Riserva di Vendicari.
- Portopalo's historic *tonnara* (tuna factory)

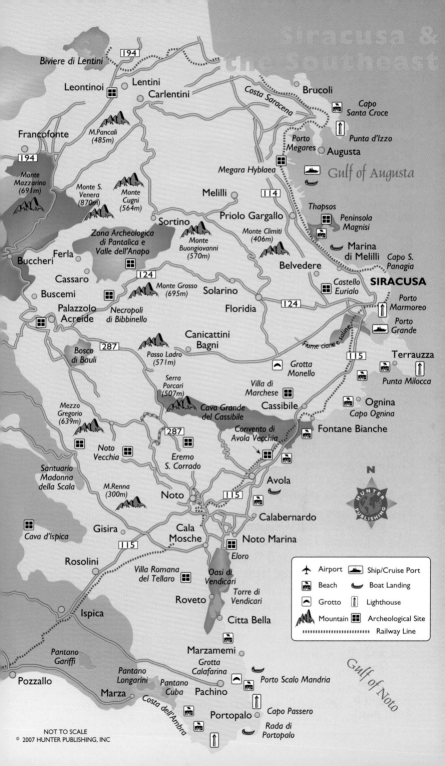

Siracusa & the Southeast

Biviere di Lentini

194

Leontinoi

Lentini

Carlentini

Costa Saracena

Brucoli

Capo Santa Croce

Punta d'Izzo

Porto Megares

Augusta

Gulf of Augusta

Francofonte

194

M. Pancali (485m)

Monte Mazzarino (691m)

Monte S. Venera (870m)

Monte Cugni (564m)

Megara Hyblaea

Melilli

Priolo Gargallo

114

Thapsos

Peninsola Magnisi

Sortino

Monte Buongiovanni (570m)

Monte Climiti (406m)

Marina di Melilli

Capo S. Panagia

Zona Archeologica di Pantalica e Valle dell'Anapo

Belvedere

Buccheri

Ferla

Cassaro

124

Monte Grosso (695m)

Solarino

Castello Euríalo

SIRACUSA

Buscemi

Palazzolo Acreide

Necropoli di Bibbinello

Floridia

124

Porto Marmoreo

Porto Grande

Bosco di Bauli

287

Passo Ladro (571m)

Canicattini Bagni

Fiume ciane e saline

115

Terrauzza

Punta Milocca

Serra Porcari (507m)

Villa di Marchese

Grotta Monello

Mezzo Gregorio (639m)

Cava Grande del Cassibile

Cassibile

Capo Ognina

Ognina

Convento di Avola Vecchia

Fontane Bianche

287

Noto Vecchia

Eremo S. Corrado

Santuario Madonna della Scala

M. Renna (300m)

Noto

Avola

115

Calabernardo

Cava d'Ispica

Gisira

Cala Mosche

Noto Marina

N

Rosolini

115

Villa Romana del Tellaro

Eloro

Oasi di Vendicari

Roveto

Torre di Vendicari

Citta Bella

HUNTER PUBLISHING

Ispica

Marzamemi

Pantano Gariffi

Grotta Calafarina

Pozzallo

Pantano Longarini

Pantano Cuba

Pachino

Porto Scalo Mandria

Marza

Costa dell'Ambra

Portopalo

Capo Passero

Rada di Portopalo

Gulf of Noto

✈ Airport	⛴ Ship/Cruise Port
🏖 Beach	⛵ Boat Landing
🕳 Grotto	🗼 Lighthouse
⛰ Mountain	▦ Archeological Site
┈┈┈┈┈ Railway Line

NOT TO SCALE
© 2007 HUNTER PUBLISHING, INC

■ Siracusa

Siracusa should be on your travel itinerary. Many agree it's Sicily's most beautiful city – stunningly located on a small peninsula with sea views from almost every winding street. These alleys are punctuated with piazzas and age-old churches. There are also fantastic markets, fine seafood dining and access to innumerable archaeological sites.

History

Siracusa was once the cradle of Greek civilization in Italy and a rival to Athens as the most important city in the Western world. The archaeological treasures here date back 2,700 years. The Greeks and Romans left their mark and there's also a fair amount of Spanish and Byzantine. The island of Ortigia was settled in the 13th century BC by Siculian tribes. Its two natural harbors, fresh springs and access to fertile plains on the mainland naturally attracted other settlers. The Corinthians seized Ortigia in 734 BC and expanded inland, eventually breaking its colonial relationship with Corinth and trading in its own right. As it grew in power it became a rival to the Mediterranean powers of Athens and Carthage. Gelon, the tyrant of Gela, seized the city in 485 BC and continued the city's expansion. Gela, Akragas (Agrigento) and Siracusa inflicted a heavy defeat on the Carthaginians in 480 BC. By 415 BC the Greeks had been provoked enough by the city's ambitions and sent an enor-

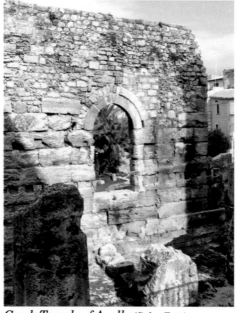

Greek Temple of Apollo (Galen Frysinger, www. galenfrysinger.com)

mous fleet to deliver Siracusa into Athenian hands. However, the fleet was destroyed and the prisoners were incarcerated in quarries that still exist today. The cruelty of this drew condemnation from the Hellenistic world.

Many of Siracusa's great public works were constructed during this time and the King's went to great lengths to invite the greatest minds of the time to the city. Mostly, Siracusa was ruled by tyrants, although there were occasional short experiments in democracy. After Dionysius II's death, the city continued in unsteady alliances to face the emerging power of Rome. But it eventually fell to the Romans in 211 BC and was ransacked. Siracusa remained the capital of Sicily but languished under Roman rule. It was briefly the capital of the Byzantine empire in 663 but was sacked by the Saracens in 878 and reduced to a fortified provincial town. Famine, plague and earthquakes decimated the town over the next 800 years. And it wasn't until the Val di Noto earthquake in 1693 that Siracusa saw a resurgence in building projects. A program began to reconstruct and restore old buildings in the new Baroque style, including the famous Duomo façade. After the unification of 1865 Siracusa became the provincial capital and began to grow again. With 20th-century development the region has been blighted by some ugly industrial development, but the historic city remains intact.

Getting Here

By Bus

 Buses stop much nearer the historical center than trains and are much faster. The bus stop is on Piazza della Posta just over the Ponte Nuovo in Ortigia. **Interbus** (Via Trieste 28, ☎ 0931-66710, www.interbus.it, €4.50) and **AST** (☎ 0931-462-711) operate a service from Catania to Piazza della Posta. Local AST buses also operate from here (see *Getting Around*).

Interbus connections from Siracusa also go to Palermo (3.25 hours, €14), Avola (40 mins, €2.20), Noto (55 minutes, €2.60), Pachino (80 minutes, €4.20) and from there a connection to Portopalo (€4.40). AST services go to Avola, Noto, Rosslini, Canicattini, Palazzolo Acreide and Modica.

By Train

 The train station in Siracusa is some distance from the historic center at the end of Via Francesco Crispi. Connections are available for all of Sicily (www. trenitalia.com) and mainland Italy, but they require a change in Catania. Train access to areas farther south like Modica and Ragusa are available, but the services are very slow and bus access is much faster.

By Car & Motorcycle

 The principle road linking Siracusa to the rest of Sicily is the SS114 from Catania, which becomes the SS115 south of Siracusa towards Noto and Ispica. During the summer, it's a long hot road into the city with long lines of traffic on the narrow roads. Better attempted in an air-conditioned bus!

Getting Around
By Bus

Much of Siracusa is walkable but you may want to use the AST city buses for routes to and from Ortigia to the mainland. The main stops on Ortigia are in Piazza della Posta, Piazza Archimede, Piazza Pancali/Largo XXV Luglio. Mainland stops are predominantly along Corso Umberto, Piazza Marconi (also called Foro Siracusano). Bus No 1 and 2 make the trip from Piazza della Posta to the archaeological park. Get tickets and information from the Piazza della Posta office.

Other useful routes from Piazza della Posta follow. The route # is at right:

FS station 10
Isola 29
Arenella 23
Fontane Bianche and Cassibile 21, 22, 27, 28
Floridia and Solarino 30
Belvedere 11, 14

By Taxi

 If you need a taxi in Siracusa you can try any of the following companies:

■ **Autoservizi**, Via Elorina 130, ☎ 0931-462-244

Siracusa

- **Central Taxi**, Via Niscemi 20, ☎ 0931-492-356
- **Con.t.a.s**, Contrada Pizzuta 1, ☎ 0931-4902-505
- **Radio Taxi**, Via Ramacca 1, ☎ 0931-757-557

By Car

 You can rent cars from these offices:

- **Allakatalla**, Via Roma 10, ☎ 0931-167-452, www. allakatalla.it.
- **Autoservizi Sixt Rent a Car**, Via Elorina 130, ☎ 0931-21413, sr@autotravel.it.
- **AVIS**, Via dei Mille 9, ☎ 0931-122-420, www. avisautonoleggio.it.
- **Europcar**, Corso Umberto 54, ☎ 0931-483-627.
- **Maggiore**, Via Pausania 6, ☎ 0931-66548.

Information Sources

 The **APT** office for the city and the entire province is in Via S. Sebastiano 45 (☎ 0931-481-200, www.apt-siracusa.it, Mon-Fri 8:30 am-1:30 pm, 3:30-6 pm, Sat 9 am-1 pm). The **AAT** office is in Ortigia on Via Maestranza 33 (☎ 0931-464-255, www.aatsr.it, Mon-Fri 8:30 am-1:45 pm, 3-5:30 pm, Sat 8:30 am-1:45 pm). Another useful information source is the Comune of Siracusa website, **www.comune. siracusa.it**.

Syrako Porta Marina Tourist Point (Via Ruggero Settimo, ☎ 0931-24133) has an excursion program operating from 1 July 1 to September 4 to places all over the city and province. Tours range from €7-20.

THE SIRACUSA WELCOME CARD

This card allows the holder a discount on excursions, rental cars, bikes, boats, hotels, restaurants and some museums in and around Siracusa. It cannot be transferred and costs €10 for five consecutive days. It is sold in travel agencies, newsagents and tourist offices in Siracusa and can be used anywhere the card badge is shown in a window. See www.comune. siracusa.it for more information.

Sightseeing

★★★Ortigia

The island of Ortigia is connected to the mainland via a bridge and is essentially the heart of Siracusa. There are 2,500 years of history to explore in a space barely one km in length, and yes, it's best undertaken on foot. From Piazza della Posta continue up the main road towards Largo XXV Luglio where the remains of the Temple of Apollo grace the square. This Doric temple is thought to date from the seventh century or early sixth century BC. The narrow streets are filled with a daily market selling luscious fruits, sea foods and other

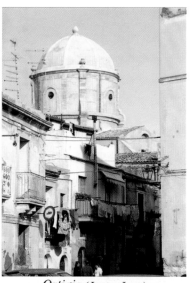

Ortigia (Joanne Lane)

paraphernelia. Continue along Corso Matteotti to Piazza Archimede, an elegant square with a 20th-century fountain bordered by cafés and *palazzi* (mansions) built in Catalan-Gothic style. It's a fine spot to take a break but the real treasure of Ortigia lies a little farther on in Piazza del Duomo – one of Sicily's great squares.

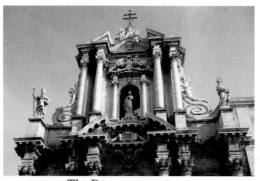

The Duomo (Joanne Lane)

★The **Duomo** (8 am-12 pm, 4-7 pm; free) is a fine example of the mix of architectural styles evident in the entire city. The ancient acropolis of the Greek city once stood here and there are still vestiges of

Following page: Siracusa's Duomo (Joanne Lane)

Siracusa

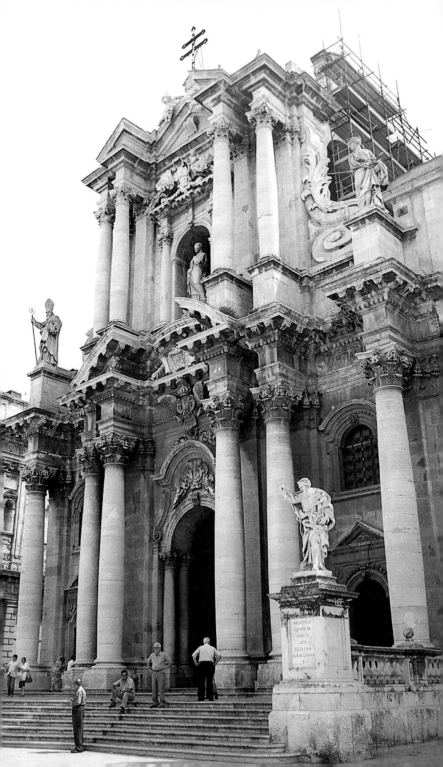

this time in the stout Doric columns inside the Duomo, part of an Ionic temple dedicated to Athena from the fifth century BC. The temple was Christianized in the seventh century and alterations were made. The central nave was split into three aisles and the columns inside were walled off. During the 12th century the interior was adorned with mosaics but these were destroyed during the earthquakes of 1545 and 1693. The Norman façade also collapsed in the second earthquake and was replaced by a Baroque front. Similarly, all the mansions bordering the square were built after the earthquake of 1693 in Baroque style.

South of Piazza del Duomo on the waterfront is **Fontana Aretusa**, populated by ducks and papyrus plants. It's a popular spot for tourists to take a break and for Siracusans on their evening stroll. The fountain is actually a 1,000-year-old

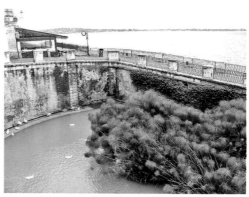

Fontana Aretusa (Galen Frysinger)

freshwater spring and there are a number of myths linked to it. The most colorful is that the goddess Artemis transformed her handmaiden Aretusa into the spring to escape the attentions of the predatory river god Alpheus.

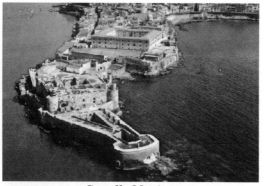

Castello Maniace

Turn away from the seafront and head down Via C a p o d i e c i, where at number 14 is the 13th-century **P a l a z z o Bellomo**, housing the Museo R e g i o n a l e d'Arte Medio-

Siracusa

evale e Moderna (closed at the time of writing), with medieval and modern art.

Around the corner in Via San Martino is one of Siracusa's oldest churches. The church of **San Martino** was a sixth-century basilica and rebuilt in the 14th century. Continue along the road down towards the 13th-century **Castello Maniace**. The castle is used as a barracks and off-limits but the views along the walk make it worth the effort. Turn back and follow the sea front around the far side of Ortigia, but make sure you explore the interior alleyways where you can find all sorts of hidden treasures. There are some interesting shops, including **Il Bazar delle Cose Vecchie** (Via Consiglio Reginale 7/30/4, ☎ 093-124-191, 10 am-1:30 pm, 5-9 pm; free) full of puppets, statues and ceramic plates. Another place to see is the **Museo Teatro dei Pupi** (Via della Giudecca 17, ☎ 0931-465-540, Tues-Sat 9:30 pm, www.pupari.com). Drop by for their nightly puppet shows.

DISCOUNTS

Three Siracusan museums operate under a *biglietto cumlativo* to help you save euros. The combined ticket costs €10 and provides entry to:
- Museo Archaeologico Paolo Orsi
- Parco Archaeologico della Neapolis
- Museo di Palazzo (closed at the time of writing).

The ticket can be purchased from the offices at each site. The APT is also proposing to introduce an archaeology combined ticket for sites like Megara Iblea and Palozzolo Acreide.

The Mainland

The mainland quarters of Siracusa are not as picturesque as Ortigia but are worth exploring, especially the Neapolis and archaeological park, the renowned **Museo Archeologico Paolo Orsi** and the city's extensive catacombs.

The Arachidna quarter lies directly across the bridge from Ortigia. It was heavily bombed during WWII and retains little of its former charm. However, it's an area you're likely to pass through at some stage and worth a stop for a couple of key sites. The first is the park known as the **Foro Sirucsano**

(Siracusan Forum), once the site of the *agora*. Little remains of it now, except a few columns. The area is a busy one with bus stops and major traffic intersections. Not far away is the little-visited but far more interesting **Ginnasio Romano in Via Elorina** (☎ 0931-481-111, 9 am-1 pm, free). The name is confusing as it was never a gymnasium but a small Roman theater from the first century AD. To the east lies **Porto Piccolo** and the ancient **Arsenale**, where ships were set into pits for refurbishing. There's also the **Edificio Termale** (Thermal Building), a Byzantine bathhouse where the Emperor Constans was supposedly killed by a soap dish in 668 AD. North of the arsenal is **Piazza Santa Lucia**, the modern city's most pleasant square. It is named after the 17th-century church of Santa Lucia at the northern end. The church was built in 1629, supposedly marking the spot where Siracusa's patron saint, St Lucy, was martyred. Under the church is the largest system of subterranean tombs in Italy after Rome. They are the oldest in Sicily but unfortunately generally closed to the public.

Tyche is another district of Siracusa that stretches north from Santa Lucia. It is riddled with catacombs, some of which are open to the public. During Roman times Christians were not allowed to bury their dead within the city limits (which in those days was Ortigia). So they went to the outlying areas of Tyche and its system of aqueducts that had been unused since Greek times. The **Catacomba di San Giovanni** (9:30 am-12:30 pm, 2:30-6 pm; €4) lies below the **Basilica di San Giovanni**. This church was abandoned in the 17th century and is open to the sky. It was once the city's cathedral and built over the crypt of St Marcian, the first bishop of Siracusa, who was flogged to death here in 254. The catacombs are gloomy, dank and not just a little spooky. Don't come alone! There are thousands of niches along the walls and tunnels lead off from the main gallery, culminating in round chambers used by the faithful for prayers. Most of the treasures buried with the bodies have been pillaged, but one was unearthed in 1872 and the **sarcophagus** is now on exhibit in the Museo Archeologico Paolo Orsi.

The **Museo Archaeologico Regionale Paolo Orsi** (Tues-Sat 9 am-7 pm, Sun and holidays 9 am-1 pm, €6) is just around the corner on Viale Teocrito and is Sicily's most extensive archaeological museum. It was named after the archaeol-

Siracusa

ogist Paolo Orsi who arrived in Siracuse in 1886 and devoted 45 years to uncovering its ancient treasures. There are three sections to the museum – a bit of a maze. The first begins with a geological overview of Sicily and covers artifacts from the Palaeolithic period to the early Greek settlements. Section B deals with the Greek settlement of Sicily, particularly in Megara Hyblaea and Siracuse. The museum's most famous exhibit is here, the **Venus Anadiomene** or **Landolina** (named after the archaeologist who found her). The name Anadiomene means "rising from the sea" and the Venus does appear to be doing that while trying to protect her modesty. Section C concentrates on the Siracusan outposts at Eloro, Akrai, Kasmenai and Kamarina.

Also on Viale Teocrito at number 66 is the **Museo del Papiro** (☎ 0931-61616, Tues-Sun 9 am-1:30 pm, free), about the history and techniques of processing the papyrus plant – now a symbol of the city – for use in baskets, boats and paper. **L'Angolo dei Papiro** (Via Giuseppe Agnello 11, ☎ 0931-782-788, www.angolodelpapiro.com, 9:30 am-6 pm) near the entrance to the Parco Archaeologico is a good place to see where papyrus is grown. The owner Angelo cuts and slices the papyrus to make paper products. It takes three hours to make the paper and three days to press it.

Opposite the Museo del Papiro is the **Santuario della Madonna delle Lacrime** (8 am-12 pm, 4-7 pm, free). The Sanctuary of Our Lady of the Tears was commissioned to house a statue of the Madonna that allegedly wept for five days in 1953. The monument is rather prominent, reaching a height of 330 feet and designed to re-

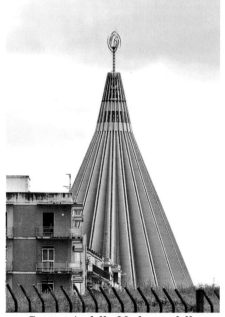

Santuario della Madonna delle Lacrime (Galen Frysinger)

semble a giant teardrop. You can make up your own mind how it fits with the rest of the city's skyline.

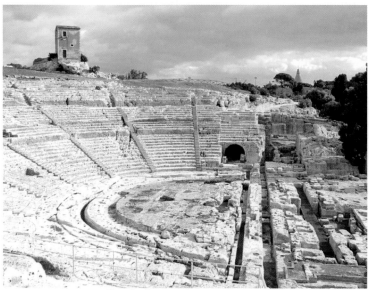

Greek theater (Galen R Frysinger)

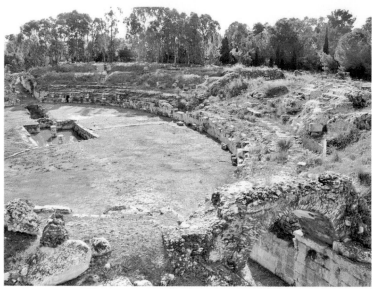

Roman amphitheater (Galen R Frysinger)

The **Parco Archaeologico della Neapolis** (Viale Paradiso, ☎ 0931-65068, 9 am-7 pm, €6) is to the west of here. It's fairly extensive and, not surprisingly, the most visited site in Siracusa. The Neapolis contained the ancient city's social and religious amenities such as theaters, altars and sanctuaries, so it was never, actually inhabited. The third-century BC **Greek theater**, completely hewn from rock, is a masterpiece. When the Romans took the city they adapted it for gladiatorial combat. Today the theater is still used but without the bloodshed! In May and June concerts and Greek dramas are performed. Ask at the ticket office for details.

The other areas of interest in the park include the **Latomie del Paradiso** (Garden of Paradise) and the second-century AD **Roman amphitheater**. The Latomie was a limestone quarry run by the Greeks and also a prison. In the garden is a remarkable cavern known as the **Orecchio di Dionisio** (Ear of Dionysius). There is a story about the tyrant king Dionysius building it to listen to

Orecchio di Dionisio (Galen R Frysinger)

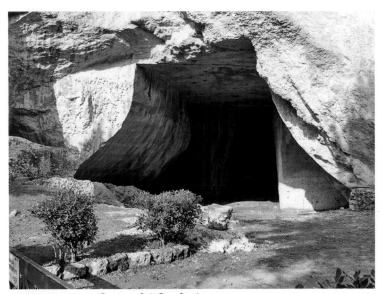

Grotta dei Cordari (Galen R Frysinger)

conversations of conspirators, but it was more likely dug as a quarry and later used as a sounding board for the theater performances nearby. It still has a great sound-enhancing effect. Feel free to test it out. The second cave, **Grotta dei Cordari** (Rope-makers' Cave) was used for the manufacture of rope. There are two other quarries in the park. One has a passage to the **Necropoli Grotticelle**, a Greco-Roman burial ground with a tomb thought to contain the remains of Archimedes. The Anfiteatro Romano (see above) is actually across from the main entrance to the park but is covered by the same ticket. It was built for gladiator combat and is the third-largest in Italy after the Colosseum and the Verona amphitheater.

Other Sights

If you've still got time in Siracusa you could visit the **Museo del Cinema** (Via Alagna 41, ☎ 0931-65024, Wed 8:30 am-12:30 pm, €5) with its large film library; the **Aquarium** (Villetta Aretusa, Ortygia, 10 am-10 pm, €3); and **Latomie dei Cappuccini** (Largo Latomia, Mon-Fri 9 am-1 pm, €1).

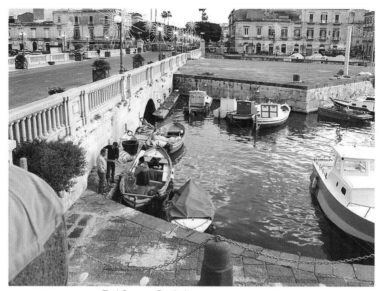

Bridge to Ortigia (Galen R Frysinger)

Adventures

On Foot

Ortigia

If you are walking around in Ortigia watch out for water thrown from balconies. See the sightseeing section above for an itinerary.

- **Riserva di Ciane**

There are several walking routes through the pleasant papyrus-fringed Riserva di Ciane. At the time of writing **Ente Fauna Siciliana** (☎ 338-488-8822) was providing free half-hour guided walks both from the river mouth near where boat tours embark and near the Villa dei Papiri on the Canicattini Bagni road. However, it is unclear if their services will continue long-term. At the river mouth there are special bird, plant and fish species they can point out to you on a route down to the beachfront where you can see the salt marshes and the city of Ortigia. Bird-watching is best from the end of September through to November. From the Villa dei Papiri entrance you can follow a pedestrian route along the Ciane

River to the source (30 minutes round-trip) or continue along the full length of the weir for about five km.

Sudestremo (☎ 335-808-5862, www.sudestremo.com) organizes walking trips in the Riserva di Ciane. **Siracusa Homecoming** (☎ 0931-946-657, www.siracusahomecoming.it) has two-hour itineraries through the Riserva for €11.

On Bicycles

 The area in and around Siracusa is very flat and you could easily cycle to the **Riserva di Ciane**. The best access route to the paths is from the Villa dei Papiri. Inside the Riserva follow the walking route outlined above along the weir all the way down to the entrance at the Porto Grande. Alternatively, head south on the SS115 to the pleasant, flat coastal areas around Ognina or Arenella.

The southern coast of Siracusa right around to the bottom point of Portopalo is very flat and easily completed in just two days with a stop in Noto.

Bike Rental Agencies Include:

- **Internet Train** (Via Roma 122, Ortigia, ☎ 0931-468-797, 10 am-10 pm).

- **TV&L Service** (Piazza Pancali ☎ 348-950-6338) have electric and standard bikes, scooters, cars, boats and canoes.

- **Sudestremo** (☎ 335-808-5862, www.sudestremo.com) arranges biking trips in the Riserva di Ciane and south to Capo Murro di Porco.

In Archaeology

There are a sprinkling of archaeological sites in the region around Siracusa. It is far more convenient to reach them by car, though it is possible to get there via public transport (with a bit of walking). **Megara Hyblaea** (9 am-one hr before sunset, free) is an ancient Greek colony to the north of Siracusa (10 km from Augusta), now located amidst a horrific sprawl of refineries and factories, but conveniently reached by local train via the Megara-Giannalena station. Alternatively, drive 25 minutes north of Siracusa on the SS114. The ruins are basically three cities built on top of each other, which were twice razed to the ground by successive rulers: Gelon, the tyrant of

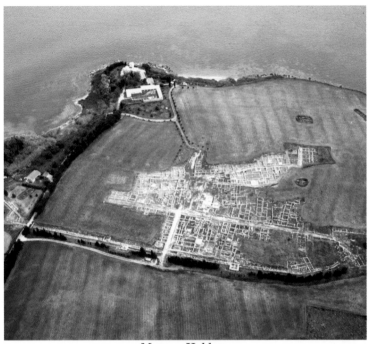

Megara Hyblaea

Gela, in 483 BC and by the Romans in 213 BC. The remains of the *agora*, various houses, baths and defence towers remain looking out to sea, although much has been pillaged for the museums of Siracusa.

Castello Eurialo (9 am-6:30 pm, free) in Belvedere is seven km west of Siracusa and the last major Greek fortification in the Mediterranean that's still standing, complete with moats and immense walls. The castle was part of a defense system that included 27 km of walls. To get here, take AST buses 11, 25 or 26 from Piazza della Posta.

The ancient village of **Thapsos** (☎ 0931-

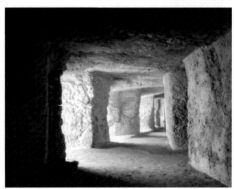

Castello Eurialo

481-111, free), dating back to between 1400 and 800 BC and housing a settlement and prehistoric necropolis, was discovered by Paolo Orsi. The Thapsos people had rock-cut tombs, which are scattered around the site, allowing experts to study the funerary habits of people in the late Bronze Age. There are also defensive structures. Thapsos is located on the Penisola Magnisi, off the SS114 north of Siracusa. The closest railway station is Priolo-Melili, a five-minute ride from Siracusa. Interbus has bus connections from Via Trieste (25 minutes, three daily) to Priolo Gargallo.

★The **Necropoli del Cassibile** is an 11th- to 9th-century BC cave necropolis encompassing over 80,000 tomb sites – located north of the seaward reaches of the reserve of Cava Grande. The Necropoli are on the SP73 Cugni-Stallaini road from Cassibile. There is no public transport direct to the Necropoli, but AST buses travel from Siracusa to Cassible, from where you can access the SP 73 on foot. A guide can transport you to the Necropoli from either Siracusa or Cassibile (☎ 0931-946-657, www.siracusahomecoming.it). For information on exploring Cava Grande del Cassibile, see *Avola*.

On Horseback

The bargaining price for tours around Siracusa by horse and cart start at €30 for a half-hour ride. The carts usually wait around Largo XXV Luglio near the remains of the Temple of Apollo. **Siracusa Homecoming** (☎ 0931-946-657, www.siracusahomecoming.it) runs horse-and-carriage tours of Ortigia or from the archeological area to Porto Grande (two hours, €20).

For a more naturalistic experience, you can attend riding lessons at **Circolo Ippico Fonti del Ciane** (☎ 0931-717-141, closed Mon), a third of a mile from the Villa dei Papiri.

Single lessons are €20 with a €10 fee for insurance and temporary license. Package trips of two or three lessons per week are €65/€100.

The Villa Messina Agriturismo (see *Where to Stay*) conducts horseback trips along the Ciane spring (Contrada Isola, ☎ 0931-68236, www.siracusa.com/messina).

In Golf

 Villa Messina Agriturismo (see above) has a mini-golf course for pitching and putting near the Peninsula della Maddalena (Contrada Isola, ☎ 0931-68236, www.siracusa.com/messina).

The **Canottieri Farina Sports Center** (Viale Pantanelli, ☎ 0931-22800, open 4-8 pm) has a nine-hole course near the Fonte Ciane and Villa dei Papiri. The holes are 55-109 yards, on a course set in a big orange grove. They also have a comfortable clubhouse.

On Water

 If you have your own snorkel you can explore the rocks below **Lungomare Vittorini**, the back road along the coast of Ortigia.

From March to November, the **Vela family** (☎ 368-722-96040, 368-316-8199) runs excursions on the Ciane River (€8, 8:30 am-7 pm). The trip takes you two km up the Ciane and then on a pleasant half-hour walk through the woods to the source pool, with its by papyrus plants. It's a relaxed journey perfect for children and older people. Guides accompany the boats from 8:30 am-1:30 pm. To get there, take Via Elorina towards the SS115 and turn left after the bridge.

Numerous companies operate from the Ortigia port, offering tours around the island and its caves. Tours of the island cost about €10 for an hour-long journey. day-trips that include meals or stops are more expensive. Most run all year but in winter there can be delays while the weather settles or they wait for enough people to fill the boat.

Ortigia Tour (☎ 368-317-0711, www.ortigiatour.com) departs from Riva della Posta, 8 am-8 pm daily (70-minute tour of caves and swim, €10.50).

Selene (☎ 347-1275-5680) have mini-cruises along the

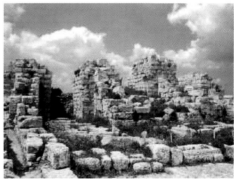

Castello Eurialo

coast of Ortigia departing from Porta Marina (€8, 40 minutes).

Siracusa Homecoming (☎ 0931-946-657, www.siracusahomecoming.it) has tours of Porto Grande (€5.50, 1½ hours), the Isle of Ortigia (€8, two hours) and the Grotta dei Fiori (€8, two hours).

If you want to be a little more independent and adventurous, you can explore the Ciane and Anapo rivers by canoe. The rivers are only navigable for an hour upstream and you access them from the south on SS114 just before the Ponticello Cinese bridge. Look for a small dirt road heading to sheds by the water where the **Associazione Sportiva Anapo** (Via Elorina 97, ☎ 093-122-393, 338-778-0820, 8 am-1:30 pm and 2:30-7:30 pm) rents canoes (€3/hr each). You could ask local buses to drop you off just after the Agip gas station. Other rental places include the **Canottieri Club** (Via Elorina 45, ☎ 0931-24777) or **Canottieri Farina** (Contrada Pantanelli, ☎ 0931-22800, 4-8 pm).

Under Water

Pianeta Blu Diving (Viale Teracati 158a, ☎ 0931-493-739, www.pianetablu-siracusa.it) has snorkeling (€25, 9:30 am-1 pm), diving and courses around the Penisola della Maddalena.

Capo Murro Diving Center (Traversa Sinerchia 4/3, Capo Murro, ☎ 0931-711-837, www.capomurrodivingcenter.it).

By Rail

★★The **Treno Barocco del Val di Noto** is a historical train driven by an old steam engine that operates on summer weekends linking historic towns in the southeast Baroque region. The train runs from the end of June until late September with two itineraries – 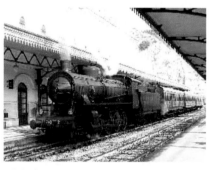 one from Siracusa to Noto, Modica and back; another from Siracusa to Ragusa, Scicli and back to Siracusa. Tickets are €20. For information, contact the Treno Barocco office (Via

dei Lilla 76, Scicli, ☎ 0932-832-458, www.trenobarocco.it). The Siracusa Welcome Card gives a 10% discount on this service.

ITINERARY A				
	Siracusa	Noto	Modica	Siracusa
Arrival		10:20 am	3:55 pm	8:15 pm
Departure	9:25 am	2:20 pm	6:20 pm	
ITINERARY B				
	Siracusa	Ragusa	Scicli	Siracusa
Arrival		12:05 pm	4:55 pm	8:15 pm
Departure	9:25 am	4 pm	6:30 pm	

Where to Eat

 There is no lack of places to eat in the streets of Siracusa. You will be limited only by your budget. For atmosphere, the small streets brimming with *trattorie* and *ristorante* from obscure arches and alleys in Ortigia can't be beat, but you'll pay a little more for them.

DINING PRICE CHART	
Price per person for an entrée, including house wine.	
€	Up to €12
€€	€13-€25
€€€	€26-€35
€€€€	Over €35

Ortigia Dining

■ *Pizzerias*

Al Ficodindia (Via Claudio Maria 7, ☎ 0931-493-900, 8:45 am-3 pm, 6-12 pm, €-€€) is a budget option for pizza in rooms with stone walls and arches.

La Siciliana (Via Savoia 17, ☎ 0931-68944, €€) is another no-frills pizzeria popular with locals.

■ *Trattorias*

Nuovo Ro (Piazza Duomo 16, €-€€) is set in a rustic courtyard with pictures of ships and murals on the walls. It's basic and low-priced with a €10 tourist menu, or you can order *alla carte*.

Trattoria Archimede (Via Gemmellaro 8, ☎ 0931-69701, www.trattoriaarchimede.it) is named after Siracusa's famous philosopher and is often full ,so book ahead. One of the house specialties is *pesce all'acqua di mare* (sea bass poached in sea water).

Ristorante Darsena da Ianuzzo (Via Riva Garibaldi 6, ☎ 0931-61522, 0931-66104, €-€€) is adjacent to the old bridge leading to Ortigia. Main courses are €6-8.

La Tavernetta (Via Cavour 44, ☎ 0931-61107, €€) is an unassuming place, rather like a humble family kitchen but with good Siracusan seafood such as *spaghetti alla margellina* (pasta, cherry tomatoes, clams and mussels).

Osteria Mariano (Viccolo Zuccola 9, ☎ 0931-67444, www. osteriadamariano.it, €€), near Via Capodieci, is a local place with no written menu featuring *antipasto* from the Monti Ibeli region. The service is fast and the ricotta is more than notable.

Trattoria Kalliope (Via del Consiglio Reginale 26, ☎ 0931-468-008, www.trattoriakalliope.com, 12-3 pm, 7-1 am, €€€) is down a narrow alleyway between two squares, with a mainly seafood menu. Eat outside during the summer.

Trattoria Taverna dei Cordari (Via dei Cordari 9, ☎ 0931-22410, www.trattoriadeicordari.com, closed Thurs, €€) is a *casalinga*-style place with seafood specialties like *ricci* and *cozze*. Main courses are €7-8.

Don Camillo (Via Maestranza 96, ☎ 0931-67133, www. ristorantedoncamillosiracusa.it, €€€€) is one of the classiest dining spots in the city, with vaulted ceilings and renowned Sicilian recipes. Sea urchins are served here, hundreds of wine varieties and fresh fish.

■ *Bars & Cafés*

Libreria Biblios Café (Via Consiglio Reginale 11, ☎/fax 0931-21491, 10 am-1 pm, 5-9 pm, €) is a café cum bookshop with Internet, books, Italian language and culture courses.

Bar della Marina (Largo Porta Marina 8) is, as its name suggests, a bar on the marina just over the bridge in Ortigia. Seats in a small roadside garden allow you to soak up the portside location.

Fermento (Via Crocifisso 44/46, ☎ 0931-60762, closed Tues) is a hip little wine spot in Ortigia. You can order pasta dishes and salads or check your e-mail.

Siracusa

★★★THE BEST GRANITA IN SICILY

The author's quest for the best granita in Sicily ended at a tiny kiosk across from Bar della Marina in Ortigia. The kiosk (☎ 380-528-1396) is manned by a large man who could well be asleep at his stall but don't worry about waking him up for fresh granita with real pieces of lemon. He'll be pleased you came by. *Che buono!*

Mainland Dining

Ionico (Riviera Dionisio il Grande 194, Santa Lucia, ☎ 0931-65540, closed Tues, €€€) has a seaside location with a terrace and veranda.

Gambero Rosso (Via Eritrea 2, ☎ 0931-68546, €€€) offers a variety of Italian food, not just Sicilian, and a range of fresh seafood.

Minosse di Visetti (Via Mirabella 6, ☎ 0931-66366, €€€€), just off Corso Mateotti, was visited by the Pope in 1993 and is famous locally as a result. The atmosphere is formal.

Ristorante La Tavernetta da Paladino (Via Tripoli 6, ☎ 0931-461-066, closed Tues, €€-€€€) is run by Antono and Salvatore Paladino. Main courses are €13-16.

Ristorante Pizzeria "Paradiso" da Pinello (Largo Anfiteatro 2, ☎ 093-161-099), on the way up to the theater, has a tourist menu. Try fresh seafood or steak and local wines.

Where to Stay

Hostels & Campsites

Ostello della Gioventu (Viale Epipoli 45, ☎ 0931-711-118, €) is the only hostel option in Siracusa. Take bus number 11 or 25 from Piazzale Marconi. The nearest campsites are **Fontane Bianche**, **Brucoli** and **Augusta**. See the *Outside Siracusa* section previously in this chapter for details. There is also **Agritourist Rinaura**, five km

HOTEL PRICE CHART	
€	Up to €25 per day
€€	€26-€55
€€€	€56-€85
€€€€	Over €85

from Siracusa, offering camping (SS 115, loc. Rinaura, ☎ 0931-721-224, €).

Bed & Breakfasts

B&B Vittoria (Via Mirabella 18, ☎ 0931-462-119) has two apartments to rent.

B&B La Corte degli Angeli (Ronco S.Tommaso 15, ☎ 338-742-2407, www.lacortedegliangeli.com, €€€) has three rooms and a central piazza.

B&B Caravaggio (Via Cairoli 8, ☎ 0931-465-932, www.bbcaravaggio.com, €€€) has simple rooms conveniently located near the bridge to Ortigia.

B&B Eurialo (Viale E Pipoli 251, €€) is six km from Ortigia, a few minutes walk from the castle Eurialo.

Apartments

Siracusa Homecoming (☎ 0931-946-657, www.siracusahomecoming.it) has excellent apartments in the center of Siracusa near Piazza Duomo and Piazza Archimede. All have color TVs, washing machines, bathrooms and kitchens. The helpful Maria Paola Uccello can also help with personal itineraries around the province.

Il Cortilletto (Via Nizza 55, ☎ 0931-60259, www.ilcortiletto.com, €€€-€€€€) has three elegant apartments that open onto an airy courtyard, and with a common lounge for reading and Internet.

Agriturismi

★**Agriturismo Limoneto** (Via del Platano 3, ☎ 093-171-7352, fax 093-171-7728, www.emmeti.it/Limoneto, €€€-€€€€), outside of town, offers traditional rural hospitality in simple settings on a lemon farm. The elderly owners, Alceste and Adelina, are all advice and helpful-

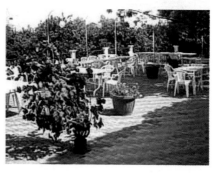

ness. They eat three meals per day with their guests, using fruits and vegetables from their garden. The 10 rooms are

simple and clean, with air conditioning. You'll have the dogs Tina and Leo for company as soon as you venture out your door.

Villa dei Papiri (Contrada Cozzo Pantano, ☎ 093-172-1321, 348-512-1829, fax 093-172-1321, www. villadeipapiri.it, €€€€), on the Ciane River Reserve, is a luxurious farm setting three km from Siracusa. It is surrounded by the wonderful Egyptian papyrus plant and there are walks, biking, horseback riding, canoeing and other activities arranged by the managers. The five doubles and 10 suites are named after Greek gods.

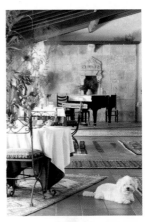

Hotels

Villa Politi (Via M. Politi Laudien 2, ☎ 0931-412-121, www. villapoliti.com, €€€€) is uniquely located in the ancient quarries of Siracusa.

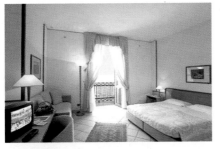

Albergo Domus Mariae (Via Vittorio Veneto 76, ☎ 0931-24845, www. sistemia.it/domusmariae) is run by an order of Ursuline nuns, with a chapel and contemplative reading room. However, it's run as a business establishment. Rates include breakfast and there's also a restaurant.

Grand Hotel Ortigia (Viale Mazzini 12, ☎ 0931-46400, www.grandhotelsr.it, €€€€) is a graceful four-story building constructed in 1905 but renovated in the 1990s, with glass chandeliers, curving staircases and wrought iron.

■ The Siracusan Interior
★★★Pantalica

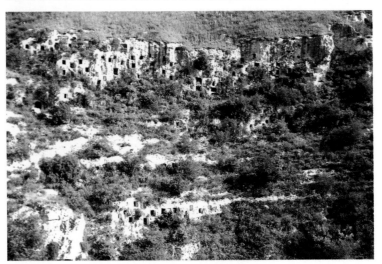

Pantalica *(Joanne Lane)*

The 5,000 tombs hewn out of limestone cliffs in a magnificent series of gorges makes Pantalica not only Sicily's greatest necropolis but one of the most magnificent walking and natural areas on the island. Itineraries can be undertaken on foot or bike, incorporate some swimming or something a little more extreme like canyoning or rock climbing. It is sure to be a highlight of a visit to the southeastern corner of Sicily.

Pantalica was first used between the 13th and 10th century BC by Sikel refugees from the coast. After the eighth century BC it is thought to have been the site of Hybla. There are some remains from this era, but they pale in significance compared to the tombs, which were later converted into cave dwellings – several skeletons have been found in each tomb suggesting a few thousand people once lived in the vicinity.

Getting Here

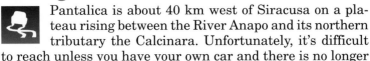

Pantalica is about 40 km west of Siracusa on a plateau rising between the River Anapo and its northern tributary the Calcinara. Unfortunately, it's difficult to reach unless you have your own car and there is no longer

any bus service operating through the park. You can hitch-hike, walk or order a taxi from Sortino or Ferla to the reserve entrances (five-six km both ways) but you're probably better off taking a tour arranged from Siracusa or call the **Corpo Forestale dello Stato** (☎ 093-167-450) to set up a free tour and they can probably organize transport on your arrival.

AST (☎ 0931-462-711) services connect Sortino to Catania and Siracusa, as well as to nearby towns Palazzolo Acreide, Carlentini and Lentini. There is also a local bus company called **Anapo Societa Cooperativa** (Via Tartaglia 32, ☎ 0931-954-333).

Information Sources

i The **Corpo Forestale dello Stato di Siracusa** (☎ 093-167-450) manages the reserve and provides two guides who are available at the reserve entrances for free guided itineraries to the necropolis. The best time to catch them is on Saturdays and Sundays, but call first to ensure they have not taken another group. They can also be available on weekdays. **Fabio Giaccotto** (Via 1 Maggio 2, Sortino, ☎ 0931-953-2777, 338-874-3831, wwfsortino@tin.it), at the Sortino entrance, has taken tourists through the reserve for 12 years.

Siracusa Home Coming (☎ 0931-946-657, www.siracusahomecoming.it) offers two-day itineraries through the reserve. One is a walk along the old railway at the bottom of the canyon with a swim in the little lakes of the river. The other includes trekking up to the Necropolis of Pantalica (three-four hours, €20).

Syrako Porta Marina Tourist Point (Via Ruggero Settimo, ☎ 0931-24133) operates tours to Pantalica on Mondays from Siracusa, also including a visit to Eurialo castle (8:30 am-7 pm, €20).

Pantalica Ranch (Contrada Chianazzo, SP 28 Solarino-Fusco, ☎ 0931-924-130, www.pantalicaranch.it) offer three-hour/half-day/full-day guided walks (€50/€75/€110 per group) through the Valle dell'Anapo.

Sudestremo (☎ 335-808-5862, www.sudestremo.com) has canyoning, trekking, climbing and mountain bike itineraries through Pantalica.

Mandala Tour (☎ 095-508-959, www.mandala-tour) has a number of itineraries that take in routes through Pantalica, including *Nature and Culture in Sicily* (eight days).

CicloFree (☎ 0931-465-396, www.ciclofree.com) has a cycling tour of southeastern Sicily.

Sortino Tourist Office (☎ 0931-917-433, www.comune. sortino.sr.it).

Sortino Pro Loco (☎ 0931-956-007).

 Pro Locos are local tourist offices.

Pro Loco Ferla (☎ 0931-870-142).
Pro Loco Tourist Office (☎ 0931-870-136).

Adventures

On Foot

 There are a number of walking itineraries in the gorge. If you don't have a map you should go to one of the two major entrances first, either five km below Sortino or six km below Ferla. You can get a map there from the Forestry Office and see if a guide is available to accompany you. The guides are free and provide amazing insights into the history of the valley and its flora and fauna. The entrance below Sortino gives you the best chance of seeing the *necropoli*. If you plan to walk, you should take plenty of water and food, good shoes, a hat, map and sunscreen. There are no facilities and no refreshments anywhere in Pantalica. Sortino and Ferla are your best local options for any resources.

The route along the valley running through the gorge is 13 km, including a series of galleries with pools for swimming, the old railway stop Stazione Pantalica and a museum (if it's open) and some wonderful scenery. It is only an easy 20-minute walk to the first gallery from the Sortino entrance; it's suitable for children and the elderly. The route along the valley floor, shady in spots, is ideal for picnicking and swimming.

The *necropoli* are actually up in the hills above on the other side of the river. Signs will point you towards the remains of a **Villagio Bizantino** with a church (about 15 minutes from the river and a steep climb), **Palazzo del Principe** (foundations of ancient Hybla: the Anaktoron or Prince's Palace – another 15 minutes farther on) and a cemetery. It's a steep climb but make sure you catch your breath by looking behind you down into the gorge – spectacular! Past the Palazzo del Prin-

cipe, turn right on the main road to reach the **Necropoli Nord** (a good half-hour round-trip), probably the best set of tombs, with the path taking you down to the water's edge and some pools and cascades to cool off in. It is possible to drive to this section from Sortino or shortcut back down to a path near the Sortino entrance (you'll need the Forestry map to find this route). Otherwise, head back the way you came.

If you plan to see the Stazione Pantalica, swim in some of the pools and visit the *necropoli* or some of the archaeological remains, you need at least a good half-day. Talk to the guides or forest workers about the best use of your time.

On Wheels

 It is possible to cycle the disused railway through the gorge, a route of just 13 km, but you do need to get permission from the Forestry Department in advance (☎ 093-167-450 or in Sortino ☎ 0931-953-695). Permits are checked at the reserve entrance but cannot be issued there. Allow a few days for processing these permits. If you use one of the guides mentioned above they should sort out the permits for you.

Siciliando (☎ 0932-942-843, www.siciliando.it) from Modica (see Tetti di Siciliando in *Where to Stay*) has a guided biking itinerary along the *ex-ferrovia* (former train line) to Pantalica. Also see **Chiaramonte Gulfi** (Ragusa and the southeast) for details of routes towards Pantalica on the *ex-ferrovia*.

On Horseback

 The **Pantalica Ranch** has half-day and full-day guided horseback tours (€13/€25/€40/€56) from their ranch on the SP 28 Solarino-Fusco (Contrada Chianazzo, ☎ 0931-924-130, www.pantalicaranch.it).

Siracusa Homecoming (☎ 0931-946-657, www. siracusahomecoming.it) does a horseback ride along the river for €15.

Where to Stay

 There are some limited options for staying near the necropoli: **Pantalica B&B** (Via Roma 98, Ferla, ☎ 0931-870-147), and **Pantalica Ranch Agriturismo** (Contrada Chianazzo, SP 28 Solarino-Fusco, ☎ 0931-924-130, www.pantalicaranch.it, €€).

Palazzolo Acreide

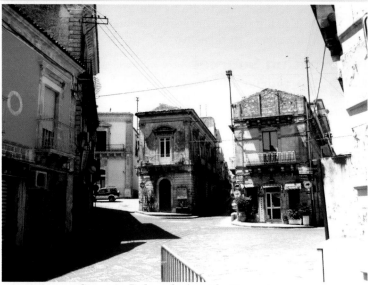

Street in Palazzolo Acreide (Clemensfranz)

Palazzolo occupies the higher slopes of a promontory that would once have given it a strategic command over the routes inland, but has now left it somewhat stranded inland from the main road and rail links. The modern town – well, it dates from the 12th century – is the successor of Akrai, a Greek colony built in the middle of the seventh century BC.

Palazzolo has been described as "dead as a doornail" at night by other guidebooks but it seems the locals take a lot of offence to that, as we found out! To be fair, a lot goes on in Palazzolo throughout the year, although outside the summer months the evenings can be quiet. But even then the Baroque town noted in Unesco's World Heritage list has its own charm. The winter months feature the Carnivale celebrations, among the most colorful in Sicily. And an excursion here at any time of year can take in the ancient ruins, classic theater and interesting museums. In all it's a pleasant excursion away from the coast.

Siracusa

Getting Here

 Bus connections to Palazzolo are via Siracusa with AST (11 daily). There are no buses on Sundays to Palazzolo from Siracusa or Catania.

Information Sources

 The **tourist office** is in Corso Vittorio Emanuele near the town hall (☎ 0931-871-280). A useful website on Palazzolo is www.palazzolo-acreide.it.

Sightseeing

The Piazza del Popolo is the heart of the town. It is dominated by the church of **San Sebastiano** and the town hall. It's commonly full in the early evenings with people enjoying *passeggiata* and the *aperitivo* hour. In the summer a series of cultural events like music, concerts, shows and exhibitions are held in the piazza. Streets and lanes from the piazza lead to a series of fine Baroque churches, including the **Chiesa Madre**, **Annunziata**, **San Paolo** and **Immacolata**.

The **Casa Museo Antonio** Uccello (Via Machiavelli 19, ☎ 093-188-1499, casamuseouccello@regione.sicilia.it, 9 am-1 pm and 3:30-7 pm, free) draws the immediate attention of most visitors. The museum celebrates the rural life and traditions of Sicily and is the lifetime collection of Antonio Uccello. There are kitchen objects, agricultural tools, shaving equipment, clothes, bird cages, jam dishes, saddles, muzzles and religious paintings. Everything is a must-see. Only 10 visitors are allowed in at a time and you visit the rooms with a guide (Italian only).

The **Akrai Archaeological Park** (☎ 093-087-6602, Tues-Sun 9 am-6:30 pm, to one hour before sunset in winter, free, www.akrai.it) contains the ruins of the ancient town and lies just outside the modern settlement. The **Greek theater** is the most complete of the ruins. It could seat 600 people and is still used today in May by high school students who come from all over Italy and Europe to perform tragedies and comedies by classical authors. At other times the *comune* presents classical museum concerts and theater productions. Next to the theater is the **Bouleuterion** or senate-house. Other fragmentary ruins include the Roman **Tempio di Persefone** and **Tempio di Afrodite**. Beyond are the two quarries from

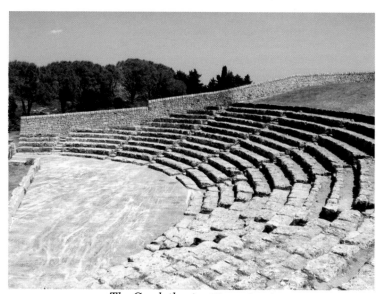

The Greek theater (Clemensfranz)

which the stone to build the city was taken. The quarries were later converted into *necropoli* (burial places). There's also a stretch of road that connected the two gates of the city. Ask the custodian about seeing a lower quarry, the **Templi Ferali**, for more niches and chambers, and the **Santoni**, 12 rock-cut sculptures of the fertility goddess Cybele that are worth the 15-minute walk. They were carved in about the third century BC.

Adventures

On Foot

The *strada panoramica,* tracing a ring road route around the Akrai Zona Archaeologica, is a pleasant three-km circuit with lovely views of the town and valley beyond.

On Wheels

Trekking Bike "Iblei Center" (Via Duca d'Aosta 3-6, ☎ 0931-881-532, www.ibleitrekkingbike.it) runs biking, trekking and mini-van excursions in and around Palazzolo. Two mountain bike itineraries operate, one to Monte Grosso and the Valle dell'Anapo (three-four hours,

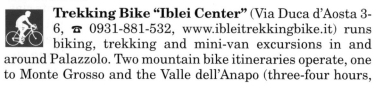

28 km, €10) and the other to Noto Antica and Noto (35 km, €40), including the cost of the bikes and guides. Mini-bus excursions to Buscemi (€40) and Noto (€48), and trekking at Pantalica (€40) and Cava Grande, are other alternatives.

Mandala Tours (Viale A. Doria 69, ☎ 095-508-959, www.mandal-tour.com) has a 10-day self-guided bike tour, *The Secrets of Sicily*, through Siracusa and the southeast, starting from Palazzolo. They arrange accommodations, bike rental, dinner and baggage transportation.

Where to Stay

Hotel Santoro (Via San Sebastiano 21, ☎ 0931-883-855, €€€) has 15 rooms with breakfast in an establishment below the Piazza. Ask in the *tabacchi* below for information. Singles/doubles/triples/quads go for €35/€55/€75/€90.

The Senatore (Largo Senatore Italia, ☎ 0931-883-443, www.hotelsenatore.it) has 21 hotel-style rooms.

Akraio B&B (Via Giuseppe Fava 7, ☎ 333-356-2360, www.akraion.it, €€) has just one room, with bathroom and kitchen. Children are welcome. It was undergoing renovation at the time of writing.

Where to Eat

The choices for eating are located around the Duomo, with **Eden Bar** and **Café Sicilia** facing each other off for positions in the square. Each has its own tables and fair share of

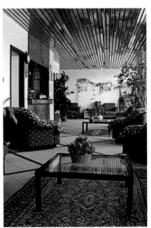

The Senatore

old men sipping drinks in the afternoon. This square is also where summer concerts are held and buses arrive. Eating options include **Ristorante Il Barocco** (Via Nicolo Zocco 27), **Trattoria La Casareccia** (Via Duca D'Aosta 19, Ronco Cananarella 13, ☎ 0931-875-962), near Piazza del Popolo, and **Il Portico** (Via Orologio 6, ☎ 0931-881-532, www.ristorante-ilportico.it, closed Tues, €€€) restaurant and wine bar. Il Portico has elegant fresco ceilings and a variety of menu choices. Come for dinner or simply to taste the wines, cheeses, cold cut

meats, honey and marmalade at the wine bar. Tourist menus are €35 for five plates.

■ The Southeastern Corner

Avola

This agricultural town has an old Baroque center, which was rebuilt after the earthquake of 1693. There are a few crumbling *palazzi* to admire and **Avola Marina** two km away is a pleasant divergence, with sandy beaches, the usual bars and *pizzerie* by the waterfront. If you're looking for cheap accommodations, there are a few campsites between here and Siracusa (see *Where to Stay*). Both buses and trains serve Avola and connect it with Siracusa and Noto, al-

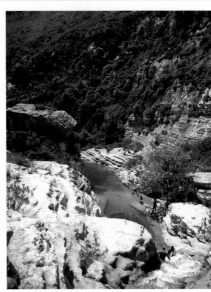

Cava Grande at Avola

though buses arrive more conveniently in Piazza Vittorio Veneto closer to the town center.

However, the main reason you might come to Avola is to visit the magnificent gorge and nature reserve of ★★**Cava Grande**. If you're driving, take the main road north out of town for 15 km past the signpost for Convento di Avola Vecchia. Then follow signs for Belvedere. A local city bus from Avola supposedly runs to the gorge, but we were unable to confirm this. A footpath at a small reserve shack and accompanying food outlet takes you right down to the River Cassibile and along the gorge. The gorge is peppered with small pools and cascades that are delightfully cool and popular in the summer months. The walk to and from the valley floor is steep, with no shade. Reserve workers will try to dissuade you, and they're justified, from attempting the journey in the midday sun during summer – it is hot! Take plenty of food and water with you as there is none down in the gorge.

Siracusa Homecoming (☎ 0931-946-657, www. siracusahomecoming.it) offers a 3-4 hour itinerary through this area for just €20. The guide can meet and transport you from Avola or Siracusa. They can also help you reach the Necropoli del Cassibile from the other side of Cava Grande (see *Archaeology Adventures* in Siracusa).

Where to Stay

 Agriturismo Masseria sul Mare (Strada Statale 115 Siracusa- Noto Km 391,600, C. da Gallina, Avola, ☎ 0957-831-232, www.masseriasulmare.it, €€-€€€) is part of the Albergabici (www.fiab-onlus.it) program in Sicily offering discounts to cyclists. Accommodation is in small cottages. Trekking and biking in the region can be arranged. There are several campsites between Avola and Siracusa on the coastal road. **Camping Sabbia D'Oro** (☎ 0931-822-415, www.campeggiosabbiadoro.com, €) is on the SS115 south of Cassibile towards Avola.

Camping Paradiso del Mare (☎ 0931-822-435, www. paradisodelmare.it) is seven km from Avola north towards Siracusa in Contrada De Gallina Fondolupo

Camping Pantanello (☎ 0931-823-275) is rather unhelpful but has a pleasant garden and is just 100 yards from the seafront.

Noto

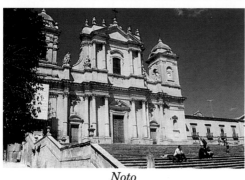

Noto

Noto has been called the "garden of stone" and is known as the capital of Sicilian Baroque. Its famed honey-colored sandstone town is often referred to as the "new town," although it dates from the 17th century. The previous town that had existed for centuries was flattened by the 1693 earthquake. The architect Giuseppe Lanza was commissioned to rebuild the town and did so 15 km away from the original site, much to the townspeople's

dismay. He created two quarters, one for political and religious administration, the other a residential area. Both were built incredibly quickly, with an emphasis on harmony, and Noto replaced Siracusa as the region's provincial capital for a time.

However, by the 20th century, much of the town had deteriorated, largely due to traffic that damaged the local soft Iblean stone. Traffic is now diverted around the outskirts of town and restoration work began in 1987. However, authorities delayed repair of the cracked cathedral dome and it collapsed in 1996! At the time of writing it was a mass of scaffolding covered by a large canvas showing tourists what it normally looks like. It's hardly the same but at least renovation work is underway.

Noto's beauty has not gone unnoticed. It is a tourist town and you'll find the cafés and bars lining the streets humming with other visitors.

Getting Here

 AST (☎ 0931-464-820) buses link Noto with Avola, Catania, Comiso, Ispica, Modia, Pozzallo, Ragusa, Rosolini, Siracusa, Vittoria and Gela. **Interbus** (☎ 0931-66710) connects Noto with Siracusa (seven daily), Portopalo, Pachino (via Riserva di Vendicari), Avola, Cassibile and Catania. Information and tickets in Noto can be obtained from Bar Efirmedio, Largo Pantheon in Giardini Pubblici (☎ 0931-835-023). **Intercity** buses pull in at the Giardini Pubblici (public gardens). The bus for Pachino leaves from the train station. A **Caruso** bus links Noto to Riserva di Vendicari.

Noto is linked with the principal Sicilian cities by the **train** (www.trenitalia.com). The train station is a 10-minute walk from the historic center along Via Principe del Piemonte. The **Treno Barocco del Val di Noto** historical train also runs to Noto. See the *Adventures by Rail* section later in this chapter. By **car**, take the A18 Messina-Catania-Siracusa or A19 Palermo-Catania-Siracusa. Exit at the Bivio Cassibile and follow the SS115 to Noto.

Getting Around

 This and That (Corso Vittorio Emmanuele 123, ☎ 338-739-4391, 9 am-1:30 pm, 3-8 pm) rents cars (€35-45), bicycles (€8/day) and motos (€28). **Caruso**

buses to Noto Marina leave from Giardini Pubblici (Via G. Borsi, ☎ 0931-836-123).

Information Sources

 APT tourist office, Piazza XVI Maggio, Villetta Ercole (☎ 0931-573-779, fax 0931-836-7445, Mon-Sat 8:30 am-1:30 pm, 3:30-6:15 pm, Sun 9 am-12:45 pm).

Associazione Turistica Pro Noto (Via Gioberti 13, ☎/fax 0931-836-503, pronoto@tiscali.it, Tues-Sun 9 am-1 pm, 3-6 pm).

Events

Events worth coming to Noto for include the **Primavera Barocca** festival in May when the entire street of Via Nicolaci is covered in flowers, and the **Val di Noto** festival (www.valdinotofestival.it) from July to September.

Sightseeing

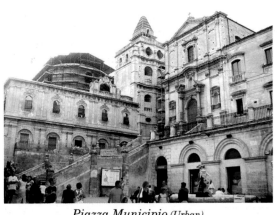

Piazza Municipio (Urban)

Noto is one of Sicily's easiest towns to explore because more of the honey-rich monuments lie along Corso Vittorio Emanuele. This road runs through the heart of the lower, patricians' quarter and is easily reached from Giardini Pubblici where you get off the bus by walking through Porta Reale. The **Museo Civico** (Corso Vittorio Emanuele 149, ☎ 0931-836-462, Tues-Sun 9:30 am-1:30 pm, 4-8 pm, €1.50) is one of the first buildngs along the Corso, inside the **Convento del Santissimo Salvatore**. It contains the **Galleria Pirrone** and finds from Greek coastal sites and material from Noto Antica. The museum was closed for a number of years but has finally reopened to the public.

☞ The €3 join ticket or *biglietto cumulativo* allows the ticket holder entry to Museo Pirrone, Sala degli Specchi and the Teatro or pay €1.50 for the individual entrances. Tickets are available at the entrance counters or the APT.

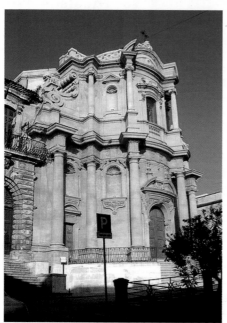

San Domenico (Stefano Mortellaro)

The **Piazza Municipio**, about halfway along the Corso, is a pretty square and arguably the heart of the town. Across from it lies the **Duomo** at the top of a staircase. The cathedral is still impressive but a long way from being unveiled from scaffolding as restoration works continue. The **Palazzo Landolina** next to it once belonged to Noto's oldest noble family. Opposite is the town hall, **Palazzo Ducezio**, which houses **La Sala degli Specchi** (☎ 0931-896-943, Tues-Sun 9 am-1 pm, 4-8 pm in summer, 9 am-1 pm and 3-7 pm in winter). For €1.50 you can see the "hall of mirrors" – a palatial room with 19th-century frescoes. The **bell tower** (10 am-1 pm, 3-8 pm, €1.50) of **Chiesa di San Carlo** is the best place to view the town. A narrow staircase leads to the top for a view over the

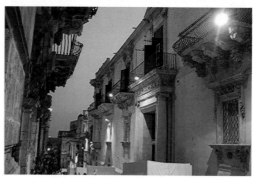

Via Nicolasi in Noto (Urban)

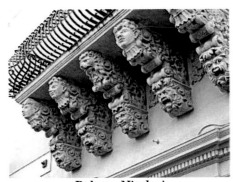
Palazzo Nicolaci

rooftops. It's one of the best photos of Baroque Sicily. On the street across from the Chiesa di San Carlo is **Palazzo Nicolaci** (Via Nicolaci, ☎ 093-183-5005, 10 am-1 pm, 3-7:30 pm, €3). If you don't want to go inside it's still worth a stroll by to see the fancy balconies where chubby sculpted beasts stare down from above. The **Teatro Comunale** (Piazza XVI Maggio, ☎ 093-189-6655, Tues-Sun 9:30 am-1:30 pm and 4-8 pm, €1.50) is opposite the APT office. It is used to host dramatic and musical performances, cultural encounters, international congresses and meetings but happily the three tiers of gilded seating are open to tourists at other times.

Around Noto

Noto Antica

The 15-km drive up to Noto Antica is long and winding through spectacular rocky country with crumbling bridges. The only way up here is by car. It can be biked, but it's a steep climb. Noto Antica is the location of the original town before it was flattened by the earthquake of 1693. There's some good walking through this country and good picnic spots, but it is remote. There is no water or sustenance available and many paths require some bush bashing. However, there are archaeological highlights, including the impressive ramparts of the medieval castle at the entrance and modest necropoli. There is also a Hellenistic gymnasium and a long-abandoned Cappuchin Convent. If you want to stay up here, try **Agriturismo Fattoria Monte Alveria** (☎ 0931-810-183) just past the castle.

Adventures

By Rail

The **Treno Barocco del Val di Noto** operates to Noto. See *Adventures by Rail* in Siracusa for details.

Where to Stay

Accommodations used to be limited in Noto but there are now many B&Bs offering affordable choices right in the historic center. The only real budget choice is the **Hi Hostel Il Castello** (Via Fratelli Bandiera, ☎ 392-415-7899, €) for €15 per person, including breakfast. The closest camping is **Il Forte** at Marzamemi-Spinazza (☎ 0931-841-132) and **S. Lorenzo** at Contrada San Lorenzo (☎ 0931-841-064) near the Vendicari Riserve.

B&Bs

Centro Storico B&B (Corso Vittorio Emanuele 64, ☎ 093-157-3967, www.centro-storico.com, €€-€€€) is a good central choice with elegant spacious rooms, wrought iron bed headboards and private bathrooms.

B&B Meridies (Via Roma 39/41, ☎ 338-954-6548, www.bbmeridies.com) has three rooms and rents scooters, cars and bikes.

B&B Teatro (Piazza XVI Maggio 10, ☎ 0931-838-503, www.bbnoto.com) is right near the Teatro.

Villa Catera Liberty B&B (Via Ferruccio 2, ☎ 338-230-4042, www.villacatera.com, €€) is 50 yards from Porta Reale just after the fontana on the main corso. A kitchen and balcony make this a good choice.

Hotels

Hotel della Ferla (Via A. Gamsci, ☎ 0931-576-007, www.hotelferla.it, €€€€) is on the higher end of the scale. Rooms look out over blossoming gardens. It is part of the Albergabici group, which gives discounts to cyclists.

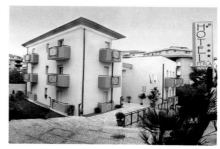

Agriturismo

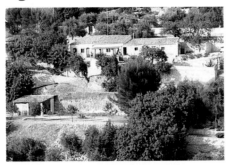

La Suma Sumalia (C. da San Giovanni, ☎ 093-189-4292, www. lasumasumalia.com, €€€) is one km from Noto, set on a hillside overlooking a valley with almonds, olives and carob trees. The building was an old rural mansion and has been refurnished. The terrace offers fine views and is the ideal place to relax for breakfast.

Where to Eat

Noto offers some great locations and excellent prices.

Il Giglio (Piazza Municipio 8-10, ☎ 093-183-8640, fax ☎ 093-183-7973, €) has one of the best locations in town opposite the Cathedral. Ask to sit outside for a view of the piazza or enjoy the pictures of Noto on the walls inside. Tourist menus €8. Finish off your meal by wandering down the stairs outside to **Gelateria Costanzo** (Via Silvio Spaventa 7-11) for dessert.

Ristorante Il Barrocco (Via Cavour Ronco S. Gadari, ☎ 093-183-5999, €) is another good option housed in old 17th-century stables. Tourist menus €8. The seafood is notable and you can read the messages of previous guests on the walls.

Trattoria Al Buco (Via Zanardelli 1, ☎ 093-183-8142, closed Sun, €) near Porta Reale is another inexpensive option. Tourist menus €8, plates from €5.

Trattoria Giufa (Vico Pisacane 3, ☎ 320-487-7456, 329-732-5431, closed Wed, €€), in a narrow lane way halfway down the Corso, makes fresh pasta and serves seafood dishes.

Neas Ristorante (Via Rocco Pirri 30, ☎/fax 093-157-3538) specializes in marine food cooked Sicilian-style.

Caffe Sicilia (Corso Emanuele 125), right near the Duomo, has the best views of the church, with refreshing *granite*, cactus pear jam and *gelato* mixes like jasmine flower and orange.

Bar Penguino (Corso Emanuele 135) is another good option for snacks, gelati and coffee.

Bar La Vecchia Fontana (Corso Emanuele 150 , ☎ 338-230-4042) is popular for evening drinks with a good choice of cocktails and granite.

★★Riserva Naturale di Vendicari

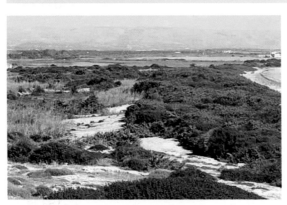

This beautiful natural oasis on the coast south of Noto is a stunning wetlands reserve made up of three separate marshes and a splendid sandy beach. If you are spending any time in the south you should get here. Entry to the reserve is free (open 8 am-10 pm), but you do pay for parking, usually €5 for a motorhome, €2 for a car and €1 for a motorbike depending on what entrance you go to. There are three entrances, one near Eloro, the second from Agriturismo Roveto and the third near the village of San Lorenzo. Caruso runs a bus from Noto to Eloro Marina, a short distance from the northernmost perimeter of the reserve and SAIS buses (Noto-Pachino) can stop at the Roveto.

A walking track runs the whole length of the Riserva – you can get a map at the main entrance. From Cittadella (San Lorenzo) in the south, it's 7.7 km (two hrs) to the Roveto entrance and another 11.8 km (three hrs 20 mins) to Eloro. The tracks are well signposted and even the plants are named. If you have limited time, use the main entrance at Roveto, passing the birdwatchers' lagoons to the 15th-century *tonnara* and the picturesque **Torre Vendicari**, one of the numerous defensive towers on the southerly coastline. There's a lookout point over the **Pantano Piccolo lake**, often alive with jumping fish, and the cove of **Calamosche**, where you can swim. If you still have time, continue on to **Eloro**. To the south of the main entrance are more lagoons and the remains of the curious Trigona church marked as **Torre Cittadella**. The site

was once a Byzantine-era settlement dating to the fourth and fifth century. Birds are most plentiful during the migration period (October-November or Febuary-March). In autumn, the lakes are full, while in summer they can tend to be very dry.

Where to Stay

Azienda Agrituristica San Lorenzo (San Lorenzo, ☎ 084-1064, fax 0932-9423-9652, €) is open year-round and within walking distance of the southern entrance to the Vendicari Reserve. It is family-run and is currently camping-only, although there are plans to prepare on-site caravans for €20 each. Camping is currently €10/€12 in low/high season. Outdoor cooking facilities are available in the pleasant garden or ask in advance for a half- or full pensione. If you don't have a car call ahead for a pick-up from Pachino.

Agriturismo Tenuta Arangio Vendicari (C. da San Lorenzo, ☎ 0931-599-092, www.vendicari-agriturismo.com, €€) is three km from the reserve entrance. It's literally a blue oasis like something on a Greek island.

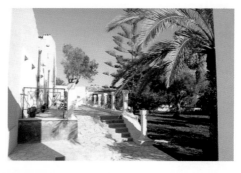

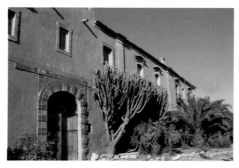

★**Agriturismo Roveto** (Contrada Roveto, Vendicari, ☎ 0931-66024, www.roveto.it, €€€) is a handsome choice right near the central entrance to the reserve. Dating from 1762, the rustic farmhouse on 140 acres has been restored with old barns and lodgings now used for doubles (€65), quads (€85) and self-contained apartments. The restaurant uses home-grown produce like oil, vegetables

and fruits and home-made fresh pasta. They can arrange horseback riding, tennis and other excursions.

Agriturismo Calamosche (Spiaggia Calamosche Noto, ☎ 347-858-7319, www.parcheggiocalamosche.com, €€) is at the northern entrance to the reserve, only 10 km from Noto and part of the Albergabici

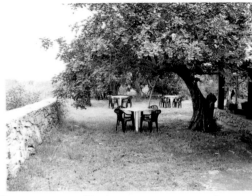

system, offering a discount to cyclists.

Where to Eat

There are a few options for eating in San Lorenzo, including **Residence Le Onde Bar and Restaurant** (☎ 093-184-1112), **Pizzeria San Lorenzo** on the road to Marzamemi and a small *alimentari* near the Camping San Lorenzo.

Marzamemi

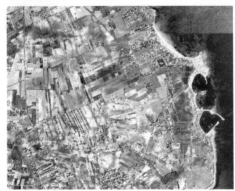

Aerial view of Marzamemi

The southern corner of Sicily has a vaguely North-African atmosphere and indeed the town of Marzamemi's name rings oddly of of Arabic origins. At first glance it appears nothing more than a rather low-key resort or fishing port, and if you arrive at the wrong time of day or on a Tuesday (when many shops close) it can seem almost like a ghost town. But on summer evenings there can be a really active nightlife and the friendly population is bound to invite

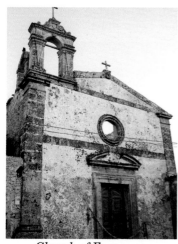
Church of Francesco

you along to something. In summer the town hosts a film festival and bars sing until the dawn breaks.

There's a faintly fishy smell in Marzamemi, not surprising as the whole town is right on the sea, but particularly down at the port. There's a 17th-century *tonnara* (fish processing factory) here with a couple of rustic bars and pizzerias, where someone's usually having a quiet drink or a game of cards. In Piazza Regina Magherita is the old **church of Francesco** built by the Princes of Villadorata, some fantastically derelict doorways and another great bar and restaurant.

Information Sources

In late July or August every year the international festival **Cinema del Frontiera** (www.cinemadifrontiera.it) is held in the town square.

Il Paguro (c/da Porto Fossa, Marzamemi, ☎ 338-541-8373, www.ilpaguro.it) is a scuba center offering dive courses and excursions to warships and relics. Snorkeling is from €15/ €40 for half/full days, diving from €25/€45 for short/day-long submersions.

Getting Here & Around

Marzamemi is out on a limb in terms of public transport. There are two bus connections to Portopallo every day that leave from the school at 8 am and 3 pm. From there, you can travel on to other places in the province (see *Portopalo*).

Drago Mar (Via dei Mille 125, Pachino, ☎ 0931-594-454, www.dragomar.sr.it) offers boat itineraries from Marzamemi to Vendicari or to Isola di Capo Passero, Isola delle Correnti and Spiaggia Granelli.

Where to Stay

 Camping Forte Village (Contrada Spinazza, ☎ 0931-841-011, www.fortevillage.net) is on the road north to San Lorenzo. The unusually shaped **Hotel Celeste** (Viale del Lido 7, ☎ 0931-841-244), near the port, and **Hotel Conchiglietta** (Via Regina Elena 9, ☎ 0931-841-191), on Lungomare, are the hotel options. Both have restaurants.

Where to Eat

 For such a small town, there is a surprising choice of places to eat. For snacks try **Via Regina Elena**. There's **Stuzzco**, selling panini, cheese, salami and snacks. **Crêpes Maria** (Via Regina Elena 28, open from 8 to late, closed Tues) is

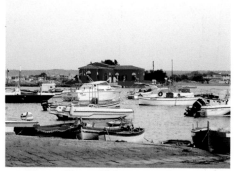
Port of Marzamemi

a pub on the other side of the street with crêpes and bruschetta. It is usually open very late, until about 6 am in summer.

Cialoma Bar (Piazza Regna Margherita, 7 am-5 am) is a good place to get a glass of *vino*, *granita* or *cremolata di frutta* at sunset.

Giramapao (Via Marzamemi 77, ☎ 0931-841-149, www. giramapao.it, closed Mon, €€-€€€) is a popular spot for a pizza and widely recommended by locals.

Down at the fishing port is **Bar La Balata**, with a café/bar and game room, as wll as Pizzeria La Balata serving pizza at night in a rustic atmosphere with a wood-fire oven. It's atmospheric to say the least. **Taverna La Cialoma** (Piazza Regina Margherita 23, 7:30 am-2:30 pm and 7-1 am, closed Tues) is in the church piazza – a great place to try fresh fish and regional plates.

L'Aquario, near La Conchiglietta (Via Jonio, closed Mon), is also recommended.

Portopalo

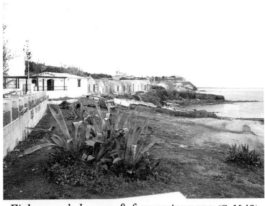

Fishermen's houses & former tonnara (G. Melfi)

Portopalo is the southern most town in Sicily. It's a lot more lively than Marzamemi with several bars, hotels and an active fishing and boating life. There are two islands in the town's vicinity. The **Isola di Capo Passero** has a 17th-century castle, **Il Castello Fortezza di Carlo V**, and you can get over there by a boat or fishing tour or persuade someone to row you over. Locals say you can swim to the island in summer. There are plans to make the castle into a museum by 2007. You can see the island from the Piazza Terrazza dei Due Mare. The **Isola delle Correnti** is Sicily's southernmost point just a km or two out of town and part of a pleasant walking itinerary (see *Adventures on Foot*).

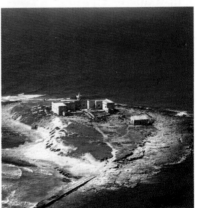

Isola delle Correnti

About one km north of the town towards Pachino is a picturesque 17th-century ★*tonnara* or fish processing facility (Via Tonnara SP Marzamemi-Portopalo, ☎/fax 093-184-4333, open 9 am-7 pm) beautifully located on the sea from where you can see Noto on a clear day. The *tonnara* has been decked out with statues, nets, ropes, towers and Greek-style columns among its crumbling ruins. There is a chapel, diving center inside (see *Adventures on Water*) and a restaurant (see *Where to Eat*) open to members only.

Getting Here

 Interbus runs two daily buses from Catania via Avola (Corso V Emanuele), Noto (Via Ppe di Piemonte) and Pachino (Via Unita) to Portopallo (Via Tasca) at 9 am and 2 pm. One weekday service at 1:35 pm leaves Siracusa for Portopalo. Three services through Avola (via Noto and Pachino) run direct to Portopalo.

Information Sources

 Associazione Proloco Portopalo di Capo Passero (Via F. Garrano 9, www.prolocoportopalo. org).

Events

The **Portopalo Film Festival** (www.cortopalo.it) is held in October every year, with the program starting about 9 pm every night in the Piazza Terrazza dei Due Mare, featuring regional and national artists. The other major event is the **Palio del Mare** (August 12-14), with boat races.

Adventures

On Foot

 ★**Isola delle Correnti** is Sicily's southernmost tip. There's nothing between here and Africa except boats of illegal immigrants! It's not strictly an island as it is still joined to land by a submerged neck or eroding causeway. It can be reached by half-walking and half-wading at low tide. Do not attempt it at high tide when currents can make it more dangerous. The island is tiny and you can complete the cross-ing and explora-tion in under an hour. There's an old lighthouse and outhouses but it's usually deserted, except for the occasional fisherman, wild rabbits and plants. During the summer

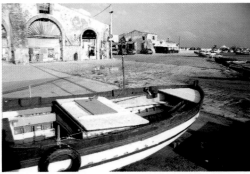

Portopallo (Joanne Lane)

months you can join other tourists in a mud bath on the island. The island is six km south of Portopalo, an uninteresting route on tarmac with little traffic for hitchhiking. There is no public transport.

On Bikes

Free Biking (Via N. Costa 60, ☎ 093-184-4329, 338-941-8266) rents bikes and scooters.

On & Under Water

Contact **Gabriele** from the Gabriele Hotel for **fishing** excursions (☎ 0931-842-701).

Tre Anelli (Via V. Emanuele 88, ☎/fax 093-184-2026, www.treanellisport.it) rents **diving, snorkeling and fishing** equipment.

El Cachalote is the **diving** center inside the Tonnara di Portopalo (☎/fax 0931-844-333, 334-317-9341, www. elcachalote.com). The center is open year-round and arranges excursions above and below the water, with night dives followed by snacks and music. They offer snorkeling and diving courses and group packages. Trips can take in a war plane, war ship, salt ship, Spanish galleon, caves and coves around the *tonnara*.

Cabana & Nabana (Isole delle Correnti, ☎ 338-322-5319, 333-625-7910, www.cabananabana.it) is a long stretch of **beach** right near the campsite where you can rent pedal boats, canoes, windsurf, surfboards and sailing boats. The center is open from June to September.

Surfing and windsurfing at Portopalo is favorable when the *Sirocco* (from Africa), *Grecale* (from the Balkans and Greece) or *Tramontana* winds hit Portopalo. During the Sirocco the best areas are **Porto Pescherecci**, the beach near **Carratois** and **l'Isola delle Correnti**. During *Grecale* or *Tramontana* winds, **Morghella** or **Scalo Mandrie** are preferable locations. You can get equipment or information from **Pensione Scala** (Via Carducci 6, opposite Albergo Perseo, ☎ 0931-784-2701, www.pensionescala.com).

Where to Stay

Camping Captain (Isola delle Correnti, Portopallo di Capo Passero, ☎ 0931-842-595, www. campingcaptain.it, €) is on the southernmost point of

Sicily in front of the Isola delle Correnti. It's basically the last dunes of Europe before the waters leading to Africa and is unparalleled for views. To get here follow signs to the Isola delle Correnti, and turn left at a small shop two km out of town.

Gabriele Hotel (Via Europa 36, ☎ 0931-844-159, www.gabriele-hotel. com, €€¥€€i) is run by a friendly family and named after its owner. You'll probably spot Gabriele in his beret in a bar before you get to the hotel. The family arranges surfing, fishing and other itineraries.

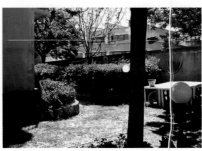
Gabriele Hotel garden

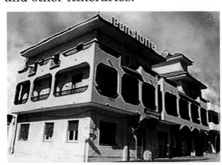
Pensione Scala

Pensione Scala (Via Carducci 6, opposite Albergo Perseo, ☎ 0931-784-2701, www.pensionescala.com, €€-€€€) is run by the same family as the Gabriele Hotel. The modern building is just out of the epicenter, with sea views from the balconies and rooftop.

Where to Eat

The choice place to eat in Portopalo is at the *tonnara* (12:30-2:30 pm, 8-10:30 pm) if you can convince them to serve non-members or at least a drink. Book first.

There are a number of bars in the main street, including the popular **Bar Blu** and **Caprice**, opposite each other in the main street. The **Koala Bar** (Via Carducci 17, ☎ 0931-843-170) is also popular for coffee and snacks.

Da Mauri (Via Tagliamento 22, ☎ 0931-842-644) is highly rated by locals for its fine food.

Ristorante Al Faro da Corrado (Via Emanuele 205, ☎ 0931-842-772, closed Mon) serves fish specialties near the port. **Tavernetta del Porto la Giara** (ContradaPorto, ☎ 0931-843-217) is right at the port with sea and boat views.

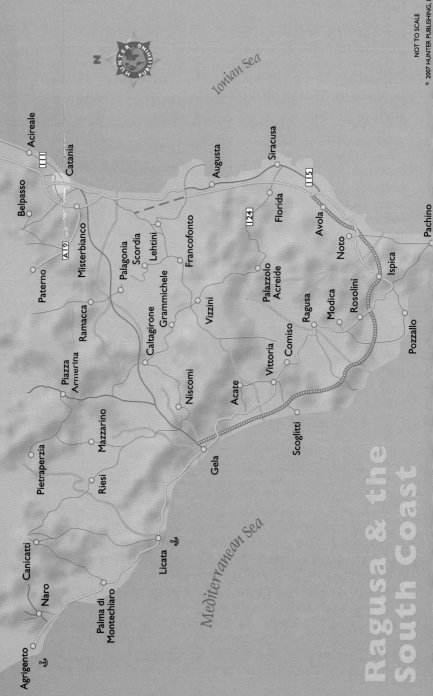

Ragusa & the
South Coast

NOT TO SCALE

© 2007 HUNTER PUBLISHING, INC

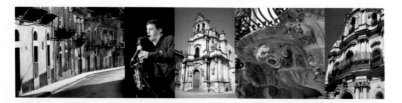

Ragusa & the Southeast

The province of Ragusa is notable for its pockets of Baroque grandeur in **Ragusa** (the capital of the same name), **Modica** to the south, **Comiso** and **Vittoria** to the west, and **Scicli** and **Ispica** nearer the coast. The bare hills and deep valleys of the region, known as the Iblei, are varied and change depending on the seasons, making for inter-

esting country excursions by foot, bike or horseback. Drystone walls and stone *masserie* (homesteads) are also a feature of Ragusa – a characteristic that developed in the 17th and 18th centuries as the land was cleared of stones for cultivation. The **Cava d'Ispica** is one of the great geographical formations in this region, a gorge lined with rock-cut tombs like the country-side around Chiaramonte Gulfi. The Ragusan coast has pleasant holiday towns, a few ancient sites and good beaches.

RAGUSA HIGHLIGHTS

- **Ragusa Ibla**: Climbing the torturously steep streets in this Baroque hamlet.
- **Montalbano locations**: The southeast corner of Sicily is where the famed TV detective series *Montalbano* was filmed.
- **Chiaramonte Gulfi's "balcony"** over Sicily.
- The stunning walk through **Cava d'Ispica**.
- Listening to Vittoria's jazz sensation **Francesco Cafiso**.
- Modica's famed **spicy chocolate**.

■ Ragusa

Like other towns in southern Sicily, the old town of **Ragusa Ibla** was flattened by the 1693 earthquake and rebuilt in planned Baroque style above the original settlement. However, unlike Noto, the old town was also rebuilt, creating a curious mix of medieval and Baroque. Rivalry developed between the two towns and lasted until 1926 when they were united. However, the unification served only as an impetus to move all business and industry to the new Ragusa, leaving Ragusa Ibla depopulated. Today Ragusa Ibla is still where most of the sights are and where tourists want to spend their time. It's also one of my favorite places in Sicily and a good base for seeing the region.

Getting Here

All transport arrives in the new town. Buses stop outside the train station in Piazza del Popolo. **Interbus** connects Ragusa with Catania (€6.60, two hours). **AST** (☎ 0931-46271) has connections with Siracusa, Gela, Vittoria, Modica, Palermo and Chiaramonte Golfi. Schedules are posted on the wall by the bus park.

The following bus lines link Ragusa to the rest of the province:

COMPANY	PHONE	ROUTES
Tumino	☎ 0932-623-184, 0932-651-967	Ragusa, Marina di Ragusa, Villaggio Gesuiti, Casuzze, Punta Secca, SC Camerina, Kamarina
		Ragusa, S. Croce Camerina, Punta Braccetto, Punta Secca, Casuzze, Marina di Ragusa
		Ragusa, Cda 100 Pozzi, Bivio Donnafugata, S Croce Camerina, Kamarina
AST	☎ 0932-681-818, 0932-752-538	Ragusa to Ragusa Ibla
Etna Trasporti	☎ 0932-623-440, 095-532-716	Marina di Ragusa, S Croce Camerina, Ragusa, Coffa, Aeroporto, Catania
		Ragusa, Giarratana, Monterosso Almo, Vizzini, Francoforte, Lentini, Catania
Giamporcaro	☎ 0932-981-632, 0932-869-612	Vittoria, Comiso, Ragusa

		Vittoria, Comiso, S. Croce Camerina, Marina di Ragusa
SAIS	☎ 0932-623-440, 0935-524-111, 091-704-1211, 095-536-168	Vittoria, Comiso, S. Croce Camerina, Marina di Ragusa and further afield to Catania, Messina and Florence
		Ragusa, Pisa (Fri & Sun 3:45 pm)
SIMILI	☎ 0933-981-894, 0933-981-251	Modica, Ragusa, Annunziata, Castiglione
OMNIA	☎ 092-259-6490	Ragusa, Gela, Agrigento
SENA	☎ 0932-623-440	Ragusa, Bologna (Tues & Sun 7:45 pm)

There is a train station that connects Ragusa with the western coast towards Gela, Agrigento and beyond. Trains are useful for short journeys to Modica (20 mins), Ispica (one hour), Noto (1½ hours). However, buses are generally considered the best option for getting around on the eastern coast and, if you're traveling farther afield, the quickest option is a bus to Catania (two hours), then journey on from there.

The **Treno Barocco del Val di Noto** historical train also passes through Ragusa (see *Adventures by Rail*). Traveling by car to Ragusa takes you through some splendid countryside, especially from Comiso. You'll have a lot of fun negotiating Ragusa Ibla's narrow streets.

Getting Around

Local buses are operated by **AST** and tickets cost €0. 85. Buses 1 and 3 run from outside the Ragusa train station in Piazza del Popolo up to Giardino Ibleo in Ragusa Ibla three times hourly during the week and hourly on Sunday.

You can rent a car for just €25 per day from **Pluchino**, Via M Rapisardi 80, ☎ 0932-621-687 in Ragusa's new town.

Information Sources

The information offices are both in Ragusa Ibla. There's the **Pro Loco** (Largo Camerina 5, ☎ 0932-124-4473, Tues-Sat 10:30 am-12:30 pm and 4-9 pm, Sun 10:30 am-12:30 pm, www.prolocoragusa.it) and the very

helpful **AAPIT Ragusa** (Via Capitano Bocchieri 33, ☎ 0932-221-511, www.ragusaturismo.it, Mon-Fri 9 am-2:30 pm).

Local guides include:

- **Dr Francisco Cannt** (☎ 338-767-774) and **Dr Tumino Simone** (☎ 338-422-3237), who run group tours and cooking courses.

- **Ragusani Volanti** (www.ragusanivolanti.it) is a group of passionate cyclists from Ragusa who do mountain bike trails around Ragusa.

- **Club Green Bike** (☎ 338-749-6406, www.greenbiker. com) can accompany cyclists on routes around the province. Or see their online itineraries for Ragusa, Modica, Chiramonte Gulfi and Monti Iblei.

See *Adventures on Wheels* for more details.

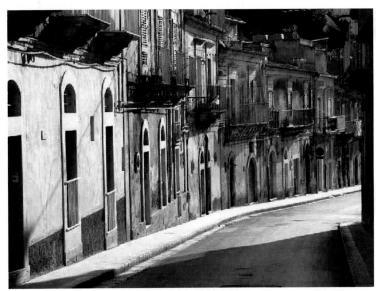

Street in Ragusa

Sightseeing

The Upper Town

All transport drops you in the new town in Piazza del Popolo. From here walk straight down Viale Tenente Lena through Piazza della Liberta across the Ponte Nuovo bridge spanning

the ridge. Most of the sights are on the other side of Ponte Nuovo, also marked as Ponte Pennavaria on maps. The parallel Ponte dei Cappuccini is motor-free and a good place to get a good view of the town. The **Museo Archeologico Ibleo** (Via Natalelli, ☎ 0932-622-963, 9 am-1:30 pm, 4-7:30 pm) is just after Ponte Nuovo, containing finds from prehistoric sites, including the Greek site of Camarina on the coast beyond Punta Braccetto.

The **Duomo di San Giovanni Battista** in Piazza San Giovanni is farther along Via Roma and the liveliest spot in the commercial town, particularly around *passeggiata* time. The Duomo is dedicated to John the Baptist and was finished in 1774.

There isn't a lot else to see in the upper town, although it does have its fair share of elegant *palazzi*. If you have limited time, head straight for Corso Italia and Via XXIV Maggio. From the terrace of the 15th-century church **Santa Maria delle Scale**, or at other places along the stairs below it, you get a phenomenal view of Ragusa Ibla. If you're ascending from Ragusa Ibla, make sure you look behind you! From the terrace, you can see the layers of streets, houses and churches all piled on top of each other atop the outcrop of rock on which the town perches. It's one of the most glorious town views in Sicily!

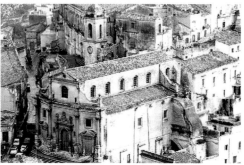

Santa Maria delle Scale

★★★Ragusa Ibla

A UNESCO World Heritage site, Ragusa Ibla is a fabulous town with tortuously steep, narrow streets where you have to breathe in just to pass another vehicle or person. Every step feels like it's either up or down but every twist and turn of the many narrow streets also hints of another church or piazza to marvel at, a secluded restaurant, a fantastic Baroque man-

Following page: Ragusa Ibla (Joanne Lane)

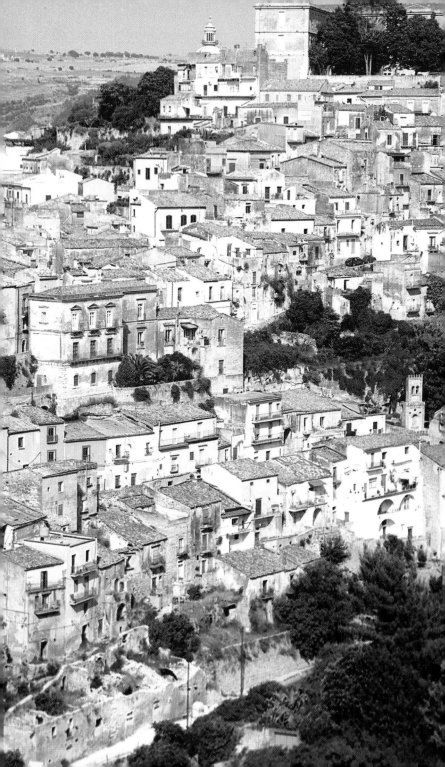

sion or quiet garden. If you're entering the town via Santa Maria della Scala keep descending on foot past the Chiesa del Purgatorio, now reopened after restoration. There is a pleasant piazza here and a good café/bar for evening life. Head into the set of narrow streets beyond the church and you'll eventually hit the sloping, palm-lined ★**Piazza del Duomo** and ★★**Cattedrale di San Giorgio**. Fans of Montalbano should immediately recognize the church and piazza. The

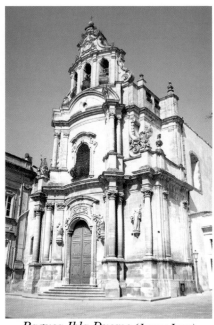

Ragusa Ibla Duomo (Joanne Lane)

Ragusa & the Southeastern

Duomo was built in 1744 by Rosario Gagliardi, who took nearly 40 years to complete it. The three-tiered façade is considered a Sicilian Baroque masterpieces. If you're just passing

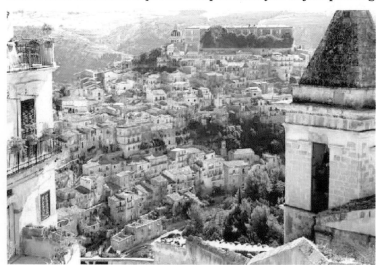

Looking down on Ragusa

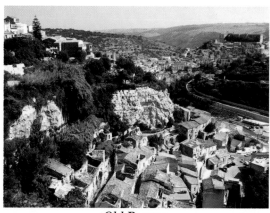

Old Ragusa

through, you could come to Ragusa Ibla for this church and piazza alone.

If you like Gagliardi's work, have a look at the façade and balconies of the **Chiesa di San Giuseppe** in Piazza Pola to the east of Piazza del Duomo on Corso XXV Aprile. Continue away from the Piazza del Duomo to the eastern end of town and the Giardino Ibleo (8 am-8 pm). This is a peaceful corner with flowerbeds, picnic spots, medieval churches and fountains. The other thing to do here is to wander, making sure you stroll down Via del Mercato at some point to look out over the valley below.

Adventures

On Foot

Follow the route described between Ragusa and Ragusa Ibla in *Sightseeing*. It is best attempted descending from the upper town to Ragusa Ibla. It takes 40-50 minutes from Corso Italia to Piazza del Duomo.

See *Adventures on Wheels* for joint walking/biking routes from the Eremo della Giubiliana.

On Wheels

The countryside surrounding Ragusa is fabulous for mountain biking. **Club Green Bike** (☎ 0932-644-449, 338-749-6406, www.greenbikerg.com) rents bikes (€13 per day) and lists numerous itineraries on their website Their routes take in the area around Ragusa and the wider province, and also to Mt Etna and Nebrodi. They recommend the **Cava Misericordia** near Ragusa Ibla, **Il Bosco di**

Calaforno, Il Bosco di Canalazzo and **I Boschi di Chiaramonte Gulfi**.

Ragusani Volanti (www.ragusanivolanti.it) is another cycling group from Ragusa with similar route suggestions. Contact them for details.

The **Eremo della Giubiliana** (see *Where to Stay*) is the start of a number of bike and walking routes that are indicated with a small white sign containing the direction, the route and the red turret (the symbol of the Eremo). Bikes are provided free of charge for guests. If you are cycling from Ragusa, follow signs to Marina di Ragusa. The Eremo is indicated on your right-hand side about seven km out of town.

ROUTE	TIME	DIFFICULTY	SIGHTS
1 - Eremo – Torre Renna	40 minutes walking, 15 minutes biking	easy	Renna Cave, necropolis, Renna fountain and tower of the 15th and 16th century
2 - Eremo – Villa Pozzilo	40 minutes walking, 20 minutes biking	easy	A typical 18th-century farm, views over the Irminio River Valley and southeastern coast
3 - Eremo – Castello di Donnafugata	5 hours walking, 2 hours biking	hard	Typical 18th-century farms, paths and caves of naturalistic interest, Donnafugata castle (see *Donnafugata* later in this chapter)
4 - Eremo – Zinnafondo – Cavalusi – Minnulidi – Torre Renna	3 hours walking	hard	Typical 18th-century farms, Cavalusi cave and fountain, paths and caves of naturalistic interest, 16th-century water fountain of Renna Tower
5 - Eremo – Pozzillo & Pozzillo di Sotto	1 hour 40 mins walking, 20 minutes biking	easy	Typical 18th-century farms, Royal Borbons paths, Nifosi Villa, view of the Irminio River Valley and southeastern coast
6 - Eremo – Irminio Valley, private beach and nature reserve	4 hours walking, 1 hour biking	medium	Typical 18th-century farms, Royal Borbons paths, view of the Irminio River valley and southeastern coast, private beach, tides and dunes and the natural reserve of the Irminio river

On Horseback

 The **Eremo della Giubiliana** (see *Where to Stay*) has horseback riding for guests around the farmland surrounding it. Routes pass old masserie (homesteads) and plenty of the drystone walls common in the region.

In the Air

 The **Eremo della Giubiliana** (see above) has its own airfield and offers scenic flying tours in a Cessna of the southeast and other parts of Sicily like Etna, the islands and even into north Africa.

By Rail

 The **Treno Barocco del Val di Noto** is a historical train driven by an old steam engine that operates on summer weekends linking historic towns in the southeast Baroque region. The train runs from the end of June until late September with two itineraries, one from Siracusa to Noto, Modica and back; another from Siracusa to Ragusa, Scicli and back to Siracusa. Tickets are €20. For more information, contact the Treno Barocco office (Via dei Lilla 76, Scicli, ☎ 0932-832-458, www.trenobarocco.it). The Siracusa Welcome Card gives a 10% discount on this service.

ITINERARY A			
	Siracusa	**Noto**	**Modica**	**Siracusa**
Arrival		10:20 am	3:55 pm	8:15 pm
Departure	9:25 am	2:20 pm	6:20 pm	
ITINERARY B			
	Siracusa	**Ragusa**	**Scicli**	**Siracusa**
Arrival		12:05 pm	4:55 pm	8:15 pm
Departure	9:25 am	4 pm	6:30 pm	

Where to Stay

Hotels

 In Ragusa Ibla the choice place to stay is ★**Locanda Don Serafino** (Via XI Febbraio 15, Ragusa Ibla, ☎ 093-222-0065, fax 093-266-3186, www.

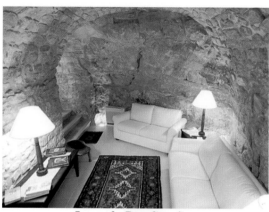

Locanda Don Serafino

locandadonserafino.it, €€€€), with unique rooms excavated out of the rock. The family owns a fabulous restaurant of the same name.

Il Barocco (Via Santa Maria La Nuova 1, Ragusa Ibla,

Ragusa & the Southeastern

☎ 0932-663-105, www.ilbarocco.it, €€€-€€€€) is in an 18th-century building once used as a horse manger and carpenter's workshop.

The **Jonio** (Via Risorgimento 49, ☎ 0932-624-322) is conveniently

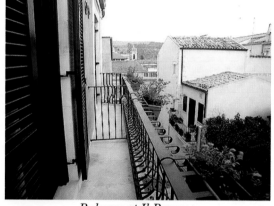

Balcony at Il Barocco

located near the train station.

Mediterraneo Palace (Via Roma 189, ☎ 0932-621-944), near the museum, is a Best Western with features typical of the chain.

B&Bs

The well located **Le Fioriere B&B**, (Maria Paterno Arezzo 104, Angolo Piazza Duomo, Ragusa Ibla, ☎ 0932-621-530, www.bblefioriere.it, €€€) has two triples.

HOTEL PRICE CHART	
€	Up to €25 per day
€€	€26-€55
€€€	€56-€85
€€€€	Over €85

From the bedrooms of **All'Idria B&B** (Corso Mazzini 159/b, ☎ 0932-651-418, www.bedandbreakfastallidria.it, €€) you get a view of the cupola of the Duomo of San Giorgio.

Il Cantuccio B&B (Via A. Oriani 15/a, ☎ 0932-641-869, vivianalatona@virgilio.it).

Il Giardino dei Sospiri (Via dei Sospiri 24, ☎ 093-265-1418, www.ilgiardinodeisospiri.it, €€) is 150 feet from the legendary 13th-century Chiaramonte castle. These are among Ragusa's most economical rooms.

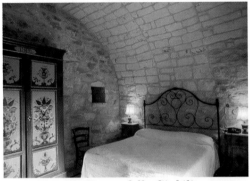
Room in Eremo della Giubiliana

Just outside of town is the ★**Eremo della Giubiliana** (C. da Giubiliana SP per Marina di Ragusa 7½ km, ☎ 093-266-9119, fax 093-266-9129, www.eremodella-giubiliana.it), a renovated, fortified house owned and managed by a noble Sicilian family. Tower suites and rooms with antique furnishings from the family's history provide a unique setting.

Where to Eat

All these listings are in the old town, which is the most atmospheric place to eat.

★★The **Locanda Don Serafino** (39 Via Orfanotrofio, ☎ 0932-248-778, €€€€), run by the same family as the hotel, is a gastronomical experi-

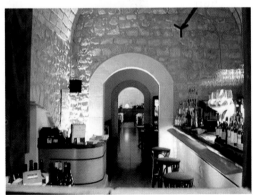
The restaurant in Locanda Don Serafino

ence. The dishes are immacu-
lately presented, featuring
local produce. In the evening
they light candles at little tables in the streets under
flowering trees. A full meal
costs €50. The family heads
a group calle Le Soste di
Ulisse (www.lesostediulisse.
it), which includes great eating places around Sicily.

DINING PRICE CHART	
Price per person for an entrée, including house wine.	
€	Up to €12
€€	€13-€25
€€€	€26-€35
€€€€	Over €35

Duomo (Via Capitano Bocchieri 31, ☎ 0923-651-265, www.
ristoranteduomo.it, closed Monday and Sunday night) is a
strong rival for taste and style and part of the same group
above.

Trattoria La Rusticana (Corso XXV Aprile 68, Piazza Pola,
☎0932-227-981, €€) appears regularly in the Italian TV series, *Inspector Montalbano*, as the detective's favorite eatery.

**Ristorante Il Bar-
occo** (Via Orfano-
trofio 29, ☎ 0932-652-
397, www.ilbarocco.
it), with a hotel of the
same name, is run by
the Cabibbo brothers
and a favorite for
Ragusan dishes. Also
try their traditional
sweets and gelati at
the **Gelateria Il
Barocco** (Largo S.
Domenico, Angelo Via Giardini, ☎ 0932-246-149, closed Mon).

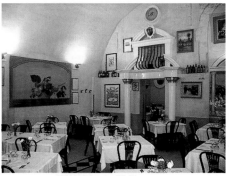

Ristorante Il Barocco

There are a number of bars and cafés below the Duomo on
Piazza San Giovanni including the swish Caffe Italia.

At **Creperia Antoci** (Via Risorgimento 13), pick up a sweet
or savory crêpe for as little as €1.40-€3.40. The crêpes are almost like pizzas, with mozzarella, tomato and basil toppings.

One of Ragusa's notable culinary products is *le focacce di
ricotta e salsiccia*, warm bread filled with ricotta and spicy
sausage. Delicious. Try it at **S. Giorgio Forno-Biscotteria**
(Corso XXV Aprile 84, ☎ 0932-652-489).

Ragusa & the Southeastern

The other Ragusan favorite is *caciocavallo ragusano*, a tasty cheese formed into a parallel-piped shape made from Modica cow's milk and used for *antipasti* and desserts. It can be sweet or spicy and is often used in Ragusan restaurants.

■ Marina di Ragusa

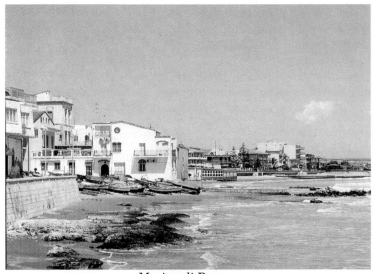

Marina di Ragusa

This beachfront town, 24 km from Ragusa, is packed in summer, particularly August, but is quiet and pleasant at other times of year. There is a tourist office in Piazza Duca degli Abruzzi 8 (9 am-1 pm and 3-10 pm in summer, 9 am-12 pm and 3-9 pm winter). **Tuminio** (☎ 0932-623-184) and **Etna Trasporti** (☎ 0932-623-440) connect it with Ragusa. **SAIS** (☎ 0932-623-440) and **Giamoporcaro** (☎ 0932-988-300) connect with Vittoria, Comiso and S. Croce Camerina.

During high season, you'll find food everywhere in Piazza Duca degli Abruzzi, where bars and restaurants crowd the square. **Pizzeria di Serafino** (Lungomare Andrea Doria, ☎ 0932-239-522) is owned by the same family that owns the classy Locanda Don Serafino Hotel in Ragusa Ibla and considered the seafood choice of the town.

There's a campground on Lungomare Andrea Doria called **Baia del Sole** (☎ 0932-230-344, www.baiadelsole.it). It's a km or two out of town but there's eating nearby.

■ Modica

Modica lies 30 km south-west of Noto and 10 km south of Ragusa. Like its neighbours, Modica has the same elegant Baroque buildings that rival Ragusa for charm, an upper and lower town, magnificent churches – it's been described as the city of 100 bells and 100 churches – and it's another good base for travelling around the region. You could happily spend a half-day here in the UNESCO World Heritage Site. Highlights include the fantastic Chiesa di San Giorgio and the exquisite Modican chocolate.

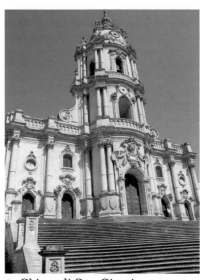

Chiesa di San Giorgio (G. Melfi)

Getting Here

Buses pull in at Piazzale Falcone Borsellino on Corso Umberto at the opposite end from the train station. You can get tickets and timetables from Bar Centro opposite or Café Sicilia (2 Corso Umberto I). **SAIS** goes to Ragusa, Comiso, Catania, Messina and Rome; **SITA** to Perugia, Siena, Florence, Pisa, La Spezia, Geneva and Bologna. **AST** (☎ 0932-752-538) connects Modica with Donnalucata, Acate, Avola, Ispica, Pachino, Palermo, Pedalino, Rosolini, Sciicli, Pozzallo, Chiaramonte, Noto and Siracusa. There are direct departures for Catania and its Fontanerossa airport daily from Modica Bassa.

The train line also connects Modica with the rest of the island, although bus travel is generally faster. The **Treno Barocco del Val di Noto** historical train arrives in Modica. See *Adventures by Rail*.

Ragusa & the Southeastern

Information Sources

Tourist offices include the **APT** (149 Corso Umberto I, ☎ 0932-753-324) and the **Pro Loco Modica** (Via de Leva 3, ☎ 0932-905-221, www.prolocomodica.it)

Sightseeing

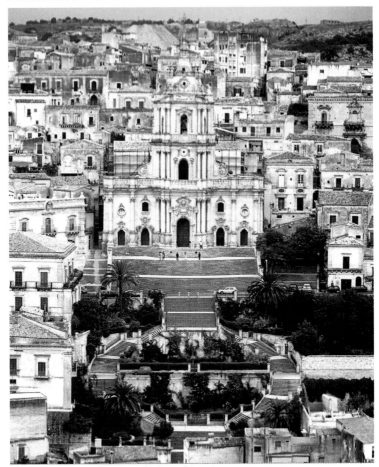

Duomo di San Giorgio (Joanne Lane)

Modica lies in a gorge formed by four hills in the south of the Iblei Mountains. It is divided into the upper town (**Modica Alta**) and the lower town (**Modica Bassa**). Most of the sights

are in Modica Alta. Modica Bassa is traced by Corso Umberto I, along which are a number of churches, including the fine **Duomo di San Pietro**, with imposing statues of the apostles, old *palazzi* and interesting balconies.

Historically, Corso Umberto was a river and Modica was considered the Venice of the South for the many bridges that crossed it. However, after a flood of 1902 the rivers were covered up and Corso Umberto became the main street.

The best place to start in Modica Alta is via the ★★**Duomo di San Giorgio**, about halfway along the Corso, which rivals its namesake in Ragusa Ibla. Actually, few sights match the approach to it up twin staircases of 250 steps, giving you a view over the honey-colored rooftops of the town. The staircases are flanked by gardens, with lawns, fresh lavendar, roses and bougainvillea. The 18th-century façade is attributed to Rosario Gagliardi with his trademark belfry. The interior is enriched by stuccoes and gildings, decorations and paintings.

★MODICAN CHOCOLATE

Modica is famed for its chocolate known as *lolli modicani*. The tradition of chocolate making was brought to Sicily by the Spaniards, who controlled the island from the 13th to 15th centuries. Their tradition was handed down from the Aztecs in Mexico, who drank chocolate liquid and added vanilla, chili pepper, cinnamon, coffee and citrus fruit to their crushed cocoa rather than sugar, making a spicier kind of chocolate. The **Antica Dolceria Bonajuto** (159 Corso Umberto 1, ☎/fax 093-294-1225, www. bonajuto.it) has been making chocolate in Sicily since 1880, when Francesco Bonajuto, following in his fathers footsteps, qpened a small shop producing Arab and Spanish delicacies. Today the shop is still a point of reference for Modican chocolate. Chocolates are no longer made on the premises, but you can taste an array of chocolates and sweets made according to Aztec tradition and the unusual 'Mpanatigghi, a typical Modican biscuit like an empañada combining meat and chocolate – a common Spanish culinary practice!

Eurochocolate is held for a week in March to celebrate chocolate.

Adventures

On Foot

The best viewpoint of Modica is a bit of a walk but worth the effort. Follow Corso Umberto I to the end past the bus station and turn left, following the road to Ragusa. Turn left and follow signs for Belvedere and you'll see views of the town from along the road. It's a good half-hour from the end of the Corso.

I Quattro Colli (four hills) is an easy trekking route of four hours around the four Modican hills, led by **I Tetti di Siciliando B&B** (Via Cannata 24, ☎ 0932-942-843, www.siciliando.it). The B&B provides details on the route for their own guests; otherwise, you can undertake it with a group (maximum price €75).

On Wheels

The countryside around Modica is hilly but spectacular. Rent a bike and head out on your own or contact the following operators for itinerary suggestions.

I Tetti di Siciliando B&B (Via Cannata 24, ☎ 0932-942-843, www.siciliando.it) has four-five mountain bikes for €10/day, or less for several days. They list a lot of itineraries on their website (www.siciliando.it) with varying grades of difficulty. They can also arrange guided tours. Their routes include the *ex-ferrovia* (see *Chiaramonte Gulfi*), Cava d'Ispica (see *Ispica*, *Capra d'Oro* (towards Ragusa Ibla) and the *Fiume Tellesimo* (towards Noto).

Club Green Bike from Ragusa (☎ 0932-644-449, 338-749-6406, www.greenbikerg.com) has bikes for €13/day, but less for longer periods. They are based in Ragusa but also recommend itineraries into the region surrounding Modica (they can also accompany you). If you want to venture out, see their online itineraries of Irminio Valley, Servi Gorge, Magnesi Gorge, Frigitini, Conca del Salto and Ceci-Streppennosa and Piano Ceci-Streppennosa.

By Rail

The **Treno Barocco del Val di Noto** historical train also services Modica. See *Adventures by Rail* in Ragusa for details.

Where to Stay

Modica Bassa

La Terrazze di Modica B&B (Via Mantenga Idria 9, ☎ 0932-941-531, www.laterrazzadimodica.com, €€) has rather plain rooms but scores for its superb location across the valley from Modica. The views of the town are unparalleled, especially from the terrace at night. Follow the signs for Belvedere.

Pineta Monserrato B&B (Via Nazionale 106/120, ☎ 093-294-6908, www.pinetamonserrato.it, €€-€€€) is built into the hillside, made completely from natural stone. There are two separate apartments with kitchens.

Hotel Principe La'Aragon (281 Corso Umberto 1, ☎ 0932-756-041, www.hotelprinicpedaragona.it, €€€€) has simply furnished clean rooms near the bus terminus.

Casalbergo Garibaldi (Via Ritiro, ☎ 0932-751-140, www.casalbergogaribaldi.it, €€€) is in a small alley off the main Corso. Singles, doubles and quads.

Hotel Relais Modica (Via Tommasso Campailla 99, ☎ 093-275-445, www.hotelrelaismodica.it, €€€-€€€€) near the tourist office has spacious rooms and breakfast.

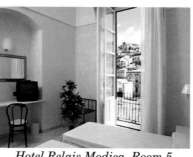
Hotel Relais Modica, Room 5

Modica Alta

B&B Dei Ruta (Via Moncada 9, Modica Alta, ☎ 093-275-5600, www.deiruta.it) is adjacent to San Giorgio and, if you don't mind the pealing of bells, a good place to stay.

I Tetti di Siciliando (Via Cannata 24, ☎ 0932-942-843, www.siciliando.it, €€-€€€) is one of the best choices near the Duomo with fantastic views of the city from its balconies and cheerful, sunny rooms. They are part of the "Cooperative Siciliando," which

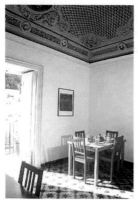
I Tetti di Siciliando

organizes art courses, bike itineraries and excursions through the Ragusa province.

B&B del Duomo (Via San Michele 2/a, ☎ 333-106-54995, paolodd@tiscalinet.it) is adjacent to the Duomo – you can see it from your bedroom windows.

Villa Raineri B&B (Via Caitina 74, ☎/fax 093-290-4777, 339-468-4388, saverinocassone@jumpy.it) has a ninth-century garden with jasmines, almonds, carobs, olives, bagolas and prickly pears. There are two triples and one quad.

★**La Gazza Ladra** (Via Blandini 11, ☎ 0932-755-655, www.palazzofailla.it, €€€€), in a 17th-century building, is a bit of a climb through Modica Alta, but well worth it. There are just seven rooms with original pavements, frescoes and antique furnishings, which have been recently restored. Service is exemplary, with Modican chocolate left on your pillow. There is also a bar, restaurant and café and WiFi Internet connections. A gazza ladra is a bird that steals things – no reflection on the staff.

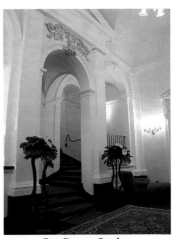

La Gazza Ladra

Where to Eat

 Modica is renowned for its rich culinary tradition (not just chocolate!), reflecting both its Arab and Spanish invaders with a range of sweet and savory dishes. Some dishes you might come across include:

- cavatieddi – fresh pasta dish with a sauce based on pork stew.
- scaccie modicana – a pastry roll stuffed with seasoned cabbage.
- salsiccia di pecora – grilled lamb sausages.
- biancomangiare – a creamy almond dessert.

★**Antica Dolceria Bonajuto** (159, Corso Umberto 1, ☎ 093-294-1225) and **Caffe dell'Arte** (114 Corso Umberto 1, ☎/fax 093-294-3257, www.caffedellarte.it) are the places to come for Modican chocolate and sweets.

For snacks with a view, try the **Bar del Duomo** (Via S. Michele 6, closed Mon, 8 am until late), behind the Duomo, for panini, toast, gelati, rullini. There's also **Pizza Pazza in Piazza** (Pizza Matteotti 3, ☎ 0932-752-407, €€), meaning "mad pizza in the piazza." They serve pizza and panini. **Ideal Pizza** (Via Nazionale 10, ☎ 0932-945-272, €€) has a combination of snacks and meals, with everything from pizza, panini and waffles to *antipasto* and other dishes.

At **Il Cortiletto degli Antichi Sapori Modoceni** (275 Corso Umberto I, ☎ 333-844-0116, closed Mon, €€) you can try specialties such as tripe, lamb and rabbit at economical prices. For something really special, ask for *turciniuna* (sheep bowels) or *mpanata di agnello* (a savory cake or pie made from bread dough and filled with lamb).

Gargantara (Corso Umberto I, ☎ 0932-752-927, closed Mon, €€€€) serves Ibleo food plates but is a little more expensive. Ask for their specialty – cheese with ibleo honey and pear.

La Gazza Ladra (Via Blandini 11, ☎ 0932-755-655, www.palazzofailla.it) is a hotel and restaurant. On Fridays there's a piano bar. The restaurant serves traditional Modican food. The **Café Blandini**, also on the premises, is a good spot for a cocktail, typical liquors and tea/coffee.

Fattoria delle Torri (Vico Napolitano 14, ☎ 0932-751-286, closed Mon, €€€) is a favorite with the locals in Modica Alta.

Taverna Nicastro (Via S. Antonino 28, ☎ 0932-945-884, closed Mon and Sun, €€-€€€) is also recommended by locals and features some of Modica's best home cooking.

■ Ispica

Ispica lies at the head of a wide gorge in the Iblei Mountains. The ★**Cava d'Ispica** is an extravagant gorge near the town stretching for 13 km to the northeast with rock-cut dwellings and tombs scattered along it. Potentially it could make one of the most interesting walking itineraries in the province, though only four or five km of it are navagable from the southeast end near Ispica and about three km from the northeast end. A project is underway to clear the gorge of vegetation, but there is no clear idea when this will be finished.

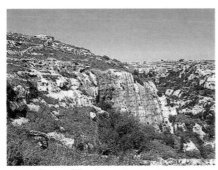

Cava d'Ispica (Affinità Elletive)

The caves in the gorge served as shelter for prehistoric settlers. Inside they had all they needed, with food and water supplies. According to the helpful Pro Loco office on-site (9 am-8 pm summer; Mon-Sat 9 am-1 pm, 3-5 pm, Sun 9 am-1:45 pm winter), 8,000 people visit this site every year, although 2,500 people visited the Cava in August 2006 alone, so the numbers are growing.

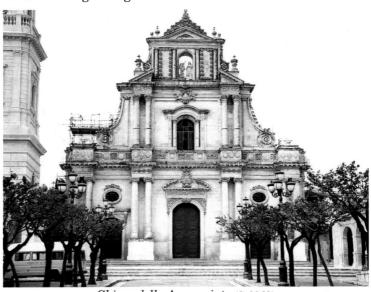

Chiesa della Annunziata (G. Melfi)

From the Pro Loco office in the Forza Park there is an easy 20 minute walking itinerary starting counter-clockwise past the **Marquess' Palace**. This 15th-century site has cobbles and rings outside to tie up horses. It was once considered one of Sicily's most beautiful palaces. Some of the rooms have original tiles; there is also a kitchen with three granaries. Continuing on after the Palace, drop down to the **Chiesa della Annunziata**, also built in the 15th century. There is a great

view into the gorge from near the church. The path turns to the left after the church past several caves used as cemeteries and later modified for stables, storerooms and working areas. These date to a much older period. The Scuderia (main stable) has a long manger on the right wall and archaeologists have found old graffiti on the left wall representing men and horses – if you can make it out you did better than I did! A little museum farther on is closed and appears empty (ask at the Pro Loco office if you want to get in). Outside the museum are the "One Hundred Steps," now closed. They may have once been a well, since at one time a river flowed in the bottom of the valley.

I Tetti di Siciliando (see *Modica - Where to Stay*) offers a biking itinerary through the Cava d'Ispica.

In August, music concerts are held in the park. At other times it's always a good spot for a picnic. Outside the Forza Park beyond the parking lot, a steep slope goes down into the gorge. The interesting little church of **Santa Maria La Cava** down here has a chapel and side altar. Frescoes inside date back to Byzantine times. From here you can walk into the gorge. It is isolated and hot so you won't want to attempt it alone or without water and food supplies.

The other entrance to the Cava di Ispica is six km off the road halfway to Modica. The signage is rather poor but, if you do make it, you'll find most of the gorge is closed while they continue work on repairing tombs and cleaning out the bramble. You can see part of the eerie catacombs for €2.

AST (☎ 0932-681-818, 0932-752-538) buses come here from Donnalucata, Acate, Avola, Pachino, Palermo, Pedalino, Rosolini, Scicli, Pozzallo, Chiaramonte, Modica, Noto and Siracusa. The **Pro Loco** in town is at Corso Umberto 32 (☎ 0932-951-133), although you may get more information from the one at the Forza park. To get to the Forza park follow signs from the main piazza. It's about one or two km out of town.

■ **Pozzallo**

There's not a great deal to do or see in Pozzallo, though it could make a useful base for visiting the region, with a smattering of hotels and campgrounds. It is also the place to get ferries for Malta that leave year-round from the port. Tickets

are €83 one-way or €108/€126 round-trip in low/high season. There are discounts for youth and children. The journey takes only 1½ hours but it can be rough in bad weather. Tickets are available from **Virtu Ferries** (Via Studi 80, ☎ 0932-954-062, www.virtuferries.com, 9 am-1 pm, 4-7 pm). Check the Virtu site for current schedules. At the time of writing, boats were departing Pozzallo at about 9 am and 9:30 pm, with a third service on Fridays at 3:30 pm. The harbor office opens one hour before every departure.

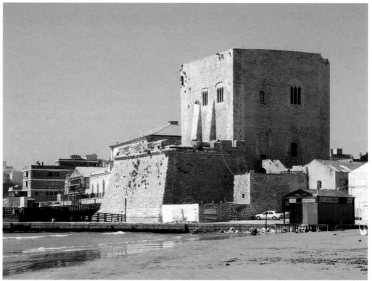

The Torre Cabrera in Pozzallo was used against the Turkish invasions in the 14th and 15th centuries (G. Melfi)

AST buses (☎ 0932-681-818, 0932-752-538) come here from Donnalucata, Acate, Avola, Pachino, Palermo, Pedalino, Rosolini, Sciicli, Ispica, Chiaramonte, Modica, Noto and Siracusa. AST buses also stop at the port. Pozzallo is on the train line linking it to other cities.

Where to Stay

The King's Reef (SP Pozzallo-S Maria del Foccallo, ☎ 093-295-7611, www.kingsreef.com, €) is a few km out of town, offering campsites and small bungalows with bunk beds. A restaurant and bar operate in season. Bikes cost €2 to rent. You can also use the kitchen for €2,50.

L'Agave B&B (Via Matteotti 15, ☎ 093-295-3046) is in the historic center. It has a variety of rooms with private bathrooms and breakfast.

Garden House B&B (Via Luigi Sturzo 106, ☎ 0932-957-961) is also on the port end of town.

Hotel Continental (Contrada Danielle, ☎ 0932-958-858, www.pozzallo.it/hotelcontinental, €€€) has no-nonsense rooms 500 yards from the port.

Hotel Villa Ada (Corso Vittorio Veneto 3, ☎ 0932-954-022, www.hotelvillaada.it, €€-€€€€), open all year, is smart and modern.

■ Scicli

Scicli was the only UNESCO World Heritage Site listed in Sicily a few years ago and has undergone a tourist transformation since then. Old guide books may describe the town as having a geriatric population and quiet squares, but no more! The town has woken up with the UNESCO listing and there are summer festivals in the square, bustling restaurants and lots of accommodation choices. It's a popular choice for tourists because it's one of the

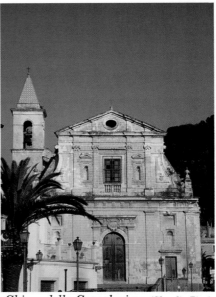

Chiesa della Consolazione (Claudio Zisa)

few *flat* Baroque cities to walk around (although it's not without its steep streets) and day-trippers come in hordes – Germans, French and Americans. However, at night it becomes a local hangout again with the usual clubs of old men in the streets, but a strong youth population too and a number of popular bars and restaurants.

The early settlement of Scicli on the hill of San Matteo goes back to the time of the Sikels, who lived in Sicily between 1000 and 1200 BC. The name Scicli may come from the Greek word *sikla*, meaning milk pail. Archaeological findings testify to the presence of human beings from early times, including the Arabs, Normans and Aragonese. Between the 14th and 16th centuries, it expanded into the valley, then was also re-built after the 1693 earthquake. The modern town now lies at the bottom of a bluff and is surrounded by rocky hills. It too has the warm honey-dew colored buildings, beautiful 18th-century churches and elegant balconies of all the Baroque towns.

Getting Here

 SAIS buses (☎ 0932-623-440) leave for Rome at 6:10 pm via Modica and Ragusa. **AST** (☎ 0932-681-818, 0932-752-538) connects Scicli with Donnalucata, Acate, Avola, Ispica, Pachino, Palermo, Pedalino, Rosolini, Pozzallo, Chiaramonte, Modica, Noto, Gela and Siracusa.

The **Treno Barocco del Val di Noto** historical train is another option for getting to Scicli. See *Adventures by Rail*.

Information Sources

i **Compagnia del Mediterraneo** (Piazza Italia 23, ☎ 0932-932-510, www.compagniadelmediterraneo.it, Mon-Sat 10 am-1 pm, 3-8 pm, Sun 10 am-1 pm) is a busy, privately run tourist company that provides tourist information and organizes events, guided tours, and accommodations, plus house rental, car rental and advice on restaurants. Guided tours of the *Centro Storico* leave from the office at 6 pm on Saturday (€10 per person). Book ahead. Other guided tours cost €125 (four hours, groups of 1-54), or €205 (eight hours, groups of 1-54). The **Pro Loco** (Via Castellana 5, ☎/fax 0932-932-782, open 10 am-1 pm, 4-8 pm) is another option for information, down the little lane behind the Compagnia del Mediterraneo. They have information on places to stay but not much else.

Useful Websites

■ www.siciltravel.com
■ www.barycentro.it (Corso Umberto 4620470, ☎ 093-275-3375) – dining and tourist information.
■ www.soggiornareinsicilia.it – lists B&Bs.

Events

 Scicli's religious festivals and events are also worth seeing. **Easter** and **Christmas** celebrations are colorful, there's the horse parade in honor of **San Giuseppe** in March that travels to Donnalucata, and the great **Battle of the Militia** in May.

Sightseeing

As with the other Baroque cities of the Val di Noto, the reconstruction of Scicli enriched the city with many wonderful churches and palaces built between 1700 and 1800. These include the **Church of Santa Teresa**, the **Chiesa di San Giovanni**, the **Chiesa di San Bartolomeo** and **Palazzo Beneventano**, which are all included on the UNESCO World Heritage List. Other interesting churches include **Chiesa e Convento del Carmine**, **Chiesa della Consolazione** and **Chiesa di S. Maria la Nova**, which houses a Byzantine cypress statue of Madonna della Pietra.

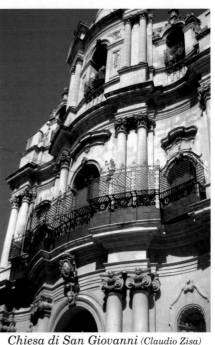

Chiesa di San Giovanni (Claudio Zisa)

The main **Piazza Italia** is a huge open space great for the evening *passeggiata*, the impressive 17th-century mother church **Chiesa di S. Ignazio** and with a bunch of bars and restaurants.

The town hall, **Palazzo Spadaro**, and **Palazzo Beneventano** (see *Adventures on Foot*) all boast Baroque decorations.

Ragusa & the Southeastern

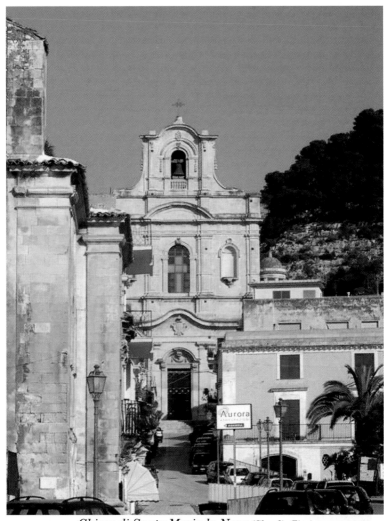

Chiesa di Santa Maria la Nova (Claudio Zisa)

Adventures

On Foot

 Walk past the 17th-century Palazzo Beneventano's grotesque sculptures (Via Francesco Formino Penna) and up to **Piazza E Dandolo**, passing women hang-

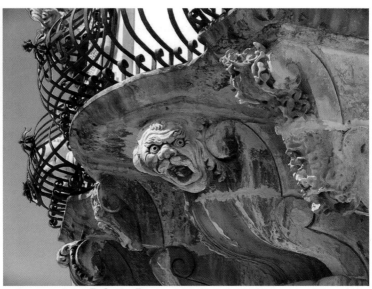

Palazzo Benevntano (Ignazio Caloggero)

ing laundry. This is an increasingly steep slope and soon takes you out of the busy streets to places only bikes and small cars can pass. A little cobbled path leads up to the empty church of **San Matteo**, which is now in ruins. At one time this was the

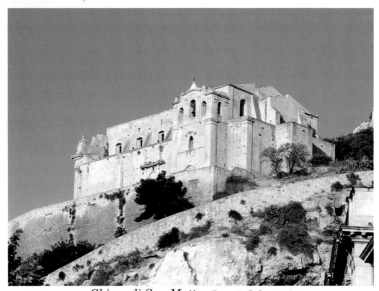

Chiesa di San Matteo (Ignazio Caloggero)

Ragusa & the Southeastern

principal church of Scicli. Peek inside the gates to see columns and graffiti inside. There's also a fantastic view over the town. You will easily make out the main piazza. Beyond the church, a path leads to another church another 10 minutes up and farther still to a small lookout in the remains of an old castle. From here you can easily see how Scicli folds around the ridges that overshadow it from above. You can also see a series of abandoned cave dwellings littering the hills. Nativity scenes called *presepe* are placed in these caves at Christmas time. The caves, known as Chiarafura, were dug out in the tufa cliffs. Some were inhabited by poor local people as recently as 1958. Lights illuminate the caves and rock walls above the town at night.

By Rail

 The **Treno Barocco del Val di Noto** also operates to Scicli (see *Adventures by Rail* in Ragusa).

Where to Stay

 Gli Arancini di Montalbano (Via Bovio 39, ☎ 0932-931-321, www.arancinidimontalbano.com, €€) is one of the best budget options in Scicli and promises that you'll want for nothing. Two rooms and *arancini* for breakfast!

Casa Corinne, also in the Centro Storico, is handled by Compagnia del Mediterraneo (☎ 0932-932-510, €€). There's just one double room.

If you want to book something by the week or month, **Casa Malisa** (☎ 0932-932-510), near the Chiafura caves, is a house that can sleep up to seven people. Weekly rates range from €320-€500, depending on the season.

Loggia dell'Accanto (Contrada Balata, ☎ 0932-932-701, 347-607-6210, €€-€€€) is a family-run B&B in the home of the delightful English-speaking couple Andrea and Giovanna Tomasello. It is a few km out of town with a beautiful view of Scicli from the terrace. Make sure you try Giovanna's *granita* if she has some available.

Where to Eat

 You will probably notice **I Sapori del Vicolo** (Via Pluchinotta 2, ☎ 0932-841-984, closed Tues in winter, €€) if you're here at night. Candles mark the way

down the laneway at night and there is outdoor seating on wooden platforms during the summer. Rock walls, a fish tank and black and white pictures of the region complete the interior. They serve pizza and seafood.

In Piazza Italia are a number of bars and cafés, including **Café Italia** near the cinema , Gran Caffe with a garden area and **Café Sicilia** (closed Tues).

At the other end of the square, opposite Chiesa di S. Ignazio and past the tourist agency, is **Antico Café**, a friendly place serving all kinds of pastries, arancini and pizza. Look at the old pictures of Scicli while you wait.

Other bars line Via Nazionale between the two main piazzas. **Bar Popolo** and **Art Café** are popular with young crowds. There's another good night spot at **Iguana Ristorane/Pub** (Via Musso, closed Tues) 50 yards down a lane at the left-hand end of Piazza Italia.

∎ The Coast

The Ragusan coast from Pozzallo to Gela has some nice stretches and makes a pleasant itinerary change from stomping around the inland Baroque towns. At **Sampieri** is a pleasant undeveloped beachfront with open sands. There's an old *tonnara* (fish processing facility), a small boat harbor and locations used for the TV series *Montalbano*. There's a camp-

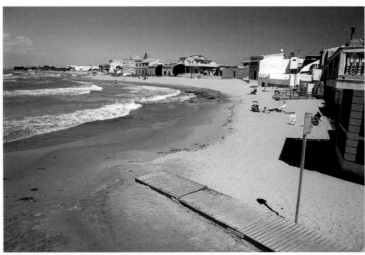

Montalbano Beach (Joanne Lane)

ground here, **La Spiaggetta** (Miramare 50, ☎ 0932-939-737, www.la-spiaggetta.com, €) with its own beachfront.

Kaukana is an archaeological site (9 am-2 pm) on the main road just before Punta Secca. If it is locked, cut through to the beach road to see the ruins and foundations belonging to houses and stores. Kaukana was an important trading harbor in late Roman/Byzantine times. However, it's not terribly exciting and if you have limited time you'd be better off continuing down to see the ruins at Camarina.

Punta Secca is almost deathly quiet out of season, with little more than a lighthouse, a few shops, the beach and a sirocco wind that blows sand through the town all day long. Bring a scarf! However, its seafront is worth a brief stop at least. The Bar Montalbano is across the road. You can get a good granite here.

Just north of Punta Braccetto are the remains of ancient **Camarina**, a Syracusan colony founded in 599 BC. The colony was devastated several times by conflicts with Gela to the north and eventually destroyed by Rome in 258 BC. The site is not as fantastic as Agrigento or Selinunte, but the open setting by the sea is wild and beautiful. The **Museo Regionale Kamarina** (☎ 093-282-6004, 9 am-2 pm and 3-7 pm, €3) contains finds from the site, including coins, helmets, columns, amphora jugs, rope and sarcophagi. Out the back of the museum are the actual site ruins. If you don't want to pay, you can get a glimpse of them from the road.

Just inland lies the **Donnafugata Castle** (☎ 0932-619-333, Tues-Sat 9:30 am-1 pm, Sun 9:30 am-1 pm, 3-6:30 pm), an ancient fortress rebuilt and embellished in the 19th century by Baron Corrado Arezzo de

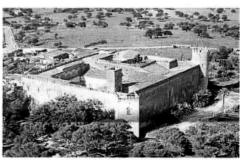

Donnafugata Castle

Spuches. The castle is privately owned and currently closed to the public for renovations. There are plans to open it for weddings and events, although details are not clear. Over the years different parts of the castle have been opened to the

public, including the stone-walled maze of gardens and some of the 122 rooms, such as the music room with painted columns on the wall, the room of mirrors with gilded freezes and the hall of the shields with wallpaper of hand-painted shield motifs.

■ Comiso

Comiso is infused with a Baroque spirit like many of the other towns in the region. It does not have the hilltop drama of Noto, Ragusa or Modica. But it is immediately appealing, with sights clustered around Castello Aragonese and Chiesa Madre. It too was destroyed by the earthquake of 1693 and rebuilt in Baroque style.

Getting Here

 AST links it to Ragusa (30 mins) and Vittoria (15 mins). **Giamporcardo buses** (☎ 0932-988-300, 0932-866-283) run to Ragusa, Vittoria, Catania, Scoglitti, S Croce Camerina and Marina di Ragusa. **SAIS** (☎ 0932-623-440) has connections to Vittoria, S Croce Camerina and Marina di Ragusa. **SIMILI** (☎ 0933-981-894) runs to Pedalino, Mazzaronello, Mazzarrone, Granieri, Regalsemi and Caltagirone.

Information Sources

 Comune di Comiso (Via degli Studi 9, ☎ 0932-748-204, www.comune.comiso.rg.it, Tues-Sat 9 am-1 pm, 4-8 pm, Sun 9 am-1 pm) is in Piazza delle Erbe.
Pro Loco Comiso (Via Di Vita 6, ☎ 0932-961-586, assprolococomiso@tiscalinet.it).

Events

 The **Centro Servizi Culturali** arranges different events in Comiso, including the **Settembre Kasmeno** (2-24 September), with music, theater, film and cabaret performed throughout the town.

Sightseeing

Comiso has easily navigable streets with helpful tourist boards outside major sites (in Italian) explaining the history

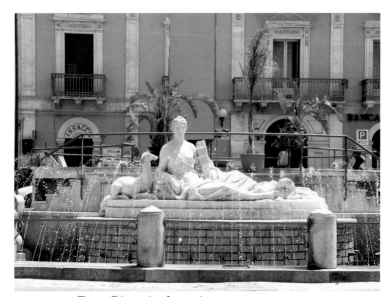

Fonte Diana in the main square (Clemensfranz)

or detail of the location with a map. But what's great about Comiso is that the important edifices can easily be spotted poking up above the other buildings, making it easy to follow your nose. Most of the churches appear to open in the afternoon.

Piazza delle Erbe is the main square in the historic center where you will find the comune and **Museo Civico di Storia Naturale** (Piazza delle Erbe, ☎ 093-272-2521, Tues-Sat 9:30 am-1 pm, 4-7 pm, Sun 9:30 am-1 pm, closed Mon, €2). Rooms are dedicated to reptiles, crustaceans, insects, mammals and birds. Kids and nature enthusiasts will love the sounds of dolphins and whales, and the variety of stuffed animals. By the side of the comune

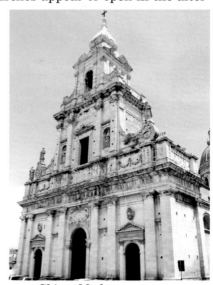

Chiesa Madre (Clemensfranz)

you will see Roman mosaics and baths discovered in the 1930s.

The **Chiesa di Santa Maria delle Stelle** also lies off the piazza. It is currently closed for reconstruction but you can look in from the gates. The **Intorno al Giardino** restaurant is outside. Behind the church veer east towards Piazza Fonte Diana and then along Via San Biagio to the 18th-century **Castello Argonese**, which now houses **Bar Castello**. You can wander in the grounds while you sip your coffee. Just up the hill is the lovely 16th-century **Chiesa di San Biagio** that is usually open in the afternoons. It's a lovely church with original paved floors, ceiling paintings and huge wooden doors. The other major church is the **Chiesa di S. Francesco** (13th century), preserving Nasellis' tomb by A. Gagini. The Nasellis were an aristocratic family that controlled the town from the 15th to the 18th century.

Adventures

On Foot

 The *comune* has laid out a walking itinerary through town marked by plaques. The route starts from Piazza Fonte Diana along Via San Biagio, then goes out to Villa Comunale, back along Via Dabormida past several churches to Piazza delle Erbe.

Where to Stay

 There aren't a lot of options in Comiso itself. **Villa Orchidea** (Contrada Rotondo, ☎ 0932-879-108, www.villaorchidea.it) and **Cordial Hotel** (SS 115 Comiso-Vittoria, ☎ 0932-967-866) are just out of town.

Where to Eat

Foccaccia with ricotta and salsiccia is a specialty in Comiso. Most eating places are on Corso Vittorio Emanuele. However, there are these other options in the historic part of town:

Bar Castello (Via S. Biagio 39, ☎ 093-272-1112, 3 am-11 pm, closed Tues), inside the castle grounds, is a pasticceria, too, with the specialty *cavoli siciliani* (Sicilian cabbage).

Ragusa & the Southeastern

Intorno al Giardino Café (Via Mons. Rimmaudo 34, ☎ 093-296-1244, intornoalgiardino@virgilio.it), outside the Chiesa Madre, is a gelateria, caffetteria, wine bar and restaurant.

Bar Ristorante Pizzeria Sport (Battaglia Salvatore, Piazza delle Erbe 5, ☎ 093-272-1016, closed Wed, €) is a fine spot to enjoy a pizza until late.

There are quite a few snack bar options in Via San Biagio, including the **Creperia, Panineria, Frutteria** (Via S. Biagio 85) and **Café Borghese** (Via San Biagio 86).

L'Antica Comiso (Via G. Di Vita 5, ☎ 0932-961-788).

■ Vittoria

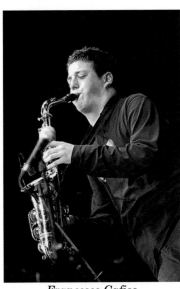

Francesco Cafiso

Leaving Comiso, you will have barely blinked and you'll be in Vittoria, home of the teenage saxophone sensation ★**Francesco Cafiso**. Make sure you hear him play if you come to Sicily. Concerts are common in the summer. Go to the website www.francescocafiso.it for details. Unfortunatelythere's not a lot else to keep you here.

The **Museo Civico Polivalente** and **Pro Loco** information office are both at Via del Quattro 16. Vittoria is linked via **Giamporcardo buses** (☎ 0932-988-300, 0932-866-283) to Comiso, Ragusa, Catania, Scoglitti, S Croce Camerina and Marina di Ragusa. **SAIS** (☎ 0932-623-440) runs to Comiso, S Croce Camerina and Marina di Ragusa.

The town features two main squares connected by Via Cavour, with the same elegant façades and paved streets you see throughout the Baroque region. **Piazza del Popolo** is the principal square, with the **Madonna della Grazia** and the later Neoclassical **Teatro Comunale**. In the smaller Piazza

Ricca is the church of **San Giovanni Battista**. In Piazza del Popolo you'll find a number of cafés.

■ Chiaramonte Gulfi ★

This hilltop town to the north of Ragusa is worth the visit for its views across inland Sicily, earning its nickname as the balcony of Sicily. It's a good spot to escape the heat of the plains and a potential lunch spot on your way through to Caltagirone or farther afield. It's a very small town and it won't take you long to explore the options. Climb Via S. Giovanni to the top for views. You can get some salami and cured hams here, mozzarella di buffala,

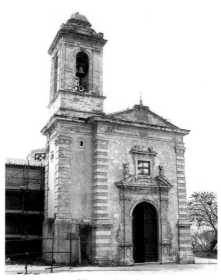

Chiesa Madre

scamorza di buffala, or formaggi di buffala. There's also a common garden. However, if you're a biker, you'll probably come here for the biking possibilities nearby. See below.

The **Antica Stazione** (C. da Santissimo Chiaramonte Gulfi, ☎ 0932-928-083, www.anticastazione.com, €€) was one of the stations on the *ex-ferrovia* (old railway) but was converted into a restaurant, with a large dining room for events. The cuisine is based on the gastronomical tradition of Chiaramonte, including stuffed pork chops, sausage, pork in aspic and homemade pasta (cavati). It's a good spot to stop after one of the bike itineraries.

Adventures on Wheels

Chiaramonte Gulfi is the starting point for a number of mountain bike itineraries. These routes all start from near the Piazzale del Santuario di Maria Santissima delle Grazie and lead into the Arcibessi forest.

A 10-km route to Monterosso called **Green Way** follows *l'ex ferrovia* (old train line) route (Ragusa-Siracusa-Vizzini) on a track from Chiaramonte to Monterosso, finishing at Pantalica. Other tracks on the route go Monterosso-Buccheri and Monterosso-Giarratana-Palazzolo – both asphalted.

A longer itinerary of 100 km (one-two days) leaves Chiaramonte Gulfi towards Monte Arcibessi and Lake Dirilla, then on to Vizzini. From here the route goes to Buccheri, Sortino, Ferla, Palazzolo Acreide, Giarratana and Monterosso, before returning to Chiaramonte Gulfi. **Green Bike MTB Ragusa** (www.greenbikerg.com) completes a 100-km itinerary from Chiaramonte Gulfi on the first Sunday in October every year. At other times of the year they may accompany you if you give them notice.

From Chiaramonte or Monterosso you could also climb the highest peak in the Ragusan province, **Monte Arcibessi** (2,972 feet).

For more details on all these itineraries contact Green Bike (☎ 0932-644-449, www.greenbikerg.com).

Siciliando (☎ 0932-942-843, www.siciliando.it) in Modica (see Tetti di Siciliando in *Where to Stay*) also offers a guided itinerary along the ex-ferrovia (former railway) to Pantalica.

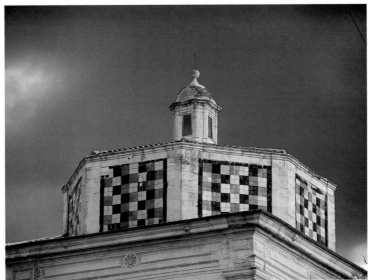

Chiaramonte Gulfi, architectural detail

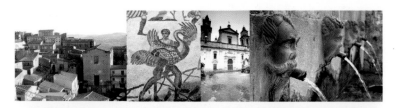

The Interior

This chapter takes in the provinces of Enna, Caltanisetta and Caltagirone, encompassing the vast central part of Sicily. If you want to see more traditional Sicilian life, this is where you should come. The mountainous interior has considerable beauty and remains substantially underdeveloped compared to the coast. There is far less tourist infrastructure, public transport or budget accommodation choices, but get your own vehicle and it will be far less problematic. However, the archaeological ruins, amazing cities and some of Sicily's best festivals make it well worth seeing.

■ Enna & the Northeast Interior

This section incorporates Enna and stretches to the northeast through Leonforte, Nicosia and the towns of Cerami, Tronia and Cesaro on the borders of the Parco dei Nebrodi. It also includes Gangi, Sperlinga and borders areas of the Parco Madonie. Enna is the major town here and the best place to base yourself.

ENNA HIGHLIGHTS

- Blustery Enna and the views from Castello di Lombardia.
- La Gran Fonte fountains in Leonforte, 24 waterspouts in a sculpted façade.
- Motor racing action at Pergusa.
- The sombre Settimana Santa in Enna.
- The castles of Cerami, Troina and Cesaro.
- A walking itinerary past Sperlinga's troglodytic houses.
- The excellent food at Gangi Vecchio.

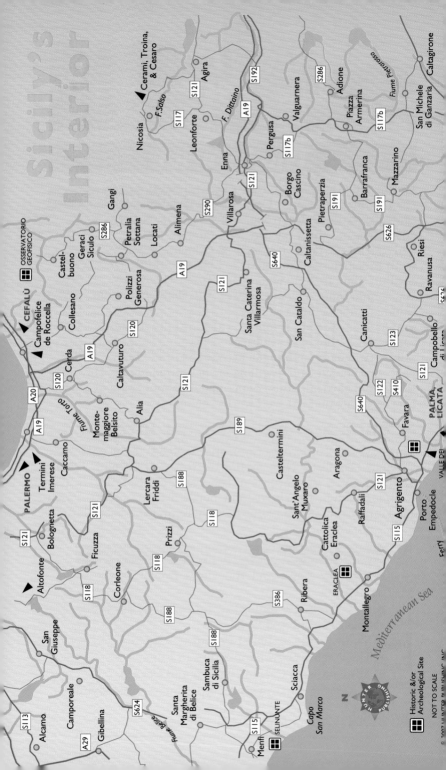

Enna

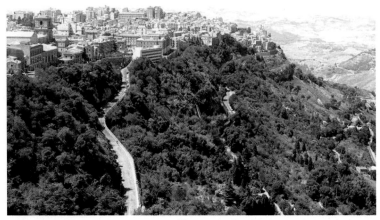

Enna

Enna is the highest provincial town in Italy at 3,110 feet above sea level. Bring a jacket even in mid-summer for the cool evenings and mornings! However, the cooler climate does make it an appealing and popular summer retreat. It's also very centrally located with good transport services to many towns.

Enna's hilltop location made it a magnet for successive invaders over the centuries, all of whom besieged and fortified it. Obviously, it was never impregnable – the Saracens climbed through the sewers in 859 AD to capture it. The medieval center remains well preserved and offset by beautiful panoramas. The climb alone to the top of the ridge sets the tone; it certainly earns its nickname as the *belvedere* (viewpoint) of Sicily.

Getting Here

 The bus terminal is in Viale Diaz in the new town, about 10 minutes walk from the historic center. **SAIS** buses (☎ 0935-500-902, www.saisautolinee.it) connect Enna with Gangi, Sperlinga, Villadoro, Calascibetta, Catania (10 times daily, one hr 20 mins), Palermo (10 daily, one hr 50 mins), Gela (seven daily, one hr 15 mins), Piazza

The Interior

Armerina (two direct services daily, one hr 35 mins) and Aidone (one direct daily, one hr). SAIS also stops in Piazza Bernini in Enna Bassa, but check the route first.

The **train station** (☎ 0935-500-910), with connections to Catania and Palermo, is five km from the town center in Enna Bassa. A local bus does connect it to town (see *Getting Around*).

Getting Around

 SAIS services and local buses run regularly between the train station and the main center. SAIS also has daily departures for Pergusa (10 daily, 20 minutes). Local bus number 1 does a city circuit from Piazza Vittorio Emanuele up to the castle.

Parking is difficult to find in Enna. There is free parking below the town in Via Pergusa, including an area for camper-vans, but it' a bit of a walk up to the center. Alternatively, buy a time ticket of €.52/hr from a *tabacchi*.

Taxis are available in Viale Diaz (☎ 0935-500-906) or Piazza Scelfo (☎ 0935-500-905). For **car rental**, you could try these agencies:

- **Bevilacqua** (☎ 333-598-6903)
- **Di Nicolo** (☎ 360-531-152)

Information Sources

 The **APT Enna** (Via Roma 413, ☎ 0935-528-228, 0935-528-288, Mon-Fri 8:30 am-1:30 pm, Sat 9 am-1 pm, 3-7 pm, Sun closed, www.apt-enna.com) has lots of information on the town and the province, including a good map.

Events

A **market** is held every Tuesday in Piazza Europa, Enna Bassa.

The Easter parade, ★★★*Settimana Santa*, is one of the most interesting in Sicily. The parades of penitents marching in absolute silence is both eerie and moving. Every day one of the 15 fraternities leaves from its church and marches to the Duomo. The parades and events start on Palm Sunday and culminate on Easter Sunday.

Sightseeing

The prize attraction in Enna is the ★**Castello di Lombardia** (☎ 0935-500-962, 9 am-8 pm summer, 9 am-5 pm winter, free, www.castellodilombadia.com), at the top of Via Roma, dominating the eastern spur. It was built by the Saracens but it was Frederick II of Aragon (1272-1337) who ordered the curtain wall be built, with towers on each side. The wall and six of the original 20 towers remain. You can climb the tallest of these, Torre Pisana, for a breathtaking view over

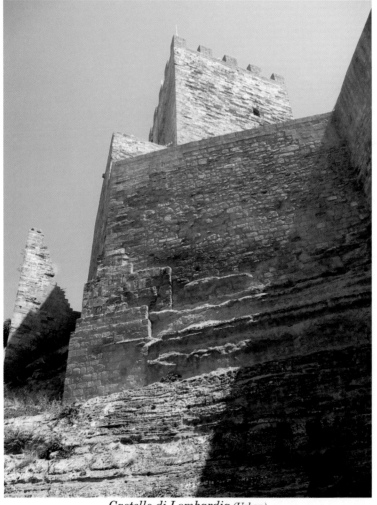

Castello di Lombardia (Urban)

the town and into the valley below, including Lago Pergusa.
You can also see across to the hilltop town of Calascibetta on a
clear day. The castle grounds include several courtyards and
gardens that can be quite deserted late in the evening. The
Rocca di Cerere is just beyond the castle, where the remains of a temple to Demeter lie on an outcrop of rock. It's a
good spot for sunrise or sunset or a lunchtime picnic. Ceres is
the Roman counterpart to Demeter, hence the name.

An interesting walking itinerary in *Adventures on Foot* is a
good way to cover the rest of the town's sights.

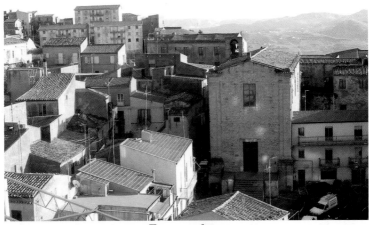

Enna rooftops

Adventures
On Foot

The best way to explore the town is to catch local bus
number 1 up to the Castello di Lombardia (see *Sightseeing*) and walk back down Via Roma. Along the way,
music lovers should not miss the **Museo Multimedial**e (Via
Roma 533, ☎ 0935-22429, 10 am-1 pm, 3:30-7:30 pm, €2). In
the multimedia directory of the Enna province you select a
town, city, ruins or nature reserve to explore with photographs set to music. There's an excellent painting section of
Enna artists, including Caravaggio, and on the *Settimana
Santa*. The **Duomo** (☎ 0935-500-940, 9 am-1 pm, 4-7 pm,
free) is the next stop on Via Roma and the central point of

Settimana Santa celebrations. The Duomo dates from 1307, but has been rebuilt several times, combining Gothic-Catalan, Renaissance and Baroque influences. The interior is completely encrusted with ornamentation. It's quite spacious inside with dark grey columns, a carved wooden ceiling and wooden balconies by the altar. The **Museo Civico Alessi** (☎ 093-550-3165, 8 am-8 pm daily, €2.60) is next door, containing the cathedral's treasury with Canonical robes, ornaments and silverware. There is also a picture gallery with Enna painters of the 19th century. Across the road in Piazza Marconi is the **Museo Archeologico Varisano** (☎ 0935-528-100, 9 am-6:30 pm daily, €2.07), with fascinating finds relating to the life of native people during the Hellenization of the territory. One hundred yards farther down Via Roma is **Pallazzo Pollicarini**, a Catalan-Gothic palazzo that is now apartments. Stroll past the APT beyond Teatro Garibaldi to the main square, **Piazza Vittorio Emanuele**. This is the central square, with a number of bars. The piazza beyond Francesco Crispi has a pleas-

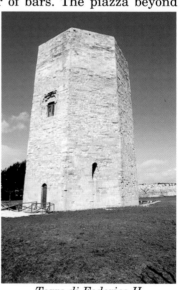

ant fountain and a good view out from Enna beyond. The church of **San Francesco** flanks the piazza with a massive 16th-century tower. If you enjoy the views, continue along Viale Caterina Savoca back up to the castle to complete a round-trip.

The other end of Via Roma leads to the modern part of the city. The **Torre di Federico II** (9 am-5 pm daily, free) in the Giardino Pubblico is 72 feet high and part of the city's defences. It was linked by a secret passage to the Castello di Lombardia.

Torre di Federico II

On Wheels

If you feel the need to rev up your holiday in the Sicilian interior you can watch the motorsports at the Autodromo di Pergusa (www.autodromopergusa.it) from May to September. Pergusa is nine km south of Enna and the racetrack circles the Lake.

The Interior

Where to Eat

 Ristorante La Fontana (Via Volturo 6, ☎ 0935-25465, €€), in Piazza S Francesco Crispi, has a covered area outside for eating. The other restaurant in Piazza S Francesco Crispi is **Da Gino** (Via Lombardia 2, ☎ 0935-25878), currently undergoing restoration and closer to the castle.

DINING PRICE CHART	
Price per person for an entrée, including house wine.	
€	Up to €12
€€	€13-€25
€€€	€26-€35
€€€€	Over €35

Trattoria La Botte (Via Roma 488, ☎ 0935-502-331, closed Mon, €) serves local dishes and has a music and piano bar. €13 fixed menu.

Ristorante Centrale (Piazza VI Dicembre 9, ☎ 0935-500-963, www.ristorantecentrale.net, €€€) serves typical Ennese food.

Good local bars include **Extra Bar** (Via Roma 31) and **Caffe Roma** (Via Roma 312).

Where to Stay

 Accommodation is fairly limited in Enna. You may need to travel to Pergusa or other nearby centers for more options. There is a camper service off to the right on Via Pergusa as you climb up to the town.

HOTEL PRICE CHART	
€	Up to €25 per day
€€	€26-€55
€€€	€56-€85
€€€€	Over €85

Grande Albergo Sicilia (Piazza N. Colaianni 7, ☎ 0935-500-850, www.hotelsiciliaenna.it, €€€€) is well located, but pricey.

B&B Domus (Via delle Magnolie 14, Enna Bassa, ☎ 0935-531-364, €€) is the lower town, not far from the train station.

Leonforte

The small town of Leonforte is about a half-hour drive away (SAIS connections from Enna) and sits facing Enna on a hillside, giving a superb view over the 18 km between the two towns. If you have a car you will find the one-way system of streets annoying – you have to double back all the way around

if you miss something. Leonforte was founded in 1610 and was once renowned for its horse breeding. Most of the action is around the central square. Of interest is the **Duomo**, particularly atmospheric at night when flickering candles create eerie shadows inside, **Palazzo Branciforti** (1620) and the **Chiesa di Cappuccini** (1630). But the key sight is the ★**Gran Fonte** – 24 waterspouts gushing from a sculpted façade built in 1651 by Nicolo Branciforte. The fountain is below the cathedral in a small square. At night it is evocatively lit up and you could enjoy drinks and snacks at the rustic bar across from it. There's also **La Lanterna Trattoria** in Piazza 4 Novembre or the **606 Cocktail Bar** (Corso Umberto 148) if you need something to eat.

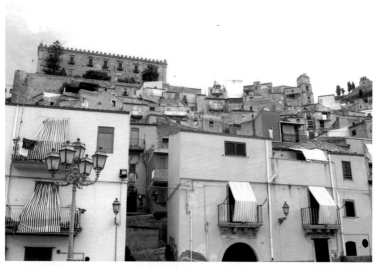

Leonforte (Urban)

The ★★**Villa Gussio Nicoletti** (Contrada Rossi CP 126, ☎ 093-590-3268, fax 093-590-3627, www.villagussio.it, €€€-€€€€), just out of town, is an amazing setup over eight acres. This is the ultimate in deluxe accommodations, with tennis courts, two swimming pools, a golf course and club house, SPA, trattoria and pizzeria, enoteca, anthropological museum, congress center, wine tasting, cooking courses and other excursions. This complex was originally the property of Baron Francesco Gussio. Spa packages (☎ 093-903-268,

10 am-1 pm, 5-8 pm) are very affordable. Treatments include chocolate facials €40, anti-aging €55, hot stones €50, manicures €10 and pedicures €15. Wine tasting takes place in the Baron's old wine *cantina* (cellar). The nine-course golf course will open in 2007.

Cerami, Troina & Cesaro

If you're making a beeline back to Taormina or into the Parco dei Nebrodi you could follow the S120 through Cerami (21 km), Troina (46 km) and Cesaro (66 km) and do a castle tour. All three towns have battered castle fragments set into rocks above the town. The landscape along the route is mostly agricultural, with tractors ploughing the fields.

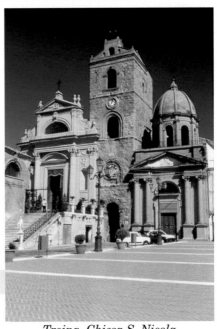

Troina, Chiesa S. Nicola

★Sperlinga

Following the road from Nicosia the other way on the SS 120 towards the Monti Madonie is the interesting town of Sperlinga (10 km). This western route on the S120 has several daily services from Nicosia. The name of the town derives from the Latin *spelunca*, meaning cave. This is a direct reference to the many cave dwellings on the sandstone slopes of the town. These cave dwellings or *troglodytic* houses and the castello (☎ 093-564-3025, 9:30 am-1 pm, 3-7 pm, €2) above the town make an interesting itinerary.

The original settlement dates back to Sicel times (12th-18th century BC), but the main part of the castle was constructed by the Normans about 1000 AD. The underlying town was founded in 1597. The entrance to the castle passes the **Museo della Civilta Contadina** (same opening hours) where old

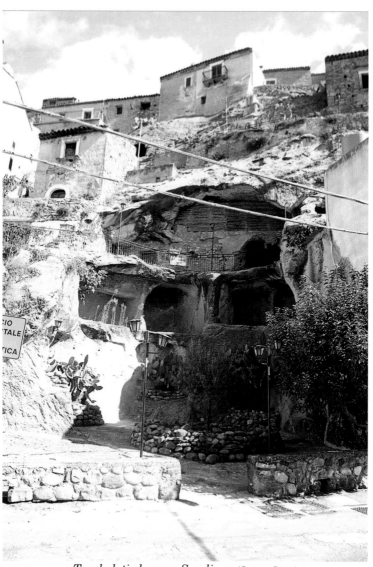

Troglodytic houses, Sperlinga (Joanne Lane)

farming equipment, weaving and other household items are displayed. Women from the community are often here, demonstrating how they make carpet from bits of fabric. You can buy their products for as little as €5. Farther up in the castle is a guard room, meeting room, the stables, an area for metal work, a kitchen and even a church. From the highest points

The Interior

you can see views of the town. There are also various old pictures and paintings of the castle, nobles and nearby towns.

To see the *troglodytic* houses take the small road that heads down opposite the Bar Al Castello. Some of the old grottoes are boarded up; others are full of wood or chickens. Some appear inhabited and those closer to town have pleasant gardens. The route will take you down to the main road.

Gangi

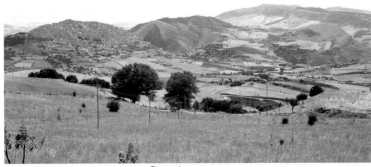

Gangi (Archenzo)

Farther along the SS120 just before the Madonie Park, Gangi seems oddly reminiscent of Ragusa Ibla, sitting on the same kind of symmetrical mound. Archaeologists have identified Gangi as the ancient city of Engyum, a Greek colony founded by colonists from Minoa. It started to develop in the 14th century and retains much of its medieval quality. If you're looking for a base in this region or a bite to eat, try the marvelous ★★**Gangi Vecchio** (Contrada

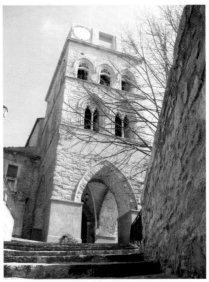

Torre Civica, Gangi (Marco Sauro)

Gangivecchio snc, ☎ 0921-689-191, paolotornabene@ interfree.it) about four km out of town. Run by the friendly owners Paolo Tornabene and partner Alda, it was the Benedictine Monastery of Santa Maria Annunziata in the 14th century. It was converted into a summer residence by the Barons of Bongiorno in the 18th century. Next to the informal agriturismo is a restaurant run by Paolo's sister Giovanna. Wanda and Giovanna Tornabene run the restaurant out of the abbey and have produced cook books, *La Cucina Siciliana di Gangivecchio* and *Sicilian Home Cooking*. If you've seen or read the books, you'll want to taste the famed homestyle cooking too. They also offer cooking classes.

■ Caltanisetta & the Northwest Interior

This is another of Sicily's less populated inland provinces, with less going for it than the northeast or southern parts. More than likely, you'll pass through much of it without a cursory glance at the towns. Public transport in this region is rather awkward, although it is possible to reach the gems of the province. These include the beautiful hill town of Sant'Angelo Muxaro, where you can trek to ancient tombs and eat ricotta with shepherds, sleuth for Mafia connections in Corleone, marvel at the grand piazza of Palazzo Adriano, used for one of Italy's most famous movie sets, and trek in the wonderful woods of Ficuzza.

CALTANISETTA HIGHLIGHTS

■ **Sant'Angelo Muxaro** – Trek, bike or horseback ride around the hilltop town to ancient tombs, drop into caves and enjoy the traditional foods and festivals.

■ **Palazzao Adriano** – The famed piazza used in *Cinema Paradiso* is Sicily's biggest and best.

■ **Corleone** – Famous for its Mafia associations.

■ **Ficuzza** – Explore the woods of Ficuzza on foot, bike or horseback.

The Interior

Caltanisetta

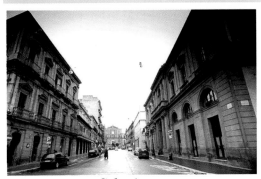
Caltasinetta

The president of Italy visited Caltanisetta in 2004 but did not do too much to put it on the map. You'll find pictures of the visit in the Gran Café Romano on Corso Umberto. But there's not a whole lot else going on here and the bar is as good a place to hang out as any. Caltanisetta is a transit zone for wherever else you want to go. If you're traveling through by car your best option is to get some cash, *benzina,* food for the journey and continue on. There's really not a lot to keep you.

Getting Here & Getting Around

 SAS (☎ 0934-456-072, www.saistrasporti.it) connects to Enna (50 minutes, €3.30) and Villarosa (30 minutes, €2.50). The bus station is at Piazza Republicca off Via Turati. **Trains** (☎ 0934-23016) connect Caltanisetta to Catania, Palermo and Agrigento. They arrive at the station in Piazza Roma near the Museo Civico and the staff are incredibly friendly if you're stuck here for a few hours. Say hello to the station master from us!

SCAT is the local urban bus (Umberto Drv 110, ☎ 0934-29576).

Information Sources

 The **APT Tourist Office** is opposite the Gran Café at Corso Umberto 109 (☎ 0924-530-411, www.aapit.cl.it, Tues-Fri 10 am-1 pm). The tourist office is at Viale Conte Testasecca 20 (☎ 0934-21089, Mon-Fri 9 am-1 pm, Tues 9 am-6 pm).

Sightseeing

Caltanisetta boasts a few meagre attractions to fill in time if you're waiting for a bus or train. It's unlikely you'd come here seeking them out. The **Museo Archaeologico** (Via Colaianni 3, Mon-Fri 9:30 am-12:30 pm, 4-8 pm, Sat and Sun 9:30 am-12:30 pm) contains some early Sicilian finds, including vases and Bronze Age figures. The main square is **Piazza Garibaldi** (head straight up from the train station, turn left into Via Crispi and right onto Corso Vittorio Emmanuele). It con-

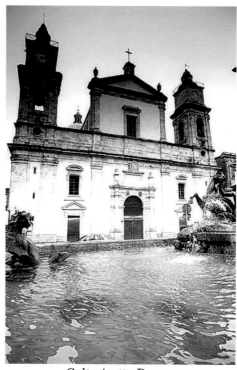

Caltasinetta Duomo

tains the **Duomo** and **Chiesa di San Sebastiano**. Once you've exhausted these sights there's also the **Castello di Pietrarossa** (head out on Corso V. Emanuele) balanced on an outcrop of rock.

Where to Stay

Hotel Giulia (Corso Umberto 85, ☎ 093-405-42927), in Venetian style, has 18 bedrooms with all comforts.

Near the Duomo you can try **Antico Café del' Duomo** for snacks or stroll down to the **Gran Café Romano** opposite the tourist office. This is where the President visited and is a rather elegant establishment. Dine in style on rounded soft-seated lounges in a saloon-style bar. There are snacks and hot meals. **Trattoria La Scalincuta** (Via Mons Gutta Duria) serves couscous.

The Interior

Ristorante L'Archetto (Via Nicolo Palmeri 10, closed Thurs, €-€€) is down a narrow lane full of laundry near Hotel Gulia. It's known for handmade pasta dishes, seafood and pizza. Tourist menus are €10-15. **Al Teatro Ristorante** (Via Arco Calafato 25) has lunch and dinner menus.

■ Toward the Coast

★★★Sant'Angelo Muxaro

This small agricultural center is on a hilltop in the pictur-esque Platani River Valley and one of the most important pre-historic Sicilian villages. Museums in Agrigento, Palermo and Florence have thousands of Minoan and Mycenaean ceramic pieces from here. Around the base of the hill are numerous tombs or *tholos* hewn out of the rock dating from the fifth to ninth century BC. It's also a good place to try some kayaking, trekking or biking and well worth a day-trip from Agrigento. If you stay overnight you can also see Sant'Angelo's main sights when the town, the hill and necropolis are illuminated (after 8 pm).

Getting Here

 Lattuca (☎ 0922-36125) buses make the trip from Agrigento daily at 9 am (arrives 10:30 am), 2 pm (arrives 3:30 pm) and 5 pm (arrives 6:30 pm). Buses for Agrigento depart at 7 am, 11 am and 4 pm. Cuffaro buses from Palermo leave at 5 am; those leaving Sant'Angelo for the Palermo airport leave at 5 am and 7 am.

Information Sources

i Your first port of call should be to **Val di Kam** (Via Liberta 1, ☎ 0922-919-670, www.valdikam.it, 9 am-1 pm, 3-8 pm), in the main square, who can fill you in on everything you need, from itinerary planning to food and accommodation. The friendly Pier Filippe and his wife MariElla also arrange biking, walking, caving, horseriding and other itineraries around town. But if you want to be inde-pendent, they can also suggest itineraries to follow.

- **Pro Loco** (Via Vittorio Emanuele 15, ☎ 0922-801-309)
- **Comune Sant'Angelo Muxaro** (☎ 0922-919-506)
- **Cave guide Giovanni Buscaglia** (☎ 0922-919-068)

Events

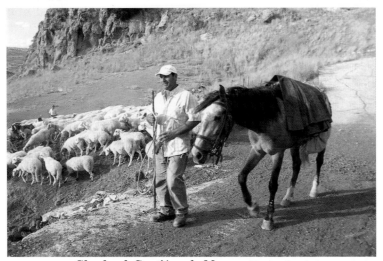

Shepherd, Sant'Angelo Muxaro (Joanne Lane)

Regular festivals are held in the town, including the **Mercatino della Sicana** (September), selling typical products. The **Sagra del Ricotto** on January 6 is when the local *pastori* (shepherds) come into the piazza with their traditional ricotta cheese.

Sightseeing

You can see the main *tholos* (tombs) on foot. Head out of town the way you came in and you'll find them signposted to the right on the last stretch down to the main road. Alternatively get the bus to drop you at this junction on your way in. A path drops down to the **"beehive" caves**. The biggest of these is the *tombe del principe*, which has a funerary bed and vault. It is believed the tomb was for a king or famous man. Two golden rings (in the Paolo Orsi, Siracusa) and four gold cups (one in the British Museum, London) were found here. Continue on the path to other *tholos* around the base of the hill; there are actually six tomb sites.

The Interior

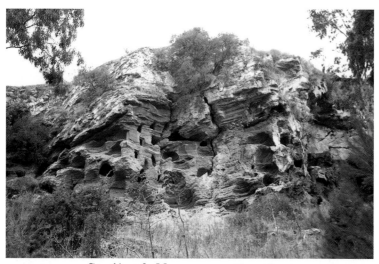

Sant'Angelo Muxaro caves (Joanne Lane)

Adventures

Underground

The cave formations around Sant'Angelo Muxaro can be explored with the right equipment and guide – they should not be attempted alone. The guides are born in this area and know the country well. **MariElla** of **Val di Kam** (Via Liberta 1, ☎ 0922-919-670, www.valdikam.it, 9 am-1 pm, 3-8 pm) is a particular natural at caving and often goes out exploring to find new caverns. The mountains around Sant'Angelo Muxaro are made of chalk and there are caves everywhere. Some are very deep. Caving requires a minimum or two people and costs €20-€25. You are given shoes and helmets. The Grotte delle Necropoli and Vallone del Ponte are two key caving sites.

On Foot

Follow the sightseeing routes above to visit the principal caves. Or wander the narrow lanes of the town. There are two churches hidden in the streets and a small cheese factory where you can taste soft ricotta cheese.

Val di Kam (Via Liberta 1, ☎ 0922-919-670, www.valdikam. it, 9 am-1 pm, 3-8 pm) has half-day and full-day trekking itineraries that include a buffet lunch, a cappuccino made from

goats' milk by a local shepherd and the opportunity to collect wild asparagus. Alternatively, they can give you maps and you can coordinate your own itinerary.

One of their routes starts out from the base of the hill into Sant'Angelo. Turn right onto the main road and follow it out past the village beyond the Grotte delle Necropoli (too deep to explore alone) and Vallone del Ponte (good for caving) and then turn through the forestale (forestry) gate into **Bosco Castello** after about four km. On the left are an interesting set of caves and you can find wild asparagus here in the right season. The forest track is a dirt road that winds through for another four km down to the main road at the back of town. Turn right on this and follow the rough, rocky path, with wonderful views of the river below past almond, olive and *ficchi di India* (prickly pear) trees. The round-trip is 12-13 km. It could also be attempted on a mountain bike or by car.

Val did Kam can arrange for you to spend a day with shepherds and get them to make the popular soft cheese ricotta. Or they can involve you in local harvests of almonds, tomatoes, grapes and olives.

On Water

 The **Platini River** below town is suitable for kayaking tours of about 10 km. Organize boat rental and transportation with **Val di Kam** (see above).

On Horseback

 Contact **Val di Kam** (see above) for horseback riding itineraries for up to four or five people in the local woods and necropolis or farther afield towards the Valley of Temples (Agrigento), the sulphur mines of Comitine and the Naro dam. Overnight excursions are also possible.

Where to Stay

 Val di Kam (see above) has also developed B&B accommodation around town with local people as part of an initiative called **Orange Juice** (www.orangejuice.it). They can bed up to 50 people (with notice). Prices range from €28-€35 per person.

Where to Eat

 For a small place Sant'Angelo has a surprising number of places to eat.

The Interior

Il Cappriccio (Main Piazza 33, ☎ 092-291-9634, closed Mon) is open for lunch and dinner with pizza and main meals. **Eden Pizzeria** (Piano Croce, Piazzetta Belvedere, ☎ 0922-919-392, closed Thurs).**Ristorante Villa Gioiosa** (Piazzetta Belevedere, ☎ 0922-919-042, closed Tues) serves lunch and dinner. **Bar Sant'Angelo**, in the main square next to the *gelateria* ,can provide snacks.

Palazzo Adriano

This has to be Sicily's best square and is immediately recognizable to visitors as where *Cinema Paradiso* was filmed – the fabulous 1988 classic about a young boy growing up with the local cinema. The young Toto – now in his 20s – is actually from Palazzo Adriano and works locally (the writer's secret) so you might see him around!

The square is an attraction in its own right but the quiet streets, classic churches, good eating and beautiful surrounding countryside add to its charm. Surprisingly, it still seems little visited, except by film aficionados – mostly Japanese and some Italians, Germans and Dutch, who come to relive the magic of the film.

There are two major ethnic groups in Palazzo Adriano that still guard their religions, costumes and traditions. One group

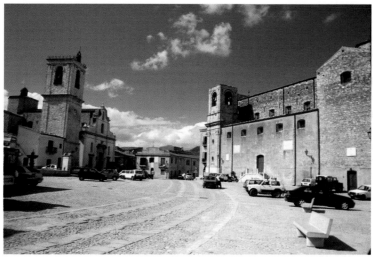

Piazza Umberto in Palazzo Adriano (Joanne Lane)

is Greek/Albanese (Byzantine) and the other Italian/Latin.
The Albanese arrived in the 1400s.

Getting Here

Palazzo Adriano is served by **AST** buses (☎ 091-680-0011, www.aziendasicilianatrasporti.it). Access to
Palermo is possible via four direct services or a
change in Corleone (7:15 am), from where you could make six
connections to the capital. Buses for Palazzo Adriano leave
Corleone at 1:30 pm.

Information Sources

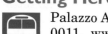

Tourist Office (Via Francesco Crispi 31, ☎ 091-834-8423 or 091-834-9051). **Pro Loco Ufficio Turstico**
(Piazza Umberto I, ☎ 091-834-9911, Mon-Fri 8 am-
2 pm, Tues and Thurs 3-6 pm).

Sightseeing

The key sights are clustered around the famed ★★★**Piazza
Umberto**. There's really nothing like this in all of Italy – a
vast space that immediately grabbed director Giuseppe
Tornatore's attention and which is jokingly described as the
piazza that won the Oscar. It is still used by cars and, during
the day, looks like a grand parking lot. If you're hoping for
good photos, get here very early or wait for midday when people go home. Unlike other piazzas in Italy that are round or
square, this one has no real form and there is no central point,
just a fountain to one side (the **Fontana Ottagonale**, dating
from 1608). The movie theater used for the film was constructed and destroyed for the movie. The interior of the
theater was shot in Chiesa Santa Maria del Carmelo near the
supermarket, past the *carabinieri*. It is open on Saturday afternoons for mass. If you wander the few streets of the town
you may recognize other filming locations.

In the main square are two churches for each of the religious
groups of Palazzo Adriano. The Byzantine church, **Chiesa
Maria SS Assunta**, was built in the 16th century. Inside is a
beautiful wooden altar. The **Chiesa Maria SS Lume** of the 18th
century is *Romano*. Both are open in the mornings until 1 pm.

In the Municipio, to the left side of the Assunta church, is the
Pro Loco tourist office and a photographic exhibit from the
filming of *Cinema Paradiso*. There are also black and white
photographs of the town's past and the Museo

Geonaturalistico with fossils found in the area, particularly from Pietra di Salamone.

If you have extra time in Palazzo Adriano, follow some of the *sentieri* by the Club Alpino Italiano to Pietra di Salamone – the tourist office can give you a map.

Where to Stay & Eat

 Albergo del Viale (Viale Vittorio Veneto 2, ☎ 091-834-8164, 333-445-2231, www.albergodelviale.it, €€) is close to the center and offers weekend specials from Saturday morning to Sunday night, including two lunches and one dinner for €50. The restaurant has a good view of the piazza and serves local food and grilled meat.

Albergo a Casa Vecchia (Via Cartiera 1, ☎ 091-834-9051, €€) is an old house recently restored with elegant rooms and a restaurant. The food is typically Sicilian, using old recipes, with local seasonal vegetables such as asparagus and fennel. Grilled lamb, sausage and veal are also offered.

★Corleone

The notorious town of Corleone seems to be one of those that time forgot. The approach to the town tends to prepares you for the experience, taking you along some of Sicily's worst

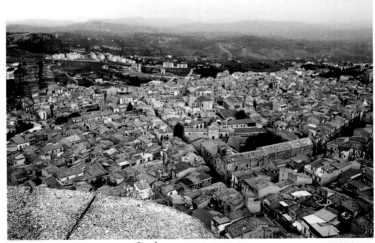

Corleone (Michael Urso)

roads – and that's saying something – with huge potholes, piles of rubbish and a large population of stray cats. The town is set beneath a cliff, an ominous spectre somewhat symbolic of the control the Mafia must exercise over this town. There is something heavy in the Corleone air that is almost palpable. Nothing seems to be open or to function, and the locals even joke openly about it. There are probably interesting things to see and do, if only you can find them. This town was among the most difficult to research in all of Sicily. If you're with a guided tour you'll probably have a better chance of getting something out of it. Expect museums, restaurants and tourist offices to be closed. Having said that, Corleone is certainly an interesting place to linger for a few hours.

THE MAFIA

What exactly is Corleone's association with the Mafia? Well it has had one of the highest murder rates per capita in the world and the fire brigade found a whole bunch of corpses in a crevice near Corleone in 1948, including a "missing" trade union leader. Mario Puzo chose the name Corleone for the central character in *The Godfather* because the town was renowned as a stomping ground for Mafia leaders. In 1993, the alleged Mafia boss, Salvatore Riina, was actually arrested and it was discovered that he lived in Corleone with his family for over 20 years. It has been the birthplace of Mafia bosses Michele Navarra, Luciano Leggio, Leoluca Bagarella, Salvatore Riina and Bernardo Provenzano. In 2003 an unsuccessful referendum was held to change the name of Corleone to its ancient name of *Cuor di Leone* (Lion Heart). The idea was to shed its association with Mafiosi. Interestingly, the grandparents of Al Pacino (who plays Michael Corleone in *The Godfather*) emigrated from the town, part of the same generation as Don Vito Corleone from the film.

Getting Here

 AST buses go from Palermo to Corleone (10 daily, two hrs 15 mins) and **Ficuzza** (five daily, 25 minutes). You can also get to Palazzo Adriano from Palermo.

Information Sources

i Corleone's tourist offices appear to be permanently closed and if you question the locals about it you will likely be met with either gales of laughter or helpful suggestions that they *might* open next summer! Among the offices that were closed when I visited are the Pro Loco in Piazza Nasce, the Ufficio Turistico (☎ 091-846-3655) and a second Pro Loco in the Villa Comunale. The best place for information is the Central Bar, opposite the Villa Comunale. The friendly manager felt sorry for the number of tourists turning up seeking information from perpetually closed offices and made a map of town that he distributes free of charge. It's worth stopping here for coffee anyway.

Corleone locals are surprisingly engaging and you'll find them willing to help you.

Sightseeing

The **Villa Comunale** or public gardens are a pleasant, large space popular with the aging population and foreign tourists trying to get into the Pro Loco. From Villa Comunale, walk

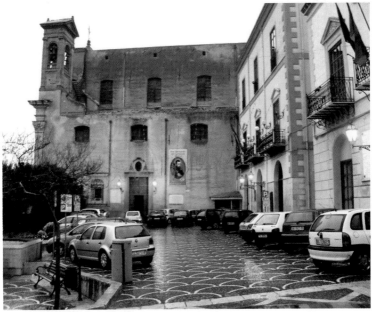

Chiesa Madre, Corleone (Galen R Frysinger, www.galenfrysinger.com)

straight up Via Francesco Bentivegna to the **Chiesa Madre** in Piazza Garibaldi. There were reportedly once 100 churches in Corleone. Now there are 40, but it's unlikely you'll find too many open. However, this one usually is.

To the right of the church are two of Corleone's three museums. They may not necessarily follow their official hours, however! The **Museo Anti Mafia** (Via Orfanotrofio 7, ☎ 091-845-2487, cidmacorleone@yahoo.it, Mon-Sat 9 am-1 pm, 3:30-7:30 pm, Sun 10 am-12 pm, 4-8 pm), near Piazza Giuseppe Garibaldi, has documented the progress of the Mafia movement since the 1960s. Exhibits include photographs of those who have been killed, such as Borsellini (the judge) and known Mafia members. They offer guided tours in English. **Museo Civico** (Via Orfanotrofio 7, ☎ 091-846-8084, Mon-Fri 9 am-1 pm, 3:30-7:30 pm, Sat and Sun 10 am-12 pm, 4-7 pm), in the same building, has finds from the Neolithic, Norman, Hellenistic and Roman ages, all found near Corleone. Exhibits include ceramics, mosaic stones and amphorae.

The third museum is **Museo Etnografico del Corleone** (Piazza Asilo), which was closed at the time of writing. Well placed signs across from Piazza Garibaldi mark the route down rubbish-lined streets.

Beyond the museum you can see the **Castello di Saraceni**, also known as **Castello Sottano**. Corleone was built between two rocks on which two Saracen fortifications were built. In this one is a monastery with barefoot Franciscan friars wearing long beards. It's an impressive entrance to the castle up the side of a rock face. Everyone can visit (9 am-12:30 pm, 5-7 pm), but women are only allowed inside the chapel. There's a good view from the top.

If you return to Piazza Giuseppe Garibaldi and turn left on Via Roma to Piazza San Domenico, you can follow directions to **La Cascata delle due rocche**, where the defensive walls that once connected the Castello Soprano and Castello Sottano fell down.

Where to Eat

 The **Central Bar**, across from the Villa Comunale, is your best bet for snacks and food. There are some other options along Via Francesco Bentivegna. Or try **Trattoria Gennaro** (Via Verde, ☎ 091-846-4767), which is

also a hotel. **Al Capriccio Restaurant** (☎ 0918-467-938) or **A'Giarra** (☎ 091-846-4000) have pizza and local dishes.

Where to Stay

 Belvedere (☎ 0918-464-000) in Contrada Belvedere or **Agriturismo a Casa Mia** in Loc. Malvello (☎ 091-846-7529).

Ficuzza

Ficuzza is a small, misty hamlet in the mountains south of Palermo where the old *ferrovia* (train line) to Corleone used to pass through. Ferdinand I of the Two Sicilies Kingdom (comprising Naples and Sicily) lived here too and built a royal residence for hunting. The **Bosco della Ficuzza** is a natural park and the largest wood in western Sicily that Ferdinand used in his exile as a royal game reserve. The wood is protected by the imposing Rocca Busambra and is an ideal place for those keen on wild orchids. Horseback riding, trekking and cycling are possible in the park.

The few streets of Ficuzza town are near the hunting lodge, with a few shops and bars, an army of dogs and cats (some of which were lying dead in the street when I was last there) and graffiti that say *vogliamo la luce* (we want the light). Whether there is light at night or not we don't know but on first appearances the town does appear a little scabby and deserted. However, hang out for a bit and you will see other people around. It's a popular route for walkers and bikers and at any moment a group of German cyclists could pull in to the Bar Caveretta to liven it up. Or you may get stuck with just the dead dog. In any case, it's worth a visit.

Information Sources

Antica Stazione Ferroviaria di Ficuzza (☎/fax 091-846-0000, 338-574-1023, www.anticastazione.it) is the best option and usually has maps and information at any time of year. The *Forestale* (☎ 091-846-4062), the local forestry department, which is behind the hunting lodge, should be able to provide details of Bosco di Ficuzza, although they had run out of maps when we visited late in the season. **Bar Cavaretta** also sells books and maps when they're in print. They often run out at the end of the season.

The **APT** in Palermo (www.palermoturismo.com) produces a
sentieri map, *Corleone Bosco della Ficuzza* (1:50,000), and a
smaller brochure with 15 itineraries in the province.

To get a guide call the Centro Guide Naturalistiche (GAIE)
☎ 091-846-0107.

Getting Here

 AST buses (☎ 091-688-2783) run from Ficuzza to
Palermo (five daily, one hr 20 mins) and Corleone
(five daily, 25 mins).

Sightseeing

The **Palazzina** or **Palazzo Reale Borbonico** (☎ 091-846-
0107, 9 am-1 pm, 3-7 pm; €2), dating from 1802-1806, looks
more like a stately English manor and completely dominates
the town across a broad stretch of lawn. Staff provides a
guided tour as part of the entrance fee. The king only lived
here for 2½ years and came to hunt in the woods nearby. Local
stones were used to build the lodge and the entrance pavement looks like a fish spine. There are two corridors on the
bottom floor. To the left the servants lived – easily noted by
the kitchen and uneven floor. To the right is the Cappareale,
made of a red marble from Corleone. The house was robbed

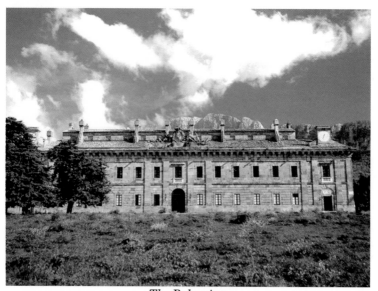

The Palazzina

many times but there are still vestments and old books. The nobles lived on the first floor. In the bedroom are original frescoes – all hunting scenes – and the original furnishings include a *bidea* (toilet). The king's bedroom was lit by a fire from the room underneath. In the cellars below the ground floor the horses were kept. There's an old Sicilian cart here, a military telegraph room used in the war and a cantina for making oil, wine and cheese. Another room was used for conserving the meat that was hunted. Across the lawn outside the palace are a series of arches where horses were kept and now home to the Guardia Medica.

Adventures

On Foot

Walks of varying distances are signposted from the town if you don't have any maps or information with you. At the Antica Stazione Ferroviaria (see *Where to Stay*) you can follow the former railway track for 21 km. It's actually a mountain bike course (see *Adventures on Wheels*). Another walking track, *sentiero 5*, passes through here to a bridge and cave. Contact them directly about their other itineraries.

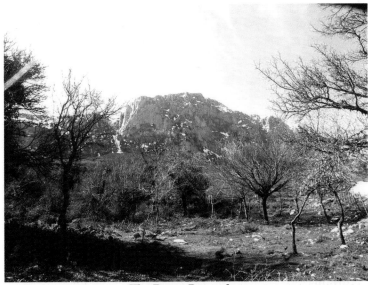

The Rocca Busambra

The APT Palermo lists nine *sentieri* of varying difficulty through the park. Most are ring routes so you can return to your starting point. The most panoramic and spectacular is the one along the ridge of **Rocca Busambra** (six hours), but it is recommended you take a guide. The route from the **Alpe Cucco** hostel is considered the finest valley walk. The paths starting at **Gole del Drago** allow you to visit the places where the king used to hunt and fish.

On Wheels

 You can rent mountain bikes from the **Antica Stazione Ferroviaria** for €5/hr and complete the 21-km ride on the old railway track.

There are two other official mountain bike routes from Ficuzza to Alpe Cucco and Valle Agnese, along the antica ferrovia and back to Ficuzza. A second starts in Massariotta and goes to Ficuzza, Alpe Cucco and Pizzo di Casa.

Another itinerary of 35 km (3½ hours) starts from the main gate of Regia di Ficuzza. It continues via the former rail line to Santa Barbara, Gorgo del Drago, Alpe Cucco and back. The Palermo bike group, Bokos, promotes this itinerary, which is described in full at www.bokos.it/bikeaffair.

On Horseback

 The APT Palermo lists four horseback itineraries through the park:

- Ficuzza to Lago dello Scanzano
- Rifugio Val dei Conti to Bosco Manca
- Ficuzza to Godrano
- Azienda Gorgo del Grago to Fanuso and Cozzo Tondo

The **Forestale**, or forestry department (☎ 091-846-4062), can provide horseback tours of the forest if a request is made to their Palermo office. Or contact these groups:

- Bolognetta (Valle degli Elfi C. da Stallone SP 77, km 13,370, ☎ 091-829-1406).
- Gorgo del Drago (C. da Cannitello, ☎ 091-820-8000, 091-820-8303).
- Villa Russo (C. da Pilastri, Chiosi, ☎ 091-846-4925).
- Antica Stazione Ferroviaria can organize special rides for groups of at least eight persons, lasting two days or more.

The Interior

Where to Stay & Eat

 The **Antica Stazione Ferroviaria di Ficuzza** (☎/ fax 091-846-0000, 338-574-1023, www.antica-stazione.it, €€) is one km before town on the old railway station of the narrow gauge line that ran from Palermo to Corleone. Ficuzza was a place to break the journey and was actually used for filming *The Godfather* scene when Michael Corleone arrived in Sicily. The old railway track is still used (see *Adventures*). Inside, the old station is now a refined restaurant (closed Mon) and a lively wine hall. In July and August there are jazz and blues concerts.

Bar Pizzeria Cavaretta (☎ 091-846-3915) is a good central spot in town to stop for a bite. They've been operating since 1953 and on some days they make fabulous cannolli.

■ The Southern Interior

This part of the interior has far more going for it, featuring two of the island's biggest drawcards, the towns of Piazza Armerina and Caltagirone. There are also the extensive ruins of Morgantina and the incredible mosaics of Villa Romana del Casale. The southern interior is also well served by train and bus, and features one of the island's few hostels.

HIGHLIGHTS

- **Palio dei Normanni**, Piazza Armerina – This colorful festival re-enacts medieval battle scenes and horseback riding skills from centuries past.
- **Villa Romana del Casale** – The ancient mosaics at the villa outside Piazza Armerina.
- A *fragola con panna* (strawberries and cream) flavored *granita* in Piazza Armerina.
- **La Scala** – Caltagirone's staircase with beautiful ceramic tiles is one of Sicily's most visited and photographed sights.
- **Butera's balcony** over Sicily.
- The ancient ruins of **Morgantina**.

Piazza Armerina

The lively 17th-century town of Piazza Armerina is one of the highlights of a visit to inland Sicily. It is well served by public transport and has a number of key attractions, including the exquisite mosaics at Villa Romana del Casale and one of the island's most interesting horseback riding festivals. There are plenty of accommodations and enough to see to keep you at least a day or two.

Getting Here & Getting Around

Most buses stop at Piazza Senatore Marescalchi on the main road, Via Generale Ciancio. There is a bus office here that is almost always closed. Fortunately, route times are posted outside or you can ask at Bar della Stazione next door. There are **AST buses** (☎ 095-723-0511) from Siracusa and Caltagirone, **Etna Trasporti** (☎ 093-556-5111) to/from Aidone (eight daily, 15 minutes), Enna and Catania (six daily, €7); and **SAIS** to Caltagirone (45 minutes, €2.50).

Traffic in Piazza Armerina's one-way system can be a nightmare so avoid driving through if you can. **Buses** to Villa Romano leave between 10 am and 3 pm from the station; watch for their orange bus. The service stops running after October. If you're looking for **car rental** the friendly staff – especially Giuseppe – at **Maxicar** (C. da Cicciona 16, ☎ 093-585-426, 334-140-0239) will help you out and even pick you up from town. Thanks to all of them for their hospitality and service – including some very good *granite* and impromptu tour guiding. If you need a **taxi**, call ☎ 0935-680-501.

Information Sources

The **Centro di Informazione Turistiche** (Via Cavour 15, ☎ 093-568-3049, Mon-Fri 9 am-1 pm, 3-7 pm in summer, mornings only in winter) is uphill from Piazza Garibaldi towards the Duomo. They should be able to give you a map of the town and information about the Roman Villa at Casale.

Comune Piazza Armerina (Piazza Garibaldi, ☎ 0935-683-049, www.comune.piazzaarmerina.en.it).

Events

Major festivals in Piazza Armerina include the **Palio dei Normanni** held over three days from August 12-14 and a **religious festival** on May 3 when the image of the Madonna is taken around the town.

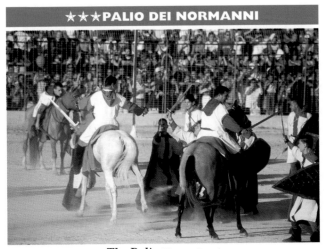

★★★**PALIO DEI NORMANNI**

The Palio (Joanne Lane)

This medieval pageant (www.paliodeinormanni.it), from August 12-14, celebrates Count Roger's capture of the town from the Moors in 1087. Festivities culminate on August 14 with historical parades, reenactments of the final battle and a joust with armor, lances and horses. The horsemen undertake four trials, competing for the *contrade* (districts) of the town: Monte, Castellina, Canali and Casalotto. The whole town celebrates good naturedly. If you're anywhere in Sicily during this time make your way over here.

There's a permanent taste of the Palio at the **Mostra Permanente Palio dei Normanni** (Palazzo Senatorio, Via Cavour 1, ☎ 0935-982-257, Mon-Sat 10 am-1 pm, 4-7 pm, mornings only in winter) up from Porta Giovanni. Pictures and costumes are on display explaining the 50-year history of the festival that was founded by the two brothers Angelo and Giuseppe Urzie to revive medieval horsemanship.

Sightseeing

★★★**Villa Romana del Casale** (☎ 0935-680-036, 8 am-6:30 pm, €8) is actually five km out of town (see *Getting Here & Getting Around*). It's Sicily's most important Roman ruin and probably *the* reason you're in Piazza Armerina. The beauty of the mosaics and the sheer size of the villa is astounding. It was most likely the property of a Roman dignitary and used as an occasional retreat and

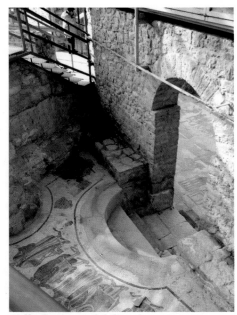

Villa Romana del Casale (Galen R Frysinger)

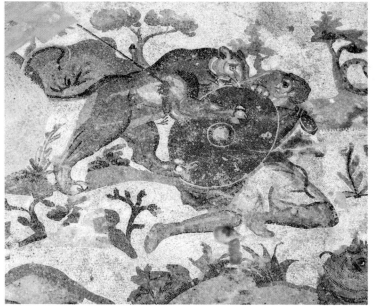

Mosaic from Villa Casale (Galen R Frysinger, www.galenfrysinger.com))

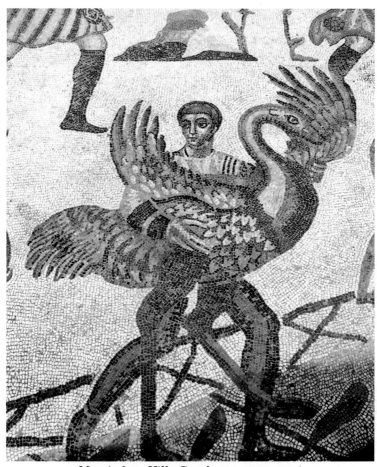

Mosaic from Villa Casale (Galen R Frysinger)

hunting lodge – as the many mosaics attest. There are four groups of buildings which date from the early fourth century. It was used until the 12th century, when a landslide left it covered in mud and probably protected it from vandalism and the adverse effects of nature. The ruins were noticed again in 1761 but not excavated until 1929, then more comprehensively in the 1950s. They are now under a protective structure and have raised walkways. There are Roman baths near the entrance, a latrine area, a courtyard, gymnasium and the central area contains the hunting scenes mosaic – among the

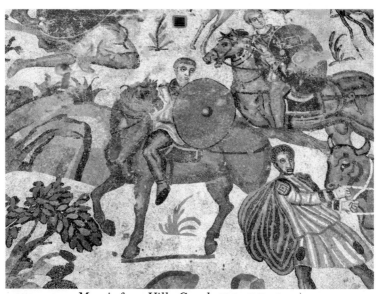

Mosaic from Villa Casale (Galen R Frysinger)

largest ever found – and the famed mosaic of 10 girls wearing bikinis.

Back in town much of the action and sights center around **Piazza Garibaldi**. The **Museo Archaeologico** (☎ 093-568-8510, 8 am-6 pm, €6) in the square contains findings from the Villa Romana. Up the hill on Via Cavour, past the tourist office, is the **Piazza del Duomo** and the 17th-century **Duomo**, where celebrations for the Palio are held. It took nearly three centuries to build this church, with its majestic portal and tortile columns. Inside, the interior is blue and white. This is the town's highest point and the square beyond has great views over the town. Adjacent to the Duomo is the 18th-century **Palazzo Trigona**. The area around the Duomo is known as the Castellina district because there was a medieval castle where the monastery of St Francis now stands (off Via Cavour).

Narrow alleys behind the Duomo lead into older parts of town known as **Il Monte**. The fishbone streets and narrow alleys are fun to explore. Via Monte was once the town's main street; you can veer off down to the churches of San Martino and Crocifisso. Or head down Via Floresta from near Palazzo Trignona to a 14th-century Aragonese castle. Follow Via V. Emanuele back to Piazza Garibaldi.

The Interior

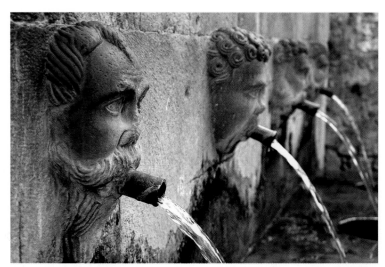

The Fonte dei Casale (Joanne Lane)

The **Canali district** is in the lowest part of town, once inhabited by Jews. An abundant fresh water supply was provided by the ★**Fonte dei Canali**, which fed the medieval washhouse near the small church of St Lucy. Casalotto is the district the other side of Via Liberta and the fourth part of town.

Where to Stay

Hostel

The friendly ★**Ostello del Borgo** (Largo S. Giovanni 6, ☎ 093-568-7019, www.ostellodelborgo.it, €) has 20 rooms in the cells of an 18th-century convent right in the historic center of town. It's one of Sicily's few and best hostels.

B&Bs

B&B Giucalem (La Casa Negli Orti, C. da Belvedere snc, ☎ 093-589-801, www.giucalem.com, €€) is near the Villa Casale on the road to the mosaics.

B&B Marconi (Via Marconi 26/28, Via Sette Cantoni 8, ☎/fax 093-568-2989, 329-090-8075), in the center, has five plain rooms, a terrace and a café downstairs where you can breakfast on typical Sicilian *cornetti*, *granite*, *cannoli* and *latte di mandorle*.

La Locanda del Normanno B&B
(Via Orfanotrofio 76, ☎ 333-337-08919, 333-972-8317, www.locandadelnormanno.com, €€), in the Monte quarter, with four rooms and attached baths. There's also a small terrace with views of the old roofs in the quarter.

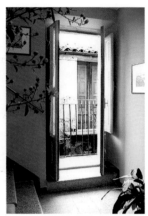

Locanda del Normanno

La Casa sulla Collina d'Oro B&B (Via Mattarella snc, ☎/fax 093-589-680, ☎ 333-466-8829, www.lacasa-sullacollinadoro.it,

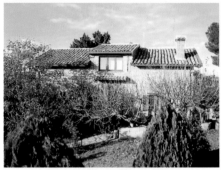

Casa sulla Collina d'Oro

€€€) is a little way from the center. It has bright, cheerful rooms and equally colorful names.

Hotels

Hotel Gangi (Via Generale Ciancio 68/70, ☎ 0935-682-737, fax 0935-687-573, www.hotelgangi.it, €€€-€€€€) has reasonably spacious hotel rooms.

Hotel Villa Romana (Via A. De Gasperi 18, ☎/fax 0935-682-911, www.piazza-armerina.it/hotel-villaromana) is Piazza Armerina's largest and grandest hotel, with three restaurants and 55 rooms, used by business travelers and for local receptions.

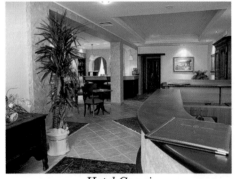

Hotel Gangi

The Interior

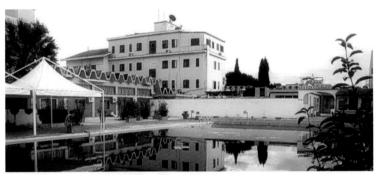

Park Hotel Paradiso

Park Hotel Paradiso (Contrada Ramaldo, ☎ 0935-680-841, www.parkhotelparadiso.it, €€€€) is a four star with a swimming pool. Rooms are tastefully decorated and it attracts both business people and tourists.

Agriturismi

Two agriturismi 10-15 km out of town offer a unique experience in the area. The ★★**Agriturismo Gigliotto** (C. da Gigliotto SS 117 bis Km 60, ☎/fax 0933-970-898, 335-838-0324, 337-889-052, www.gigliotto.com, €€€€), on 840 acres of land, produces a range of cereals, grains, wine and oil. It offers opportunities to watch the harvests, walk, ride horses etc. A swimming pool is fantastically located with a view of the hillsides around. The rooms use traditional furniture from the owner's family collection. Gigliotto was a 14th-century monastery. You can also do horseback riding and walking excursions. They allow camping on site.

The nearby **Vecchia Masseria** is another good choice (☎/fax 093-568-4003, 335-534-9141, 333-875-573, www.vecchiamasseria.it, €€).

Where to Eat

Cafés

Caffeteria Marconi (Via Marconi 26/28, ☎ 093-568-2989) is a sala a the or tea room.

The **Cattedrale Café** is a good local option opposite the tourist information office in Via Cavour.

★**Café Sport** has Piazza Armerina's best *granite* – try *fragola con panna* – outside the Comune offices (Via Marconi

2, Piazza Garibaldi, ☎ 093-568-0081). You'll spot its mosaics above the door outside Chiesa S Rocco.

The **Bar Duomo** in the piazza behind the church has seating out in the square, but you could also take food across to benches by the belvedere.

At **Café des Amis** (Via Marconi 22, ☎ 0935-680-661, www. cafédesamis.net) you can find typical sweets like *cannolli*.

Enotecas

Vilma Wine Bar (Via Garibaldi 89, ☎ 093-568-4609) is an English-speaking place, good for an evening drink and with free Internet.

Restaurants

Garibaldi 62 (Via Garibaldi 62, ☎ 093-568-8537, www. garibaldi62.it, closed Mon) is a classy spot combing modern elegance and old charm. It has an interior garden. You need to reserve ahead.

Pizzeria Teatro (Via Teatro 5, closed Tues, €€-€€€) has seats overlooking the teatro and has copied mosaics from the Villa Romano for the floors and walls. Pizza is cooked *forno a legna*, other specialties include *pappardelle al teatro* (with cream, ham, mushrooms, tomatoes and brandy) and *pappardelle della Sicilia* (with tomatoes and ricotta).

Ristorante Tavernetta Almonte (Via Cavour, ☎ 093-568-5883) specializes in seafood.

Pizzeria da Toto (Via Mazzini 29, ☎ 0935-680-153, 9:30 am-4 pm, 6-12 pm, closed Mon) is recommended.

Pepito (Via Roma 140, ☎ 0935-685-737, closed Tues) serves grilled fish and meat.

Aidone

Aidone is a small provincial town that you'll probably visit only on the way to seeing **Morgantina**, the noteworthy remains of an extensive Greek city. The town itself is rather quiet with a central square and a few bars. **Etna Trasporti** (☎ 093-556-5111) runs from Piazza Armerina eight times daily (15 minutes). The only tourist office, the **Aidone Associazione Turistica Pro Loco** (☎ 0935-865-57), appeared closed at the time of writing and, if you're only here to visit Morgantina, go straight out to the site office for informa-

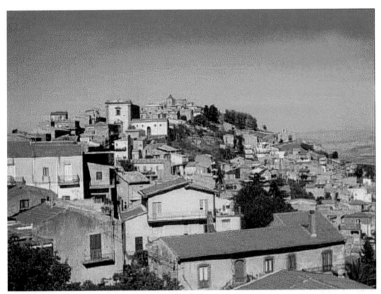

Aidone

tion. **Museo Archeologico di Aidone** (Piazza Torres Truppia, ☎ 0935-87307, 8 am-6:30 pm, €3.10) was closed at the time of writing, with plans to open shortly. It contains aerial photos and finds from Morgantina. There is no public transport to Morgantina so you'll have to hitch, walk or use your own vehicle. Locals say the SP 288 leaving Aidone is notorious for problems and best not traveled at night. It's in fairly rough condition.

The entrance to the **Morgantina ruins** (☎ 093-587-955, 8:30 am-one hr before sunset, €3) is five km from Aidone, then another km beyond the entrance off the SP 288. Morgantina was founded by the Morgeti about 850 BC, a pre-Hellenic Sikel population. It was not identified again as Morgantina until the 1950s, and archaeologists are still working to uncover more of it.

From the main entrance, the path takes you straight to the *agora* used for public meetings. The small *teatro* to the right was built in the third century BC and the Enna province organizes events here every year in August. Behind the *teatro* is a fourth-century BC *santuario* of Demeter and Kore, as well as a granary and square slaughterhouse.

If you need some-
where to stay, there
is the **Albergo
Morgantina** (Via
Adelasia, ☎ 0935-
86074) or the nearby
**Agriturismo Cam-
marata** (Contrada
Pintura S Giovanni,
☎ 0935-88144). Turn
left just before the
site entrance on the
SP 288. They have
mountain bikes and
can recommend trek-
king and horseback
riding excursions.

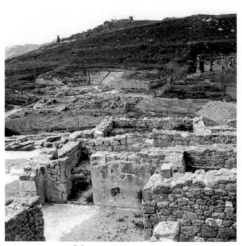
Morgantina ruins

For food try the cafés and bars in the main piazza of Aidone or
La Torre Ristorante (Via Adelasia) off the piazza. At
Morgantina there are some cafés along the road near the site
entrance. Be wary of sheep dogs on this road if you are on foot.
The best spot to eat is **Restaurant Eyexei** (Contrada
Morgantina, ☎ 0935-87074, www.ristoranteeyexei.com, €),
run by a local family who serve their own cheese, oil, meat and
vegetables. They are open every day from April to September.
They also have maps of the area.

Caltagirone

Caltagirone has a well-earned reputation for its fine ceramics, which have been produced here for over 1,000 years. Earlier Greek settlers were more inclined towards terracotta, but
with the arrival of the Arabs in the 10th century ceramics really took off. The Arabs also gave it the name Caltagirone,
which comes from *kalat* (castle) and *gerun* (caves). After the
1693 earthquake, Caltagirone was rebuilt in Baroque style
and the ceramics industry continues to flourish until this day.
The famed *scala* of Caltagirone, encrusted with ceramic designs, is one of Sicily's best-known attractions; it is even more
beautiful during the annual *Illuminata* on July 24 and 25 every year.

The Interior

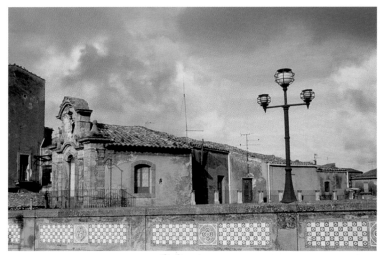

Caltagirone

Getting Here & Getting Around

AST (☎ 095-723-0511) runs between Siracusa, Piazza Armerina and Caltagirone once daily. **SAIS Autolinee** goes to Enna (one hr 25 mins, €4.40), Palermo (two hrs 50 mins, €11) and Piazza Armerina (45 minutes, €2.50). **Etna Trasporti** has services to Catania (one hr 30 mins, six daily), Piazza Armerina (60 mins, one daily). Trains also come from Gela and Catania.

Take **Linea 1** from the train station to get to Piazza Umberto.

Information Sources

3 G Tourist Service (Piazza Umberto 1, ☎/fax 093-357-781, 3gtouristservice@tiscali.it, closed Wed). **Informazioni Ufficio Turistiche Comune di Caltagirone** (Via Duomo 7, ☎/fax 093-334-191, 093-335-1073, Mon-Sat 9 am-7 pm, Sun 9 am-1 pm, 3-7 pm). **Servizi Cultura e Turismo** (☎ 093-334-191, 351-073, 41809, www.comune.caltagirone.ct.it, servizio-turismo@comune.caltagirone.ct.it). **Pro Loco Azienda Autonoma Soggiorno e Turismo** (☎ 0932-53809, Mon-Sat 8 am-2 pm, 3:30-6:30 pm; Mon and Fri-Sat mornings only in winter, closed Sun) has hotel lists, ceramic guides and maps, plus a display of ceramics and puppets.

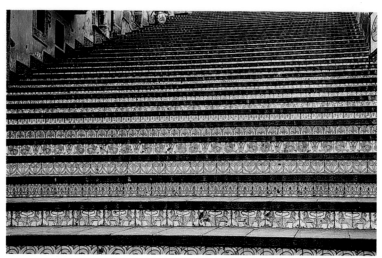
La Scala in Caltagirone

Events

 On the third Sunday of every month is **A Truvatura**, a market of antiques and handmade goods, with concerts and exhibitions.

La Luminaria or **La Scala Illuminata** is on July 24-25. In May, it's covered in flowers on the third Sunday in May.

Sightseeing

From the moment you enter Caltagirone you'll be passing endless numbers of ceramic workshops and bridges, street signs, shops and hotels lined with ceramic flowers and emblems. Even the Giardini Pubblici (public gardens; 8 am-9 pm) have ceramics as you enter. However, the 142 steps of ★★★**La Scala**, rising from Piazza Municipio to the Chiesa di Santa Maria del Monte, is the biggest drawing card of all. No two stairs are the same and you can browse in and out of rows of ceramic workshops on the way up. They sell everything from ashtrays to vases, plates, house numbers and animals. Little gifts start from just €3. The staircase was built at the turn of the 17th century but the ceramic tiles were only a recent addition in the 1950s. On July 24 and 25 every year they are made even more colorful when thousands of colored paper lamps light the stairs as part of celebrations for the feast of St James. At the top of *La Scala* is the church of

The Interior

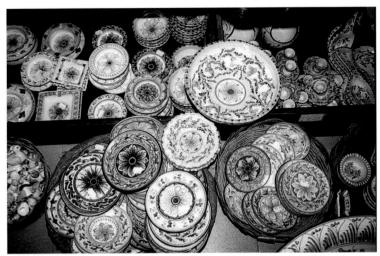

Caltagirone ceramics (Joanne Lane)

Santa Maria del Monte, where you can look down over the stairs and into the town.

You can fill your suitcases with ceramics anywhere in town. One huge warehouse is the **Ceramica di Caltagirone Mostra Mercato Permanente** (Via Vittorio Emanuele 7/9, ☎ 093-356-444, fax 093-358-749, www.ceramicadicaltagirone. it), with rows and rows of ceramics. You can also buy them online! And if you've still not had your fill, there's the **Museo Regionale della Ceramica** (☎ 093-358-418, 093-358-423, 9 am-6:30 pm, €3) near the gardens.

The main **Duomo** is in Piazza Umberto, but it's rather plain compared to other towns.

Where to Stay

 Grand Hotel Villa San Mauro (Via Porto Salvo 14, ☎ 0933-26500, €€€€) is part of the luxury Framon hotel chain, with classic suites.

La Scala Affitacamere (Scala S. Maria del Monte 8, ☎/fax 0933-57781,

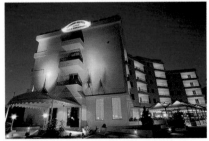

Grand Hotel Villa San Mauro

3gtouristservice@tiscalinet.it, €€) has plain rooms but a great location on the stairs.

La Pilozza Infiorata B&B (Via S.S Salvatore 95/97, www.lapilozzainfiorata.com, ☎ 0933-22162, 328-702-9543, 339-735-2861, €€€) is right in the center of Caltagirone. The 12 rooms are tastefully decorated and you get views of the higher parts of town from the breakfast terraces. Families like to use the apartment with a small cooking area.

Villino Diana B&B (Via Portosalvo 27, ☎ 0933-21175, www.villinodiana.it) has a pleasant garden and rents bikes.

Pineta San Marco B&B (Via Ottavia Penna 61, ☎ 093-360-589, 093-219-81, 339-695-3670, www.pinetasanmarco.it, €€) is a villa two km from the Caltagirone center in a green forest. They also allow parking for campers and mobile homes.

Where to Eat

Caffè dell'Arte (Piazza Umberto 1 no. 23) has good gelati.

Mario and Francesco Bar (Via Principe Amedeo 3) serves typical sweets and hot snacks. It has a garden courtyard with a view of the Duomo.

Judica & Trieste e Figli (Via P. Amedeo 22, ☎ 093-322-021) is a good spot for gelati, pastries and cocktails.

Nonsolovino Restaurant (Via Vittorio Emanuele 1, ☎ 093-331-068, closed Mon, €) serves regional foods, grilled meat and fish, as well as homemade cakes.

Pizzeria La Scala (Scala S. Maria del Monte 8, ☎/fax 093-357-781, 3gtouristservice@tiscalinet.it, closed Tues, €€) is just a few steps up the *scala* on the right in an 18th-century palace of the Princes of Reburdone. A spring-water source still flows through the restaurant and you can see it coursing through the rooms under protective glass.

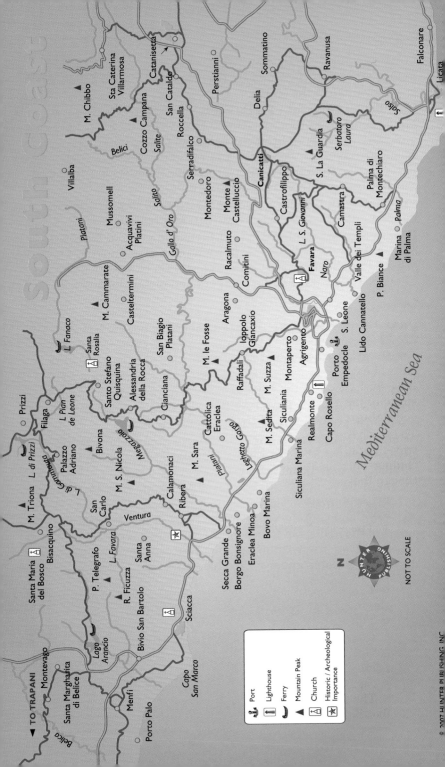

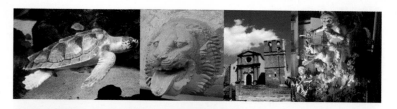

The South Coast

The south coast of Sicily runs from Gela to Sciacca and is relatively unvisited by tourists, except for **Agrigento's** splendid temples – one of Sicily's must-sees. Many people are put off by the ugly industrial development near **Gela**, but the town has some important historic remains. The

coastline also has marvelous beaches, particularly the white cliffs of **Eraclea Minoa**, north of Agrigento. **Sciacca** is a real find, with a fishing port and clifftop town, plus a fantastic summer jazz program. You could also venture out to the rugged **Pelagie Islands** or inland to see **Caltabellotta's** castles.

The south coast is easily accessible by bus and train links; boats travel regularly to the islands in season. Accommodations, including budget campsites, are plentiful along the coast, although they are scarce in the small towns of the interior.

AGRIGENTO HIGHLIGHTS

■ The **Valley of Temples** lit up at night.
■ Listening to **Sciacca Jazz** in the summer, followed by a gelato and views from **Piazza Scandaliato**.
■ **Eraclea Minoa's** Greek city ruins and a swim on the fine beach below.
■ The rocky shores of **Lampedusa**.
■ Chatting with the friar at **Monte San Calogero**.
■ **Caltabellotta's** jagged promontories and castle ruins.
■ Sunset at **Adranone**.
■ The impressive **Selinunte** temples with their 80-foot-high high columns.

■ Gela

Gela was one of the most important of Sicily's Greek cities and even rivaled Siracusa as a center of learning. But today it's surrounded by smoking industrial factories. The historical center, with its archaeological museum, is a lot better. It was founded by colonists in 689 BC and enjoyed a brief heyday until it was destroyed by Carthage in 405 BC. It was rebuilt, only to be destroyed again, thenit lay in ruins until 1230, when a new town was built. In 1927 the town took back its original

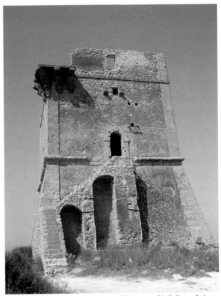

Gela's 16th-century Torre di Manfria
(LuckyLisp)

name, Gela. It was the first town in Sicily to be liberated by the Allies in 1943. The main sights in Gela are the excellent museum and the Greek defensive walls.

Getting Here & Around

Trains and buses pull in at Piazza Stazione. Services include **SAIS Autolinee** (☎ 199-720-700, 800-920-900) to Palermo, Enna, Piazza Armerina; **AST** to Siracusa and **ASTRA** (☎ 0933-923-248) to Piazza Armerina and Caltanisetta. About 10 trains operate daily between Agrigento and Gela.

From Piazza Stazione get a local bus up to the main town or, to walk there, turn right down the main road and bear right at Corso Vittorio Emanuele.

Sightseeing

The **Museo Archeologico** (9 am-1 pm, 3-7 pm, €3.10), at the end of Corso Vittorio Emanuele, contains finds from the city's

ancient acropolis, dating from the fifth century BC. Most notable is the large collection of red and black painted vases known as *kraters*. These were Gela's specialty between the seventh and fourth centuries BC. There is also a collection of ancient coins, an animated sculpture of a horse's head and the remains of necropolises from Geloan dependencies. Your ticket is also valid for the fourth-century Greek fortifications at Capo Soprano (Via Manzoni, €3.10). It's actually a three- or four-km walk to the ruins – follow Corso Vittorio Emanuele. They are fantastically preserved, probably because they were protected by sand dunes for many years before they were discovered in 1948. Protective walls of up to 26 feet helped protect them in antiquity and still exist in parts today.

Walk back through town past the two main squares containing the Chiesa Madre and down past the gardens. The **Bagni Greci** (Via Europa 50, free), near the hospital, are Greek baths that were only discovered in 1957.

The **Gela beach** is pleasant, with long sand dunes, busy lido bars and pubs. However, it is somewhat blighted by views of heavy industry.

■ Agrigento

Thousands of tourists come to Agrigento every year to see the remains of **Doric temples** on the hillock above the sea. However, it would be a mistake not to explore the sprawling medieval town above it, which contains a surprising number of interesting sights. As the capital of the province, the transport connections to Agrigento are superb and you can combine archaeological itineraries with some fabulous gastronomical experiences and good beaches at San Leone on the coast below. There's also a good range of accommodation choices.

Agrigento does have a few downsides. The massive tourism during the summer can make getting around, particularly to the temples, a traffic nightmare. Town development has also crept down the hillside towards the temples, with ugly modern buildings, highways and bridges. Unemployment is also reportedly grim and a Mafia presence is reputed in town.

Akragras was founded in 581 BC by colonists from Gela and Rhodes, designed as a lookout post over the Mediterranean to watch for the Carthaginians. They surrounded the new city

with a wall and placed the acropolis on the ridge where the modern town now lies. The southern part of the ancient city was where the temples were later built in the fifth century BC when threats of a Carthaginian invasion diminished. The temples reflected the wealth and luxury of ancient Agrigento. However, in 406 BC Carthage overcame Greek resistance, followed by the Romans in 210 BC, who named it Agrigentum. Other waves of Saracens and Normans came through and the ancient city lost its status. In the seventh century BC the bulk of the city's inhabitants moved up the hill to where the modern city now sits.

Getting Here

 Trains link Agrigento with Palermo and Catania. On other routes it could be quicker to get a bus. The train station has luggage lockers, which cost €2.50 for 12 hours. The station in Piazza Marconi lies just below the modern center of town. The valley of the temples is about one km downhill towards the coast.

Buses arrive and depart in Piazza Roselli.

Autoservizi Cuffaro (☎ 091-616-1510, www.cuffaro.info/index.htm) does nine daily trips to Palermo. **Lumia** (☎ 0922-20414, www.autolineelumia.it) travels from Agrigento to Birgi Aeroporto, Caltabellotta, Marsala, Mazara del Vallo, Sambucca, Sciacca and Trapani. **SAIS** (Via Emporium 8, ☎ 0922-412-024) connects daily with Catania, Rome and Napoli from Agrigento. It also has connections with Fontanarossa airport in Catania. The **SAL bus line** (☎ 0922-401-360) will take you direct to Falcone-Borsellino airport in Palermo. **Siremar** ferries (☎ 0922-633-6683) from Porto Empedocle access the Pelagie Islands (see *Pelagie Islands*).

Getting Around

 The local urban bus service **TUA** (☎ 0922-412-024) has five lines. All leave from Piazza Marconi. **Linea Verde** goes from the Piazza along Via Atenea and up to the Duomo. **Linea Arancione** heads out of town near the Museo Archeologico and then to Santuario di Demetra. **Linea 1** goes past the Valley of the Temple and on to Porto Empedocle. **Linea 2** goes past the temples and on to San Leone. **Linea 3** also goes past the temples and then diverts to Grand Hotel dei Templi.

Information Sources

 The best source of information is the **Ufficio Centro Turistico** in the Valle dei Templi car park (☎ 092-226-191, 333-488-2360, 8:30 am-1 pm, 3-7 pm office). The helpful Gigi Montalbano works here.

Ufficio Relazione con il Publicco at the train station (Mon-Fri 8:30 am-1:30 pm, 2:30-7:30 pm, Saturday 8:30 am-1:30 pm) actually has erratic hours.

Events

The most famous festival in Agrigento is the **Flowering Almond Festival** in February. Show, parades and meetings and a big international folklore festival enliven the town for a week.

Sightseeing

★★★Valley of the Temples

The Valle dei Templi site (8:30 am-7 pm, €6) is actually on two sides of the road, helpfully called the eastern and western zone. See *Getting Around* for information on buses. If you're driving it's a busy road in summer. Traffic wardens will show you to free spaces in the lots (€2 for three hours, 8:30 am-1 pm

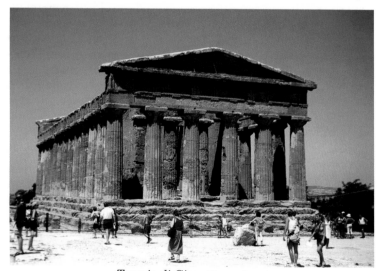

Tempio di Giove (Joanne Lane)

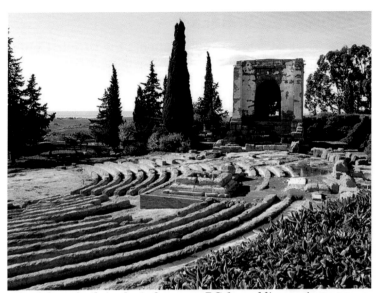

The Odeon, built in the 3rd century BC for public meetings (Galen R Frysinger, www.galenfrysinger.com)

and 4-8 pm). To avoid crowds in summer you should come early.

In the eastern zone there are no fences. The first temple is the **Tempio di Ercole (Tem**ple of Hercules). It is believed to date from the sixth century and is considered the oldest of the temples. Nine of the original 38 columns have been re-erected; you can wander the rest. The next temple is the **Tempio della Concordia** (Temple of Concord) and is the most complete. It was built around 430 BC and converted to a Christian basilica in the sixth century AD. Following the line of ancient city walls you then come to the **Tempio di Gunone** (Temple of Juno), partially destroyed by an earthquake in the Middle Ages. At the eastern end is a long altar used for sacrifices.

The western zone is where your ticket kicks in. The main feature here is the crumbling remains of the **Tempio di Giove** (Temple of Jupiter). This is the largest Doric temple ever known, but it was never completed and later was damaged by an earthquake. It once measured 367 by 184 feet with 66-foot-high columns. This temple is the most photographed site in Agrigento, although unfortunately it was covered in scaffolding at the time of writing. Other remains litter the area – fun

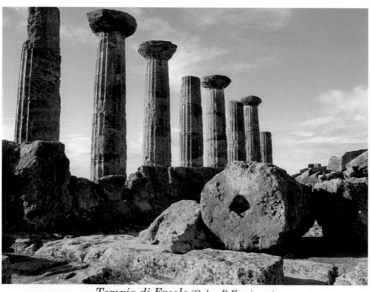

Tempio di Ercole (Galen R Frysinger)

to clamber over or piece together in your own imagination! A few hundred yards farther on is **Tempio dei Dioscuri** (Temple of the Dioscuri), built at the end of the fifth century. It was rebuilt in 1832 using materials from other temples. Behind it is a complex of altars and buildings called the **Santuario delle Divine Chtonice** (Sanctuary of the Chtonic Deities) dating from the early sixth century BC. The temples are illuminated at night from January to March and October to December, 9-11 pm. From April to September, 9:30-11:30 pm.

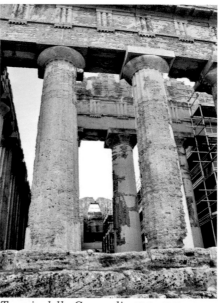

Tempio della Concordia (Galen R Frysinger)

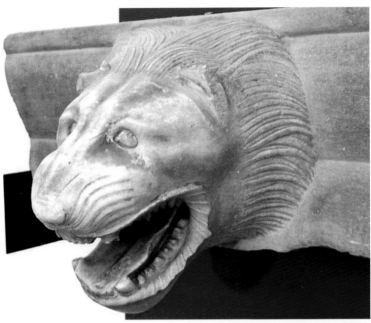

Lion rain spout in the Museo (Galen R Frysinger)

Museo Archaeologico (Tues-Sat 9 am-7 pm, Mon and Sun 9 am-1 pm, €6 or combined ticket of €10 to the Temples) is devoted to finds from the temples, the city and surrounding area. There are notes in English so you won't be completely lost. There's also a 13th-century church on the premises with a fine Gothic doorway. And across the road from the museum is the **Hellenistic-Roman Quarter** (free), with rows of houses decorated with some mosaic designs. They were inhabited on and off until the fifth century AD.

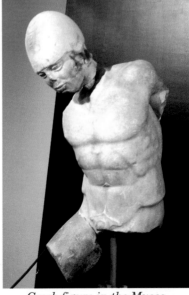

Greek figure in the Museo
(Galen R Frysinger)

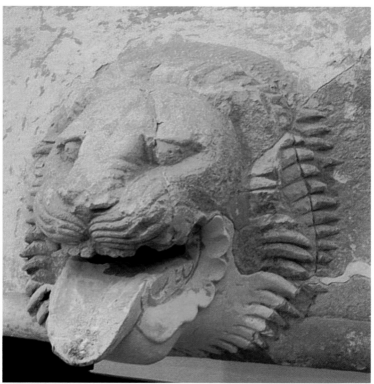

Lion ornament in the Museo (Galen R Frysinger)

The Medieval Town

Via Aetnea is the main artery of Agrigento and a pedestrian street with jewelry, shoes, designer clothes, flowers, perfume and even fish shops. The lanes coming off it are very steep but are littered with cute *trattorie*, B&Bs, old *palazzi* and a smattering of old churches. The streets are often so narrow you can hear the sounds from inside the houses – clinking cutlery at lunch time.

Via Aetnea runs from the Piazzale Aldo Moro all the way through the medieval heart of the town to Piazza Pirandello, named after Luigi Pirandello, who won a nobel prize for literature in 1934. In the piazza is the grand entrance to an ex-convent now housing the **Municipio** and a **theater** (☎ 0922-595-030, Mon-Fri 8:30 am-1 pm, Tues-Thurs 4-6 pm, €2.50). Events are held here through the year, but at other times it's open to the public. If it's not, you can ask at the desk to see the

bottom floor. You can peak through the doors to see gilded gold mirrors, marble floors, drapes and arches.

Steep streets lead from here up to the **Chiesa S M Greci** (9 am-1 pm, 3-6 pm). This is the old Greek quarter of town. It was built in the 11th century from sandstone on the site of a fifth-century Doric temple dedicated to Athena and has a similar feel to the temples in the valley below. You can see remains of the columns in the nave. Inside are Byzantine frescoes and the original Norman ceiling.

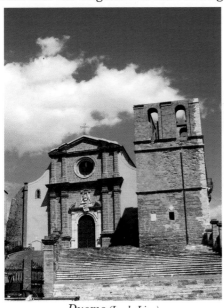
Duomo (LuckyLisp)

Keep heading up the steep streets. On Via Duomo are a line of edifices including a library or **bibliotecca** (Fri 10 am-12:30 pm) dating from 1765. You can sneak in with the public (Tues 3-5:45 pm, Thurs and Fri 8:30 am-1:30 pm). Just to the right are the ruins of the **Castello Arabo**, currently undergoing restorations. Turn left and at the end of the street is the massive **Duomo** (☎ 092-224-024, 9 am-1 pm, 3-6 pm) on a terrace at the top of the hill. It's a climb to get here but worth it (a *circolare* town bus does come up here). It was built in the year 1000 and dedicated to the town's first archbishop. Inside are wood ceilings, carved and painted columns, marble floors and a pipe organ.

Another interesting church is the **Santo Spirito** at the end of Via Fodera, built for Cistercian nuns in 1290. There is fine stucco work inside and the **Museo Civico** (Mon-Fri 9 am-1 pm, 3-5:30 pm, Sat 9 am-1 pm, €2.50), which was closed at the time of writing due to an electrical fault. It's a folk museum containing local artifacts.

LUIGI PIRANDELLO

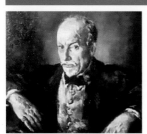 If you're interested in learning more about the Nobel Prize-winning author there are a few ports of call for you in the Agrigento region. The first is the **Library Museum Luigi Pirandello** (Via Imera 50, ☎ 0922-622-111, Mon-Fri 8:30 am-2 pm, Wed and Thurs 3-6 pm), containing documentation about the great Sicilian dramatist. It's of greatest interest to researchers and students. **Casa Natale di Pirandello** (☎ 0922-511-102, 9 am-1 pm, 2-7 pm, €2.05), in Porto Empedocle southwest of Agrigento, is the house where the famous writer was born and spent his summers. It is now a museum of memorabilia.

In November and December every year there is an international conference of Pirandello studies when scholars meet together to debate works that are still topical.

Adventures

In Air

Sicilwing (Via Provinciale 233, S. Venerina, Catania, ☎ 095-532-003, www.sicilwing.com) operates flights over the Agrigento temples at €902.50 for up to three persons in a Cessna 172. The flight is 2½ hours and departs from the Catania international airport.

On Foot

Another pleasant area to explore on foot is the **Giardino della Kolymbetra** (Valle dei Templi, ☎ 335-122-9042, 10 am-5 pm, €2). The 14-acre gardens have temple ruins, an ancient swimming pool and caves. You can call to book a guided tour.

Where to Stay

Camping

Camping options are at the beach-side resort of San Leone.

Camping Valle Dei Templi Internazionale San Leone (Viale Emporium, ☎ 0922-411-115, fax 0922-411-132, www.campingvalledeitempli.com, €€) has bungalows (€30 for two people), caravans (€20) and tenting (from €3.50-€5.50).

Lido Oasi (Viale Dune 5a Spiaggia, ☎ 092-241-6096, 339-658-3368, €) is right on the beach and open year-round.

Valle dei Templi

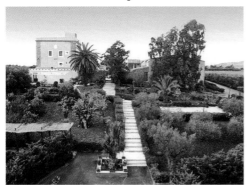
Baglio della Luna

★★**Forresteria Baglio della Luna** (Contrada Maddalusa SS640, km 4. 150, Valle dei Templi, ☎ 092-251-1061, fax 092-259-8802, www.bagliodellaluna.com, €€€€) was Ignazio Altieri's dream as an 18-year-old and realized some 25 years later when he bought and renovated this beautiful old *masseria*. Stay in the tower rooms and enjoy the temples at night.

Hotel Domus Aurea (Contrada Maddalusa SS 640, Valle dei Templi, ☎ 092-251-100, fax 092-251-2406, www.hotel-domusaurea.it, €€€€) has the

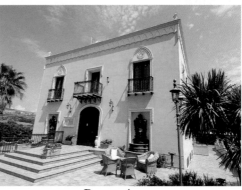
Domus Aurea

same owner as Baglio della Luna but with more hotel-like rooms and comforts and a fantastic garden.

HOTEL PRICE CHART	
€	Up to €25 per day
€€	€26-€55
€€€	€56-€85
€€€€	Over €85

The Town Center
Hotels

Bella Napoli (Piazza Lena 6, ☎/fax 092-220-435, hotelbellanapoli@tin.it, €€) is in the heart of town, with friendly management. Parking is limited nearby and it's some distance from the train station. There's a good trattoria next door.

Antica Foresteria Catalana (Piazza Lena 5, ☎/fax 092-220-435, €€) is next door to Bella Napoli, with clean pleasant rooms.

B&Bs

Atenea 191 B&B (Via Atenea 191, ☎ 092-259-5594, www.atenea191.com, €€-€€€) has seven rooms. All have terraces but only five have a view of the bay.

B&B Fodera (Via Fodera 11, ☎ 092-240-3079, 338-291-0228, www.fodera.org, €€€) is a steep climb and in a quiet location hidden from traffic. Rooms have TV and bathroom.

B&B L'Antica (Via Ficani 1, ☎ 092-259-6057, 347-139-7653, €€-€€€) is directly across from Insomnia Bar and up a small lane. It's a child-friendly establishment.

B&B Camere a Sud (Via Ficani 6, ☎ 349-638-4424, www.camereasud.it, €€€) has been recently remodeled and is located in a pleasant courtyard across from the Trattoria Athea.

Where to Eat

Café & Bars

Girasole Wine Bar (Via Atenea 70) serves breakfast and light lunches.

Caffeteria Insomnia (Via Atenea 133/135, ☎ 092-224-055) has a great selection of food, including Agrigento's best coffee, pastries and ice cream. You can also get hot meals for lunch.

Trattorias

Black Horse Trattoria (Via di Celauro, ☎ 0922-23223, €€) serves tasty, reasonably priced fare.

Trattoria de Paris (Piazza Lena 7, ☎ 092-225-413, closed Sun, €€), near Hotel Bella Napoli, serves rustic, homestyle meals.

DINING PRICE CHART	
Price per person for an entrée, including house wine.	
€	Up to €12
€€	€13-€25
€€€	€26-€35
€€€€	Over €35

Trattoria Manhattan (Salita Maddona Degli Angeli 9, ☎ 092-220-911, 12-3 pm, 6-8:30 pm, closed Sun, €€), in an atmospheric lane off Via Atenea filled with potted plants, serves fresh fish and homemade pasta. The friendly owner loved New York, hence the name, and has a an enormous tabby cat named Cicio. Eat out in the lane or inside. The chef recommends everything, but try *ravioli all'arancia* for something different.

L'Ambasciata di Sicilia (Via Giambertoni 2, ☎ 092-220-526, 034-708-71690, closed Mon, €€) has the best pizza in Agrigento. Try to get a seat here. The interior has postcards from around the world stuck on the wall, a *pupi* exhibition on the back wall and a traditional hand-painted ceiling. Their *antipasto rustico* is a favorite and they serve a long pasta called *calamaritti*.

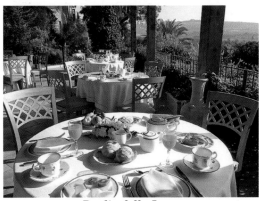

Baglio della Luna

Baglio della Luna (Contrada Maddalusa SS640, Km 4. 150, Valle dei Templi, ☎ 092-251-1061, fax 092-259-8802, www.bagliodellaluna.com, €€€€) is a more exuberant choice for dining. This Michelin-star restaurant does everything to perfection, plus you get a view of the lit-up temples at night.

Trattoria Concordia (Via Porcello 8, ☎ 0922-222-668, €€) serves good grilled fish and is well priced.

Trattoria Atena (Via Ficani 6, ☎ 0922-412-366, closed Sun, €) serves no-frills meals in a quiet piazza.

La Corte degli Sfizi (Via Cortili Contanini, €-€€) is a little *trattoria* near the top of the steps with tasty pasta, grilled sausage and swordfish.

■ Eraclea Minoa ★

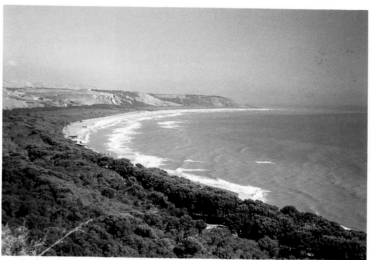
Eraclea Minoa (Joanne Lane)

This important Greek site is 35 km northwest of Agrigento and just beyond Montallegro. It was originally called Minoa after the Cretan King Minos, who founded the city where he landed. The Greeks settled here in the sixth century BC and later added Heraklea to the name. Poor old Eraclea sat right between Akragas and Selinunte and was often dragged into their border disputes. However, somehow it managed to do well. The city's most important period was during the fourth century BC and most of the ruins date from then. After that it fell into decline.

Getting Here

 Locals complain about the lack of bus service to Eraclea Minoa, saying it keeps tourism at bay and is a government conspiracy to keep money in Agrigento.

It is a pain if you're just wanting to day-trip here, but you'll wonder if the lack of tourism is a blessing in disguise. The beach remains pristine and, apart from a few busy weeks in August, it's relatively quiet. There are some good campsites here. To get here by bus, ask the driver to drop you on the SS115 at the turn-off to Eraclea Minoa. It's a hot trudge of 3½ km.

Sightseeing

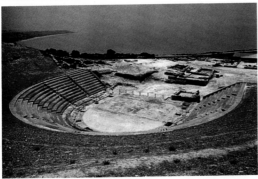
The theater

The site (☎ 092-284-6005, 9 am to one hr before sunset, €2) occupies a headland above the beach on the Capo Bianco cliff. A good part of the city remains but the main attraction is the fourth-century theater. At the time of writing it was under cover and being restored but it's still visible to visitors. There are also a number of dwellings.

Adventures

On Foot

A good walk stretches beyond the site along the cliff overlooking the splendid beach towards the Capo Bianco point. A man-made chute here should allow you to clamber down to the beach without too much trouble. Turn southeast and head back around the points to the Eraclea Minoa village. If the tide is high you may need to wade a bit or paddle around one of the promontories. Or you could continue northeast, first through the Riserva Foce del Fiume Platani. The best time to observe migratory species is from late autumn through to spring. In summer the occasional heron or egret can be seen fishing.

Where to Stay

Eracleia Minoa Village (☎ 0922-846-023, www. eracleaminoavillage.it, €-€€) is in a large pine wood that runs along the beach. It is equipped with modern facilities and plenty of space for campers beneath the trees. There are also cabins. It's at the far end of the village and open Easter to September only.

Home Holidays (Villini Marsala, SS 115 Bivio Cattolica Eraclea, ☎ 0922-840-429, 339-380-7367, www.homeholidays. com, €€€-€€€€) has small basic apartments a short distance from the beach with kitchens, TVs, phones and laundry. Prices change radically with the season from €55 in December to €100 in summer. You can usually find the owner at Lido Bellevue.

Sabbia d'Oro (Eraclea Minoa 1a Spiaggia, www.sabbiadoro-eraclea.com, €€-€€€) has apartments for just €20-€25 pp.

Throughout the town keep an eye out for *affita camere* or *casa vacanza* signs, indicating rooms or houses are for rent.

Where to Eat

The **Supermarket Tutinio** (9 am-2 pm, 5-8 pm) has ice cream, camping equipment and food.

Sabbia d'Oro (Eracleia Minoa 1a spiaggia, www. sabbiadoro-eraclea.com, €€) has a prime location right on the beach – you walk down the stairs from the restaurant almost straight into the sea. The rustic restaurant is open to the sea, made completely of wood and decorated with fishing nets. Pizza (€4-€6) and seafood (from €7) are available. To get here, keep going straight towards the sea when you enter the town.

Lido Belvedere (7 am-1 am, €€), near the Eracleia Minoa Village, is set just off the beach with a bar and restaurant serving fresh *cozze* and *spada*. Seafood tourist menus are €20, meat-based menus are €18.

■ Sciacca

If you have time for another stop on the coast it should be Sciacca to see the fabulous views from the square in the upper town. Sciacca was founded in the fifth century BC by the Greeks as a spa town for nearby Selinus. It enjoyed particular

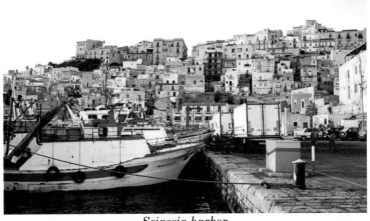

Sciaccia harbor

prosperity under the Arabs from whom its modern name is thought to derive – the Arabic word *xacca* means "from the water." During the Middle Ages a feud between rival families resulted in the death of about half the population. In the 15th and 16th centuries grander walls and *palazzo* (one or more?)were built and in the 18th century there was more construction, adding a Baroque touch to the center.

If you have a car, Sciacca is a good base to visit some of the minor inland towns nearby.

Getting Here

Buses pull up on Via Figuli at the Villa Comunale (town gardens), convenient to some budget hotels and a short walk from the main piazza. **Lumia** buses run daily between Sciacca and Agrigento. Another service goes to Trapani. **Gallo** buses run to Palermo.

Information Sources

There are two tourist offices on Corso Emanuele opposite the Piazza Scandaliato. The **APT** is at number 84 (☎ 092-240-1352) and the **AAST tourist office** is at number 94 (☎ 092-522-744). There's also an **Azienda Viaggio** at number 90.

Events

Try to time your visit for the annual **Sciacca Jazz Festival** that runs for two weeks every August (☎ 092-520-478, www.sciaccajazzfestival.com). Entry is free and concerts take place in the open-air courtyard of

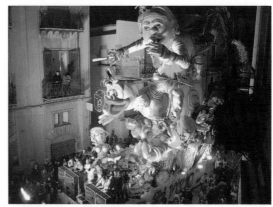

Carnival in Sciacca

Collegio dei Gesuti at number 82 of the Corso. Other events are also held here in the summer. Sciacca also has a colorful carnival in February.

Sightseeing

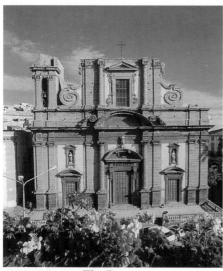

The Duomo

The main street of Sciacca is Corso Vittorio Emanuele, running right past the wonderful ★**Piazza Scandaliato**. This lovely piazza has a large terrace with several cafés and splendid views down to the port and bays below. This is really the heart of the town. At night it is filled with those taking a *passeggiata*. Back from the piazza lies the **Duomo**, first erected in 1108 and rebuilt in 1656. A sign outside it reads *Senza messa non e' Domenica* (it's not Sunday

if there's no mass). The whole town seems to have taken this idea to heart, with huge lines out the for Sunday mass. From the Duomo you could walk up through a knot of alleyways to the **Castello Conti Luna** off Via Giglio. The gates are usually open and entry is free, though it's very derelict. Wooden planking was put down a long time ago, probably as a walkway over rough ground or holes, but it's no longer safe. Continue up Via Giglio to **Porta San Calogero**, one of the five gates to the walled upper town and a smattering of churches.

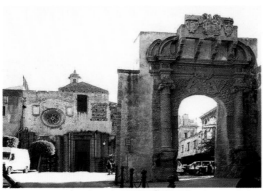

Back near the bus stop, **Villa Comunale** has good views and gardens – a pleasant picnic spot. If you drop down Via Agatocle after the gardens, you can follow the road down to the Grand Hotel delle

Ancient gate in Sciaccia

Terme. The **Piscina Parco Termale** (Mon-Sat, 9:30 am-1 pm, 3:30-7:30 pm, €4.50) next to the hotel is open to the public. In the complex next to it you can see a doctor for a health cure, physiotherapy or rehabilitation.

The Sciacca port is accessible from stairs leading off Piazza Scandaliato. The stairs are lined with ceramics and somewhat reminiscent of Caltagirone, although far smaller. Each step is different, with dolphins, fruit or sun motifs and the name of the artist, the date it was completed and where to find their work. The port has a number of good restaurants and the docks are littered with vessels – some rotting – and nets.

Where to Stay

Aliai B&B (Via Gaie di Garaffe 60, ☎ 092-590-5388, www.aliai.com, €€€) is down by the port if you want to be in a quieter part of town.

La Paloma Blanca (Via Figuli 5/7, ☎ 092-525-667, €€-€€€) has basic rooms and is a little derelict. Prices include breakfast. There's also a restaurant down near reception. It's family-run and you'll often find the children manning the reception desk.

Grand Hotel delle Terme di Sciacca (☎ 092-523-133, fax 092-587-002, www.grandhoteldelleterme.com, €€€€) has its own park and piazza.

Al Moro B&B (Via Liguori 44, ☎ 092-586-756, www.almoro. com, €€) has modern rooms in the center.

Where to Eat

 There are a lot of bars and a few restaurants along Corso Vittorio Emanuele near the piazza. Go to the **Bar del Corso** for ice cream (Corso V. Emanuele 85, ☎ 092-24489, closed Mon) during the day or visit at night for a selection of beers and wines.

At night it is rivaled by the **Caffè delle Rosse** (Corso Vittorio Emanuele 97, 7 am-1:30 pm, 4-2 am, closed Wed), serving aperitifs, panini and other bar food. Both bars have seating on either side of a fountain and there's often live music in the summer.

Trattoria Duomo (Corso Vittorio Emanuele 107, closed Thurs, €€-€€€) is directly below the Duomo. It serves paella on Tuesday and couscous and pesce on Friday.

Ristorante Miramare Pizzeria (Piazza Scaldaliato 7, ☎ 092-527-050, €€-€€€) is in the piazza with superb views down to the sea.

In Piazza S. Friscia near the Villa Comunale you can find takeout food stalls.

Portside

The best places to eat in Sciacca are the fish restaurants at the port, although you won't want to come down to these quiet streets alone.

Bar Porto San Paolo (Largo San Paolo, ☎ 0925-27482, €€) has a terrace looking down onto the port.

Trattoria Al Faro (Lungomare 25, ☎ 0925-25349, closed Sun) is right near the staircase leading down from Piazza Scandaliato above.

La Lampara (Lungomare Cristoforo Colombo, ☎ 092-585-085, closed Mon, €€) also has a good reputation for quality seafood dishes.

■ Monte San Calogero

The **Basilica Santuario di San Calogero** (Mon-Thurs 7 am-12:30 pm, 3-5:30 pm, Fri-Sat 3:30-7:30 pm) sits on a hilltop eight km from Sciacca and is an easy side-trip. Bus number five runs every 90 minutes from Sciacca's Corso Vittorio Emanuele. The bus stops right on top of the Monte, where you can enter the beautiful church. Frescoes cover virtually every inch of the ceilings and walls and a friendly bearded *padre* of the Franciscan order is usually on-hand to greet those passing through, having done so for about 55 years. San Calogero came to the **Grotta sul Kronio** below the church and lived there as a hermit for 35 years, sleeping in one of the caves. You can visit it – ask in the church. The mountain was a volcano and hot air comes through a vent in the ground. They'll show you where it is and you can put your hand in to feel the heat.

■ Caltabellotta★

This often mist-shrouded village is 20 km northeast of Sciacca. The ride itself (**SAIS** leaves three times daily from Sciacca and **Lumia** operates from Sciacca and Agrigento) is impressive and it's hard to believe the chaos of places like Agrigento is only an hour away. The town is perched on a jagged, rocky hillside with ruins of theaters, houses in the rocks, Sicani tombs, castles and fortifications. Caltabellotta was once called Camico, a fortress built by the Sicilan king Cocalo. On one of its pinnacles are the ruins of a Norman castle where the Angevins and Aragonese signed the peace treaty to end the Wars of the Vespers. Uneven rock-cut steps lead up to it behind the Chiesa Matrice. There's not much left, but the views are superb.

The **Chiesa Matrice** (10 am-12 pm) below it is a 14th-century cathedral in Norman style with Gothic arches at the end of a very wide square. Inside, huge stone columns lead down the central aisle. In the apses are frescoes and a small chapel. At the other end of the square, outside the church, is the Gothic **Chiesa di San Salvatore**. Beyond this is a stair-

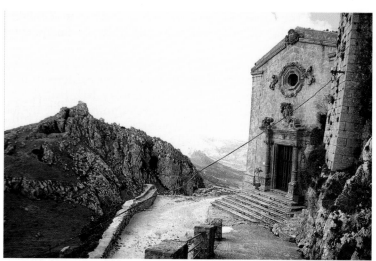
Chiesa S. Pellegrino (Joanne Lane)

case up to **Castello Nuovo**, which is currently closed for repair.

Follow the road around the back of town and turn up through a narrow entrance in the rock dropping back into town via the Byzantine/Norman **Chiesa Pietra** (closed, but worth a look). It is completely set into the rock. If you continue along the back road you eventually skirt around the town to another promontory where the **Chiesa S. Pellegrino** and the **Eremo di S. Pellegrino** (both closed) are found. The **Ristorante San Pellegrino** sits in the car park below and a path leads up behind it to the door of the church and castle. The views from here are incredible, with a profound silence broken only by birds and distant traffic. Walk back down past the Ristorante and follow the road back into town. It curls past a grassy *belvedere* (view point) with a crucifix where you can see the spread of the town including all the peaks. On the road back into town you pass the Café Morettinio and some good picnic spots.

■ **Selinunte** ★ ★ ★

The Greek city of Selinus lies half-way between Menfi and Mazara del Vallo. It's the key sight in this part of the island and one of the most captivating, with a spectacular coastal lo-

cation with the ruins of mighty temples. You can find accommodations at Marinella di Selinunte and it's easily reached by bus.

The city was colonized by Greek settlers from Megara Hyblaea in 628 BC. It grew in prestige under Siracusan protection, reaching a peak in the fifth century BC. But it was only a matter of time before the Carthaginians took notice and sacked the city in 409 BC. An earthquake razed the city and the final settlers eventually transferred to Marsala in 250 BC, just before the Roman invasion. The Arabs did occupy it briefly but the last recorded settlement was in the 13th century. It was rediscovered in the 16th century and excavations began in 1823.

Getting Here & Getting Around

To get to Selinunte by public transport you should go to Castelvetrano first, which is only 20 minutes from Mazara del Vallo by road or rail. Selinunte is a further 20 minutes from Castelvetrano. Buses mostly stop to the south of the entrance but may also drop you off at the ruins. **Salemi** (☎ 092-398-1120, www.autoservizisalemi.it) makes the journey five times daily (25 minutes, €.77) and to Palermo and Trapani (€5.16). **AST** also travels between Selinunte and Castelvetrano. From Castelvetrano there are Lumia connections to Agrigento, Sciacca, Ribera, Trapani, Menfi and Marsala.

Take a **taxi** (☎ 0923-941221, 092-394-4650) or ask at the tourist office. If you're staying at campsites or hotels on the SS 115 you can flag down a passing bus to take you into town.

Information Sources

A helpful tourist office is right at the ruins (Mon-Sat 8 am-2 pm and 2-8 pm, Sun 9 am-12 pm and 3-8 pm).

Sightseeing

Archaeological Site

Selinunte (9 am-7 pm, €6) is divided into two zones, covered by the same ticket. In the ticket office is a site model and pictures on the walls, an ATM and even Internet access! As you enter, you will see the ecotour cars and bikes that can be used

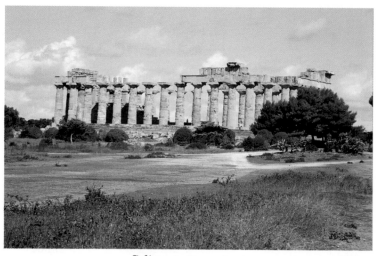

Selinunte (Joanne Lane)

if you can't or don't want to walk around. Prices range from €3 for short tours to €15 for longer journeys. The first temple you see is almost complete and is very impressive, with intact columns 80 feet high. It was probably dedicated to Hera and is part of the first group of eastern temples. The second temple is the oldest in the group, from around 550 BC. Temple G is mostly in parts, although it's fun to wander through the huge graveyard of stone and see how the columns have fallen – like being on the set of a giant jig-saw puzzle trying to work out how the pieces might fit back together.

The second set of temples in the western zone are a long way down the road. If you have a car, drive down (it's a hot 25-minute walk in summer) or use the ecotour vehicles. There are ruins of five temples here and what's left of the city streets and acropolis. Huge walls rise above the duned beach below. They were constructed after 409 BC in an attempt to protect the city. This section includes Temple C, the highest point in the acropolis, built in the sixth century BC and dedicated to Apollo. Fourteen columns were re-erected in the 1920s. Behind Temples C and D were shops, each with a courtyard. At the end of the main street is the north gate to the city, with huge blocks of stone marking a gateway 23 feet high.

The quarry where the stones were cut is at Cava di Cusa (9 am to one hr before sunset, free), about three km south of

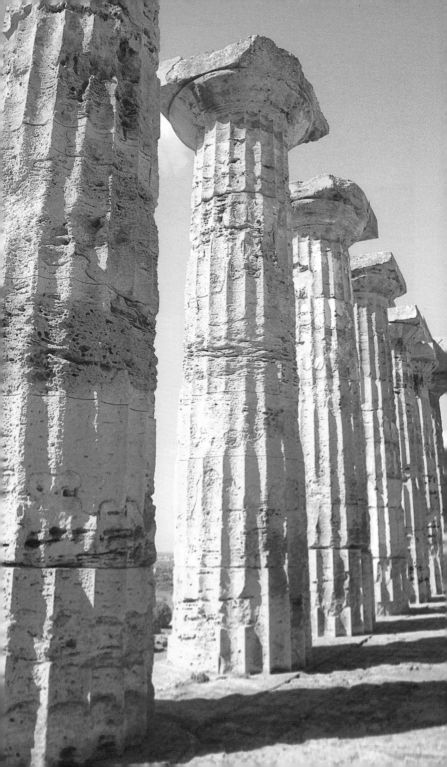

Campobello di Mazara on the road to Tre Fontane. It is reasonably well signposted. It's a very quiet place and hot in summer – bring plenty of water – which makes you realize how difficult it would have been for the ancient workers. Stone drums and columns were chiseled here and then dragged off to the ancient city on wooden carts. Some of these are still in place where they were being excavated.

Marinella di Selinunte

Marinella di Selinunte only has one main road that runs down to the small harbor at Piazza Empedocle. In the morning it's more lively when some rather characteristic locals come to bid for fish being auctioned at the pier. You can also watch them

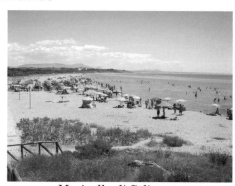

Marinella di Selinunte

bringing fresh catches into the harbor amidst a tangle of boats and nets. The beachfront is pleasant and you can rent boats to tour around (see *Adventures*).

Adventures

On Water

Albatross (☎ 328-569-3927) rents boats (€20/hr, €60/half-day, €100/all day) and windsurfing equipment.

Lido Tuxn at the port has pedal boats (€10/hr), canoes (€7/hr) and dinghies in season. You can rent an umbrella for €2/hr or €12/day. The café serves cold couscous, rice salad, fruit and drinks.

Where to Stay

Campgrounds

Camping Athena (SS 115 No. 8, ☎ 092-446-132, athenaselinunte@tin.it, €) has a restaurant and bar

Facing page: Columns, Selinunte (Joanne Lane)

and sells AST tickets. It is on the provincial road running into town. Regular buses pass every 20 minutes.

Il Maggiolino (SS 115 no. 106, ☎/fax 0924-46044, www. campingmaggiolino.it, €-€€) has bungalows and camping.

Camping Haway (Via 79, Triscina di Selinunte, ☎ 0924-84101, €-€€) is at the beach of Triscina and open June to September. Easter, May and October are possible with reservations only. They have small bungalows, tents (you can also rent) and camper spaces.

B&B

Villa Anna (SS 115 No. 136, ☎ 0924-46881, www. gattopardobb.it, €€€) is 1½ km from the archaeological park but easily reached via regular public buses.

Il Pescatore (Via Castore e Polluce 31, ☎ 0924-46303, €€) has four double rooms and use of a fridge.

The Holiday House and **Porta del Sole** (Via Apollonio Rodio 23/32, ☎ 0924-46035, €€), across the road from each other, are owned by the same family. Simple rooms have fans and balconies. There's a common lounge and fridge.

Hotels

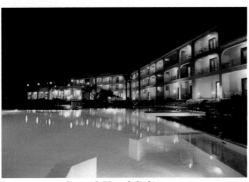

Grand Hotel Selinunte

Grand Hotel Selinunte (C. da Trentasalme, ☎ 0924-941-056, €€€-€€€€) has a large central swimming pool and frigobar-equipped rooms.

Hotel Garzia (Via A. Pigafetta 2, ☎ 0924-46024, www.hotelgarzia. com, €€€) also has a restaurant. Its rather grand yellow-brown brick exterior leads to simple rooms.

Hotel Miramare (☎ 0924-46666, www.garziahotel-miramare.com, €€€) is recognizable by its yellow concrete Arab-style flat rooftop. It has lots of balconies and flowers, plus access to a beach.

Albergo Lido Azzurro (Via Marco Polo 98, ☎ 0924-46256) has a sea view, parking and air-conditioned rooms.

Where to Eat

 Via Marco Polo is the best place to eat above the west beach. In Piazzale Efebo there's the **Oped Errante** (☎ 092-490-6457) that's almost perpetually open, serving everything from coffee to pizza and paninis.

Hotel Garzia (Via A. Pigafetta 2, ☎ 092-446-024, €€€).

Albergo Lido Azzurro (Via Marco Polo 98, ☎ 0924-46256, €€-€€€), in a whitewashed building, has pictures outside attesting to the freshness of the lobster and seafood. It's small and busy.

The **Calannino Rocca** (Via Marco Polo 49, ☎ 092-494-1025), with similar prices, has a antipasto buffet, local fish and wine.

Ristorante Pizzeria del Calannino (Via Marco Polo 53, ☎ 092-446-721, €€) serves couscous, *zuppa di pesce*, pizza and other specials for €12. You can watch the pizzas being made and have a clear view to the sea.

Lido Tuxm (☎ 0924-932-240), on the beachfront, has a snack bar serving salads and *gelati*.

Centro Nautico (☎/fax 092-44622) is on a terrace right over the sea, beyond the harbor, with a North African flavor to its menu and serving couscous.

■ Islands off the Coast

Pelagie Islands

These beautiful islands lie 240 km south of Agrigento and in many respects have more in common with the nearer African nations of Tunisia or Libya than Italy. Only Linosa is on the Sicilian continental shelf; the other two are part of the submerged African land mass. The archipelago was often abandoned or uninhabited throughout history, although it played an important role during WWII and again in 1987 when Gaddafi of Libya threatened the US base on Lampedusa. During the Fascist era Lampedusa was used to exile political enemies and later Mafia prisoners were also sent here.

Lampedusa is the largest of the islands and popular with Italians in the summer months. It has good scuba diving and

snorkeling. **Linosa** is of volcanic origin and a lot rockier. **Lampione** is uninhabited and less visited. Accommodation on the islands is noticeably pricier during summer. Come slightly out of season for discounts. At all times call ahead to book accommodations, but especially during the summer. You probably wouldn't want to visit here in winter. Services shut down and winds whip the islands.

Getting Here

 Flights arrive in Lampedusa from Palermo with either **Air Sicilia** (☎ 800-412-411) or **Alitalia** (☎ 147-865-641, www.alitalia.com). Flights are twice daily. **Air One** also flies here. However, most people come by **ferry** from Porto Empedocle, six km southwest of Agrigento (regular buses go to the port from the train station). In summer daily ferries leave for Linosa (five hrs 45 mins) and Lampedusa (eight hrs 15 mins). Contact **Siremar** (☎ 0922-633-6683) in Porto Empedocle for current schedules and fares. Their office opens from 9 am-1 pm, 4-7 pm, 9-12 pm. **Ustica Lines** (www.usticalines.it) has a daily hydrofoil to Lampedusa for €49.

Getting Around

 You can rent vehicles on the islands very easily and are advised to leave your car behind. Ustica Lines operates a hydrofoil between Lampedusa and Linosa year-round (€18, one hour).

Information Sources

 There is a useful website, www.lampedusa.to, for information about Lampedusa.

Linosa

Linosa is a submerged volcano that has been extinct for nearly 2,000 years. There are four extinct craters to poke around in, with some black beaches and rocky coves. It's not as exciting as Lampedusa, but has slowly built a tourist trade. It's a good day-trip from Lampedusa if you don't want to stay overnight.

Linosa was a haven for pirates in the 16th century and wasn't settled until the mid-19th century. It's still only sparsely populated and very small – just five square km. If you do stay, try:

Linosa Club (Contrada Club, ☎ 0922-972-066, €€€). Closed Oct-May, with a pool and restaurant.

Da'Errera (Via Scalo, ☎ 0922-972-041), also with rooms to rent, and there's a bar and pizzeria nearby.

Algusa (Via Alfieri, ☎ 0922-972-052, €€-€€€).

Adventures

On Foot

Tracks leading from either side of the port allow you to climb around the cliffs and coves to reach some black sand beaches. The island exudes tranquility and you can really get away from it all. The lava rocks can be hot in the midday sun so take water and wear shoes!

In Water

To do scuba diving, see the **Linosa Diving Center** (Via Scalo Vecchio, ☎ 0922-972-061, www.linosadivingcenter.cjb.net) or **Mare Nostrum Diving** (Via Re Umberto 84, www.marenostrumdiving.it). Dives start at about €32 for a single dive and €40 for a night dive.

Linosa has about 10 dive sites, with several underwater itineraries through shoals, archaeological routes, walls and some small caves as well. There is enough for all levels of experience: shallow and colorful depths for beginners, breath-

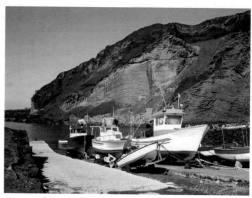

Linosa fishing boats (Hans Bickel)

taking deep dives for experts. Underwater flora and fauna are similar to tropical waters, but what really makes Linosa marvelous underwater are the strange shapes and tunnels created by lava. A wreck of an English airplane from WWII, a

Bristol Beaufighter, was found by Mare Nostrvm Tek Divers at 213-230 feet, not far from the coast.

Lampedusa

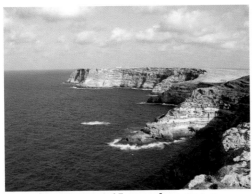

North coast of Lampedusa (Bickel)

Lampedusa lies on the continental shelf of Africa and has some unmistakable features: beaches and little inlets with fine sand, a crystalline sea, breathtaking views, high cliffs, steep bays, caves and underwater crannies. It's a popular spot for vacationing Italians. There's good diving and swimming, with some fine walks. Lampedusa is larger than Linosa with about 5,000 inhabitants.

Orange minibuses run regularly from Piazza Brignone to different beaches around the island. You can also rent bikes, scooters and cars around the town. Many hotels and campsites will provide a courtesy bus when you arrive and depart. Taxis are also available. Ferries arrive in the town of Lampedusa. The old town is a 15-minute walk, or it's 15 minutes west to the harbor at Porto Nuovo where most hotels are located. In summer a minibus meets the ferry.

There's a **Pro Loco** on Via Vittorio Emanuele 89 (☎ 0922-971-390, www.lampedusaproloco.it) or the **Ente Turismo** (Via Andrea Anfossi 3, ☎ 0922-971-171).

Spiaggia della Guitgia is the main beach and where many hotels cluster. The town activity centers on Via Roma and is the focus for the *passeggiata*.

Adventures

On Foot & Wheels

The island is only 11 km long so getting around on foot is an option. Cala La Croce is the next bay west of town. Cala La Francese is rockier and 10 minutes walk east of town. The Grotta del Teschio (the Skull Grotto)

South Coast

has a 45-foot-long sandy beach that can be reached by boat or along a rough path. From the center of Lampedusa head eastward for the airport. The unpaved road running alongside the landing strip passes by the many bays on the

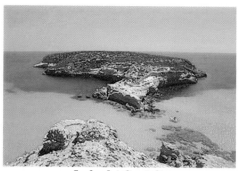
Isola dei Conigli

southern side of the island. Other points to head for include Lampedusa's highest spot, the Albero del Sole (the Sun Tree), at 400 feet above sea level.

The **Isola dei Conigli** (Rabbit Island) is seven km west of town and you could walk to it if the tide is out (or it's an easy

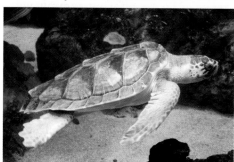
Caretta (Strobilomyces)

swim). The island contains a small nature reserve where the *caretta* (loggerhead sea turtles) lay their eggs between July and August. You can rent bikes and scooters in town and cover the same itinerary. You should easily be able to circuit the island in a day by bicycle. Take provisions with you as there are no shops on the way.

In Air

Sicilwing (Via Provinciale 233, S. Venerina, Catania, ☎ 095-532-003, www.sicilwing.com) has day flights to Lampedusa at €1,600 for up to five persons in a Seneca PA-34. The flight is round-trip from the Catania international airport. They also have flights over Agrigento, the Aeolian Islands and over Mt Etna.

The **Eremo della Giubiliana** (see page 402) also has flying trips to the Pelagie islands. The flight to Lampedusa includes a boat tour.

In Water

There is good swimming at **Cala Croce**, the first bay west of the town. You can see dolphins or the sperm whale migration (March).

Boat trips up the coast from **Cala Galera** to the lighthouse at **Capo Grecale** are a popular excursion. On the way you stop at small inlets, including **Cala Calandra** (known for the depth of one of its caves) and **Cala Francese** in the southern part of the island. Go down to the quayside to see what boat tours are on offer. Most cost about €15 for a half-day trip. Full-day trips usually have lunch thrown in. The tours depart at 10 am and return at 5 pm.

Licciardi Group (Via Siracusa 18, ☎ 0922-970-678) rents motor vehicles, motor-scooters, motorized rubber dinghies, motor boats and other types of boats, offering great weekly rates on cars (€163), scooters (€ 90) and rubber boats (€300).

Lampedusa is a paradise for snorkelers and divers, who can enjoy a rich and unspoiled submerged world inhabited by corals, sponges, *madrepores* (colored parrot-fish) and lobsters by Capo Grecale at only 150 foot depth. Its mostly sandy seaground suddenly turns into a dark-green due to the *posidonia*, a marine plant that is known as the "Mediterranean lung" for its releasing of oxygen in the water, giving life to beautiful underwater plants. You can rent gear for snorkeling in town. For diving, contact:

Lo Verde Diving (Via Sbarcatoio, ☎ 0922-971-986). **Mediterraneo Immersion Club** (Via A Volta 8, ☎ 0922-971-526). Both are at the harborfront and arrange gear rental and diving trips.

Moby Diving Center (Via delle Grotte 6, ☎ 333-956-4543). Expect to pay €33/€40 for single/night dives.

On Horseback

For horseback riding on Lampedusa, contact **Club Gli Amici del Cavallo** (C/da Cala Pisana, ☎ 0922-971-197). They also have tours by Land Rover.

Where to Stay & Eat

There are two official campsites. One is **La Roccia** (☎ 0922-970-055) at Cala Greca, three km from the town center. **Cala Francese** is nearer to Lampedusa (☎ 0922-970-720). Both are open from June to September.

Albergo Le Pelagie (Via Bonfiglio 7, ☎ 0922-970-211, €€€€) has a compulsory half-board in summer. Room rates are cheaper outside of August.

Vega (Via Roma 19, ☎ 0922-970-099, €€) is right in the town itself at the harbor end.

Belvedere (Piazza Guglielmo Marconi 4, ☎ 0922-970-188, €€) overlooks the harbor.

Club Gli Amici del Cavallo (C/da Cala Pisana, ☎ 0922-971-197, €€€-€€€€) has six rooms with half-pension and breakfast.

Hotel Guitgia Tommasino (Via Lido Azzurro 13, ☎ 0922-970-879, €€€-€€€€) is open year-round.

Cafés and restaurants compete along Via Roma serving lots of seafood and couscous. Try **I Couchini** (Via Vittorio Emanuele 37, ☎ 0922-973-080, €€-€€€) or **Al Gallo d'Oro** (Via Vittorio Emanuele 45, €).

The **Trattoria-Pizzeria Da Nicola** (Via Ponente, ☎ 0922-971-239, €€) by the Rabbit Islands Bay is also recommended. Serves typical homemade Lampedusan food.

Ristorante Il Balenottero (Via Sbarcatoio 40, ☎0922-971-025, closed Thurs, €€) has some great cooking, including shellfish salad, linguine with young whale, swordfish with lemon. They also have apartments for rent.

Le Mille e Una Notte (Via Siracusa 18, ☎ 0922-970-678) is right at the port, serving typical Sicilian cuisine with a touch of the Arabian. They also have small villas where you can stay in some of the most beautiful coves: Cala Francese and Cala Creta.

Lampione

Lampione is uninhabited and a good day-trip from Lampedusa. There is little vegetation on the island but some good offshore fishing and diving. To get there you'll have to go with a dive center, rent a boat or persuade someone to take you.

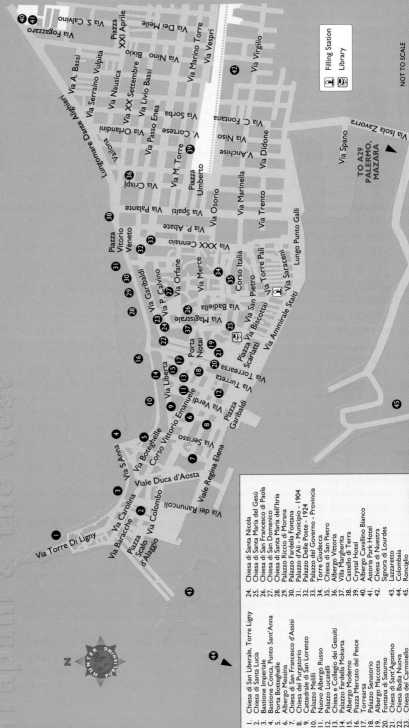

Trapani & the West

1. Chiesa di San Liberale, Torre Ligny
2. Chiesa di Santa Lucia
3. Bastione Imperiale
4. Bastione Conca, Punto Sant'Anna
5. Porta Botteghelle
6. Albergo Messina
7. Chiesa di San Francesco d'Assisi
8. Chiesa del Purgatorio
9. Cattedrale di San Lorenzo
10. Palazzo Melilli
11. Nuovo Albergo Russo
12. Palazzo Lucatelli
13. Chiesa e Collegio dei Gesuiti
14. Palazzo Fardella Mokarta
15. Albergo Moderno
16. Piazza Mercato del Pesce
17. Torrearsa
18. Palazzo Senatorio
19. Albergo Maccotta
20. Fontana di Saturno
21. Chiesa di Sant'Agostino
22. Chiesa Badia Nuova
23. Chiesa del Carminello
24. Chiesa di Santa Nicola
25. Chiesa di Santa Maria del Gesù
26. Chiesa di San Francesco di Paola
27. Chiesa di San Domenico
28. Chiesa di Santa Maria dell'Itria
29. Palazzo Riccio di Morana
30. Palazzo Fardella Fontana
31. Palazzo d'Alì - Municipio - 1904
32. Palazzo Delle Poste - 1924
33. Palazzo del Governo - Provincia
34. Torre Giudecca
35. Chiesa di San Pietro
36. Albergo Vittoria
37. Villa Margherita
38. Castello di Terra
39. Crystal Hotel
40. Albergo Cavallino Bianco
41. Astoria Park Hotel
42. Chiesa di Nuestra Signora di Lourdes
43. Lazzaretto
44. Colombaia
45. Ronciglio

Filling Station

Library

NOT TO SCALE

© 2007 HUNTER PUBLISHING, INC.

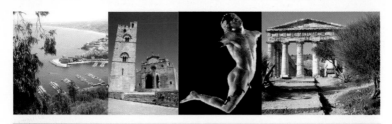

Trapani & the West

For some reason most travelers visit Sicily's eastern coast and forget about one of its most beautiful corners in the west. Happily, this area has been largely free of industrial

development, unlike other parts of Sicily, and many areas are now protected as part of marine or natural parks. There are some beautiful stretches of coastline, including fabulous offshore islands, historic towns that will inspire your imagination, the splendid ruins of Segesta, the cute village of Scopello, medieval hilltops like Erice, great wine in and around Marsala and plenty of adventure activities from biking to walking and diving.

HIGHLIGHTS OF TRAPANI

- The guts and gore of **Trapani's fish market**.
- The dramatic heights of medieval **Erice**.
- **San Vito Lo Capo**'s white sands.
- Walking through the beautiful **Zingaro Reserve** and swimming in the turquoise bays.
- Cycling to the salt dunes in **Mozia**.
- Exploring the caves on one of the **Egadi islands** under or on the water.
- Sipping the ruby-red wine of **Marsala**.
- **Segesta**'s fabulous temple.
- Trapani's Easter procession, *I Misteri*, with its wooden scenes from Christ's life carried through town.
- Staying just feet from the sea in a unit of **Scopello**'s picturesque *tonnara* (where tuna fish processing once took place).

Historically, the region has been more influenced by Phoenician and Arab culture, rather than the Greek and Norman traditions of other places. Housing, in particular, is reminiscent of North Africa. The A29 *autostrada* from Palermo into the west has made this region more integrated with the rest of the island. There are lots of accommodation options with bed and breakfasts filling in the lower end of the scale where campsites and hostels are still sometimes lacking.

■ Trapani

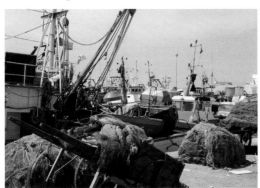
Trapani harbor

This is the administrative capital of the province of the same name. The elegant old center lies in a jumbled maze of streets on a thin peninsula. There are things to see here but none hint at any of the real grandeur of Trapani's past. Trapani flourished once as a Phoenician trading center and was the key port for Eryx (Erice). When Eryx was sacked by Hamilcar in 260 BC some of the population moved down the hill and the port became a city. The town was ensured an enduring role throughout the Middle Ages because it was an important stopover on sea routes linking Tunis, Naples, Anjoy and Aragon. In recent years Trapani has thrived on the salt, fishing and wine trades.

As a touring base for the rest of the west it's superb. There are a lot of accommodation possibilities in the old town and regular trains connect it to Marsala and Marzara; buses to Erice, San Vito Lo Capo and Segesta; and hydrofoils to the offshore islands. The best time to visit is at Easter to **see *I Misteri,*** a procession of 18th-century wooden images representing the last days of Christ's life.

Getting Here

The small national airport of **Birgi** (☎ 0932-842-502, www.airgest.com) is just 16 km south of town. **Air One** (☎ 800-900-944) flies to Roma Fiumicino, Milan,

Turin, Venice, Bari, Catania, Lampedusa and Pantelleria. **AST** buses in Trapani (☎ 0923-21021) connect to the airport (20 minutes). **Segesta** also makes a trip to the Palermo airport.

Buses arrive and depart from Piazza Montalto in the modern town, although some will also drop you at the ferry terminal, Stazione Marittima. Time tables are posted at the bus station. **Segesta** (☎ 0923-20066) runs to Palermo Borsellino (9 am daily) and the city (15 departures); **Lumia** (☎ 0922-20414) to Agrigento via Sciacca; **AST** to Erice, Castellammare del Golfo, Castelvetrano, Marsala, Mazzara del Vallo and San Vito lo Capo, as well as to Segesta and Calatafimi. **Salemi** (☎ 0923-981120) goes to Marsala.

Trains arrive at the station in Piazza Umberto from Palermo, Castelvetrano, Marsala and Marzara del Vallo. **Ferries** for Pantelleria, the Egadi Islands, Ustica, Naples, Cagliari, Tunis and Kelibia leave from the Stazione Marittima at Molo di Sanita (☎ 0924-545-433).

Getting Around

Trapani has a small center and is easily walkable. The only place you might want to consider taking a bus to is the new museum. **AST** (☎ 0923-21021) buses from Piazza Montalto go to the Birgi airport and to Erice. **Taxis** are often waiting by the port near Trattoria del Porto, or call for one at ☎ 092-321-099. **Top Transfer** (☎ 337-896-010, 349-866-2200, fax 092-355-9556, www.toptransfer.it) is a taxi service to/from Palermo P. Raisi airport (€18.50) or Birgi (€10.50). They also rent cars and run guided excursions.

Information Sources

The **APT** (Piazza Saturno, Mon-Fri 8 am-8 pm, Sun 9 am-12 pm, 4-7 pm) has excellent information on the town and province. The other helpful office is in Piazza Scarlatti I (Mon-Sat 8 am-8 pm, Sun 9 am-12 pm, ☎ 092-329-000, fax 092-324-004).

Sightseeing

All points of interest are in the old town. Immediately appealing, Corso Vittorio Emanuele runs through the

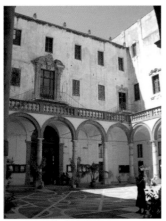
Jesuit cloister

pedestrianized heart of the city. At one end is the Palazzo Senatorio, with twin clocks. The cattedrale, farther along the *corso*, has a Baroque portico, cupolas and a vast interior. It is dedicated to San Lorenzo. The *corso* continues past balconied *palazzi* to **Torre di Ligny** right at the end of the promontory. This is an old Spanish fortification with a squat tower. Inside is a collection of prehistoric finds in the **Museo di Preistoria e Museo del Mare** (☎ 0923-22300).

Via Torresara by the Palazzo Senatorio is the other main thoroughfare leading down towards Stazione Marittima at one end and to a morning fish market at the other in ★**Piazza Mercato di Pesce**. You might need a strong

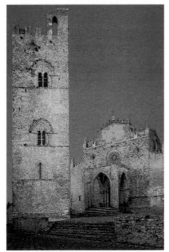
Trapani duomo

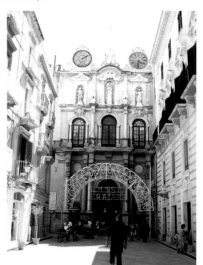
Palazzo Cavaretta

stomach for the sights and smells. It's a colorful market with the cries of vendors and characteristic locals. Come in the morning or you'll miss all the action. For a pleasant walk, stroll along **Lungomare Dante**

Alighieri or head out on the peninsula towards Punta S. Anna and Torre Ligny.

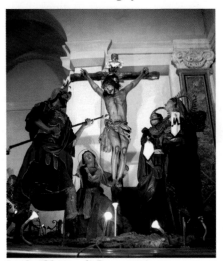

Don't miss the **★★Chiesa di Purgatorio** (Via Generale Domenico Giglio, 10 am-1 pm, 4:30-7:30 pm) for the life-size wooden statues depicting scenes from the Passion. Each is explained by multilingual signs. The statues were made from cypress wood and cork in the 18th century. Each is associated with one of the town's trades and representatives carry them through the streets on Good Friday.

In the Chiesa di Purgatorio (Joanne Lane)

The festival at that time, *I Misteri*, is one of the best in the province.

The **Santuario dell'Annunziata** (Via Conte Agostino Pepoli, ☎ 0923-539-184, 8 am-12 pm, 4-7 pm, free) is some distance east of the city center. The convent was built between 1315 and 1332 and then remodeled in Baroque style in 1760. Inside are a series of chapels and the **Cappella della Madonna**, with the beautiful smiling Madonna and Child statue attributed to Nino Pisano. There's usually a crowd of worshippers in here. The church also houses the town's main museum, **Museo Regionale Pepoli** (Tues-Sat 9 am-1:30 pm, Sun 9 am-12:30 pm; €2.50). It has an archaeological collection, statues and coral carvings.

Adventures

On Water

Journey out to the **Egadi Islands** or **Pantelleria** as part of a longer trip. Or you could see the small islands used in salt production on a day-trip (see *Mozia*) by boat or canoe.

If you want to do a fishing excursion, contact **Michele Basirico** (☎ 329-723-347) or rent a boat from **MG Nautica**

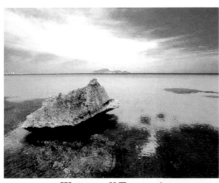
Waters off Trapani

(Via Natale Augugliaro 1, ☎ 0923-24020). You can rent a boat from **Sail Adventures** (Via Pantelleria 10, ☎ 333-898-4818, www.sail-adventures.com) or take their cultural excursion to Mothia (€41).

Sosalt (☎ 349-404-1390) does a day-long excursion for €60 to the **Riserva Naturale delle Saline di Trapani**'s uninhabited islands. A chef on board cooks your lunch.

On Wheels

At the time of writing, the bicycle path between Trapani and Mozia was being developed, with a couple of km already completed. Even if it's not completed when you are there, you can take the same trip on the main road (15 km) – an easy trip with little traffic. Alternatively, the *lungomare* east of the city is good for biking, with an easy 10-11 km route to the scenic Tonnara di Bonagia. There's also a good route at Monte Cofano (later in this chapter).

You can rent bikes at:

- **Maiorbike** (Via Alcamo 92/94, maiorbike@libero.it, ☎ 0923-542-437).
- **T.V. & L. Service** (☎ 348-950-6338).
- **Noleggio Scooter/Bike** (☎ 329-840-6209).
- **Relais Antiche Saline** (Via Giuseppe Verdi).

Lombardo Bikes sells all kinds of bicycles (Via Roma 169, Buseto Palizzolo, www.lombardobikes.com, ☎ 092-385-1181). They are in Buseto Palizzolo, not far from Trapani.

Where to Stay

Hostels & Camping

Ostello per la Gioventù G Amodeo (Viale della Pineta, Contrada Raganzili, ☎ 0923-552-964, €) is three km north of town on the Erice road. Take bus

number 23 from Via GB
Fardella to the Ospedale
Villa dei Gerani. It's 500
yards from the bus stop: take
the second right and walk up
the hill.

HOTEL PRICE CHART	
€	Up to €25 per day
€€	€26-€55
€€€	€56-€85
€€€€	Over €85

Villa Maria (Via Torre di
Mezzo 71, Marausa, ☎ 092-
384-1363, www.villamaria.marausa.it,) is near the salt lakes
12 km south of Trapani, with camping and apartments.

Hotels

Crystal (Piazza Umberto 1, ☎ 0923-20000, €€€€) is part of
the luxury Framon hotel chain.

Messina (Corso Vittorio Emanuele 71, ☎ 0923-21198, €€) is a
good budget choice in the center of town.

Vittoria (Via Francesco Crispi 4, ☎ 0923-873-044, www.
hotelvittoriatrapani.it, €€€).

Baglio Costa di Mandorla (Via Verderame 37, Paceco,
☎ 0923-409-100, www.costadimandorla.it, €€€-€€€€€) is
near the salt lakes south of Trapani.

B&Bs

Il Sole Blu B&B (Via Orlandini 7, ☎ 349-536-5768,
ezioricevuto@libero.it, €€€).

Il Cortiletto B&B (Vicolo dei Compagni 2, ☎ 0923-872-625,
€€€, www.ilcortilettotrapani.it) has four rooms behind the
post office.

Ai Lumi (Corso Vittorio Emanuele 71, ☎ 0923-872-418, www.
ailumi.it, €€€-€€€€€) is a five-minute walk from the train
station on the main street of Trapani in an 18th-century palace. Modern rooms and multilingual staff.

Where to Eat

Bars & Cafés

Café Bar a Nannini (Piazza Lucatelli) has a cool
garden.

Talon Café (Corso Vittorio Emanuele 39) is near the
cathedral with a good view of the *passeggiata* through the
centro storico.

Picadilly (Via Torresara 19, closed Sun) serves snacks and drinks in the street.

Birreria Italia (Via Torrera 5-7) is one of several bars in this corner. You can get beer and snacks here while you enjoy the *passeggiata*.

There are a few bars and cafés opposite the Stazione

DINING PRICE CHART	
Price per person for an entrée, including house wine.	
€	Up to €12
€€	€13-€25
€€€	€26-€35
€€€€	Over €35

Marittima where you can get *panini* and café or other snacks for your voyage.

Restaurants

Taverna Paradiso (Via Lungomare Dante Alighieri 24, ☎ 0923-22303, closed Sun, €€€) has a great location in a warehouse by the seafront. Ask to sit at a table in the street where they have put plants to form a small green courtyard. Most plates are about € 9: spaghetti with sea urchins, pasta with lobster and fresh artichokes.

Il Pilota (Via Ammiraglio Staiti, ☎ 092-354-8488, €) is an easy fast food joint near the ferry terminal.

I Sapori d'Oriente (Via S. Francesco D'Assisi 31, ☎ 320-053-4983) is in the *centro storico*.

Trattoria da Felice (Via Ammiraglio Staiti 45, ☎ 092-354-7822, closed Mon, €€-€€€) serves couscous with fish.

Antichi Sapori (Corso Vittorio Emanuele, ☎ 0923-22866, €€) has a couscous and fish special.

Tavernetta ai Lumi (Corso Vittorio Emanuele 75, ☎ 0923-872-418, €€) is a favorite with the locals. There's a long dining room with medieval brick arches. Specials include roast lamb in citrus sauce, larded and roasted rabbit and fresh seafood.

Cantina Siciliana (Via Giudecca 32, ☎ 0923-28673, €€€), with traditional *pupi* (Sicilian puppets) and other Sicilian bric-a-brac, has good regional plates.

Ristorante da Pepe (Via Spalti 50, €€) is a one-room restaurant with bright murals and serves average meals.

■ Islands off the Coast

The Egadi Islands

This group of three islands is very accessible, which unfortunately also means they swarm with visitors during the summer. However, if you come out of season they are less affected. The islands have been inhabited since prehistoric times. Initially there was a Phoenician-Punic settlement of Aegades, which later came under Roman control. During the Middle Ages sailors passed by on trading routes that included the Egadis. The islands actually only came under Italian ownership again in 1937.

Tuna fishing has long been a major element in the local economy. Tuna congregate here to breed at the end of spring and they are slaughtered through an ancient process known as *La Mattanza*. You'll have seen pictures of this at the museum in the Tonnara di Bonagia (see *Bonagia*).

Favignana is the largest of the three islands and the most developed. It has more options for accommodation and eating and is perfect for touring on bike, thanks to the flatness of the terrain. **Levanzo** is less developed, with a much smaller stable population. It is named after a section of the city of Genova (it was once sold to Genovese businessmen). It also shelters the **Grotta del Genovese**, a cave in which prehistoric cave paintings were discovered. Walking opportunities are good on Levanzo, but rugged, mountainous **Marettimo** is the real walking paradise. This westernmost island has far more wild beauty, and is the best choice for peace and quiet.

You could easily visit the islands on a day-trip. If you stay overnight, book ahead during summer and be prepared to pay higher prices for rooms and food than on the mainland. Out of season accommodation prices drop dramatically.

Getting Here

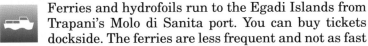

Ferries and hydrofoils run to the Egadi Islands from Trapani's Molo di Sanita port. You can buy tickets dockside. The ferries are less frequent and not as fast as the hydrofoils but you'll save money on the tickets. For example, **Siremar** (☎ 0923-545-455) operates ferries for Favignana (€3.20), Levanzo (€3.20) and Marettimo (€7.10) from Trapani. By comparison, hydrofoils with **Ustica Lines**

(☎ 0923-22200) run to Favignana (€5.30, 20 minutes), Levanzo (35 minutes, €5.30) and Marettimo (€11.80, 70 minutes). Siremar also operates more expensive hydrofoils. **Ustica Lines** also operates from Ustica to Favignana and Levanzo. It's possible to get to the Egadi Islands from Marsala (see *Marsala*). Generally, ferries call at Favignana, Levanzo and Marettimo, in that order.

Favignana

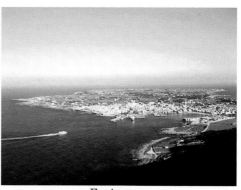

Favignana is only 25 minutes from Trapani by hydrofoil and the mostly flat island is dominated by the windswept Mt Santa Caterina (1,030 feet). Boats arrive at the port in Favignana town. The two distinctive features at the port are the Palazzo Florio (the town

Favignana

hall) and the tuna fishery, Stabilmento Florio. The tuna processing port was abandoned in 1977 due to a general crisis in the local fishing industry. It's impressive to wander around. Tuna products are available in shops everywhere. You can find a tourist office in Piazza Madrice (Pro Loco, ☎ 0923-921-647).

Getting Around

Due to the flat terrain and good road surfaces you'll find it easiest to get around by bike. Bike rental is available all over town; look for the words *noleggio bici*. **Favignana Tp** (Piazza Europa 12, ☎ 0923-922-171) rents scooters, mountain bikes and cars. **Rita** (Piazza Europa 12, ☎ 0923-022-171) also rents bikes. You can also get around via a bus service that operates from the port in summer and makes circuits on three routes. Boat tours are offered by fishermen down at the port.

Adventures

On Wheels

 Long distances and lack of shade make it difficult to walk, but the roads are good for biking. An easy route of 90 minutes starts along the road east from the ferry harbor. Five minutes along, where the asphalt bears inland, you take the dirt road straight ahead and then keep left along the coast. There are plenty of coves for good swimming and you get great views of Levanzo and the mainland. The track passes near the cemetery on Punta San Nicola and you can explore an abandoned quarry at **Scalo Cavallo**. At the next t-intersection, get a snack in the bar and then turn left for Cala Rossa (30 minutes). Leave your bike at the top and wander down to the waterside. Back on the path keep left past an old house and a shrine to a 17th-century friar. The next landmark is **Cala Blue Marino** – worthy of a photographic stop. Take the next lane branching left and stick to the coastline for a rather bumpy stretch heading towards the lighthouse at **Punta Marsala**. From here you can follow a surfaced road west around the point past Cala Azzurra and a snack bar. Keep left to Punta Fanfalo. A dirt track leads around its sea side and rejoins the road. On the road you will pass **Grotta Perciata**, a natural rock bridge. Then you will soon pass **Lido Burrone**, the island's main beach. The road back to the harbor is the next right turn. If you don't want to go by bicycle, you could walk the route in three hours.

There is also a track up Monte S. Caterina and its Norman castle overlooking the harbor area.

On Water

 Favignana has crystal-clear waters ideal for snorkeling and swimming. A particularly good spot is **Cala Rossa**. Other recommendatons are **Punta Marsala**, **Secca del Toro**, the submerged reef between Cala Rotonda and Scoglio Corrente and the depths of **Punta Ninfaio** and **Punta Ferro**. To rent a boat contact:

- **Seataxi** (Contrada Calamoni, ☎ 0923-921-011).
- **Blue Egadi** (Largo Marina, ☎ 328-058-0577).
- **Nautilia Service** (Largo Marina).
- **Il Delfino** (Via Calatafimi 7, ☎ 338-960-0310).

Where to Stay

 Camping Egad (☎ 0923-921-567, www.egadi.com/egad, €) is a campsite on the eastern side of the island. **Miramar** (☎ 0923-922-200, www.villaggiomiramare.it, €) is another one to the west. Both have cabins available.

Quattro Rose (Localita Mulino a Vento, ☎ 0923-921-223, €€€) is close to town and handy for beaches to the east.

Hotel Bougainville (Via Cimabue 10, ☎ 0923-922-033, €€-€€€) and **Hotel Aegusa** (Via Garibaldi 11, ☎ 0923-922-430, www.aegusahotel.it, €€€€) are both in town.

Al Giardino dei Limoni B&B (Vicolo Cimarosa 12, ☎ 0923-921-394, www.algiardinodeilimoni.it, €€€-€€€€€)

Elisir (Via Madonna, ☎ 0923-555-256, www.casevacanzaelisir.it) is a complex of apartments 100 yards from the port.

Where to Eat

 El Pescador (Piazza Europa 38, ☎ 0923-921-035, €€€€) requires reservations. It's right in the center, serving good spaghetti and *couscous di pesce*.

La Bettola (Via Nicotera 47, ☎ 0923-921-988, €€€) is a little cheaper and also in the center.

La Tavernetta (Piazza Madrice 61, ☎ 0923-921-939, €€) is an economical choice with an all-fish menu.

Levanzo

Levanzo town is a small cluster of square houses and holiday homes around the port with more limited accommodation and eating options than Favignana. The prime attraction is the prehistoric cave paintings at the **Grotta del Genovese**. The paintings date from 7,000-8,000 BC but are predated by the engravings believed to be from 12,000-13,000 BC. Twenty-nine animals and three masked human figures grace these walls. They were only discovered in 1994 when a Tuscan woman artist chanced upon them. Other attractions in Levanzo are the interesting birdlife and fine swimming in many small coves and caves. Levanzo was once joined to the mainland by a bridge.

South Coast

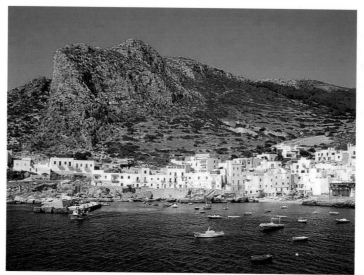

Levanzo

Adventures

On Foot

There are three great spots for swimming. The first is **Faraglione**. To get there, take a left through town and walk west along the road for one km to the rocks offshore. An option farther along is **Capo Grosso**, on the northern side of the island at the lighthouse. If you turn right out of town along the dirt road, a rocky path drops down to the sea after 300 yards to **Calo Minnola**.

To get to Capo Grosso via the lovely interior, head towards Faraglione but turn right up the steep road marked Comunale Strada Capo Grosso. It becomes a stone and dirt track once it reaches the upper part of the valley. It's around an hour round-trip to the lighthouse at Capo Grosso.

Another route heads east around the coast past the cemetery on a broad dirt track to **Cala Fredda**. Follow the path along the coast for Cala Minnola (25 minutes). It's a great spot for a picnic. Then head for the signed path for **Cala Calcara**. Take the right fork north on Sentiero Calcara through a light wood to emerge at the open ridge, with great views. You can zig-zag down to swim in the Cala Calcara (one hour). Ascend up the valley at the rear of the bay to a lane due south between dry stone walls. You pass the derelict 19th-century **Villa Florio**

and can detour up to the square-based tower **Torre Saracena**. Follow the dirt road west and turn left back down to town.

■ *Grotta del Genovese*

You can approach the famous cave by foot, Landrover or boat. It is locked so you will have to arrange with the custodian (Signor Natale Castiglione, ☎ 0923-924032, nacasti@tin.it) to visit it (10 am-1 pm, 3-6 pm, €5). Entrance is by reservation only and they can take you there by boat or Landrover (€13). The price includes the entry fee to the cave. If you want, you could arrange to be dropped there first by boat or Landrover and hike back. It's a 10-km walk of roughly two hours. The route to the cave can follow the track past Faraglione, then past some old stone buildings and cisterns up a gradual ascent to a signpost for the Grotta del Genovese. It's a tiring climb over some boulders to pick up the route to the cave. Another route follows the inland path to Capo Grosso but veers left at the signs to Grotta Genovese past a stone enclosure labeled Loc. Carvunere.

On Water

There are a number of caves around the island where locals used to hide. To visit them you can rent a boat at the port or get someone to take you. A boat ride is also a good way to save your legs and see some of the same good swimming bays from a different perspective.

■ **Egadi Snorkelling** (Via S. Scaletta 16, ☎ 0923-924-030).

■ **Franco il Pescatore** (Via Salita Chiesa, ☎ 339-679-1645).

Under Water

The clear waters around Levanzo make it good for diving. Contact **L'Isola** (Contrada Case, ☎ 320-180-9090, www.lisolasrl.it).

Where to Stay

Pensione dei Fenici (Via Calvario 18, ☎ 0923-924-083, €€€-€€€€) and **Paradiso** (Lungomare, ☎ 0923-924-080, www.isoladilevanzo.it, €€€-€€€€) are in the center of town.

L'Isola Residence (Contrada Case, ☎ 320-180-9090, www. lisolasrl.it), is outside the center and also offers tours by Landrover, boat and diving.

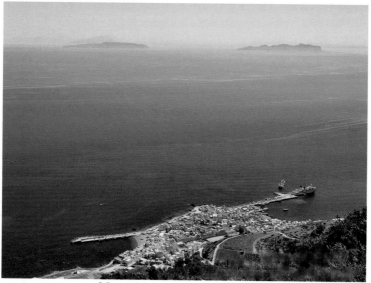

Marettimo (Residence Isola del Miele)

Marettimo

The westernmost of the islands is also the least developed, but a good spot for swimming and walking. Samuel Butler claimed this was the island of Ithaca and home to Ulysses. It certainly fits the scene, although most agree the idea is far-fetched. Even in high season it's quieter, with just some low-key development. Marettimo town has flat-roofed houses with blue shutters. There's one main street, a square with a church, and a fishing port. The fragmented coastline is pitted with rocky coves and beaches, presenting quite a different perspective than the flatter Favignana.

Adventures

Under Water

Visibility around Marettimo is 100-130 feet deep. Most of the centers offer a variety of single dives (€35) off rubber boats or full-day excursions (€65) with two dives and lunch aboard (€8). Contact:

- **Diving Center Medma** (Via Gavino Campo 3, ☎ 0923-923-414).
- **Diving El Merendero** (Via G. Pepe 9, ☎ 0923-923-149).
- **Marettimo Diving Center** (Via Cuore di Gesu, ☎ 0923-923-083, www.marettimodivingcenter.it).
- **Voglia di Mare Diving Center** (Via Mazzini 50, ☎ 339-421-3845, www.vogliadimare.com).

On Water

 Boat tours are offered from the port. In three hours you can easily do a *giro dell'isola* (tour of the island) to see the more inaccessible parts and enjoy some good snorkelling. There are a number of interesting caves around the island, including Grotta del Cammello, Tuono, Perciata and Presepio.

Alta Marea (☎ 092-392-3243, www.altamareasub.com) has excursions around Marettimo. There are daily tours by day or night or you can rent a boat with equipment for up to a week. For good swimming spots see the suggestions in *Adventures on Foot*. Other good beaches can be found right on either side of town.

On Foot

 Due to the absence of roads, there is quite a skeleton system of paths that were once used by hunters and herdsmen and are now being upgraged by the Forestry Department.

■ *Case Romane (30 minutes)*

A simple walk to the Case Romane leaves from the road by the side of CaffeTramontana. At the top you'll find the signpost for the start of the walk. The remains of the Roman defensive works are half an hour from there, next to an old church thought to have been built by Byzantine monks in the 12th century. You can extend this walk by continuing on the path to Pizzo Falcone (two-three hours round-trip) to your left. Or continue straight on a narrowing path signposted for Taurro. There are views of the Punta Troia headland and castle as the path descends gradually via outcrops honeycombed with caves. It drops right down to the junction (one hour 50 minutes) where a left variant can lead on to Cala Bianca on a rough path, or take the right fork to Punta Troia.

- *Cala Nera (two hours)*

Cala Sarda and Cala Nera are two good swimming spots on the southern coast and form a pleasant walking itinerary. Follow the road south of the port and then inland after about one km. Here the path divides. Climb for about half an hour past a pine forest and a small outhouse. Cala Sarda is beneath you (another half-hour by the smaller path to the left). If you don't go down to the bay, you could continue for an hour on the main path along the rocky west coast. There's a lighthouse here and then a route down to Cala Nera.

- *Punta Troia (three hours)*

The walk to Punta Troia follows a footpath all the way to the northeastern tip of the island. The hike takes about three hours. To get there, pass the fishing harbor with the sea on your right and continue on the coastal path for 10 minutes until the terrace wall on your left stops. A sign to Castello Punta Troia points to the left. Cut up to find the main path above you. The path stretches along the entire length of the island about 300 feet above the sea. About 30 minutes along, a signed fork uphill indicates a *sorgente* (water spring). It ends at Scalo Maestro (concrete steps) that you take down to a secluded beach. The castle is perched on a rocky crag 20 minutes along the cape. The fortification was built by the Saracens, enlarged by Roger II and later extended by the Spanish in the 17th century. The Spanish used it as a prison. The swimming here is excellent and the setting very panoramic.

Other walks to Punta Libeccio and Carcaredda are also worth exploring.

Where to Stay

Ask at the café in the main square for rooms or at any of the restaurants. Or try these options:

Marettimo Residence (Via Telegrafo 117, ☎ 0923-923-202, €€-€€€€) has 40 apartments.

Il Corallo (Via Chiusa 11, ☎ 333-699-9298) rents apartments and can arrange boat excursions.

I Delfini B&B (Via Umberto 1, 34, ☎ 0923-932-137, www. idelfinimarettimo.it, €€€), in the center, has a view of the sea.

La Perla B&B (Via Campi 13, ☎ 0923-923-206).

Rosa dei Venti (Contrada Crocilla, ☎ 0923-923-249, ☎ 0923-923-249).

Where to Eat

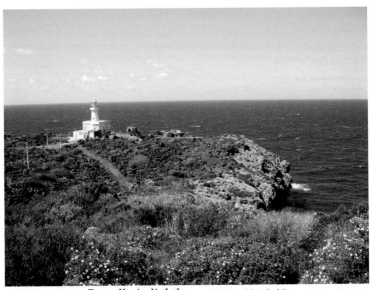

Il Timone (Via Garibaldi 18, ☎ 0923-923-142, €€), on *lungomare*, serves good fresh pasta.

Il Pirata (Scalo Vecchio 27, ☎ 0923-923-027, €€) is another good choice.

For good soups and couscous try either the **Trattoria Pizzeria Hiera** (Via Gaetano Maiorana 12, ☎ 0923-923-017, €€) or the similarly priced **Trattoia Il Veliero** (Via Umberto 22, Marettimo, ☎ 0923-923-274) on *lungomare*.

Pantelleria lighthouse (Michael Leithold)

Pantelleria

This is the biggest of Sicily's islands and actually closer to Tunisia than to Sicily. The island is a quasi-dormant volcano that last erupted in 1891 and has burned black soil. Coves and inlets line its shores, good for swimming. The largely mountainous interior is good for walking or riding around on mopeds, which you can rent at the port. It was used to film part of *Il Postino*.

Pantelleria was settled by the Ses, Neolithic people from Libya. Over time the controlling powers of the Mediterranean all took control, including the Phoenicians, the Greeks, Carthaginians, Romans and Moors. The 400-year Moorish occupation made an impact on the population, who still use a local dialect laced with Arabic words. The typical houses, *dammusi*, are also Arabic and *zbibbo* is the grape used to produce the local wine.

Getting Here

 Air One (☎ 800-900-966) flies from Trapani to Pantelleria about four times daily (30 minutes). Flights usually stop at the end of October and recommence in January.

Year-round **ferries** arrive from Trapani (2½ hours) via **Ustica Lines** (€36) which is the faster and more expensive option than night ferries with Siremar.

Getting Around

 The ferries arrive right near the center of town allowing easy access to Pantelleria town. However, given the size of the island, you will need transportation to move around. Buses connect the airport (five km southeast of town) to Piazza Cavour and other local services depart from here at regular intervals to major points around the island. Seven buses connect the southwest coast to both Scauri and Rekake. And six daily buses make the northeast trek to both Kamma and Tracino. You can also rent a moped for getting around. The island is small enough that you could get around in about four hours. You can rent scooters from **PantelRent** (Via Napoli, ☎ 0923-973-636) near the port. For mountain bikes and scooters try **Auto Noleggio Consolo** (Piazza Castello 8, ☎ 0923-912-716). For cars and scooters, try **Policardo** (Via Messina 31, ☎ 0923-912-844).

Information Sources

 There's a tourist office in Piazza Cavour (☎ 0923-911-838) that can give you a map. The website, www.pantelleria.it, is also useful.

Sightseeing

Pantelleria town was flattened during the last war and so much of the town has a modern appearance. The 16th-century

South Coast

Castello Barbacene (6 am-8 pm, free) remains on the far side of the harbor, a legacy of the Spaniards. **Gadir** on the northeastern coast is an idylic spot with a small harbor perfect for swimming. There are also numerous thermal pools. Many of the towns have options for accommodations and eating.

The other sights are around the island. There are 24 ancient craters of red volcanic rock around the main volcano **Mt Grande** (2,742 feet). This volcano dominates the center of the island. See *Adventures on Foot* for walking itineraries to the top.

The island was once dotted with *sesi*, massive neolithic funeral cairns with low passages leading to the center. Most have now been dismantled and the stones used to construct *dammusi*. **Sese del Re** is the most interesting and 15 minutes walk south of the Cuddie Rosse on the northwestern coast. *Dammusi* are Moorish in appearance with thick white-washed walls and shallow cupolas to keep the inside cool. Ridges on the top catch the rain. You will see these dotted all over Pantelleria and used in construction of hotels also. Another thing to look out for are *giardini arabi*, Moorish gardens that were built into the mountainside and protected from fierce winds by stone walls. Many houses have them.

Adventures

In Air

 Sicilwing (Via Provinciale 233, S. Venerina, Catania, ☎ 095-532-003, www.sicilwing.com) has day flights to Pantelleria at €1,600 for up to five persons in a Seneca PA-34. The flight is round-trip from the Catania international airport. They also have flights over Agrigento and Lampedusa, the Aeolian Islands and over Mt Etna.

On Water

 To visit the isolated coves of the southeastern **Dietro Isola** you need to rent a boat. There are good swimming spots here. Check out the agencies along the harbor, hotels or the boats themselves for the best prices.

On Foot

 You could catch a bus to Scauri or Rekale (25 minutes) and walk back to the Sesi (couple of hours) past the **Cuddie Rosse** prehistoric cave settlement. Fifteen

minutes farther, a track on the left leads up 1,000 feet to the first of the strange **Sesi**, Neolithic funeral mounds. These are thought to be products of the first settlers. The main one is 19 feet high. It's an hour on foot from Sesi to **Sataria**, where concrete steps lead down to a small sea pool. In the cave behind are warm water bubbles supposed to be good for skin diseases. From here it's two km (30 minutes) to Scauri. The town is tiny, with a church and few shops. **Rekale**, at the end of the bus line, is even smaller. From here you can reach the southeast of the island, including **Dietro Isola** and the hot springs at **Punto Nika**. This is accessible on foot but more easily reached by boat.

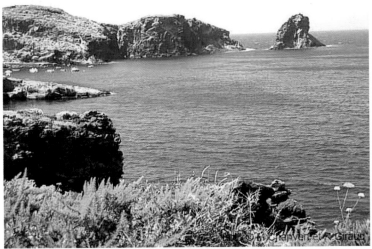

Pantelleria

Catch a bus to **Siba**, perched on a ridge above the main volcano, **Monte Grande**. Four buses climb up here daily. To climb the peak, keep left at the telephone sign by the *tabacchi* and strike off the main road. The slopes are pitted with volcanic vents marked by threads of vapor. From Siba, another path on the left brings you in around 20 minutes to a natural sauna (**Sauna Naturale**). It's a slit in the rock face where you crouch until beads of sweat break out.

The road through Siba becomes a track that descends back to the coast midway between Scauri and Rekale into the **Valle**

Monastero past an abandoned monastery. Start early to avoid too much heat on the sunless route.

On Wheels

 Six daily buses link the northeast coast to Kamma and Tracino. **Bue Marino** is the first stop where you can swim. **Cala dei Cinque Denti** has rocks shaped like teeth jutting out of the sea. There's a lighthouse at **Punta Spadillo** just beyond. However, at the first road junction you could walk 10 minutes up to the island's small lake, **Specchio di Venere** (Venus Mirror) in a former crater. It is aquamarine in the middle. Apply the mud on the edges of the lake to your body until they bake hard and then dive into the warm water and wash it off.

Gadir is the next bus stop, an idyllic harbor town with just a few houses against the volcanic rocks. From here you can walk to Cala Levante (one hour) and a tiny fishing harbor. Five minutes farther down is the **Arco dell'Elefante** (Elephant Arch), a formation of rock that looks like an elephant having a drink. You can climb to Tracino (20 minutes) past old *dammusi* and lovely gardens. Buses run back to Pantelleria.

If you want a longer walk, you can start at Tracino for Piano Ghirlandia. A track beyond Tracino eventually winds its way over to Rekale.

Under Water

Diving on Pantelleria is almost a must as the volcanic sea beds around the island are spectacular. Many diving schools

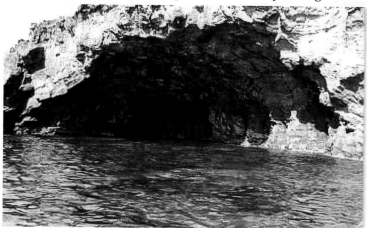

Pantelleria grotto

and centers offer trips around the island to discover different subaquatic landscapes. Some good spots include Cala Diving in Pantelleria Levante, Cala Gadir, Cala Tramontana, Punta Tracino and Punta Limarsi. Contact **Dive-X** (Via Milano e Loc. Gadir, ☎ 339-105-1878), **Cala Levante** (Loc. Cala Levente), **Green Divers** (C. da Mursia, ☎ 0923-391-1217), **Aquasub** (Cda. Scauri Porto) or **TGI Diving Center** (Loc. Punta Farm, www.tgidiving.com, ☎ 0923-911-424).

South Coast

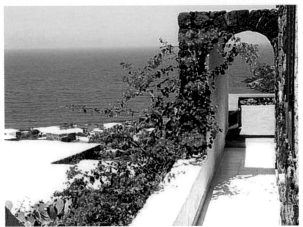

Villa Dammuso rental (www.agriturismo.net)

Where to Stay

There are other options for accommodation in Cuddie Rosse, Punta Fram and Blu Marino.

In Pantelleria town the options include:

Khamma (Via Borgo Italia 24, ☎ 0923-912-680, €€-€€€) at the end of the dock on the harborfront. Central and comfortable.

Myriam (Corso Umberto I, ☎ 0923-911-374, €€-€€€) is at the far end of the port near the castle. It's a cheap option.

Port' Hotel (Lungomare Borgo Italia 71, ☎ 0923-911-299, €€-€€€€).

The charming **Zubebi Resort** (Contrada Zubebi, www. zubebi.it, ☎ 092-391-3653, €€€€) has accommodations in

traditional *dammusi* dwellings. A wonderful pool sits on the edge of the property overlooking the sea. Family-run and friendly. The restaurant is open to the public and rooms are open by week-long rental only.

Where to Eat

 Make sure you try the Moscato wine while you are here. This sweet, amber-colored dessert wine is particularly good. It's made from zibibbo grapes that grow well in the volcanic soil. You can often buy the local wine and other foods from local producers. Look for signs that say *azienda agricola*.

The **Zubebi Resort** (Contrada Zubebi, www.zubebi.it, ☎ 092-391-3653, €€€) is open to the public for evening dining. Come a little early and they may let you swim in the pool.

Trattoria Dammuso (Via Borgo Italia, €€) has cheap meals right in the harbor.

Il Cappero (Via Roma) has medium-priced food and is poplar with the locals.

Zabib (Porto di Scauri, ☎ 0923-916-617, €€€) is in Scauri on the southwest. Good seasonal restaurant with simple dishes.

La Vela (Scauri Scalo, ☎ 0923-916-566, €€€) is just a few feet from the sea. Try the fish with ammoghiu (pesto, tomato and basil).

■ South of Trapani: Mozia to Mazara del Vallo

★ Mozia

The coastline between Trapani and Marsala is known for its salt production and the uninhabited Stagnone islands off the coast have been given over to salt extraction since the 15th century. If you take the secondary road west of the SS115 you can see the heaps of drying salt and the Dutch-style windmills. It's a picturesque region and there are opportunities to tour the islands by boat and on foot. A pleasant biking itinerary can also get you here from Trapani (see *Trapani*).

The **Museo del Sale** (☎ 360-656-053, 9 am-1:30 pm, 3:30-6:30 pm) at Nubia is just five km south of Trapani in a 17th-century salt mill. **AST** buses link Trapani and Nubia four

times daily in summer at 6:30, 8:30, 10:30 am and 1:30 pm. Two buses return from Nubia to Trapani at 9:40 am and 2:40 pm. In winter, there are just two services each way. Get on at Piazza Montalto and you'll have to walk about one km from the bus stop in Nubia.

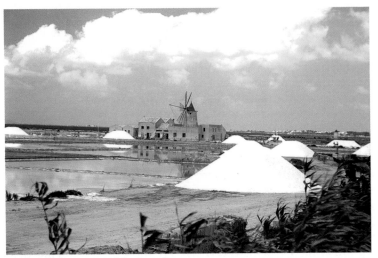

Mozia saltpans (Joanne Lane)

The **Stagnone Islands** are another 10 km south, where you can visit the ancient Phoenician settlement of **Motya** (Mozia). Along with Palermo and Solus (Solunto), Motya was one of the three main Phoenician bases in Sicily. It was settled in the eighth century BC and completely razed to the ground in 397 BC by Dionysius I. To reach the island, go to the Mozia ferry landing. **AST** buses from Piazza del Popolo in Marsala go here eight times daily (€2.58). From Trapani you first get a train to Marsala and catch the bus connection. Alternatively, a slow train will stop at either Ragatissi-Birgi or Spagnuola train station and you can hike from there to the ferry landing.

Boat operators from the ferry landing at the Saline Ettore e Infersa (salt pans) run out to the island. **Mozia Line** (☎ 0923-967-062, April-October 9 am-1 pm, 2:30-7 pm; November-March 9 am-1 pm, www.mozialine.com, €3) and **Arini e Pugliese** (9 am-1:30 pm, 2:30-7 pm, www.ariniepugliese. com) leave every 30 minutes. The boat ticket does not include entrance to the museum.

Museo Saline Ettore e Inferza (10 am-1 pm, 3:30-6:30 pm, €2, www.salineettoreinfersa.com/home.html, ☎ 0923-966-936) is similar to the one at Nubia. It's free to browse the shop and salt products but you pay €3.50 for a tour.

Very little remains of ancient Motya but it is fun to explore as part of a walking itinerary around the island. From the mueum you can head inland to a villa of the sixth-fourth century BC with moaic floors. Then return to the shorefront and follow the path southwest to an ancient guardhouse and a harbor of the fifth century BC. Round the point and head north to a sanctuary where cinerary urns containing the remains of infants and domestic animals were found. Turn right inland to a vineyard lined with olive trees and a sanctuary where furnaces made ceramic vases. The next place is a northern gateway perhaps for a defense system. Close by is the start of a sixth-century dual carriage causeway used until recent times to take produce from the grape harvest. Farther on is the eastern gateway and 10 minutes beyond is the landing stage. The whole itinerary should take less than 45 minutes.

There are no refreshments on the island but you can get food at **Mamma Caura Jazz Café** (☎ 092-373-3063, closed in winter, €€€) at the ferry landing. They have a bar, with snacks, and they sell the fantastic *pane cunzato* bread. Or try a sit-down meal in the restaurant, serving seafood and pasta. In summer they have jazz concerts. If you have a car, it's a good option to come here from Trapani for the night to dine and watch the sunset. They also have four double rooms with TV and bathrooms for €130 a night, including breakfast.

Marsala

Marsala is best known for its sweet dessert wines of the same name. It's not on a lot of tourist itineraries but it does have a pleasant town and historic quarter. In summer there are frequent traditional events and you can enjoy the famed wine everywhere you go or visit the numerous *enoteche* and *cantine*.

Marsala was founded by the survivors of the island-city Moya and was originally called Lilybaeum. It was the main city of the Phoenicians in Sicily and the only one to resist the Greek push westwards, but it succumbed to Rome in 241 BC. It was

named Marsah Ali, Arabic for the "port of Ali," by the Saracens.

One of the best times to come to Marsala is in the autumn, when the wine harvest takes place. Tractors and trucks carting loads of grapes are a regular feature on the roads, particularly out towards Salemi, dripping red juice all over the road. It can be a bit slippery! You will see teams of workers in the field.

Getting Here

Train is the best way to get here from Trapani. The station is in Via A. Fazio, a 15-minute walk from the center. **Buses** do arrive more centrally at Piazza del Popolo near Porta Garibaldi. **AST** and **Lumia** head to Trapani. Lumia runs to Agrigento also. **Salemi** (☎ 0923-981-120) buses go to Palermo airport (four daily, €7.10).

During the summer months, a hydrofoil links to the Egadi Islands via **Sandokan** (☎ 0923-712-060) and **Ustica Lines** (☎ 0348-357-9863).

Getting Around

Marsala is easy to plod around on foot. Or take bus 16 from Piazza del Popolo to Cantina Florio.

Information Sources

The **Pro Loco Marsala** is at Via XI Maggio 100 (☎ 0923-714-097, Mon-Sat 8 am-2 pm, www.prolocomarsala.org).

Sightseeing

Piazza della Republicca is the heart of the city. This giant square is fronted on one side by the **Duomo** and on the other by the **Palazzo Comunale** (town hall). Both are 18th-century buildings. The **Museo degli Arazzi** (Tues-Sun 9 am-1 pm, 4-6 pm, €1.60) is behind the Duomo on Via Garraffa 57. It contains a series of eight Flemish tapestries made in Brussels in the 16th century. On Via XI Maggio is the **Monumentale San Pietro** (Tues-Sat 9 am-1 pm, 4-8 pm, Sun 9:30 am-1:30 pm, 4-8 pm, €2), a 15th-century monastery now a cultural center. You can check the Internet here in the

South Coast

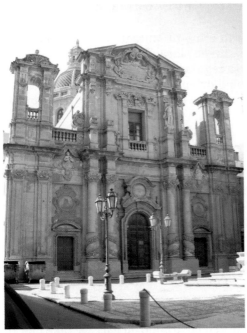

Marsala Duomo (Archenzo)

Biblioteca Comunale (Mon-Fri 9 am-12 pm, Tues and Thurs 3:30-5:30 pm).

Keep going on Via XI Maggio to the **Porta Nuova**, one of the original gates, which leads down to the municipal gardens. **Capo Boeo** is the westernmost point of Sicily (turn left onto Via Lungo Mare Boeo at the end of Via Vittorio Veneto). This was the first settlement of the survivors of annihilated Motya. The town's ancient sites are located here, including the **Insula Romana** (9 am-1 pm, 4 to one hour before sunset; free), a third-century Roman villa. It's actually in an entrance off Via Vittorio Veneto. There's also the *edificio termale* (bathhouse) and some good mosaics.

The **Museo Archeologico** (Mon-Sun 9 am-1:30 pm, Wed and Fri-Sun 4-6:30 pm, €2.30) contains all the other finds. There's a Phoenician or Punic warship that was brought here in 1977. It was

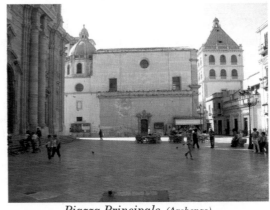

Piazza Principale (Archenzo)

probably sunk during the First Punic War in the great sea battle off the Egadi Islands that ended Carthage's rule of the waves. Amphorae, anchors, photographs and other finds from Motya and the sea are also on display.

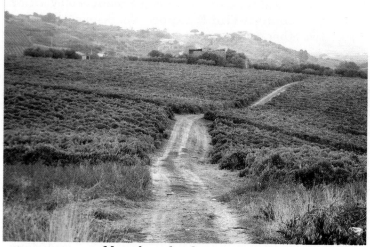

Marsala orchards *(Joanne Lane)*

Adventures

★With Wine

Thanks to its climate, Sicily produces some good wines, but one of the best-known vintages is Marsala, a dessert wine with amber and ruby tones. The British particularly enjoyed this wine, especially Lord Nelson, and they spurred local vintners to produce large qualities. Marsala is the best place to taste wine and make some purchases. There are a lot of *enoteche* in the city (see *Where to Eat*) who are particularly helpful, but you can also visit the *cantine* directly. The **Cantina Florio** (Via Lungomare Florio 1, ☎ 0923-781-111, www.cantineflorio.it) is on the Salemi road to Baglio Biesina. Call to make an appointment. This is *the* place to buy Marsala's wines and the oldest – established in 1832. Visitors can taste wines and they explain the process of production. Tours cost from €3-7. Bus 16 from Piazza del Popolo goes here.

Cantina Pellegrino (Via del Fante 37-39, ☎ 0923-719-911, www.carlopellegrino.it) and **Rallo** (Via Florio 3, ☎ 0923-721-

633) are two other options. Rallo, established in 1860, makes a top-of-the-line Marsala, Rallo Marsala Vergine, that combines older vintages aged at least 12 years. Pellegrino allows you to see the wine being bottled.

There are enoteca souvenir shops in Via Lungomare Boeo by the archaeological museum. **Enoteca Sombrero** (Via Garibaldi 32) or **Enoteca Vini & Sapori** (Via Scipione l'Africano 25) are two other good spots to stop.

Where to Stay

 There aren't a lot of options. If you have a camper there's a pull-in spot down along Viale Vittorio Veneto.

Albergo Garden (Via Gambini 36, ☎ 0923-982-320, www.albergogardenmarsala.it, €€) is one of the best budget places in town. **Hotel Centrale** (Via Salinisti 19, ☎ 0923-951-777, www.hotelcentralemarsala.it, €€€) is in the center, not far from the sea. **Hotel Carmine** (Piazza Carmine 16, €€€) is a new hotel in the city center. **Stella d'Italia** (Via Mario Rapisardi 7, €€€) faces the central piazza. **Villa Favorita** (Via Favorita 27, ☎ 0923-989-100, www.villafavorita.com, €€€-€€€€) is the priciest option in town.

Where to Eat

 For a small place, Marsala has a surprisingly good nightlife. It may appear deserted at first, but you just need to know where to head. There are some good options down at the port in summer or along Via XI Maggio, away from the Duomo and the sea.

Caffeteria Grand Italia in the main piazza serves drinks and snacks next to a good bookshop. Concerts are held in the square in summer.

★**Merkaba Caffe Letterario** (Via Amendola 57, ☎ 338-504-7509, closed Mon) is a caffeteria with a book twist. Come to read or buy books and enjoy the surroundings. There's a gramophone on the bar and the coffee machine is French, dating from the 1930s. The bathrooms are worth a peek and upstairs are comfortable seats where you can look through rare books from the 1900s or enjoy the good *aperitivi* and food.

Bier Platz Birreria (Via XI Maggio, ☎ 328-674-9660, 092-371-1770, closed Mon, €€) is hugely popular, with hundreds of tables – that fill – out in the street. On the walls are instruc-

tions about life on parchments. They serve food, but it's predominantly a wine bar.

★**Ca la Turca** (Via Caturca 6, ☎ 338-727-370, 092-371-1744, calaturca@libero.it, closed Mon in winter, €€-€€€) is a gorgeous candle-lit place to eat in one of the quaintest streets of Marsala, running off the Via XI Maggio near Bier Platz Birreria. It also has its own source of fresh seafood – the owner's father is a fisherman! The *tagliatelle al gamberone* (lobster) is recommended, or the *busciate con il sugo di tonno* (tuna). They also serve couscous. There's a set menu of €15. And they'll happily let you taste Marsala too!

Il Mare Colore del Vino is opposite and another good wine bar.

Mazara del Vallo

Don't let first appearances of Mazara deceive – it can appear chaotic, dissheveled and more like a North African city than a European one but, given some time, it charms most visitors. The Arab district is a labyrinth of streets, known as the Casbah, beyond the port. Coupled with the Baroque churches and fortified homes of the Norman conquest it's an interesting contrast. The *lungomare* is well shaded with a number of fine restaurants that make the most of its coastal location.

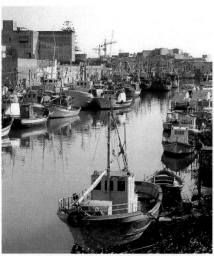
Mazara del Vallo

The port town of Mazara was one of the key cities of Saracen Sicily and its most prosperous. Actually, it is the site of the first Saracen landing in Sicily in AD 827 and it was the last place they surrendered when Count Roger took it in 1087, anxious to establish a strong Norman presence in the former Muslim powerbase.

South Coast

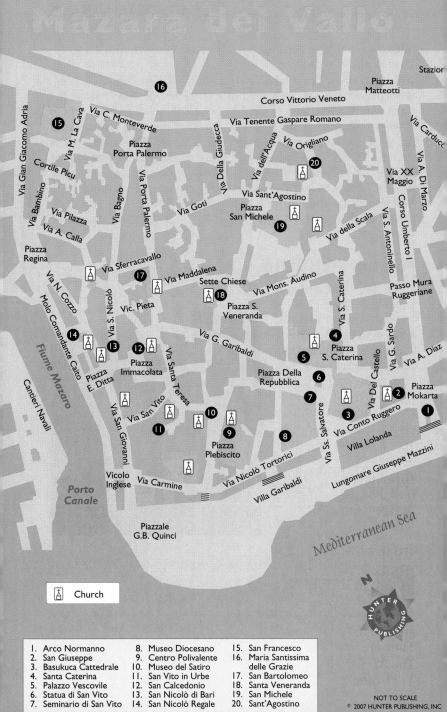

Mazara del Vallo

1. Arco Normanno
2. San Giuseppe
3. Basukuca Cattedrale
4. Santa Caterina
5. Palazzo Vescovile
6. Statua di San Vito
7. Seminario di San Vito
8. Museo Diocesano
9. Centro Polivalente
10. Museo del Satiro
11. San Vito in Urbe
12. San Calcedonio
13. San Nicolò di Bari
14. San Nicolò Regale
15. San Francesco
16. Maria Santissima delle Grazie
17. San Bartolomeo
18. Santa Veneranda
19. San Michele
20. Sant'Agostino

Church

NOT TO SCALE
© 2007 HUNTER PUBLISHING, INC

Mazara was the provincial capital until Trapani took over in 1817. Arab links have revived in recent years due to the flood of Tunisian immigrants entering Sicily here and staying on to work in the town. This has added a nice touch with Arabic newspapers, an Arabic quarter, carpet shops and some fine Arab sweets.

Getting Here

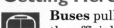 **Buses** pull in at the train station or Piazza Mateotti, the official terminus about 200 yards away. **AST** has three buses daily to/from Trapani, Marsala and Castelvetrano. **International Bus** (Via Salemi 101/a, ☎ 092-394-4650, fax 092-367-0851) has a service to/from Palermo's Punta Raisi airport and Birgi airport near Trapani (€16/€30 one-way/return).

Train connections also link Mazara with Trapani, Marsala and Castelvetrano. To/from Palermo you change at Alcamo Diramazione.

Getting Around

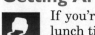 If you're driving into Mazara in the early morning, lunch time or evening, it can be chaotic. Try early afternoon, 2-4 pm, to avoid the worst rushes. There is plenty of parking down by the port. The port is on the *lungomare*, where you get boats to Pantelleria and the Egadi Islands. **Ustica Lines** departs for Pantelleria, departing at 10:15 am and returning at 4:30 pm the same day (€37.40 one-way)

International Bus (Via Salemi 101/a, ☎ 092-394-4650) offers bus excursions for a minimum of eight people to Agrigento and Sciacca, Mozia and Marsala, Erice and Segesta for €23 each.

Information Sources

i The helpful **Pro Loco tourist office** (Piazza Mokarta 14, www.proloco_mazaradelvallo.org, ☎ 0923-944-610, fax 092-393-3833, 9 am-12 pm, 4-7 pm) has the most energetic staff that can point out the real gems of the city. They may also allow you to use their Internet. They are just behind the castle ruins.

The **APT Office** is at Piazza Santa Veneranda 2, ☎ 092-384-1727, Mon-Sat 8 am-8 pm, Sun 9 am-12 pm. **Fantasy Games**

South Coast

Internet Café (C. so A. Diaz 6/8, ☎ 092-390-6549). **Futur Service** (Via Mons Audino 4, ☎ 092-390-7311, www. futureservicesnc.com) offers rental and sale of electric vehicles, bike rental, auto, car and boat, arranges excursions, rental apartments and hotel rooms (camere d'albergo).

Sightseeing

If you're at the helpful Pro Loco office, you're in **Piazza Mokarta**, named for an Arab general who lost a war here in 1075. There's also the remains of Count Roger's **Norman Castle**. This piazza links to Corso Umberto I, the main commercial thoroughfare. The piazza is a good place to get a snack or hang out at night for the *passeggiata*. Follow Conte Ruggero parallel to *lungomare* and you'll come to the excellent ★**Cattedrale del San Salvaltore** (8 am-12 pm, 5-7 pm), which was

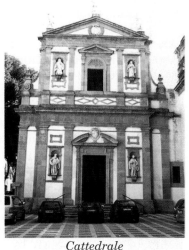

Cattedrale

originally Norman but remodelled in the late 17th century, which explains its Baroque features. This is one of the region's most beautiful cathedrals and worth coming back for if

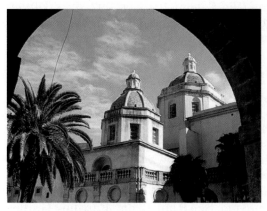

the doors don't quite open when indicated. Inside is a feast of frescoes, mosaics and stuccos on every arch and ceiling. Over the portal is a relief of Count Roger trampling a Saracen – not so politically correct today – and a

group of seven statues at the altar featuring the *Trasfigurazione*. Note the amazing carved wooden cross of 1093 too. In the square outside, Piazza Republicca, is a group of Baroque buildings. Opposite the cathedral in Via S. Salvatore is a small museum, **Museo Ornitologico** (Via San Salvatore 14, 8:30 am-12:30 pm, 2:30-6:30 pm; free), which contains a number of stuffed birds. Children might enjoy it, but there's nothing that will keep you more than a minute or two.

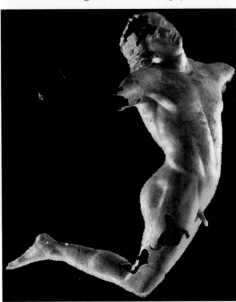
Il Satiro Danzante

Another block up is **Piazza Plebiscito** where you will find the **Collegio dei Gesuiti**, containing the **Museo Civico** (☎ 0923-940-266, closed) with two rooms of finds from the sea. In the **Museo del Satiro** (Piazza Plebiscito, ☎ 0923-933-917, 9 am-1:30 pm, 3-7 pm, €2), opposite, is the bronze statue that was found by fishermen in 1998 on Captain Franceso Adragna's boat. The statue has almost become the symbol of Mazara and is named *Il Satiro Danzante*.

To the northwest is the Casbah quarter where Arab descendants have returned with authentic restaurants and fine carpet shops, including **Amal** (Via Pescatori 10, ☎/fax 092-394-7709, 092-393-2568, 339-379-8226, www.amalsperanza.it, 9 am-1 pm, 4-7:30 pm). There is a fine selection of Tunisian carpets here and upstairs you can see women working on them.

Wind your way through to the port near Piazza Regina and you'll find Mazara's best *gelati* (see *Where to Eat*). **Roman mosaics** are visible by the **Chiesa San Nicolo Regale** from a Roman villa. The port is a busy place interesting to watch.

Walk around the corner and stroll down *lungomare* for fine seafood dining. The restaurants in this area contain parts of the original city walls inside their doors.

Something else worth checking out while you are here is the **vuccunetto**, an Arab sweet. Originally the sweet was given out by the Chiesa di San Michele as a way of enticing people to return. It's now become a specialty. You can find it at **Bar Garden** (Via Garibaldi) and **Bar Proffiterrol** (Corso Vittorio Veneto 77, ☎ 0923-939-083).

Where to Stay

Camping

 Sporting Club Camping (Localita Bocca Arena, ☎ 0923-947-230, www.sportingclub.village.com, €) is south of Mazara at the bridge.

B&Bs

Il Molo (Via Molo C. te Caito 55, ☎ 092-367-0063, €€), portside, is a good place to stay the night if you have a morning ferry. It's completely clean and comfortable and would be prime if it were not for the noisy balcony rooms and the slightly nauseating smell of boat fuel. The ticket office downstairs is run by the same people. **Sant Veneranda B&B** (Via M. Audino 4, ☎ 092-394-2106, nucciasignorello@ santaveneranda.it, €€) has just two rooms.

Stella di Mare (Via Mons A Caputo 5, Contrada Lozano 292, ☎ 092-394-6465, €€) has three rooms sharing one bathroom. Breakfast included.

La Casa al Sole B&B (Via Lorenzo Viani 2, ☎ 092-390-9664, www.lacasaalsole.com, €€-€€€) is slightly more expensive but with similar services.

Hotels

Ruggero II Hotel (Via Montevideo 20, ☎ 092-394-4643, www.ruggeroii.com, €€€€).

Kempinski Giardino di Costanza Resort & Spa (Via Salemi km. 7.100, ☎ 092-390-7763, www.kempinski-sicily. com, €€€i) is outside of town with the usual flashy resort features.

Greta Hotel (Via G Bessarione, ☎ 092-365-3889, www. gretahotel.it €€€-€€€€).

Hopps Hotel (Via G Hopps 29, ☎ 0923-946-133, www. hoppshotel.it, €€€)

Where to Eat
Bars & Cafés

 Gran Caffe (Piazza Makarta) has tables in the square and a good view of the castle, the fountains and the sea. The best gelati in Mazara is **Diademo** (Piazza Regina, 8 am-2 am, closed Thurs) near the port. They've been serving ice cream since 1943. They also have crêpes and granita. **Il Ghiottone** (36 Corso Umberto 1, €) is certainly not known for their quick service despite their claim to be *fast* food, but you can get decent hamburgers and fries. **Tunisino** (Via S. Bartolomeo), a take-out place, is like a hole in the wall, but very good. **Bar Garden** (Via Garibaldi) is the best spot for sweets.

Restaurants

Bars, cafés, restaurants and even discotecas line the full length of Via Lungomare Mazzini.

Il Gambero (☎ 0923-932-932, closed Tues, €€) actually has a three-foot-thick wall inside that once formed part of the old defensive walls of the city built in the 17th century and destroyed in the 18th century. Next door is **Zelig Disco Pub**, popular at night for their beer on tap. **Lo Scoiattolo** (☎ 0923-946-313, closed Thurs, €€) has cheap meals with a similar menu to that of Il Gambero. **Ristorante Baby and Luna** (☎ 0923-948-622, closed Mon, €€) is a popular pizzeria serving seafood and couscous.

■ Northeast of Trapani

★★★Erice

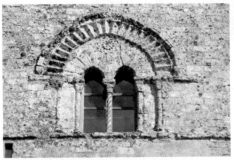
The Castello (Rosario Anselmo)

This medieval hilltop town should not be missed on any account. It's only 45 minutes northeast of Trapani by bus and you'll enjoy getting lost in the winding alleyways. The cool heights are pleasant in summer. It's

South Coast

something of a tourist trap but remains authentically medieval. Erice was settled by the Elymians, an ancient mountain people who also founded Segesta.

Getting Here

 AST buses (☎ 0923-23222) run regularly to/from Trapani (€1.81). The first bus leaves at 6:40 am. Make sure you don't miss the last one back at 8:30 pm (7:30 pm on Sunday) or you'll have to stay overnight. All buses arrive and depart from Porta Trapani. Parking is a nightmare up here in the narrow streets and rather expensive (€1/hr). You're better off coming by bus.

Information Sources

 The **tourist office** is on Viale Conte Pepoli (☎ 0923-869-388) near the bus stop.

Sightseeing

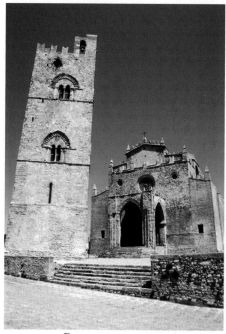

Duomo (Joanne Lane)

From Porta Trapani walk into town to the **Duomo**, to the left on Via Vito Carvini (9 am-12 pm, 3-6 pm). This is the most interesting of the Erice churches and has a lovely rose window in the façade. There's a separate bell tower with Gothic arches. **Corso Vittorio Emanuele** runs up through the center of town and is strewn with houses, shops and *pasticcerie*. At the top is the fine square, **Piazza Umberto I**, where you can get snacks and drinks. This is the heart of the little town and also where you will find the **Museo Civico**

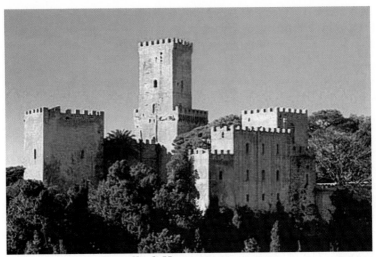

Castello di Venere (Rosario Anselmo)

Antonio Cordici (Piazza Umberto I, ☎ 0923-869-172, Mon-Thurs 8:30 am-1:30 pm, Tues, Wed and Fri 2:30-5 pm, free). They display finds from the local necropolis. To the left the road curves towards Porta Carmine. You could follow the city walls here back down to the Duomo or wander around to Porta Spada and the Quartiere Spagnolo (Spanish quarter), with a cluster of churches. Go back through Porta Carmine and left into Via Apollonis past the **Chiesa di San Giovanni Battista** on the clifftop. A path leads out to the 15th-century **Torretta Pepoli**. Back on the road, turn at the end for the Norman **Castello di Venere** (8 am-7 pm, free), built in the 12th century on the ancient temple of Aphrodite. The castle sits on a craggy outcrop with views in all directions. The panorama is stunning, to say the least. Viale Conte Pepoli drops back down to Porta Trapani.

Where to Stay

 ★**Hotel Elimo** (Via Vittorio Emanuele 73, ☎ 092-386-9377, fax 092-386-9252, www.charmerelax.com, €€€€) is the choice spot, with rooms inspired by the moustached owner's travels around the world. The common lounges contain some of his most unusual finds. The breakfast with a view to Trapani below is hard to beat. The restaurant is also first-class.

Moderno (Corso Vittorio Emanuele 63, ☎ 0923-869-300, €€€€) has a roof terrace with good views.

Ermione (Via Pineta Comunale 43, ☎ 0923-869-138, €€€) and **Villa San Giovanni** (Viale Nunzio Nasi 12,

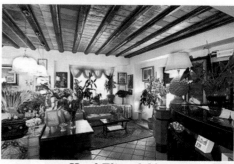

Hotel Elimo lobby

☎ 0923-869-171, €€) are the cheapest options in Erice.

Where to Eat

La Rustichella (Piazza Umberto 1 no 13, ☎ 092-869-716, €) has great takeout foods, pizza, *arancine* and pastas. Eat in the square or inside. **Enoteca Erice** (Via Guarnotti 22, ☎ 092-386-9126, www.enotecaerice.it) has typical Sicilian wines.

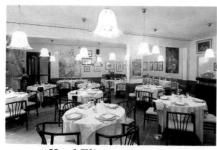

Hotel Elimo restaurant

Hotel Elimo (Via Vittorio Emanuele 73, ☎ 092-386-9377, €€€€) has fine dining on an inside terrace with a view over the Trapani Valley. **Taverna di Re Aceste** (Via R De Martini, closed Wed and Sun, €€) has decent meals at a good price. **La Pentolaccia** (Via G F Guarnotti 17, ☎ 0923-869-099, closed Tues, €€-€€€) is a popular restaurant in an old monastery.

Bonagia

Bonagia, on the coast below Erice, is a pleasant day-trip or an alternative to staying in busy Trapani. The pleasant town has a number of restaurants and a nice harbor. And there is the splendid hotel, **Tonnara di Bonagia** (Piazza Tonnara 1, Bonagia, Valderice Mare, ☎ 092-343-1111, €€€-€€€€). It's

South Coast

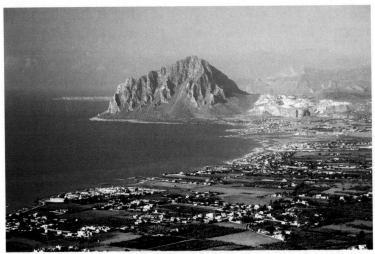

Val d'Erice *(Joanne Lane)*

now part of the Framon hotel chain but the public can visit the small museum, a shop selling tuna products and dine in the wonderful restaurant or bar. The museum is worth popping into. Steps up lead to an exhibit explaining how tuna were brought into the *tonnara* and killed using the method known as La Mattanza – basically by forming a trap with boats and nets, then slaughtering the tuna. Apartments, bed and breakfast and hotel suites are available in the hotel.

★★★San Vito Lo Capo

This small seaside town has one of Sicily's best beaches – a beautiful stretch of white sand beneath a rocky promontory. The bougainvillea-draped streets bustle with sun-worshippers in the summer months but it's quiet at other times of the year. San Vito is a symbol of the integration and mix of culture. This town was the sanctuary of San Vito, containing relics of Phoenician culture; there are also Arab and Norman objects and influences in the **Museo del Mare** and the **Couscous Festival** in August.

There's really only one strip, **Via Savoia**, running at right angles down to the beach with a few side-streets. Most are bustling with restaurants and hotels. There are only a few sights other than the beach but the northern access to the Parco dello Zingaro is just 12 km south.

Getting Here & Getting Around

 The road to San Vito Lo Capo is very scenic, especially the last stretch along the coastline. You could also bike or walk here from Scopello (see *Adventures* in that section). **AST buses** (☎ 0923-23222) arrive from Trapani's bus terminal (13 times daily, €3.91) and if you start early you could make it part of a day-trip (not including the Parco dello Zingaro). **Russo** (☎ 0924-31064) runs to Palermo twice daily and Castellamare five times daily.

It's 12 km to the Parco dello Zingaro and there are no buses. You can get a taxi (☎ 328-562-6098, 334-102-1801) which shouldn't cost too much if you split it among several people. Expect to pay about €13-€15 each way. You could also rent bikes on the *lungomare* to get there. See *Adventures on Wheels* for details.

San Vito Transfert (☎ 368-738-1189, 347-338-8608, www. sanvitotransfert.it) has daily excursions to the Riserva Naturale dello Zingaro Monday to Friday, departing at 9 am and 10 am from Piazza Marinella. The bus returns at 5 and 6 pm (€7.50). They also have trips to Erice and Segesta (€25, minimum four people), Aeroporto Falcone Borsellino (€20, minimum three people) and Aeroporto Birgi (€20, minimum three people).

Fishing and boat excursions can be organized at the tourist office. **Nautilus** (☎ 347-576-8010, €8) has a four-hour cruise to Zingaro and Scopello that runs twice daily. **Leonardo da Vinci** (☎ 333-323-7900) has a three-hour trip to Zingaro and Scopello for swimming in July and August. They depart from the port at 2:45 and return at 5:45 pm on Monday and Wednesday-Friday (€12). They sometimes run a daily ferry service from San Vito to Zingaro. See the tourist office for schedules.

The **Intrepido** mini-cruiser (☎ 339-620-8202, 339-792-3744) departs for the Egadi Islands at 9 am and returns at 6:30 pm (€35).

Small groups of up to 10 persons can go with **Escursioni Trekking** at 9 am (returns 1:30 pm) and 2:30 pm (returns 6:30 pm) to the Tonnara del Secco, Lago di Venere and Zingaro for a swim. Go down to the port or ask at the tourist office for information (€20).

Information Sources

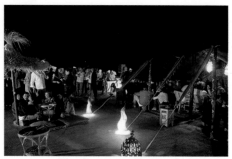

i The **APT Ufficio di Informazione** (Via Savoia 61, ☎ 0923-974-300, Thurs and Sat-Sun 8:30 am-1:30 pm or 9:30 am-1 pm, 5:30-5 pm, to 11 pm every day in summer). The **Pro Loco** (Via A Veneza 12 off V Garrico, ☎ 092-397-2464, closed Mon) lies almost directly behind the tourist office. The office is open for just one hour every day with a schedule that changes every two weeks.

A good website for tourist information is www.sanvitoweb. com.

Events

There's the famous **Couscous Festival** celebrated every August in San Vito (www.couscousfest.it).

Sightseeing

The fortress-like 13th-century **Chiesa di San Vito**, halfway down Via Savoia in Piazza Santuario, is

The Couscous Festival

dedicated to the Christian martyr San Vito. At the back is the

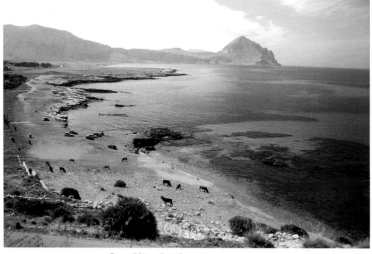

San Vito Lo Capo (Joanne Lane)

South Coast

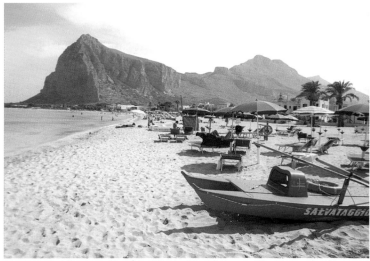

Beach at San Vito (Joanne Lane)

Museo del Mare (Piazza Santuario, ☎ 092-397-2327, www. sanviroitalia.it, 10 am-12 pm, 6-10 pm, €1), where San Vito lived, according to tradition. It contains religious objects like candlesticks, chalices, statues and sacramental robes. There are also *amphore* and ceramics from the sea, an old anchor and a canon. Go up to the top for a panoramic view from the terrace.

An easy walk could take you to the point of **Capo San Vito** itself, which is adorned by a lighthouse (closed). The harbor is generally an interesting place, with fishing boats, net mending and dogs playing.

The **Tonnara del Secco** (where tuna fish processing once took place) is two km out of town towards the Parco dello Zingaro on a flat walkable (or cyclable) road. It's in a rather secluded spot on the coast so you may not wish to come alone. It's a beautiful site, although cows have made their home in the outsheds, which creates a bit of a mess.

Adventures
On Water

 See *Getting Around* for details on itineraries you can undertake by water. **Ecodiving** operates out of the port in summer (☎ 328-142-6860, www. ecodivingservice.it).

On Wheels

 Bikes are available for rent from **Cico Camizzello** in front of Hotel Mira Spiaggia (Lungomare 6) from mid-June to mid-September for €4/hr or €6/hr (two-seater). These are really just town cruisers but you could make it out to the *tonnara* – a flat two km. Go to **Hotel Saolanto** on Via Lungomare (☎ 388-061-2352, 339-819-0816) for mountainbikes for €1.50/hr, €4/day or €15/week. To get the mountainbikes out of season you'll have to ask nicely.

Where to Stay

Camping

 ★**Camping el Bahira** (☎ 0923-972-477, €) is four km south of town on the dramatic coast at Contrada Macari. It has the most fantastic location; there are caves to explore and good snorkeling. It's also fairly rural and you could wake up to find cows with tinkling bells surrounding your camper or tent. Open only April to September for good reason. It's an exposed spot and would not be pleasant in winter. If you don't have a car, get the bus to drop you off here first.

Camping La Fata (Via P. Matarella, ☎ 0923-972-133) is in town near the bus stop. **International Camping Soleado** (Via del Secco 40, ☎ 0923-972-166, €). **Camping Village La Pineta** (Via del Secco 88, ☎ 0923-972-818, www.campinglapineta.it).

B&Bs & Rooms

Ai Dammusi B&B (Via Savoia 83, ☎ 092-362-1494, www.aidammusisanvito.it, €€€-€€€€) is close to the beach in the heart of town on the main street and handy to everything. The elegant rooms and structure are modelled after a *dammuso* (Arab house), with wrought iron bedsteads and rich rugs.

L'Agave (Via Nino Bixio 35, ☎ 092-362-1088, 328-084-8326, www.lagave.net, €€€) rents rooms with access to a fridge and allows free bike access.

Vittoria Vacanze (Via Regina Margherita 52, ☎ 092-397-4100, ☎/fax 092-397-4033, www.vittoriavacanze.com) has a variety of apartments in different places around town, some right on the beach.

Hotels

Hotel Capo San Vito (Via S Vito, ☎ 0923-972-284, www.caposanvito.it, €€€€) is right on the beach but a little shabby-looking for the price.

Miraspiaggia (Lungomare 6, ☎ 0923-972-355, www.miraspiaggia.it, €€€-€€€€) also has a seaside location.

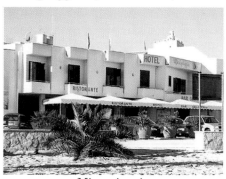

Miraspiaggia

Egitarso (Lungomare 54, ☎ 0923-972-111, www.hotelegitarso.it, €€€-€€€€), a little farther out, is cheaper. **Vento del Sud Hotel** (Via Duca Degli Abruzzi 157, ☎/fax 092-362-1450, www.hotelventodelsud.it) is about 400 yards back from the beach. The rooms are Moroccan-styled, with Islamic designs, ceramics and bright colors.

Hotel Iride (Via del Secco Villaggio Azzurro, ☎ 092-362-1414, fax 092-397-4534, www.iride-hotel.com) has funky rooms with intense colors that the owner will match according to your personality! Prices include breakfast on the veranda. They have a great deckchair area with views to the sea.

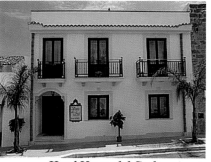

Hotel Vento del Sud

Abbadia (Via Savoia 263, ☎ 092-397-4010, fax 092-362-1771, hotelabbadia@libero.it, €€€€) is centrally located in a fairly plain building. Prices drop outside of August.

Helios Hotel (Via Savoia 245, ☎ 092-397-4418, fax 092-362-1785, www.sanvitohelioshotel.it, €€€€) has its own private stretch of sand and a shuttle to the beach. Typical hotel-style rooms. Prices drop after August.

Araba Fenice Hotel (Via Nino Bixio 16, ☎ 092-397-4154, fax 092-362-1326, hotelarabfenice@libero.it) has air-conditioned rooms with bathroom, TV, phone, and frigobar.

Where to Eat

 Via Savoia has a long line of restaurants and most set menus are €13, or you can choose from plates costing about €8-€10. Menus are shown out in the street so you can pick and choose.

★**Tha'am Ristorante** (Via Duca degli Abruzzi 32, ☎ 092-397-2836, €€) is a North African restaurant serving typical local and Arab dishes. The design is definitely north African with elegant curtains and ceramics.

La Sirenetta (Via Savoia, corner of Via Faro) overlooks the beach and port. Good ice cream choices and a shaded terrace to enjoy the views.

Ristorante Il Giardino (Via Mulin 18/20, ang. Via Savoia, ☎ 092-397-4444, €€), near the Municipio, serves a good couscous with local wines.

Dal Cozzaro (Via Savoia 15, ☎ 092-397-2777, €€) has Tunisian fare and is a notable part of the Couscous Festival. The menu even includes a dessert couscous.

★★★Scopello

Tiny Scopello is a delightful town, which is little more than a paved square and fountain with ducks. But it would be a shame to miss it. In the center of the square sits the village's 18th-century *baglio* (manor house) in which there are several restaurants, bars and tourist shops. Outside of the tourist season you get the feeling small-time traditional village life prevails. Prices drop considerably then.

Getting Here & Getting Around

 There are four services via **Tarantola** buses (info@tarantolabus.it) from Castellamare (with connections to Segesta and Caltafimi).

Four buses run down to the reserve entrance every day from the *baglio* at 9:10 am, 1:30, 3:10 and 7 pm.

Information Sources

 Cetaria Diving Center (Via Marco Polo 3, ☎ 092-454-1177, 368-386-4808, www.cetaria.com) was to become an official tourist office at the time of writing. They already provide a lot of services – diving, boat tours of Zingaro, bike rental and horseback riding.

Sightseeing

You'll soon exhaust the sites in Scopello. But there is a delightfully located ★★★*tonnara* (former tuna processing plant) just out of town. The old Tonnara di Scopello ceased operations in the 1980s. It is still privately owned and the gate is always open (free) for visitors to wander around and admire the abandoned buildings, lines of rusting anchors and ruined old watchtowers. A sign at the entrance requests that you respect the site's tranquility (no radios, dogs, beach umbrellas).

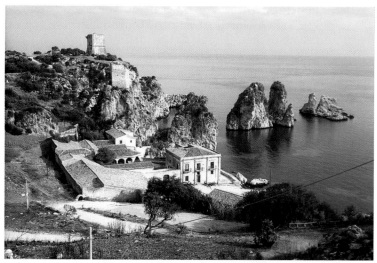

Tonnara di Scopello (Joanne Lane)

Please do so, as the owners live on the premises and have thought about removing access if there are continued disturbances. You can swim in the beautiful water and even stay down here (see *Where to Stay*). In summer it can be busy; if you want to avoid the crowds the best time is 6 am-7 am.

Adventures

On Foot

★★★**Parco dello Zingaro**. The southern entrance to the reserve (October-March 8 am-4 pm, April-September 7 am-9 pm, www.riservazingaro.it, €3) is two km from Scopello. The other entrance is 12 km from San Vito Lo Capo and has more easily accessible sights like Torre Uzzo and Tonnarella dell'Uzzo, but the beaches are good from both sides and access by bus is better from Scopello. If you're planning to walk all the way through, it won't matter where you start.

The stretch of seven km now forming Parco dello Zingaro is one of the most picturesque Sicilian coastlines. It was only made a reserve in 1980 after protests against a planned road through the area. There's a network of paths and six beaches. You'll find excellent swimming, rich plant life and at least 40 different bird species. No motorized vehicles are allowed inside; it's walking only. The tourist hut at the entrance provides maps and details of the routes through the reserve. At the entrance is a bar where you can get a few refreshments and souvenirs. Don't rely on it to be open. Coastal paths are

well signed but there are no refreshments available, so come well prepared. Spring is one of the best seasons, when orchids and other flowers are in full bloom.

Under Water

 C e t a r i a Diving Center (Via Marco Polo 3, ☎ 092-454-1177, 368-386-4808, www.cetaria. com) organizes boat excursions into the Zingaro Reserve, stopping at beaches that can only be reached by sea for swimming and snorkeling. Masks and fins are provided.

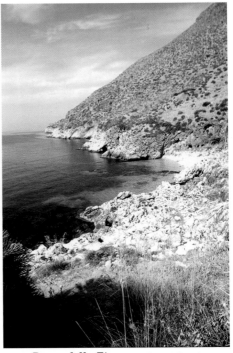

On Horseback

Parco dello Zingaro (Joanne Lane)

 Contact the **Cetaria Diving Center** (see above) to arrange a ride with the Ranch Contra da Terre Nuovo (☎ 338-777-5709). It's hard to find the ranch and best to set up the ride in advance from town.

On Wheels (bike or car)

★★Castello di Baida (seven km)

 Rent a mountain bike from **Cetaria Diving Center** (see above) for €8/€12 (half/full day) and leave Scopello heading back towards Castellammare. About one km out of town is a turn to Castello di Baida before a small market with a fruit shop and trattoria. The initial five km is a continual climb up a cliff face above the sea. At the top you drop down for about two km with views of rural fields and cows. You'll see a small clump of houses at the end of a short rise. This is the old Baida. It once had four towers and was the residence of the Barrone (Baron) of Baida. Today three families live inside. Have a poke around and you'll probably run

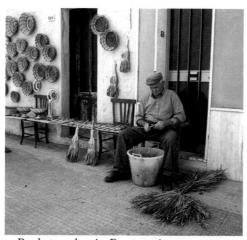

Basket-maker in Purgatorio (Joanne Lane)

into the friendly Signora Enza or her son Nino. Actually, it's more likely their little dog Nikita will come out first. The Signora speaks only Italian but Nino can manage some German. The Signora can provide accommodation (☎ 339-263-1724, 092-438-127) in summer. Bed and breakfast is €20. They can also provide *casalinga* meals or you can eat at the **Ristorante Baida** (☎ 092-433-439) where Nino works. The Signora makes some fantastic pesto, caponata, dried tomatoes and melanzane dishes. She also invented a sauce that is yet to be named. Ask for the *pesto di baida* or *pesto rosso* with pine nuts, almonds, basil, chilli pepper, dried tomatoes and nuts (€5). Delicious.

If you're here on July 26 the small community celebrates the **Festa della Madonna di S. Anna**. There's a procession and fireworks, with a communal dinner at the Baida.

If you want to try a longer cycle or drive, the road from Baida to San Vito is very beautiful but very bad. Outside the Baida, go straight ahead up a rough road along the ridge above the sea. The views are fantastic and it's completely deserted – you'll pass only an occasional herd of cows. Don't expect to see anyone else. The road eventually becomes very bad tarmac and is in fact officially closed. You eventually join the *strada* for Purgatorio and San Vito Lo Capo. Stop at the school in Purgatorio and there should be an elderly man out making grass baskets. If you've come on your bike, the only way back to Scopello is the way you came.

Where to Stay

To stay at the ★**Tonnara di Scopello** (☎ 091-304-481, 338-691-9133, 328-675-9959, 347-074-5089, 347-324-3789, www.tonnaradiscopello.com) call ahead to book basic apartments from €35pp/night. Rooms have kitchens. The *tonnara* actually has 37 owners. Three people live here from April-November each year.

Camping Lu Baruni (Localita Barone 27, ☎ 0924-39133, www.campinglubaruni.it) is open March-September. It's a little farther from town, near the Taraltola bus stop.

Camping Baia di Guidaloca (☎ 0924-541-262, closed in winter, €) is right near Cala Bianca in front of the Russo bus stop, where you can catch a bus to the reserve. Food is available at the beach front. It's about one-two km from Scopello.

★**Pensione Tranchina** (Via A. Diaz 7, ☎ 0924-541-099, €€-€€€) is the choice location in Scopello, run by a friendly multilingual couple. Their premises featured in *Salute*, a cook book about Sicily, so you know you'll be fed well. Make sure you dine there at least once. For €19-€23 you can be stuffed with pasta, fish, salad and dessert. They make their own oil, jams, marmalades (orange and grapefruit) and are open all year.

La Tavernetta (Via A Diaz 3, ☎/fax 092-454-1129, albergolatavernetta@libero.it, €€€) is next door. **Maria B&B** (Piazza Nettuno 3, ☎ 092-454-1216, www.bedandbreakfastmaria.com) is opposite the fountain and family-run.

Where to Eat

Pensione Tranchina (Via A. Diaz 7, ☎ 0924-541-099, €€) has wonderful meals but they are for guests only.

La Terrazza (Via Marco Polo 5, ☎ 092-454-1198, closed Tues, €€€) is named for its great view over the sea. It's open all year and they rent rooms too. Try *panzerotti agli scampi* – pasta and seafood with cream on top.

La Tavernetta (Via A Diaz 3, ☎/fax 092-454-1129, albergolatavernetta@libero.it, €€€) has a restaurant with meals for about €30.

Inside the *baglio* (manor house) you have the choice of **Il Baglio** (Baglio Isonzo 4, ☎ 092-454-1200, 368-665-53), serving pizza, the **Spagghetiti Fior di Mare** (closed Mon) or **Bar Nettuno** (☎ 0924-541090, open late March-November) for snacks and drinks. In winter they are open on weekends only.

La Craparia in the square serves *pane zatu*, a special local bread with oil, oregano and sardines. They also have delicious cheese, sun-dried tomatoes and *melanzane* (eggplant). A gruff signora from a bakery signposted down a small lane beyond the square also sells the same bread, where it probably originates. To find it, walk past Pensione Tranchina towards the reserve.

Castellammare del Golfo

This pretty little town nestles around a castle and small port and is entirely enclosed by surrounding hills. It once had one of the worst reputations in Sicily for Mafia violence, although that's hard to believe today, given the quietness of the quaint harbor.

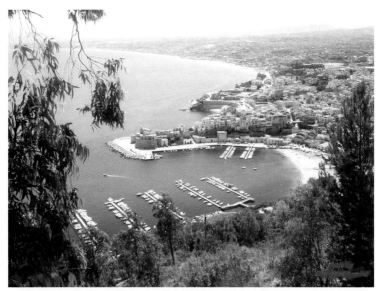

Castellamare del Golfo (Giuseppe Pitarrese)

Getting Here

There's a train station four km east of town and a shuttle bus meets most of the arrivals to take you to Castellammare. Regular buses also run to Scopello (four daily) and to San Vito Lo Capo, Palermo, Trapani, Alcamo and Calatafimi/Segesta. The only buses on Sunday go to Palermo. **AST** (☎ 0923-23222) and **RUSSO** (☎ 0924-31364) leave from Trapani to Castellammare five times daily. There are connections from here to Scopello four times daily.

Getting Around

Ecomar (☎ 338-976-8201, www.charterboats-ecomar.it) rents boats down at the port from June-September. In low season they are only €50/€70 for a half/full day but during peak season you'll pay €90/€140.

Motonave Leonardo Da Vinci (Via G. Medici 75, ☎ 0924-34222, www.motonavaleonardodavinci.com) offers excursions by boat. There are daily departures at 8:15, 9:30 and 10:40 am for San Vito Lo Capo, Zingaro and Faraglioni di Scopello, returning at 4:15, 6 and 7 pm. With lunch, it's €23.

Sightseeing

The 17th-century **Aragonese castle** sits on the walls above the harbor, nestled into a rocky promontory. Inside are two museums and the tourist office. The **Museo Annalisa Buccellato** (Piazza Castello, ☎ 0924-33533, Tues-Sat 9 am-

1 pm, 4-8 pm, free) contains old typewriters, farming utensils, water wheels, books and newspapers. It was established by the parents of Annalisa after she died suddenly. The **Museo dell'Aqua e dei Mulini ad Aqua** explains the Arab mills and irrigation systems in the Mediterranean basin. Upstairs is a tourist office (Mon-Fri 9 am-1 pm, Tues and Thurs, 3:30-7:30 pm). Ask to have a look around. There's a rather spectacular staircase that takes you up to the roof where you can get good views. There's also a model of the *tonnara* at Scopello and pictures of towers and lighthouses.

The other point of interest in town is the yellow-fronted 18th-century **Chiesa Matrice** off Via G Puccini, down an alley to your left on the way back from the castle.

The ★★**port** below the *castello* is gorgeous. Wooden boats are parked among the cars, while nets lie out to dry and to be mended. In summer, boat excursions leave from here to the Parco dello Zingaro.

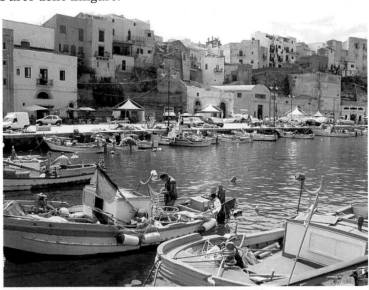

Port of Castellamare del Golfo

Where to Stay

The best accommodation is in the port.

Hotel Al Madarig (Piazza Petrolo 7, ☎ 0924-33533, www.almadarig.com, €€€€) is right on the edge of a wide piazza with sea views. The name comes from the Arab name for Castellamare.

Hotel La Piazzetta (Piazza Europa 8, ☎ 0924-35550, www. lapiazzettahotel.com, €€€-€€€€) is in the upper part of town

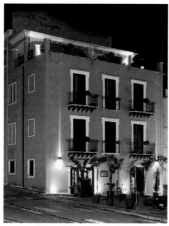

Hotel La Piazzetta

☎ 0924-30685, www.
bedrais.it, €€€) and
Camping Nausicaa
(Forgia Plaia, ☎ 0924-
33030, www.nausicaa-
camping.it €) are the
cheapest options. The
campground is two km
from the train station and
about 500 yards from town.

Where to Eat

 As with lodging. the
best place for din-
ing is in the port.
La Campana (Via Macello
12, ☎ 0924-32123, closed
Wed €€) doesn't have a
portside location but is an
economic choice.
Hotel Cetarium (Via Don
Leonardo Zangara, ☎ 0924-
533-401, www.

away from the sea, about a
block back. It's the large yellow
building in Piazza Europa.
Hotel Cetarium (Via Don Leonardo Zangara, 45, ☎ 0924-
533-401, www.hotelcetarium.
it, €€€€) is superbly located
down in the port. Beautiful
rooms and a fantastic restaurant.
Hotel Cala Marina (Via Don
Leonardo Zangara 1, ☎ 0924-
531-841, www.hotelcala-
marina.it, €€€€) is on the
beach front to the right of the
port. They can arrange scuba
diving excursions in the area.
Rais B&B (Via Tobruk 2,

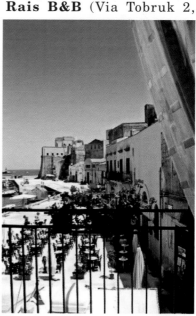

View from balcony, Hotel Cetarium

hotelcetarium.it, €€€€) has a prime location. It is also a res-
taurant with a modern menu featuring couscous with fish and
Sicilian wines.
Vogue Bar (Via Don Leonardo Zangara) is a popular, hip spot
open almost 24 hours in summer. Great ice cream and
Internet access. Next door is **La Cambusa** (Cala Marina 6,

☎ 0924-30155, €€), which displays the fish outside its doors.
€8 for pasta plates.
Ristorante L'Approdo (Lungomare, under the castle,
☎ 091-31525, €€€) serves a fine *spaghetti con uova di pesce*.

Calatafimi/Segesta

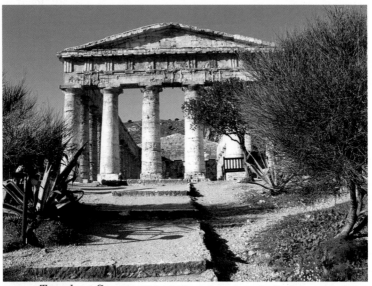

Temple at Segesta (Galen R Frysinger, www.galenfrysinger.com)

Segesta lies 15 km south of Castellamare del Golfo and the ruins of the ancient city are among the best in Sicily. The ancient Elymians (who also founded Erice and Entella) were renowned for their choice of sites. This is one of the island's most impressive. The city eventually came under Hellenic influence and sought an alliance with Athens in 426 BC. The temple dates from this time but was never finished, as Segesta was alwasy warring with Selinus and a new dispute broke out with them in 416 BC.

Getting Here

If you are driving on the Palermo-Trapani motorway you will see Segesta from the strada. If you're coming by public transport you can get here via AST buses from Trapani and Palermo. Trains from Trapani to Segesta Tempio station is only half a mile from the entrance to the ruins of the ancient city of Segesta.

Sightseeing

The site of ★★**Segesta** (☎ 092-495-5841, 9 am-6 pm, €6) contains the Doric temple itself, started in 424 BC on a low hill near the café and car park. From a distance it looks great, but as you get closer you can see the repair work. The 36 regular stone columns still stand up. It was never completed so it never had a roof. Beyond the main entrance the teatro (theater) is a 1½-km walk of 25 minutes. There is a bus to the site every half-hour (€1.20). This is the most intact of the city's ruins and concerts are held here during the summer months. Beyond are excavations of a mosque and Arab-style houses. There are also remains of a late medieval church.

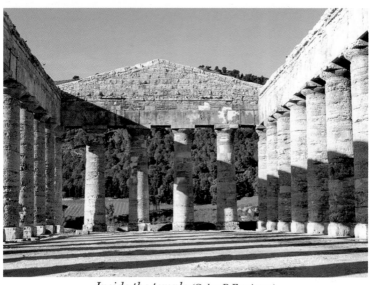

Inside the temple (Galen R Frysinger)

Language

As detailed earlier, more than 70% of locals speak Sicilian among themselves and may not be fluent in Italian. If they do speak Italian you may notice they prefer to be addressed in the formal third person (*lei* instead of *tu*). Another thing to remember is that you should not use the informal greeting *ciao* when you meet strangers. It's far more polite to use *buongiorno* or *buona sera*, depending on the time of day, to greet them and then *arriverdeci* or *arriverderla* on departure.

Italian has masculine and feminine forms, usually ending in 'o' and 'a' respectively. In this guide we have used both forms separating them with a slash and listing the masculine form first. We would advise you get hold of an Italian phrasebook for more detail on the Italian language. Sicilians are friendly and you'll find hand signals and other forms of international communication go a long way, as do your efforts to use as many local words as you can. *Buona fortuna!*

Pronunciation

Sicilians tend to pronounce vowels more openly than in mainland Italy and do not roll their r's as much, so you may actually find it more comprehensible, even if your command of Italian is limited.

Vowels

Vowels are more clipped than in English and getting these right will help greatly.

a   as in art, eg. caro (dear), amico/a (m/f) (friend)

e   as in tell, eg. mettere (to put)

i   as in inn, eg. inizio (start)

o   as in dot, eg. donna (woman), as in port, eg dormire (to sleep)

u   as the oo in book, eg. puro (pure)

Consonants

Italian consonants are not pronounced that differently from their English counterparts, but there are rules with some of them.

c   as k before a, o and u; as ch in choose before e and i

ch   hard k sound

g   like the g in get before a, o and u; like the j in job before e and i

gh   hard, as in get

gli   as the lli in million

gn   as the ny canyon

h   always silent

r   a rolled rr sound using the tongue

sc   as the sh in sheep before e and i; as sk before h, a, o and u

sch   hard sk sound

z   as the ts in lights, except at the beginning of a word, when it's like the ds in beds

If ci, gi and sci are followed by a, o or u, the i is not pronounced unless the accent falls on the i. For example the name Giovanni is pronounced joh'vahn'nee'.

Word Stress

Double consonants are pronounced as longer, forceful sounds and stress on a word most often falls on the second-to-last syllable, eg. spa-ghet-ti. If you see an accent over a word the stress is on that syllable eg cit-tà (city).

Greetings

Hello (morning) . . . . Buongiorno
Hello (evening) . . . . Buonasera
. . . . Ciao (informal)
Goodbye . . . . Arriverdeci
. . . . Ciao (informal)
Yes . . . . Si
No . . . . No
Please . . . . Per favor/per piacere
Thank you . . . . Grazie
That's fine . . . . Va bene/prego
I'm fine . . . . Bene
Excuse me . . . . Mi scusi/permesso, Scusami (informal)
Sorry (forgive me) . . . . Mi scusi/mi perdoni

Conversation

What's your name . . . . Come ti chiama?/Come ti chiami? (inf.)
My name is... . . . . Mi chiamo ...
Where are you from? . . . . Di dov'è?/Dal dov'è sei?/Dal dov'è viene?
I'm from... . . . . Sono di... (Stati Uniti, Inghilterra)
How old are you? . . . . Quanti anni ha/hai? (inf.)
I'm ... years old . . . . Ho ... anni
I (don't) like... . . . . (Non) mi piace...
Just a minute . . . . Un momento/un attimo
How are you? . . . . Come stai (inf.)/sta?
I'm here on vacation . . . . Sono qui in vacanza
I live in ... . Abito a ...

Asking for Help

I (don't understand) . . . . Non capisco
Please write it down . . . . Può scriverlo, per favor?
Can you show me (on the map) . . . . Può mostrarmelo (sulla carta/piana)?
Do you speak English? . . . . Parla inglese?
Does anyone here speak English? . . . . . C'è qualcuno che parla inglese?
How do you say ... in Italian . . . . Come si dice ...in italiano?
What does ... mean? . . . . Che vuole dire ....?
What time is it? . . . . Che ora è?/che ore sono?
Che cos'è? . . . . What is it?
Why? . . . . Perchè?
What time does it open? . . . . A che ora apre?
What time does it close? . . . . A che ora chiude?

Documentation

Name . . . . nome
Surname . . . . cognome
Mr . . . . signor
Mrs . . . . signora
Miss . . . . signorina
Nationality . . . . nazionalità
Date of birth . . . . data de nascita
Place of birth . . . . luogo de nascita
Sex (gender) . . . . sesso
Passport . . . . passaporto

Visa . . . . visto

Getting Around

What time does ... leave/arrive? . . . . A che ora ... parte/arriva?
  the aeroplane . . . . l'aereo/aeroplano
  the boat . . . . la barca
  the (city) bus . . . . l'autobus
  the (intercity) bus . . . . il pullman/corriere
  the train . . . . il treno
ferry . . . . traghetto
ship . . . . nave
hydrofoil . . . . aliscafo
I'd like a ... ticket . . . . Vorrei un biglietto ...
one-way . . . . di solo andata
round-trip . . . . di andata e ritorno
1st class. . . . . prima classe
2nd class . . . . seconda classe
The train has been canceled . . . . Il treno è soppresso
/ delayed. . . . . / in ritardo
How long does it take?. . . . . Quanto ci vuole?
What number bus is it to? . . . . Che numero di autobus per... ?
Next stop please. . . . . La prossima fermata per favore
the first. . . . . il primo
the last . . . . l'ultimo
platform number . . . . binario numero
bus station . . . . auto stazione
train station. stazione ferroviaria
ferry terminal . . . . stazione marittima
port . . . . porto
ticket office . . . . biglietteria
timetable . . . . orario
taxi . . . . taxi
on foot . . . . a piedi
hitchhiking . . . . autostop
parking . . . . parcheggio
I'd like to rent ... . Vorrei noleggiare ...
a bicycle . . . . una bicicletta
a boat . . . . una barca
a car . . . . una macchina
a motorcycle . . . . una motocicletta

Directions
Where is ...? . . . . Dov'è...?
Where are ... ? . . . . Dove'è sono ... ?
Can you tell me when to get off? . . . . . Può dirmi quando devo scendere?
Go straight ahead . . . . Si va sempre diritto
. . . . Vai sempre diritto (inf).
How far is it?. . . . . Quanto lontano è?
Turn left . . . . Gira a sinistra
Turn right . . . . Gira a destra
  at the next corner . . . . al prossimo angolo
  at the traffic lights . . . . al semaforo
  behind . . . . dietro
  in front of. . . . . divanti
  far . . . . lontano
  near . . . . vicino
opposite. . . . . di fronte a

Signs
entrance/exit . . . . entrata/uscita

```
free entrance . . . . . . . . . . . . . . . . . . . . . . . . . . ingresso libero
toilets . . . . . . . . . . . . . . . . . . . . . . wc/gabinetto/bagno
arrivals/departures . . . . . . . . . . . . . . . . . . . . arrive/partenze
open/closed . . . . . . . . . . . . . . . . . . . . . . . . . aperto/chiuso
pull/push . . . . . . . . . . . . . . . . . . . . . . . . . tirare/spingere
closed for holidays . . . . . . . . . . . . . . . . . . . chiuso per ferie
closed for restoration . . . . . . . . . . . . . . . . . chiuso per restauro
drinking water . . . . . . . . . . . . . . . . . . . . . . . acqua potabile
to let . . . . . . . . . . . . . . . . . . . . . . . . . . . . . . . . affitasi
danger . . . . . . . . . . . . . . . . . . . . . . . . . . . . . . . pericolo
do not touch . . . . . . . . . . . . . . . . . . . . . . . . non toccare
no smoking . . . . . . . . . . . . . . . . . . . . . . . . . vietato fumare
one way . . . . . . . . . . . . . . . . . . . . . . . . . . . . senso unico
no entry . . . . . . . . . . . . . . . . . . . . . . . . . . . . senso vietato
slow down . . . . . . . . . . . . . . . . . . . . . . . . . . . rallentare
no through road . . . . . . . . . . . . . . . . . . . . vietato il transito
no parking . . . . . . . . . . . . . . . . . . . . . . . . . diveto di sosta
```

Town Terminology

```
I'm looking for ... . . . . . . . . . . . . . . . . . . . . . . . Cerco ...
I want to go to ... . . . . . . . . . . . . . . . . . . . Voglio andare a ...
   a bank . . . . . . . . . . . . . . . . . . . . . . . . . . . . . un banco
   the church . . . . . . . . . . . . . . . . . . . . . . . . . la chiesa
   the city center . . . . . . . . . . . . . . . . . . . il centro (città)
   my hotel . . . . . . . . . . . . . . . . . . . . . . . . . mio albergo
   the market . . . . . . . . . . . . . . . . . . . . . . . . . il mercato
   the museum . . . . . . . . . . . . . . . . . . . . . . . . il museo
   the post office . . . . . . . . . . . . . . . . . . . . . . la posta
   a public toilet . . . . . . . . . . . . . . . un gabinetto/bagno pubblico
   the telephone center . . . . . . . . . . . . . . . . il centro telefonico
   the tourist office . . . . . . . . . . . l'ufficio di turismo/ d'informazione
   the station . . . . . . . . . . . . . . . . . . . . . . . la stazione
I want to change . . . . . . . . . . . . . . . . . . . Voglio cambiare ...
   money . . . . . . . . . . . . . . . . . . . . . . . . . . . . . denaro
   travelers checks . . . . . . . . . . . . . degli assegni per viaggiatori
beach . . . . . . . . . . . . . . . . . . . . . . . . . . . . la spiaggia
bridge . . . . . . . . . . . . . . . . . . . . . . . . . . . . il ponte
castle . . . . . . . . . . . . . . . . . . . . . . . . . . . . il castello
cathedral . . . . . . . . . . . . . . . . . . . . il duomo/la cattedrale
island . . . . . . . . . . . . . . . . . . . . . . . . . . . . l'isola
main square . . . . . . . . . . . . . . . . . . . . . la piazza principale
market . . . . . . . . . . . . . . . . . . . . . . . . . . . . il mercato
mosquela moschea
old city . . . . . . . . . . . . . . . . . . . . . . . . . il centro storico
palace . . . . . . . . . . . . . . . . . . . . . . . . . . . . il palazzo
ruins . . . . . . . . . . . . . . . . . . . . . . . . . . . . la rovine
sea . . . . . . . . . . . . . . . . . . . . . . . . . . . . . il mare
square . . . . . . . . . . . . . . . . . . . . . . . . . . . la piazza
tower . . . . . . . . . . . . . . . . . . . . . . . . . . . . la torre
```

Accommodation

```
I'm looking for ... . . . . . . . . . . . . . . . . . . . . . Cerco.....
   a guesthouse . . . . . . . . . . . . . . . . . . . . . una pensione
   a hotel . . . . . . . . . . . . . . . . . . . . . . . . . . un albergo
   a youth hostel . . . . . . . . . . . . . . . un ostello per la gioventù
   a campsite . . . . . . . . . . . . . . . . . . . . . . un campeggio
Where is a cheap hotel? . . . . . . . . . Dov'è un albergo che costa poco?
What is the address? . . . . . . . . . . . . . . . . . Cos'è l'indirizzo?
```

Could you write the address please?
. . . . Può scrivere l'indirizzo per favore?
Do you have any rooms available?. . . . .
. . . . Ha camere libere/C'è una camera libera?
... for one/two/three people . . . . per una persona, due/tre persone
... for one/two/three nights... . . . . per una notte, due/tre notti
I have a booking . . . . Ho una prenotazione
I would like .... Vorrei ...
a bed . . . . un letto
a single room . . . . una camera singola
a double room . . . . una camera matrimoniale
a room with two beds . . . . una camera doppia
a room with a bathroom . . . . una camera con bagno
to share a dorm . . . . un letto in dormitorio
hot/cold water . . . . acqua calda/fredda
a balcony . . . . una terrazzo
with a shower/bath . . . . con una doccia/un bagno
How much is it ...? . . . . Quanto costa ...?
per night . . . . per la notte
per person . . . . per ciascuno?
May I see it? . . . . Posso vederla?
Where is the bathroom? . . . . Dov'è il bagno?
I'm/We're leaving today . . . . Parto/Partiamo oggi
Big/small . . . . grande/piccolo/a
With/without . . . . con/senza
Vacant/occupied . . . . libero/occupato

Shopping

I'd like to buy .... Vorrei comprare ...
How much is it?. . . . . Quanto costa?
I (don't) like it . . . . (Non) Mi piace
May I look at it? . . . . Posso dare un'occhiata?
I'm just looking . . . . Sto solo guardando
It's cheap . . . . Non è caro/a
It's too expensive . . . . è troppo caro/a
I'll take it. . . . . Lo/La prendo
Do you accept ... . Accettate ...?
credit cards . . . . carte di credito
travelers checks . . . . assegni per viaggiatori?
more . . . . più
less . . . . meno
smaller . . . . più grande
cheap/expensive . . . . economico/caro
enough . . . . basta

Adventure Activities

Diving . . . . immersione
Trekking. . . . . trekking
Walk . . . . camimnare
Route. . . . . percorsi
Itinerary. . . . . itinerari
Path . . . . sentiero
Off-road . . . . Strade bianche
Bicycle . . . . Biciclette

Times & Dates

What time is it?. . . . . Che ora è?
It's (8 o'clock). . . . . Sone (le otto)
in the morning . . . . di mattina

Language

in the afternoon . . . . di pomeriggio
in the evening . . . . di sera
When? . . . . Quando?
today . . . . oggi
tomorrow . . . . domani
yesterday . . . . ieri
day after tomorrow . . . . dopodmani
now . . . . adesso
later . . . . più tardi
Monday . . . . lunedi
Tuesday . . . . martedi
Wednesday . . . . mercoledi
Thursday . . . . giovedi
Friday . . . . venerdi
Saturday . . . . sabato
Sunday . . . . domenica
January . . . . gennaio
February . . . . febbraio
March . . . . marzo
April . . . . aprile
May . . . . maggio
June . . . . giugno
July . . . . luglio
August . . . . agosto
September . . . . settembre
October . . . . ottobre
November . . . . novembre
December . . . . dicembre

Numbers

0 . . . . zero
1 . . . . uno
2 . . . . due
3 . . . . tre
4 . . . . quattro
5 . . . . cinque
6 . . . . sei
7 . . . . sette
8 . . . . otto
9 . . . . nove
10 . . . . dieci
11 . . . . undici
12 . . . . dodici
13 . . . . tredici
14 . . . . quattordici
15 . . . . quindici
16 . . . . sedici
17 . . . . diciasette
18 . . . . diciotto
19 . . . . dicianove
20 . . . . venti
21 . . . . ventuno
22 . . . . ventitre
30 . . . . trenta
40 . . . . quaranta
50 . . . . cinquanta
60 . . . . sessanta
70 . . . . settanta

80 . . . . ottanta
90 . . . . novanta
100. . . . . cento
1,000. . . . . mille
2,000. . . . . due mila

Health

I'm ill . . . . Mi sento male
It hurts here . . . . Mi fa male qui
I'm. . . . . Sono...
  asthmatic . . . . asmatico/a
  diabetic . . . . diabetico/a
  epileptic . . . . epilettico/a
I'm allergic to .... Sono allergico/a
  to antibiotics . . . . agli antibiotici
  to penicillin . . . . alla penicillina
antiseptic. . . . . antisettico
aspirin. . . . . aspirina
condoms. . . . . preservative
diarrhea. . . . . diarrea
medicine . . . . medicina
sunblock cream. . . . . crema/latte solare (per protezione)
tampons. . . . . tampons

Food

Basics
Breakfast . . . . (prima) colazione
Lunch . . . . pranzo
Dinner . . . . cena
Restaurant. . . . . ristorante
Grocery store. . . . . alimentary
What is this?. . . . . (Che) cos'è?
I'm a vegetarian. . . . . Sono vegetariano/a

Meats
Anchovies. . . . . acciughe
Lamb . . . . agnello
Lobster . . . . aragosta
Steak . . . . bistecca
Squid . . . . calamari
Rabbit . . . . coniglio
Cutlet or thin cut of meat . . . . cotoletta
Mussels . . . . cozze
Dentex (type of fish) . . . . dentice
Liver . . . . fegato
Prawns. . . . . gamberi
Crab. . . . . granchio
Beef . . . . manzo
Cod . . . . merluzzo
Oysters. . . . . ostriche
Swordfish . . . . pesce spada
Chicken . . . . pollo
Octopus . . . . polpo
Sausage . . . . salsiccia
Sardines . . . . sarde
Mackerels. . . . . gombro
Sole . . . . sogliola
Turkey . . . . tacccchino
Tuna . . . . tonno

Language

Tripe . . . . trippa
Veal. . . . . vitello
Clams. . . . . vongole

Vegetables

Asparagus. . . . . asparagi
Artichokes . . . . carciofi
Aubergines . . . . melanzane
Capers . . . . caperi
Carrots . . . . carote
Cabbage . . . . cavolo/verza
Chicory. . . . . cicoria
Mixed vegetables . . . . verdure
Mushrooms . . . . funghi
Onion . . . . cipolla
Potatoes . . . . patate
Peppers . . . . peperoni
Peas . . . . piselli
Pumpkin . . . . zucca
String beans. . . . . fagiolini
Spinach . . . . spinaci
Tomatoes . . . . pomodori
Zucchini . . . . zucchini

Fruit

Apples . . . . mele
Bananas . . . . banana
Cherries. . . . . ciliegie
Figs . . . . fiche
Grapes . . . . uva
Limone . . . . lemons
Melon . . . . melone
Oranges . . . . arance
Pears . . . . pere
Peaches . . . . pesche
Pineapple . . . . ananas
Strawberries . . . . fragole

Desserts

Cake . . . . torta
Cake with candied fruit . . . . cassata
Fruit salad . . . . macedonia
Ice cream. . . . . gelato
Trifle . . . . zuppa inglese
Fried pastry stuffed with sweet ricotta. . . . . cannolli
Ice cream, cake and candied fruit . . . . cassata

Soups

Broth . . . . brodo
Pasta in broth . . . . minestrina in brodo
Vegetable soup. . . . . minestrone
Egg in broth . . . . straciatella

Starters (antipasti)

Antipasto misto . . . . mixed cold meats and cheese
Caponata . . . . mixed aubergine, olives and tomatoes
Caprese . . . . tomato and mozzarella cheese salad
Insalata di mare. . . . . seafood salad
Insalata di riso. . . . . rice salad
Melanzane alla parmigiana
. . . . Fried eggplant in tomato sauce with parmesan
Prosciutto . . . . Ham

Pasta

Cannelloni . . . . large tubes of pasta
Fettuccine. . . . . narrow pasta ribbons
Gnocchi . . . . potato and dough dumplings
Lasagne. . . . . lasagne
Pappardelle . . . . pasta ribbons
Penne . . . . small tubular pasta
Ravioli . . . . stuffed square shaped pasta
Risotto . . . . cooked rice with sauce
Spaghetti . . . . spaghetti
Tagliatelle . . . . pasta ribbons
Tortellini . . . . small rings of pasta, stuffed

Pasta Sauces

Tomato and bacon . . . . alla matriciana
Meat sauce (Bolognese) . . . . al ragu'
Tomato and chili . . . . all' arrabbiata
Egg, bacon and black pepperalla. . . . . carbonara
Tomato and basil. . . . . napoletana
Cream, prosciutto and sometimes peas . . . . con panna
Basil, garlic and oil; often wit pine nuts. . . . . pesto
Clams, garlic and oil; sometimes with tomato . . . . alle vongole
Seafood . . . . marinara/frutti di mare

Pizzas

Olives, prosciutto, mushrooms and artichokes . . . . capricciosa
Mushrooms . . . . funghi
Oregano . . . . margherita
Anchovies. . . . . napoletana
Tomato, mozzarella and onions. . . . . pugliese
With four types of cheese . . . . quattro formaggi
Like a capricciosa, but sometimes with egg . . . . quattro stagioni

Drinks

Beer . . . . birra
Bottle . . . . bottiglia
Coffee . . . . café
Glass . . . . bottiglia
Fruit juice. . . . . succo di frutta
Hot chocolate . . . . cioccolata calda
Ice . . . . ghiaccio
Lemonade. . . . . limonata
Milk . . . . latte
Tea . . . . te'
Sweet . . . . dolce
Water . . . . acqua
Wine . . . . vino
Red . . . . rosso
White . . . . bianco
Dry . . . . secco
Rose . . . . rosato
Litre . . . . litro
Half-litre . . . . mezzo litro
Quarter-litre . . . . quarto

Eating Phrases

Buon apetito. . . . . good appetite/enjoy your meal
Mangia senza complimenti . . . . no need for thanks
Salute! . . . . cheers

Language

Index

Accommodations, 54; Aeolian Islands, 212-213, 219, 222, 228-229, 233, 237-238, 241; Catania, 296-299, 309, 318-322; for children, 80; Interior Sicily, 438, 439-440, 445, 449, 452, 456, 460, 466-468, 471, 474-475; Northern Ionian Coast, 250, 255, 262, 263-264, 267-268, 272; Palermo, 130-132; Palermo excursions, 137, 140, 145, 149; Ragusa and the South Coast, 402-404, 411-412, 416-417, 422, 427; Siracusa and the Southeast, 364-366, 370, 374, 376, 381-382, 384-385, 387, 390-391; South Coast, 488-489, 493, 496-497, 503-505, 511; Trapani and the West, 518-519, 524, 526-527, 529-530, 535-536, 542, 548, 551-553, 557-559, 563-564, 567; Tyrrhenian Coast, 155-156, 165-166, 172, 178, 180-181, 182, 187, 189-191, 196, 200, 202

Aci Castello, 304

Aci Trezza, 305-306

Acireale, 307-309

Acquacalda, 210

Acropolis (Himera), 155

Adrano, 336

Adventures: Aeolian Islands, 210-212, 226-228, 238-240, 241; Catania, 299-303, 306-307, 324-340; Interior Sicily, 436-437, 448-449, 458-459; Northern Ionian Coast, 249, 261-262, 271-272; Palermo, 126-127; Palermo excursions, 142-149; Ragusa and the South Coast, 400-402, 410, 420-422, 427, 429-430; Siracusa and the Southeast, 369-370, 373-374, 381-383, 389-390; South Coast, 487, 503, 507-510; Trapani and the West, 517-518, 525-526, 532-535, 541-542, 556-557; Tyrrhenian Coast, 164-165, 174-178, 186-190

Aeolian Islands, 203-241; Alicudi, 240-241; Filicudi, 238-240; highlights, 204; Lipari, 205-215; Panarea, 223-230; Salina, 219-222; Stromboli, 230-238; Vulcano, 215-219

Agrigento, 478, 479-491; adventures, 487; festivals, 481; getting here and around, 480-481; highlights, 477; information, 481; sightseeing, 481-487; where to eat, 489-491; where to stay, 488-489

Aidone, 469-471

Air travel, 62, 75; Aeolian Islands, 204-205; Catania, 276-277, 333-334; Palermo, 97; Ragusa and the South Coast, 402; South Coast, 487, 506, 509-510; Trapani and the West, 514-515, 532

Akrai Archaeological Park, 372-373

Albergheria district, 109

Alcantara Valley, 243, 268-270

Alcara Li Fusi, 190-191

Allume caves, 218

Annunziata, 372

Antica Stazione, 429

Antichi Mercati, 114-116

Apollonia, 187

Aquacalda, 211

Aquariums, 155, 355

Archaeological sites: Aeolian Islands, 208-210, 226-227, 238; Catania, 289; Interior Sicily, 436, 447, 463-465, 470; Northern Ionian Coast, 252, 267; Palermo, 92, 130; Palermo excursions, 142, 145-146, 148-149; Ragusa and the South Coast, 424; Siracusa and the Southeast, 350-355, 372-373, 380; South Coast, 478, 479-480, 481-484, 491-492, 500-503; Trapani and the West, 532, 537-538, 568-569; Tyrrhenian Coast, 152-153, 154-155, 182, 187, 193-195

Archaeology adventures, 357-359

Arsenale, 351

Art galleries and museums: Aeolian Islands, 209, 220-221; Catania, 285, 287, 304, 306, 309, 316, 337, 338; discounts, 350; hours, 49; Interior Sicily, 436-437, 440-441, 445, 455, 470; Northern Ionian Coast, 249, 254-255, 259-260, 270; Palermo, 121-123; Palermo excursions, 139, 140, 141, 146-147, 149; Ragusa and the South Coast, 397, 416-427, 428; Siracusa and the Southeast, 349-350, 352, 355, 372, 378; South Coast, 479, 484, 486-487; Trapani and the West, 516, 517, 536, 539-540, 547, 550-551, 553, 566; Tyrrhenian Coast, 153-154, 155, 163, 179, 183, 192, 202

Arts and architecture, 34-35

Assessorato Turistico, 153

Associazione Culturale Sicilia e Dintorni, 157-158

Associazione Naturalistica, 178

Atelier sul Mare Albergo Museo, 182

Avola, 375-380

Azienda Autonoma di Soggiorno e Turismo, 198

Badia di Sant'Agata, 283-284

Bagni di Cefala (Arab baths), 18

Bar Il Vitello, 254

Bars *see* Cafés and bars

Basilica di San Giovanni, 351

Basilica Santuario di San Calogero, 498

Baths: Arab, 18; Greek, 479; Roman, 210, 308; sulphur, 216-217; thermal, 88, 496

Beaches, 210, 217, 221, 226; Aeolian Islands, 232; Catania, 291; Northern Ionian Coast, 260; Ragusa and the South Coast, 406, 423-424; Siracusa and the Southeast, 375, 390; South Coast, 479, 503

Bed and breakfasts: Aeolian Islands, 237-238; Catania, 299, 319, 321-322;